# Genitourinary Cancers: Molecular Pathogenesis and Clinical Treatment

# Genitourinary Cancers: Molecular Pathogenesis and Clinical Treatment

Editor: John Simmons

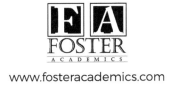

www.fosteracademics.com

www.fosteracademics.com

**Cataloging-in-Publication Data**

Genitourinary cancers : molecular pathogenesis and clinical treatment / edited by John Simmons.
     p. cm.
Includes bibliographical references and index.
ISBN 978-1-64646-578-1
1. Genitourinary organs--Cancer. 2. Genitourinary organs--Cancer--Pathogenesis.
3. Genitourinary organs--Cancer--Treatment. 4. Molecular microbiology. I. Simmons, John.
RC280.G4 G46 2023
616.994 6--dc23

Foster Academics,
118-35 Queens Blvd., Suite 400,
Forest Hills, NY 11375, USA

ISBN 978-1-64646-578-1 (Hardback)

# Contents

# Preface

Genitourinary (GU) cancers refer to the cancers which occur in the urinary system and the male reproductive system. The main parts of the urinary system are urethra, kidneys, ureters and bladder. There are various types of GU cancers such as kidney cancer, bladder cancer, prostate cancer and testicular cancer. The diagnosis of these cancers can be done by performing tests such as medical imaging and biopsy. Patients of GU cancers require special care and medication. Surgery, radiation and chemotherapy are some of the major treatment options for GU cancers. This book strives to provide a fair idea about genitourinary cancers and to help develop a better understanding of the latest advances in their clinical management. It also aims to shed light on some of the unexplored aspects related to their molecular pathogenesis. A number of latest researches have been included to keep the readers up-to-date with the global concepts related to this medical condition.

The information contained in this book is the result of intensive hard work done by researchers in this field. All due efforts have been made to make this book serve as a complete guiding source for students and researchers. The topics in this book have been comprehensively explained to help readers understand the growing trends in the field.

I would like to thank the entire group of writers who made sincere efforts in this book and my family who supported me in my efforts of working on this book. I take this opportunity to thank all those who have been a guiding force throughout my life.

Editor

# An Effective Hypoxia-Related Long Non-Coding RNAs Assessment Model for Prognosis of Clear Cell Renal Carcinoma

Han Zhang[1,2†], Chuan Qin[3†], Hua Wen Liu[2], Xiong Guo[4] and Hua Gan[1*]

[1] Department of Nephrology, The First Affiliated Hospital of Chongqing Medical University, Chongqing, China, [2] Department of Oncology, Chongqing University Three Gorges Hospital, Chongqing, China, [3] Department of Gastrointestinal Surgery, Chongqing University Three Gorges Hospital, Chongqing, China, [4] Department of Gastrointestinal Surgery, The First Affiliated Hospital of Chongqing Medical University, Chongqing, China

*Correspondence:
Hua Gan
ganhua113@sohu.com

†These authors have contributed equally to this work and share first authorship

Hypoxia is a significant clinical feature and regulates various tumor processes in clear cell renal carcinoma (ccRCC). Increasing evidence has demonstrated that long non-coding RNAs (lncRNAs) are closely associated with the survival outcomes of ccRCC patients and regulates hypoxia-induced tumor processes. Thus, this study aimed to develop a hypoxia-related lncRNA (HRL) prognostic model for predicting the survival outcomes in ccRCC. LncRNAs in ccRCC samples were extracted from The Cancer Genome Atlas database. Hypoxia-related genes were downloaded from the Molecular Signatures Database. A co-expression analysis between differentially expressed lncRNAs and hypoxia-related genes in ccRCC samples was performed to identify HRLs. Univariate and multivariate Cox regression analyses were performed to select nine optimal lncRNAs for developing the HRL model. The prognostic model showed good performance in predicting prognosis among patients with ccRCC, and the validation sets reached consistent results. The model was also found to be related to the clinicopathologic parameters of tumor grade and tumor stage and to tumor immune infiltration. In conclusion, our findings indicate that the hypoxia-lncRNA assessment model may be useful for prognostication in ccRCC cases. Furthermore, the nine HRLs included in the model might be useful targets for investigating the tumorigenesis of ccRCC and designing individualized treatment strategies.

Keywords: clear cell renal carcinoma, hypoxia, long non-coding RNA, prognosis, biomarker

## INTRODUCTION

Renal cell carcinoma (RCC) causes more than 100,000 deaths per year (1). Although target therapy and immunotherapy have improved the prognosis of RCC patients (2), the 5-year survival rate remains less than 10%. Clear cell renal cell carcinoma (ccRCC) is the main subtype of RCC, accounting for 70–75% of all RCC cases (3). In clinical practice, the prognosis and treatment of ccRCC are primarily based on the tumor stage. However, the outcomes still vary among patients with the same tumor stage because of molecular heterogeneity (4). Therefore, it is vital to identify individualized biomarkers that can identify patients at high risk of death and help stratify patients for individual treatment to optimize the therapeutic effect.

Hypoxia refers to a reduction of oxygen availability at the cell level, including in tumors (5). As a significant clinical feature, hypoxia regulates various tumor processes, including angiogenesis, cell proliferation, invasion, apoptosis, and radiochemotherapy resistance (6). Hypoxia adaption is a key factor in tumor progression and has been proven to be a cause of treatment failure (7).

Long non-coding RNAs (lncRNAs) are untranslated RNAs of >200 nucleotides in length (8). They have recently attracted increasing research attention because of their involvement in several key molecular and biologic processes (9, 10). For example, lncRNAs regulate hypoxia-related tumor processes (11). In RCC, lncRNA-SARCC can regulate tumor cell proliferation through the androgen receptor/HIF-$2\alpha$/C-MYC axis under hypoxia (12). lncRNA EGOT can also regulate autophagy under hypoxia in renal tubular cells (13). Therefore, a hypoxia-related lncRNA (HRL)-based prognostic model may be potentially useful in ccRCC.

As such, this study aimed to develop a HRL prognostic model for predicting the survival outcomes in ccRCC.

## MATERIALS AND METHODS

### Data Source

Transcriptome expression profiles for patients with ccRCC were obtained from The Cancer Genome Atlas database ((TCGA), https://cancergenome.nih.gov/) on June 29, 2020 (14). The expressions were quantified with fragments per kilobase of exon per million reads mapped. The corresponding clinical information of the patients from whom the samples were obtained was also downloaded from the database, which included age, sex, tumor grade, tumor stage, and survival (**Table 1**). Patients with incomplete information or <30 days of data were excluded because they might have died because of acute complications, rather than of the cancer itself.

Data on hypoxia-related genes were collected from the Molecular Signatures Database V7.2 (https://www.gsea-msigdb.org/gsea/msigdb, Hypoxia M10508, Hypoxia cancer M7547) (15). If the expression data of the gene are not detected in more than 50% of the samples, the gene is excluded. Immune infiltration data were collected from CIBERSORT (https://cibersort.stanford.edu/) (16), which contains abundances of 22 types of tumor-infiltrating immune cells, namely, naive B cells, memory B cells, plasma cells, CD8 T cells, naive CD4 T cells, resting memory CD4 T cells, activated memory CD4 T cells, follicular helper T cells, T cells regulatory, gamma delta T cells, resting NK cells, activated NK cells, monocytes, macrophages M0, macrophages M1, macrophages M2, resting dendritic cells,

**TABLE 1** | Baseline patient characteristics (n = 537).

| Characteristic | 537 clear cell renal carcinoma patients |
|---|---|
| **Age** | |
| <=65 years | 352(66%) |
| >65 years | 185(34%) |
| Unknown | 0(0%) |
| **Sex** | |
| Female | 191(36%) |
| Male | 346(64%) |
| Unknown | 0(0%) |
| **Tumor Grade** | |
| 1&2 | 244(45%) |
| 3&4 | 285(53%) |
| Unknown | 8((2%)) |
| **Tumor Stage** | |
| I | 269(50%) |
| II | 57(10.5%) |
| III | 125(23%) |
| IV | 83(15.5%) |
| Unknown | 3(0.5%) |
| **Pathologic T Stage** | |
| T1&2 | 344(64%) |
| T3&4 | 193(36%) |
| Unknown | 0(0%) |
| **Pathologic N Stage** | |
| N0 | 240(45%) |
| N1 | 17(3%) |
| Unknown | 280(52%) |
| **Pathologic M Stage** | |
| M0 | 426(79%) |
| M1 | 79(15%) |
| Unknown | 32(6%) |

activated dendritic cells, resting mast cells, activated mast cells, eosinophils, and neutrophils.

### Definition of Hypoxia-Related Long Non-Coding RNAs

Genes were identified as protein-coding genes or lncRNAs according to their Ensembl IDs. The lncRNAs were further screened *via* the Genecards database (https://www.genecards.org/) (17). We excluded the lncRNAs recognized as "Pseudogene," "Uncategotized," and "No results" in the database. Differentially expressed lncRNAs between the kidney and healthy renal tissue were identified *via* the differential-expression analysis using the R package "limma" (log2 fold-change [logFC] of >1 and an adjusted false-discovery rate [FDR] of <0.05) (18). Heatmaps and volcano plots were used to visualize the differentially expressed lncRNAs *via* the R package "pheatmap." (19)

We then performed co-expression analysis between hypoxia genes and differentially expressed lncRNAs based on the Spearman correlation analysis (20, 21). LncRNAs with a Spearman correlation coefficient ≥0.4 and a P-value ≤0.001 were identified as HRLs.

### Development of the Hypoxia Long Non-Coding RNA-Related Prognostic Model

All the samples were randomly divided into the training dataset and the 1st validation dataset at the ratio of 1:1. Then the samples were randomly divided into the 2$^{nd}$ validation dataset and 3$^{rd}$ validation dataset at the ratio of 3:7. The training dataset was used to construct the HRL-related prognostic model to predict the prognosis for ccRCC patients. Univariate Cox regression analyses were used to extract the hypoxia survival-associated lncRNAs *via* the R package "survival" (significant at P ≤ 0.01). A Cox proportional hazards model with a lasso penalty analysis was used to construct the HRL model with the optimal prognostic value *via* the R packages "glmnet" and "survival." (22) The risk score of each sample was calculated based on the regression coefficients from the model and lncRNAs' expression. The formula is below:

$$\text{Risk score (patient)} = \sum_{k=1}^{n} (coef \times exp)$$

with "n" representing the number of lncRNA; "k," the serial number of each lncRNA; coef, the coefficient value from the Cox proportional hazards analysis; and exp, the expression of the lncRNA (23).

## Validation of the Model

The validation datasets were used to validate the predictive power of the HRL-related model. In each dataset, patients were assigned to the low- and high-risk groups based on the median risk scores. Kaplan–Meier survival curve analyses and log-rank tests were performed to evaluate the predictive power of the model for overall survival (OS), using the R package "survival" and "survminer." Receiver operating characteristic (ROC) curves (24) and area under the ROC curves (AUC) were calculated to assess the accuracy of the model, using the R package "survivalROC." An AUC of >0.75 was judged as excellent predictive value. Univariate and multivariate analyses *via* the R

package "survival" were also performed to verify the independent prognostic predictors. The nomogram was plotted using the R package "rms." (25)

## Gene Set Enrichment Analysis

Gene set enrichment analysis (GSEA) (version 4.0.1, http://www.broadinstitute.org/gsea) was performed to identify differences in the set of genes expressed between the low- and high-risk groups in the enrichment of Kyoto Encyclopedia of Genes and Genomes (KEGG) and Gene Ontology (GO) data. Gene set permutations were performed 1,000 times for each analysis.

## Statistical Analysis

All statistical analyses were performed using the R software (version 3.6.1, http://www.R-project.org). The PERL programming language (version, 5.30.2, http://www.perl.org) was used to process data. The Wilcoxon signed-rank test was used for identifying differentially expressed lncRNAs and tumor-infiltrating immune cells. The Spearman correlation analysis was used for identifying HRLs. The Kaplan–Meier method and log-rank test were performed to compare the OS between the high- and low-risk groups.

## RESULTS

### Hypoxia-Related Long Non-Coding RNAs in Clear Cell Renal Carcinoma

A total of 14,143 lncRNAs were extracted from the TCGA database. We identified 1,926 differentially expressed lncRNAs in renal cancer specimens (n = 539) and normal renal specimen (n = 72) (logFC of >1 and FDR of <0.05) (**Figures 1A, B**).

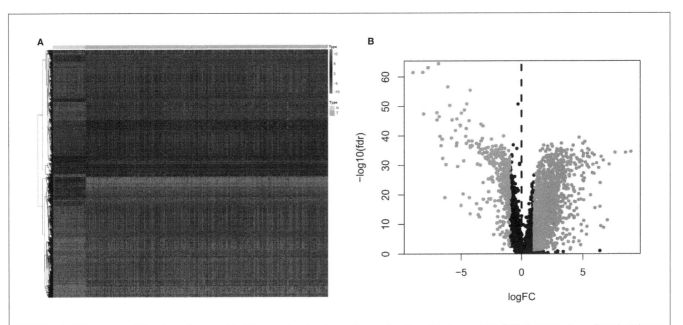

**FIGURE 1** | **(A)** Heatmap and **(B)** volcano diagram of the Wilcoxon signed-rank test showing the differentially expressed lncRNAs between clear cell renal carcinoma and normal tissue samples. The red, green, and black dots represent the upregulated lncRNAs, downregulated lncRNAs, and no difference, respectively.

Among these lncRNAs, 186 lncRNAs were excluded due to the lack of definition in the Genecards database.

Of the 137 hypoxia genes obtained from the Molecular Signatures Database V7.2, four genes (FGF3, LIN28B, MMP13, and TH) were excluded owing to a lack of over 50% expression information. In total, 598 HRLs were confirmed by co-expression analyses between hypoxia genes and differentially expressed lncRNAs (P ≤ 0.001, Spearman correlation coefficient ≥0.4).

## Construction of Hypoxia Long Non-Coding RNA-Related Prognostic Model

After excluding patients without cancer or survival data, we merged the survival data with lncRNA expression data of each patient. We then divided the remaining patients into the training dataset (n = 255) and the 1st validation dataset (n = 252) at the ratio of 1:1 and divided the patients into the 2nd validation dataset (n = 153) and the 3rd validation dataset (n = 354) at the ratio of 3:7. The risk model was developed using the training dataset and validated using the validation datasets.

Univariate cox regression analyses were first performed for the hypoxia differentially expressed lncRNAs, and the results showed that 163 lncRNAs were significantly related to the OS of ccRCC (P ≤ 0.01). A Cox proportional hazards model with a lasso penalty analysis was further performed to construct the optimal risk model (**Figures 2A, B**). Ultimately, nine optimal prognostic HRLs were obtained and incorporated into the risk model: ITPR1-DT, AC008760.2, AC084876.1, AC002070.1, LINC02027, AC147651.1, FOXD2-AS1, LINC00944, and LINC01615 (**Figure 2C**). The risk score for each patient was calculated as: risk score = (0.271 × ITPR1-DT expression) + (0.011 × AC008760.2 expression) + (0.546 ×AC084876.1expression) + (−0.514 × AC002070.1 expression) + (−0.173 × LINC02027 expression) + (−0.027 × AC147651.1

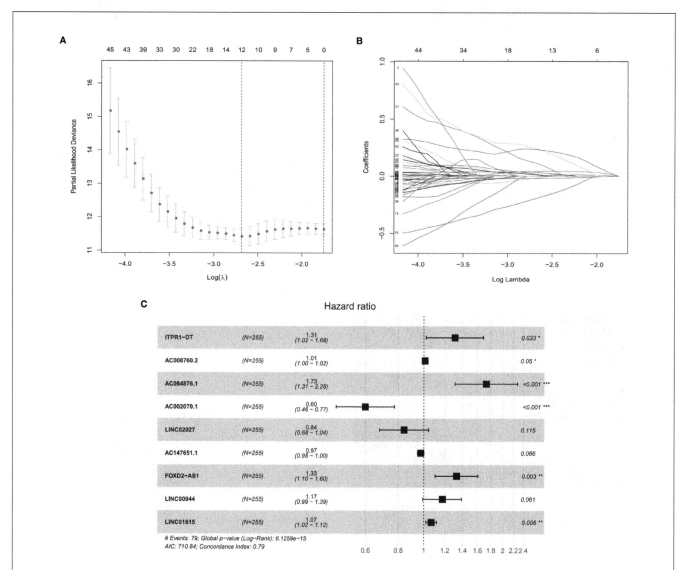

**FIGURE 2 | (A, B)** The LASSO Cox regression model to identify the most robust lncRNAs. **(C)** Forest plot of the multivariate Cox regression model showing the nine optimal prognostic hypoxia-related lncRNAs. * represents p < 0.05, ** represents p < 0.01, *** represents p < 0.001.

expression) + (0.286 × FOXD2-AS1 expression) + (0.161 × LINC00944 expression) + (0.065 × LINC01615 expression).

## Validation of the Prognostic Score

To verify the accuracy of prognostic prediction of each patient, we performed ROC in the training dataset and the validation datasets. In the training dataset, the AUCs for predicting the 3-, and 5-year survival were 0.805, and 0.802, respectively, indicating excellent prognostic power (**Figures 3A, B**). Similar results were obtained in the 1st (**Figures 3C, D**), 2nd (**Figures 3E, F**) and 3rd (**Figures 3G, H**) validation datasets.

The patients were then divided into the high- and low-risk groups using the median risk score as a cut-off. Kaplan–Meier curves were plotted in the training dataset, and the results showed poorer survival in the high-risk group than in the low-risk group (P = 1.922e-10) (**Figure 4A**). The survival analyses in the validation groups also revealed poorer survival in the high-risk groups than in the low-risk groups [3.078e-08 in the 1st

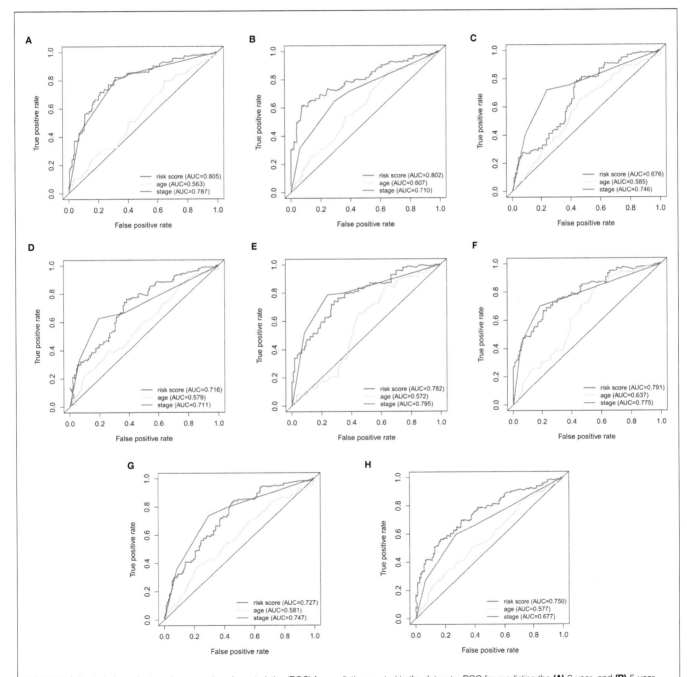

**FIGURE 3** | Survival-dependent receiver operating characteristics (ROC) for predicting survival in the datasets. ROC for predicting the **(A)** 3-year, and **(B)** 5-year survival in the training dataset. ROC for the **(C)** 3-year, and **(D)** 5-year survival in the 1st validation dataset. ROC for predicting the **(E)** 3-year, and **(F)** 5-year survival in the 2nd dataset. ROC for predicting the **(G)** 3-year, and **(H)** 5-year survival in the 3rd validation dataset.

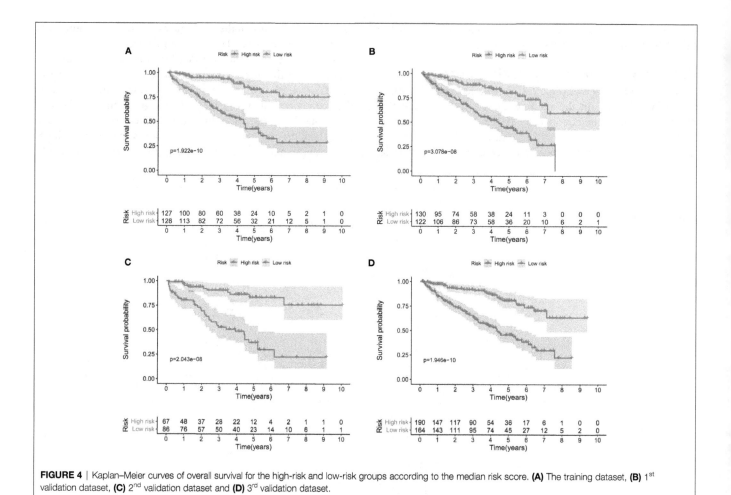

**FIGURE 4** | Kaplan–Meier curves of overall survival for the high-risk and low-risk groups according to the median risk score. **(A)** The training dataset, **(B)** 1st validation dataset, **(C)** 2nd validation dataset and **(D)** 3rd validation dataset.

(**Figure 4B**), 2.043 e-08 in the 2nd (**Figure 4C**), and 1.946e-10 in the 3rd validation dataset (**Figure 4D**)].

The risk score distributions, survival status, and risk gene expressions in each dataset are shown in **Figure 5**. The low-risk groups had obviously higher survival rate (**Figure 5A**) and lower values for the risk score (**Figure 5C**) in the training dataset. Moreover, as the risk score increased, the expressions of the protective lncRNAs (AC008760.2, LINC00944, LINC01615, ITPR1-DT, AC084876.1, and FOXD2-AS1) decreased, whereas those of the risk lncRNAs (AC147651.1, LINC02027, and AC002070.1) increased (**Figure 5E**) in the training dataset. Similar results were obtained in the 1st (**Figures 5B, D, F**), 2nd (**Figures 5G, I, K**) and 3rd (**Figures 5H, J, L**) validation datasets.

In the univariate analysis to evaluate the relationship between clinical characteristics and OS, the TNM stage was excluded because several patients had missing information. The results showed that age (P = 0.003), tumor grade (P = 0.031), tumor stage (P < 0.001), and risk score (P < 0.001) were significantly associated with prognosis (**Figures 6A, C, E, G**). Multivariate analysis confirmed age, tumor stage, and risk score as independent prognostic factors (**Figures 6B, D, F, H**). In addition to risk score, age and tumor stage could also divide patients into high- and low-risk groups effectively (**Supplementary Figure 1**). To further verify the predictive

power of our risk score in the patients with same tumor stage, we divided early stage (I and II) and advanced stage (III and IV) ccRCC patients into the high- and low-risk groups using the median risk score. Kaplan–Meier curves were plotted in two groups, and the results showed poorer survival in the high-risk groups than in the low-risk groups (**Supplementary Figure 2**).

The independent prognostic factors (age, tumor stage, and risk score) were used to develop the nomogram for predicting the 1-, 3-, and 5-year prognoses of the patients (**Figure 7A**). Similar results were obtained in the validation datasets (**Supplementary Figure 3**). In the nomogram, we can calculate the point of each factor and the total points of all factors. The 1-, 3-, and 5-year survival rates could be predicted by the corresponding value of total points.

## Clinical Utility of the Risk Score

The association among the risk lncRNAs (ITPR1-DT, AC008760.2, AC084876.1, AC002070.1, LINC02027, AC147651.1, FOXD2-AS1, LINC00944, and LINC01615), risk score, and clinicopathologic parameters (age, sex, tumor grade, and tumor stage) was analyzed in the training dataset (**Table 2**). The risk score was obviously higher in samples with high-grade and advanced-stage tumor (**Figures 7B, C**). Similar results were obtained in the validation datasets (**Supplementary Tables**).

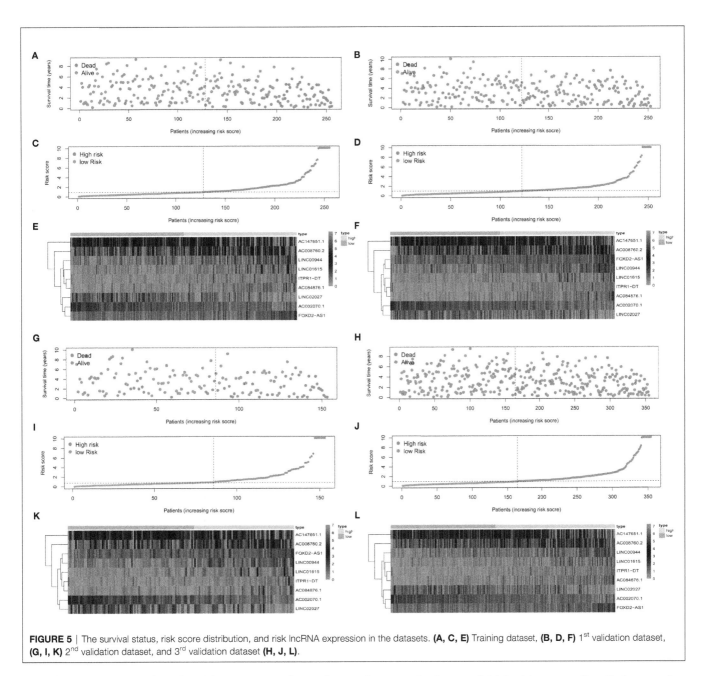

**FIGURE 5 |** The survival status, risk score distribution, and risk lncRNA expression in the datasets. **(A, C, E)** Training dataset, **(B, D, F)** 1st validation dataset, **(G, I, K)** 2nd validation dataset, and 3rd validation dataset **(H, J, L)**.

This finding supports that the risk score can also reflect tumor progression.

To explore which pathways were enriched, we used GSEA software to perform KEGG (**Figures 8A, B**) and GO analysis (**Figures 8C, D**). KEGG analysis identified multiple tumor-related signaling pathways in the high-risk group, such as homologous recombination, Base excision repair, and cytokine-cytokine receptor interaction. Surprisingly, KRGG and GO analysis identified that several immune-related signal pathways and genes were enriched in the samples.

We further analyzed the correlation between immune cell infiltration and the risk score. First, we plotted the immune landscape of all the samples, as shown in **Figure 9A**. Then, we analyzed the difference in the number of immune cells

between the low- and high-risk groups for all the samples. We identified six types of immune cells with differences in infiltration between the two groups, namely, plasma cells, follicular helper T cells, regulatory T cells, M2 macrophages, resting dendritic cells, and resting mast cells (**Figure 9B**).

## DISCUSSION

Despite advances in diagnosis and treatment, ccRCC as a lethal RCC subtype remains to have poor prognosis (26). Further, current prognostic models for ccRCC have limited predictive capability because of the complex molecular heterogeneity of this

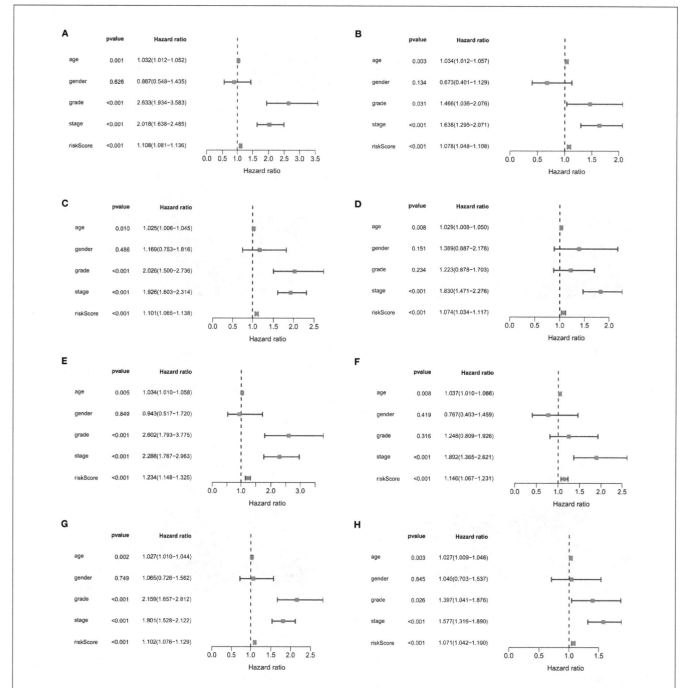

**FIGURE 6** | Forest plot of the univariate and multivariate Cox regression analysis showing that the risk score was an independent risk factor for overall survival in the training dataset **(A, B)**, 1st validation dataset **(C, D)**, 2nd dataset **(E, F)** and the 3rd validation dataset **(G, H)**.

malignancy. Hence, in this study, we identified a novel prognostic model for predicting ccRCC outcomes.

Hypoxia has been confirmed to be closely related to tumorigenesis and tumor progression of ccRCC (27). Previous studies have established that lncRNAs are involved in tumorigenesis, tumor progression, and metastasis (28–30). In this study, HRLs were related to the survival outcomes of patients with ccRCC, and thus we developed an HRL-related model to

predict ccRCC prognosis. To our best knowledge, this is the first study to develop such predictive model for ccRCC.

Previous studies suggested that lncRNAs are involved in multiple processes in ccRCC (31, 32). For example, lncRNA UCA1 plays an oncogenic role in RCC by regulating the miR-182-5p/DLL4 axis (33). LncRNA URRCC can also promote the proliferation and metastasis of ccRCC by regulating the P-AKT signaling pathway (34). Further, lncRNA OTUD6B can inhibit

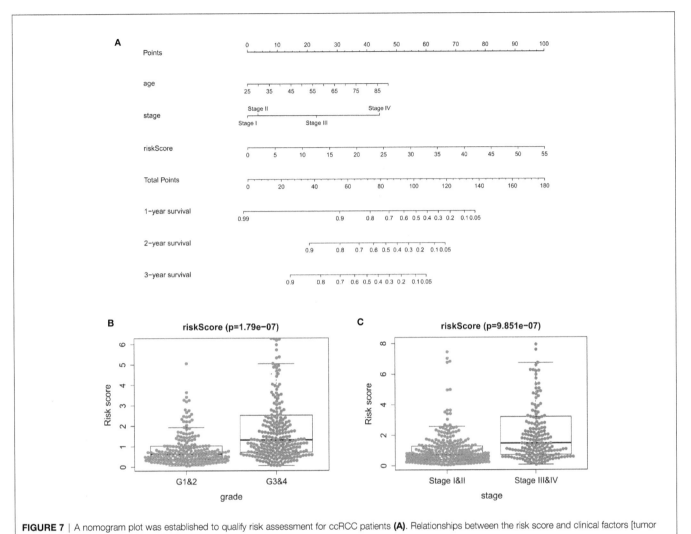

**FIGURE 7** | A nomogram plot was established to qualify risk assessment for ccRCC patients **(A)**. Relationships between the risk score and clinical factors [tumor grade **(B)** and tumor stage **(C)**] in clear cell renal carcinoma.

**TABLE 2** | Relationships of the risk score and the risk genes with clinical variables in ccRCC.

| lncRNA symbol | Age(≤65/>65) | Sex(male/female) | Tumor grade(1&2/3&4) | Tumor stage(I & II/III & IV) |
|---|---|---|---|---|
| ITPR1-DT | 0.89(0.374) | −0.152(0.879) | −1.907(0.058) | −1.454(0.148) |
| AC008760.2 | 1.779(0.077) | 1.179(0.241) | −2.858(0.005) | −1.62(0.108) |
| AC084876.1 | −1.782(0.077) | 0.062(0.951) | −2.83(0.005) | −3.251(0.001) |
| AC002070.1 | 0.86(0.391) | 0.86(0.391) | 5.216(4.132e-07) | 3.722(2.446e-04) |
| LINC02027 | −0.991(0.323) | 2.373(0.019) | 1.248(0.213) | 1.076(0.283) |
| AC147651.1 | 0.522(0.602) | 1.313(0.191) | 4.319(2.462e-05) | 2.032(0.043) |
| FOXD2-AS1 | −0.575(0.567) | 0.473(0.637) | −2.183(0.030) | −3.833(1.836e-04) |
| LINC00944 | −1.54(0.125) | −1.947(0.053) | −3.653(3.219e-04) | −4.291(2.922e-05) |
| LINC01615 | 0.994(0.321) | −1.957(0.052) | −2.12(0.036) | −2.276(0.025) |
| Risk Score | −0.563(0.574) | 0.438(0.662) | −4.646(7.756e-06) | −3.993(1.171e-04) |

*lncRNA, long non-coding RNA.*

ccRCC cell proliferation by suppressing the Wnt/$\beta$-catenin pathway and the expressions of epithelial-to-mesenchymal transition-related proteins (35). In this study, we screened 1926 differentially expressed lncRNAs in ccRCC tissue, relative to the levels in adjacent normal renal tissue. The results indicated that lncRNAs are closely related to the tumorigenesis of ccRCC, in agreement with previous findings.

Tumor hypoxia is defined as lower oxygenation in solid tumors than in normal tissues. Hypoxia can lead to resistance to chemoradiotherapy and target therapy (7, 36); increases angiogenesis and vasculogenesis (37), thus predisposing to tumor metastases; and contributes to altered metabolism and genomic instability. LncRNAs have been reported be involved in the development of ccRCC by regulating the hypoxia pathway. For

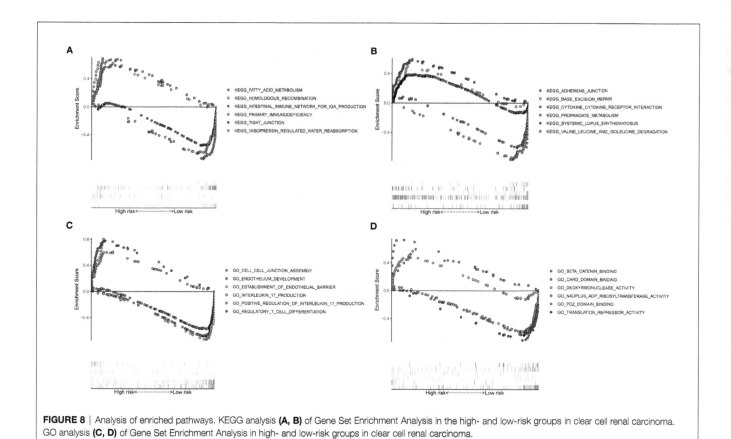

**FIGURE 8** | Analysis of enriched pathways. KEGG analysis **(A, B)** of Gene Set Enrichment Analysis in the high- and low-risk groups in clear cell renal carcinoma. GO analysis **(C, D)** of Gene Set Enrichment Analysis in high- and low-risk groups in clear cell renal carcinoma.

example, Hamilton et al. found that lncRNA HOTAIRM1 inhibited the hypoxia pathway in ccRCC (38). Zhang et al. revealed that under hypoxic conditions in ccRCC, lncRNA CRPAT4 promoted cell migration by regulating AVL9 (39). In the present study, we performed a co-expression analysis between hypoxia genes and differentially expressed lncRNAs through paired lncRNA and mRNA expression data in ccRCC patients from TCGA. A total of 598 lncRNAs were extracted and defined as HRLs. The close association between hypoxia genes and HRLs in ccRCC samples indicate that HRLs are involved in the development of ccRCC.

Among all the HRLs, nine lncRNAs (i.e., ITPR1-DT, AC008760.2, AC084876.1, AC002070.1, LINC02027, AC147651.1, FOXD2-AS1, LINC00944, and LINC01615) were identified to be independently associated with prognosis and were thus used to develop the prognostic model. ROC curves confirmed the good specificity and sensitivity of the HRL-based prognostic model. Kaplan-Meier survival curves showed excellent efficiency of our HRL-related model in stratifying patients with different risks of mortality. Multivariate analyses demonstrated that the age, tumor stage and the risk score were independent prognostic factors. We further identified the prognostic predictive power of our risk score in the patients with same tumor stage. Hence, our HRL-related model maybe useful as a supplement to the tumor stage for better stratifying patients and for providing a more individualized approach to treatment. We further developed a nomogram by integrating age, tumor stage, and risk score. From it we can easily

obtain a single number, which reflects survival when accounting for these three factors.

Tumor hypoxia also changes the interaction and cross-talk of cancer cells with the surrounding tumor microenvironment, leading to immune resistance and immune suppression, which help tumor cells escape immune surveillance (5, 40, 41). To determine whether our HRL-related model can also reflect the tumor microenvironment, we performed GSEA. The results showed that several immune-related GO terms or signaling pathways were enriched in the high-risk group. We further plotted the immune landscape of each ccRCC sample for exploring the tumor immune microenvironment in patients with ccRCC. Then, we compared the infiltration of every immune cell type between the high- and low-risk groups. Plasma cells, follicular helper T cells, regulatory T cells, M2 macrophages, resting dendritic cells, and resting mast cells were found to be differentially infiltrated in ccRCC, which are closely associated with tumorigenesis, progression, and metastasis (42–46). This finding supports that our HRL-related model can partly reflect immune infiltration and provide valuable information for immunotherapy.

The whole process of our analyses was based on the data from TCGA database, which contains complete clinical and survival data of patients with ccRCC. It also has sufficient ccRCC samples to be divided into a training dataset and validation datasets. Therefore, a prognostic model constructed using TCGA database has better statistical power than a model constructed using

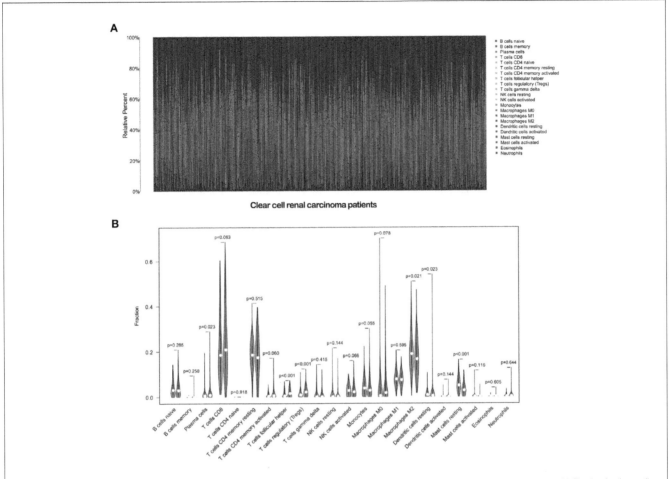

**FIGURE 9** | Immune landscape of the patients with clear cell renal carcinoma **(A)**. Relationships between the risk score and the immune cell infiltration in clear cell renal carcinoma **(B)**.

patient samples derived from a single institution. However, the current study still has some limitations. First, we haven't found an available independent lncRNA dataset to validate the usefulness of our prognostic model, and we were not able to validate in clinical practice owing to the lack of ccRCC samples. Second, the relationship between the nine lncRNAs and ccRCC remains unclear to date because of the limited number of lncRNA researches. The validity of our prognostic model should be evaluated in further research with a large number of clinical samples and with adequate follow-up duration. In addition, the underlying mechanisms by which lncRNAs influence the prognosis of ccRCC should be investigated in *in vivo* and *in vitro* experiments.

## CONCLUSION

Our hypoxia-lncRNA assessment model may be useful to improve the prognostic prediction of ccRCC patients with the same tumor stage. Furthermore, the nine HRLs included in the model might be useful targets for investigating the tumorigenesis of ccRCC and designing personalized individualized treatment strategies.

## AUTHOR CONTRIBUTIONS

HZ and HG designed the study. HZ and CQ collected and analyzed the data, and drafted the manuscript. CQ and HL made the figures and tables. XG provided critical suggestions regarding the figures and manuscript. HG led the research team. All authors contributed to the article and approved the submitted version.

## ACKNOWLEDGMENTS

We would like to thank Editage (www.editage.cn) for English language editing.

## SUPPLEMENTARY MATERIAL

**Supplementary Figure 1** | **(A)** Kaplan–Meier curves of overall survival for the young (≤50 y) and elderly (>50 y) groups. **(B)** Kaplan–Meier curves of overall survival for the early (I–II) and advanced (III–IV) tumor stage groups.

**Supplementary Figure 2** | Kaplan–Meier curves of overall survival for the highrisk and low-risk groups according to the median risk score. **(A)** ccRCC patients with early tumor stages (I–II) and **(B)** advanced stages (III–IV).

# REFERENCES

1. Hsieh J, Purdue M, Signoretti S, Swanton C, Albiges L, Schmidinger M, et al. Renal cell carcinoma. *Nat Rev Dis Primers* (2017) 3:17009. doi: 10.1038/nrdp.2017.9

2. Haddad A, Margulis V. Tumour and patient factors in renal cell carcinoma-towards personalized therapy. *Nat Rev Urol* (2015) 12(5):253–62. doi: 10.1038/nrurol.2015.71

3. Störkel S, Eble J, Adlakha K, Amin M, Blute M, Bostwick D, et al. Classification of renal cell carcinoma: Workgroup No. 1. Union Internationale Contre le Cancer (UICC) and the American Joint Committee on Cancer (AJCC). *Cancer* (1997) 80(5):987–9. doi: 10.1002/(sici)1097-0142(19970901)80:5<987::aid-cncr24>3.0.co;2-r

4. Molina A, Lin X, Korytowsky B, Matczak E, Lechuga M, Wiltshire R, et al. Sunitinib objective response in metastatic renal cell carcinoma: analysis of 1059 patients treated on clinical trials. *Eur J Cancer (Oxford Engl 1990)* (2014) 50(2):351–8. doi: 10.1016/j.ejca.2013.08.021

5. Jing X, Yang F, Shao C, Wei K, Xie M, Shen H, et al. Role of hypoxia in cancer therapy by regulating the tumor microenvironment. *Mol Cancer* (2019) 18(1):157. doi: 10.1186/s12943-019-1089-9

6. Parks S, Cormerais Y, Pouysségur J. Hypoxia and cellular metabolism in tumour pathophysiology. *J Physiol* (2017) 595(8):2439–50. doi: 10.1113/jp273309

7. Zhao C, Luo C, Wu X. Hypoxia promotes 786-O cells invasiveness and resistance to sorafenib via HIF-2α/COX-2. *Med Oncol (Northwood London England)* (2015) 32(1):419. doi: 10.1007/s12032-014-0419-4

8. Fatica A, Bozzoni I. Long non-coding RNAs: new players in cell differentiation and development. *Nat Rev Genet* (2014) 15(1):7–21. doi: 10.1038/nrg3606

9. Kopp F. Molecular functions and biological roles of long non-coding RNAs in human physiology and disease. *J Gene Med* (2019) 21(8):e3104. doi: 10.1002/jgm.3104

10. Tsagakis I, Douka K, Birds I, Aspden J. Long non-coding RNAs in development and disease: conservation to mechanisms. *J Pathol* (2020) 250(5):480–95. doi: 10.1002/path.5405

11. Choudhry H, Harris A, McIntyre A. The tumour hypoxia induced non-coding transcriptome. *Mol Aspects Med* (2016) 47–48:35–53. doi: 10.1016/j.mam.2016.01.003

12. Zhai W, Sun Y, Jiang M, Wang M, Gasiewicz T, Zheng J, et al. Differential regulation of LncRNA-SARCC suppresses VHL-mutant RCC cell proliferation yet promotes VHL-normal RCC cell proliferation via modulating androgen receptor/HIF-2α/C-MYC axis under hypoxia. *Oncogene* (2016) 35(37):4866–80. doi: 10.1038/onc.2016.19

13. Wang I, Palanisamy K, Sun K, Yu S, Yu T, Li C, et al. The functional interplay of lncRNA EGOT and HuR regulates hypoxia-induced autophagy in renal tubular cells. *J Cell Biochem* (2020) 121(11):4522–34. doi: 10.1002/jcb.29669

14. Liu J, Lichtenberg T, Hoadley K, Poisson L, Lazar A, Cherniack A, et al. An Integrated TCGA Pan-Cancer Clinical Data Resource to Drive High-Quality Survival Outcome Analytics. *Cell* (2018) 173(2):400–16.e11. doi: 10.1016/j.cell.2018.02.052

15. Liberzon A, Birger C, Thorvaldsdóttir H, Ghandi M, Mesirov J, Tamayo P. The Molecular Signatures Database (MSigDB) hallmark gene set collection. *Cell Syst* (2015) 1(6):417–25. doi: 10.1016/j.cels.2015.12.004

16. Chen B, Khodadoust M, Liu C, Newman A, Alizadeh A. Profiling Tumor Infiltrating Immune Cells with CIBERSORT. *Methods Mol Biol (Clifton NJ)* (2018) 1711:243–59. doi: 10.1007/978-1-4939-7493-1_12

17. Safran M, Dalah I, Alexander J, Rosen N, Iny Stein T, Shmoish M, et al. GeneCards Version 3: the human gene integrator. *Database J Biol Database Curation* (2010) 2010:baq020. doi: 10.1093/database/baq020

18. Ritchie M, Phipson B, Wu D, Hu Y, Law C, Shi W, et al. limma powers differential expression analyses for RNA-sequencing and microarray studies. *Nucleic Acids Res* (2015) 43(7):e47. doi: 10.1093/nar/gkv007

19. Li W. Volcano plots in analyzing differential expressions with mRNA microarrays. *J Bioinf Comput Biol* (2012) 10(6):1231003. doi: 10.1142/s0219720012310038

20. Chen S, Lin F, Zhu J, Ke Z, Lin T, Lin Y, et al. An immune-related lncRNA prognostic model in papillary renal cell carcinoma: A lncRNA expression analysis. *Genomics* (2020) 113:531–40. doi: 10.1016/j.ygeno.2020.09.046

21. Wei C, Liang Q, Li X, Li H, Liu Y, Huang X, et al. Bioinformatics profiling utilized a nine immune-related long noncoding RNA signature as a prognostic target for pancreatic cancer. *J Cell Biochem* (2019) 120(9):14916–27. doi: 10.1002/jcb.28754

22. Huang R, Chen Z, Li W, Fan C, Liu J. Immune system–associated genes increase malignant progression and can be used to predict clinical outcome in patients with hepatocellular carcinoma. *Int J Oncol* (2020) 56(5):1199–211. doi: 10.3892/ijo.2020.4998

23. Li H, Gao C, Liu L, Zhuang J, Yang J, Liu C, et al. 7-lncRNA Assessment Model for Monitoring and Prognosis of Breast Cancer Patients: Based on Cox Regression and Co-expression Analysis. *Front Oncol* (2019) 9:1348. doi: 10.3389/fonc.2019.01348

24. Martínez-Camblor P, Pardo-Fernández J. Parametric estimates for the receiver operating characteristic curve generalization for non-monotone relationships. *Stat Methods Med Res* (2019) 28(7):2032–48. doi: 10.1177/0962280217747009

25. Jiang W, Guo Q, Wang C, Zhu Y. A nomogram based on 9-lncRNAs signature for improving prognostic prediction of clear cell renal cell carcinoma. *Cancer Cell Int* (2019) 19:208. doi: 10.1186/s12935-019-0928-5

26. Shingarev R, Jaimes E. Renal cell carcinoma: new insights and challenges for a clinician scientist. *Am J Physiol Renal Physiol* (2017) 313(2):F145–54. doi: 10.1152/ajprenal.00480.2016

27. Harris A. Hypoxia–a key regulatory factor in tumour growth. *Nat Rev Cancer* (2002) 2(1):38–47. doi: 10.1038/nrc704

28. Olivero C, Martínez-Terroba E, Zimmer J, Liao C, Tesfaye E, Hooshdaran N, et al. p53 Activates the Long Noncoding RNA Pvt1b to Inhibit Myc and Suppress Tumorigenesis. *Mol Cell* (2020) 77(4):761–74.e8. doi: 10.1016/j.molcel.2019.12.014

29. Li J, Chen C, Liu J, Shi J, Liu S, Liu B, et al. Long noncoding RNA MRCCAT1 promotes metastasis of clear cell renal cell carcinoma via inhibiting NPR3 and activating p38-MAPK signaling. *Mol Cancer* (2017) 16(1):111. doi: 10.1186/s12943-017-0681-0

30. Liu X, Hao Y, Yu W, Yang X, Luo X, Zhao J, et al. Long Non-Coding RNA Emergence During Renal Cell Carcinoma Tumorigenesis. *Cell Physiol Biochem Int J Exp Cell Physiol Biochem Pharmacol* (2018) 47(2):735–46. doi: 10.1159/000490026

31. Flippot R, Beinse G, Boilève A, Vibert J, Malouf G. Long non-coding RNAs in genitourinary malignancies: a whole new world. *Nat Rev Urol* (2019) 16(8):484–504. doi: 10.1038/s41585-019-0195-1

32. Barth D, Slaby O, Klec C, Juracek J, Drula R, Calin G, et al. Current Concepts of Non-Coding RNAs in the Pathogenesis of Non-Clear Cell Renal Cell Carcinoma. *Cancers* (2019) 11(10):1580. doi: 10.3390/cancers11101580

33. Wang W, Hu W, Wang Y, An Y, Song L, Shang P, et al. Long non-coding RNA UCA1 promotes malignant phenotypes of renal cancer cells by modulating the miR-182-5p/DLL4 axis as a ceRNA. *Mol Cancer* (2020) 19(1):18. doi: 10.1186/s12943-020-1132-x

34. Zhai W, Zhu R, Ma J, Gong D, Zhang H, Zhang J, et al. A positive feed-forward loop between LncRNA-URRCC and EGFL7/P-AKT/FOXO3 signaling promotes proliferation and metastasis of clear cell renal cell carcinoma. *Mol Cancer* (2019) 18(1):81. doi: 10.1186/s12943-019-0998-y

35. Wang G, Zhang Z, Jian W, Liu P, Xue W, Wang T, et al. Novel long noncoding RNA OTUD6B-AS1 indicates poor prognosis and inhibits clear cell renal cell carcinoma proliferation via the Wnt/β-catenin signaling pathway. *Mol Cancer* (2019) 18(1):15. doi: 10.1186/s12943-019-0942-1

36. Bielecka Z, Malinowska A, Brodaczewska K, Klemba A, Kieda C, Krasowski P, et al. Hypoxic 3D in vitro culture models reveal distinct resistance processes to TKIs in renal cancer cells. *Cell Biosci* (2017) 7:71. doi: 10.1186/s13578-017-0197-8

37. Chung C. From oxygen sensing to angiogenesis: Targeting the hypoxia signaling pathway in metastatic kidney cancer. *Am J Health-system Pharm AJHP Off J Am Soc Health-System Pharmacists* (2020) 77(24):2064–73. doi: 10.1093/ajhp/zxaa308

38. Hamilton M, Young M, Jang K, Sauer S, Neang V, King A, et al. HOTAIRM1 lncRNA is downregulated in clear cell renal cell carcinoma and inhibits the hypoxia pathway. *Cancer Lett* (2020) 472:50–8. doi: 10.1016/j.canlet.2019.12.022

39. Zhang W, Wang J, Chai R, Zhong G, Zhang C, Cao W, et al. Hypoxia-regulated lncRNA CRPAT4 promotes cell migration via regulating AVL9 in

clear cell renal cell carcinomas. *OncoTargets Ther* (2018) 11:4537–45. doi: 10.2147/ott.S169155

40. Kumar V, Gabrilovich D. Hypoxia-inducible factors in regulation of immune responses in tumour microenvironment. *Immunology* (2014) 143(4):512–9. doi: 10.1111/imm.12380

41. Noman M, Hasmim M, Lequeux A, Xiao M, Duhem C, Chouaib S, et al. Improving Cancer Immunotherapy by Targeting the Hypoxic Tumor Microenvironment: New Opportunities and Challenges. *Cells* (2019) 8 (9):1083. doi: 10.3390/cells8091083

42. Zhang H, Yue R, Zhao P, Yu X, Li J, Ma G, et al. Proinflammatory follicular helper T cells promote immunoglobulin G secretion, suppress regulatory B cell development, and correlate with worse clinical outcomes in gastric cancer. *Tumour Biol J Int Soc Oncodevelopmental Biol Med* (2017) 39 (6):1010428317705747. doi: 10.1177/1010428317705747

43. Ngabire D, Niyonizigiye I, Patil M, Seong Y, Seo Y, Kim G. βM2 Macrophages

Mediate the Resistance of Gastric Adenocarcinoma Cells to 5-Fluorouracil through the Expression of Integrin 3, Focal Adhesion Kinase, and Cofilin. *J Immunol Res* (2020) 2020:1731457. doi: 10.1155/2020/1731457

44. Ling Z, Shao L, Liu X, Cheng Y, Yan C, Mei Y, et al. Regulatory T Cells and Plasmacytoid Dendritic Cells Within the Tumor Microenvironment in Gastric Cancer Are Correlated With Gastric Microbiota Dysbiosis: A Preliminary Study. *Front Immunol* (2019) 10:533. doi: 10.3389/fimmu. 2019.00533

45. Bagheri V, Abbaszadegan M, Memar B, Motie M, Asadi M, Mahmoudian R, et al. Induction of T cell-mediated immune response by dendritic cells pulsed with mRNA of sphere-forming cells isolated from patients with gastric cancer. *Life Sci* (2019) 219:136–43. doi: 10.1016/j.lfs.2019. 01.016

46. Aponte-López A, Muñoz-Cruz S. Mast Cells in the Tumor Microenvironment. *Adv Exp Med Biol* (2020) 1273:159–73. doi: 10.1007/978-3-030-49270-0_9

# 2

# The *CSRNP* Gene Family Serves as a Prognostic Biomarker in Clear Cell Renal Cell Carcinoma

*Huaru Zhang [1,2], Xiaofu Qiu [1,2] and Guosheng Yang [1,2,3]\**

[1] The Second School of Clinical Medicine, Southern Medical University, Guangzhou, China, [2] Department of Urology, Guangdong Second Provincial General Hospital, Guangzhou, China, [3] Department of Urology, Shanghai East Hospital, Tongji University School of Medicine, Shanghai, China

*\*Correspondence:*
*Guosheng Yang*
*2008yangguosheng@sina.com*

The cysteine-serine-rich nuclear protein (*CSRNP*) family has prognostic value for various cancers. However, the association between this proteins and prognosis of clear cell renal cell carcinoma (ccRCC) remains unclear. This study aimed to determine the prognostic value of the *CSRNP* family for patients with ccRCC. Therefore, the gene expression profiling interactive analysis database was used to analyze the mRNA expression of *CSRNP* family members (*CSRNPs*) in relation with survival. Combined and independent prognostic values of CSRNPs were evaluated using SurvExpress and multivariate Cox regression analyses, respectively. Potential signaling pathways impacted by *CSRNPs* were evaluated using Metascape. Associations between the *CSRNP* family and immunocyte infiltration were determined from single-sample gene set enrichment analysis. Both cBioPortal and MethSurv were used to explore whether genomic and epidemic alterations might influence prognosis. We found that when both *CSRNP1* and *CSRNP3* had a low expression, patients with ccRCC had a worse overall survival (OS). Therefore, a prognostic signature was constructed as follows: risk score = $-0.224 \times \exp_{\text{mRNA of } CSRNP1} + 0.820 \times \exp_{\text{mRNA of } CSRNP2} - 1.428 \times \exp_{\text{mRNA of } CSRNP3}$. We found that OS was worse in patients from the high- than from the low-risk groups (AUC = 0.69). Moreover, this signature was an independent predictor after adjusting for clinical features. Functional enrichment analysis positively associated CSRNPs with the acute inflammatory response and humoral immune response pathways. This was validated by correlating each *CSRNP* with 28 types of immunocytes in tumor and normal tissues. A higher expression of *CSRNP1* and *CSRNP3* was associated with a better prognosis in both the high- and low-mutant burden groups. Cg19538674, cg07772537, and cg07811002 of *CSRNP1*, *CSRNP2*, and *CSRNP3*, respectively, were the predominant DNA methylation sites affecting OS. The *CSRNP* gene family signature may serve as a prognostic biomarker for predicting OS in patients with ccRCC. The association between *CSRNPs* and immune infiltration might offer future clinical treatment options.

Keywords: clear cell renal cell carcinoma, *CSRNP* family, prognosis, immune infiltration, The Cancer Genome Atlas (TCGA)

## INTRODUCTION

Renal cell carcinoma (RCC) has multiple histological subtypes; together, they account for nearly 3% of all human malignant carcinomas (1). The incidence and mortality of RCC continue to increase, and predictions in the United States indicated that 73,750 new cases should be expected in 2020, and that these would directly result in 14,830 deaths (2). The most prevalent (70%–80%) histology of RCC is clear cell renal cell carcinoma (ccRCC) (3). However, 20%–30% of patients with ccRCC have confirmed metastasis at the time of diagnosis (4). Furthermore, although targeted therapy is promising, the 5-year survival rate of patients with metastatic ccRCC remains < 10% (5). Therefore, novel effective biomarkers should be explored to predict the prognoses of patients with ccRCC.

The cysteine-serine-rich nuclear protein (CSRNP) family members, CSRNP1, CSRNP2, and CSRNP3, have been considered as nuclear proteins (6). Their corresponding transcription factors, which are conserved from *Drosophila* to humans (7), play essential roles in many important processes, such as cephalic neural progenitor proliferation, overall zebrafish survival (8), and mouse development (6).

Interleukin-2 induces *CSRNP1* (also known as Axin1 upregulated 1; *AXUD1*) in mouse T cells; it expresses a 1.7 kb transcript with five exons in some malignant cancers, such as kidney, liver, lung, and colon carcinomas (9). Besides, a 4.1 kb *CSRNP2* transcript has been detected in numerous mammalian organs, especially in the brain, ovary, and thymus. Finally, *CSRNP3* (also known as *Mbu-1*) is a brain-specific gene (10); it is expressed in the brain and spinal cords of embryonic to adult mice only (11). These findings suggested that the *CSRNP* gene family might have great value in different cancers. However, few publications have described associations between CSRNP family members and the prognoses of patients with ccRCC.

We therefore explored the distinct expression and multilevel prognostic values of CSRNPs using integrative bioinformatics analysis tools to provide further guidance for the diagnosis and clinical therapy of patients with ccRCC.

## MATERIALS AND METHODS

### mRNA Expression of *CSRNPs* and Patient Survival

We explored whether the expression of CSRNP family members, which are involved in different clinical stages and affect the prognosis of ccRCC, differed between ccRCC and normal tissues. We therefore analyzed mRNA expression, stage-specific expression, overall survival (OS), and CSRNPs matching normal and genotype-tissue expression (GTEx) data derived from The Cancer Genome Atlas (TCGA), using the Gene Expression Profiling Interactive Analysis (GEPIA) online tool (12) (http://gepia.cancer-pku.cn/), to investigate genomic functionality. We obtained the expression profile of TCGA-KIRC from UCSC Xena (https://xenabrowser.net/datapages/?cohort=GDC%20TCGA%20Kidney%20Clear%20Cell%20Carcinoma%20(KIRC)&removeHub=https%3A%2F%2Fxena.treehouse.gi.ucsc.edu%3A443) and the expression profile and clinical features of GSE29609 from the Gene Expression Omnibus (http://www.ncbi.nlm.nih.gov/geo/).

### Prognostic Values of the CSRNP Family Signature

We aimed to construct a comprehensive CSRNP family signature to better predict the OS of ccRCC patients. The SurvExpress online tool (13) (http://bioinformatica.mty.itesm.mx:8080/Biomatec/SurvivaX.jsp) was utilized to construct and evaluate the prognostic value of the CSRNP family signature. Here, a risk score formula was obtained, and the risk score for each patient was automatically generated. Patients were assigned to high- or low-risk groups based on the median cutoff value of the risk scores. Moreover, the independent prognostic value of the CSRNP family signature was determined using multivariate Cox regression analysis incorporating age, gender, grade, stage, and the signature.

### Functional Enrichment Analysis of Differentially Expressed Genes (DEGs) Between Healthy and Tumor Groups and High- and Low- Risk Groups

We then investigated the correlations between potentially critical pathways and the risk score model. First, DEGs between normal or adjacent tissues and ccRCC ($|\log_2 FC| > 1$ and $P < 0.05$) were detected using volcano plots. Then, samples were classified as belonging to the high- or low-risk groups based on the median cutoff of the risk score model; DEGs between these two groups ($|\log_2 FC| > 1$ and $P < 0.05$) were also identified *via* volcano plots. Finally, DEGs that merged in Venn diagrams were considered as risk-related DEGs and selected for further analysis by Metascape (14) (http://metascape.org/gp/index.html).

### Correlations Between *CSRNPs* and Immune Infiltration

According to the results of the functional enrichment analysis, CSRNP family members may play a role in ccRCC immunotherapy-related signaling pathways. To further verify this finding, we calculated the immune infiltration of 28 immunocytes using a set of genes determined by single-sample gene set enrichment analysis (ssGSEA) (15). Subsequently, the correlations between each *CSRNP* family gene and the 28 immunocytes were evaluated in normal kidney and ccRCC tumor samples.

### Prognosis of Genetic and Epigenetic Changes in *CSRNP* Family Members

Since the transcriptional gene expression profile could be affected by genetic and epigenetic changes (16, 17), we examined whether CSRNP family genetically and epigenetically influenced the prognosis of ccRCC.

First, genetic alterations, which mainly comprised missense and truncating mutations, amplification, and deep deletion, were analyzed using cBioPortal (18) (http://www.cbioportal.org/).

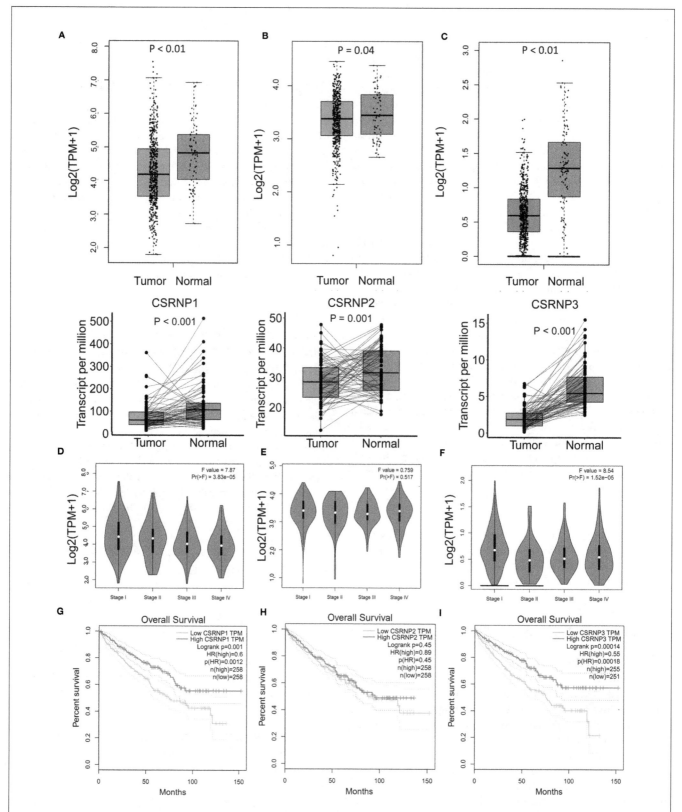

**FIGURE 1 |** mRNA expression, stage-specific expression, and overall survival of CSRNP gene family members according to GEPIA. **(A–C)** mRNA expression of CSRNP family members in tumor and normal tissues (upper image), and paired tumor and normal tissues (lower image). Green: tumor tissues; gray: normal tissues. **(D–F)** Stage-specific mRNA expression of CSRNP family members. **(G–I)** Kaplan-Meier curves of the overall survival analysis in relation to the CSRNP family.

Patients were assigned to groups with a high- or a low-mutant burden based on the median cutoff value, and their survival was analyzed using Kaplan-Meier (K-M) curves according to the genetic alterations found in each *CSRNP* family gene.

Then, we assessed epigenetic changes in the *CSRNP* family, and evaluated the relative DNA methylation site data from TCGA using the comprehensive bioinformatics platform MethSurv (19) (https://biit.cs.ut.ee/methsurv/). Moreover, the prognostic values of all methylation sites associated with CSRNP family members were assessed.

## Statistical Analysis

Univariate and multivariate Cox regression analyses of CSRNP family members were performed for assessing the OS of patients, using hazard ratios (HR) and a 95% confidence interval (95% CI). Paired t-tests were conducted to compare tumor and adjacent normal tissues from patients from the TCGA-KIRC dataset. OS was evaluated using the K-M curves. $P$ values < 0.05 were considered statistically significant.

## RESULTS

### mRNA Expression Levels of *CSRNP* Family and OS

*CSRNP1*, *CSRNP2*, and *CSRNP3* were significantly less abundant in ccRCC (n = 532) than in normal (n = 72) tissue sample data from TCGA-KIRC database (**Figures 1A–C**). Moreover, comparisons of paired tumor and adjacent normal tissues from patients generated similar results (**Figures 1A–C**). We also found that *CSRNP1* displayed significantly different stage-specific expression: the more advanced the ccRCC stage, the lower the *CSRNP1* expression (**Figure 1D**). However, the expression of *CSRNP2* did not differ between stages (**Figure 1E**), whereas *CSRNP3* showed a higher expression in stage I than in stage II-IV ccRCC samples (**Figure 1F**). We also compared the expression of *CSRNPs* across different Fuhrman grades based on GSE29609 and found no significant differences (**Figure S1**).

We then evaluated whether *CSRNP* mRNA levels affected the prognosis of ccRCC, and found that high mRNA levels of *CSRNP1* (HR: 0.60, $P$ = 0.001) and *CSRNP3* (HR: 0.55, $P$ < 0.001) were significantly correlated with favorable OS (**Figures 1G, I**). In contrast, the mRNA expression of *CSRNP2* was not significantly associated with a favorable OS (**Figure 1H**).

### Combined Prognostic Value of the *CSRNP* Family Signature

We constructed a CSRNP family signature risk score model as follows: risk score = $-0.224 \times \exp_{\text{mRNA of } CSRNP1} + 0.820 \times \exp_{\text{mRNA of } CSRNP2} - 1.428 \times \exp_{\text{mRNA of } CSRNP3}$, according to the coefficient indexes shown in **Table 1**. Differences in the expression patterns of CSRNPs were observed between the low- and high-risk (n = 234 each) groups based on the median cutoff value of risk scores. A lower expression of *CSRNP1* and *CSRNP3* was observed in the high-risk group, whereas there was a higher expression of *CSRNP2*, compared to those levels

**TABLE 1 |** Cox proportional hazard regression analysis result shows the coefficient of CSRNP family.

|  | Co-ef | Exp(coef) | Se(coef) | Z | Pr>|Z| |
|---|---|---|---|---|---|
| CSRNP1 | -0.224 | 0.799 | 0.092 | -2.429 | 0.01513 |
| CSRNP2 | 0.820 | 2.271 | 0.255 | 3.213 | 0.00131 |
| CSRNP3 | -1.428 | 0.240 | 0.442 | -3.228 | 0.00125 |

*Co-ef, co-efficient; Exp (co-ef), Expectation (co-ef); Se (co-ef), standard error (coef).*

observed in the low-risk group (**Figures 2A–C**). As expected, the low-risk group had a better OS than the high-risk group (**Figure 2D**; HR: 2.30, 95% CI: 1.63–3.24, $P$ < 0.001). Moreover, the area under the curve (AUC) of a time-dependent ROC increased to 0.69 during the follow-up period (**Figure 2E**). In addition, we compared the distribution of clinical features between the low- and high-risk groups and found similar age and sex distributions between them. However, more patients in the high-risk group had advanced tumor stages or tumor grades (**Table 2**).

Results from a multivariate Cox regression analysis suggested that the CSRNP family signature was an independent predictor for the prognosis of patients with ccRCC (**Figure 2F**; HR: 1.550, 95% CI: 1.084–2.220, $P$ = 0.0163).

### Functional Enrichment Analysis of *CSRNP* Impacted Genes

Significant DEGs between normal and ccRCC tumor tissues ($|\log_2 \text{FC}| > 1$ and $P$ < 0.05; **Figure 3A**) and between high-and low-risk groups were selected ($|\log_2 \text{FC}| > 1$ and $P$ < 0.05; **Figure 3B**). Then, DEGs that were significantly upregulated in tumor tissues and the high-risk group (481 genes) and those significantly downregulated in tumor tissues and the low-risk group (44 genes) (**Figure 3C**) were further analyzed using Metascape. The results showed that CSRNPs were associated with different pathways, including the acute inflammatory response, humoral immune response, natural killer cell differentiation involved in immune response, and regulation of immune effector process (**Figures 3D, E**).

### Correlations Between CSRNPs and Immune Infiltration

The functional enrichment analysis associated the CSRNP family with immune infiltration signaling pathways. To further verify this, we calculated the immune infiltration of 28 immunocytes between tumor and paracancerous tissues, and found that 22 out of the 28 immunocytes were more abundant in tumor than in paracancerous tissues (**Figure 4A**).

We then evaluated the correlation between *CSRNPs* and the 28 immunocytes in normal kidney and ccRCC samples. The results indicated that the immune infiltration profiles of the *CSRNPs* differed between normal and ccRCC tissues. Moreover, the CSRNP family was significantly correlated with more immunocytes in tumor than in normal tissues. We found that all three *CSRNPs* were positively associated with the infiltration of type 2 T helper cells, mast cells, and natural killer cells, and negatively associated with the abundance of CD56[bright] natural killer cells and activated CD8 T cells (**Figure**

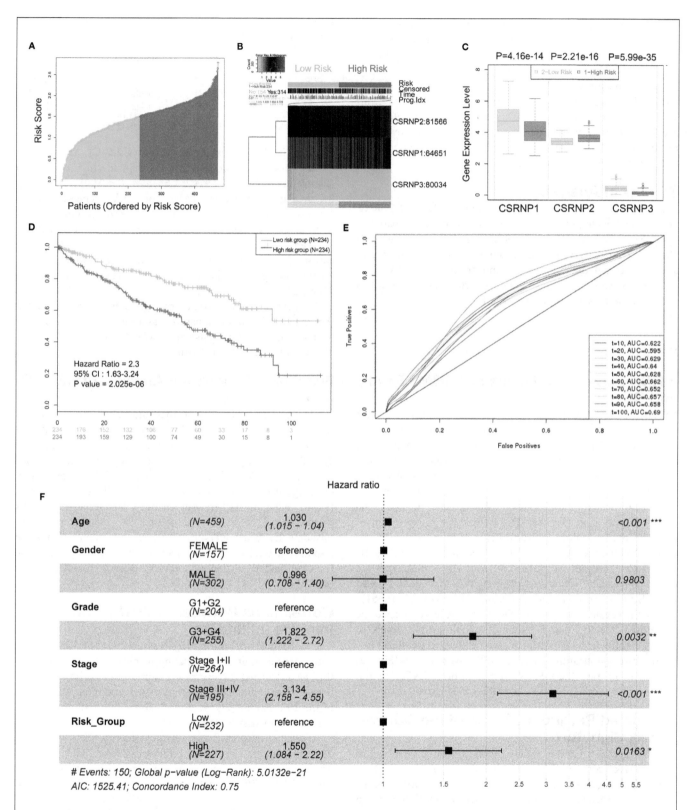

**FIGURE 2** | Prognostic values of the CSRNP family signature determined using SurvExpress. **(A)** Patients were assigned to high- and low-risk groups based on median cutoff risk scores. **(B)** Heat map of CSRNP family members expression. **(C)** Comparison of the expression of *CSRNP* genes between low- and high-risk groups. **(D)** Survival analysis of low- (green) and high-risk (red) groups. **(E)** Time-dependent receiver operating characteristics (ROC) curves. **(F)** Multivariate Cox regression analysis of variables and CSRNP family signature risk scores. *$P < 0.05$, **$P < 0.01$, ***$P < 0.001$.

**TABLE 2 |** Summarization of clinical features.

|  | Subgroup | Low risk | High risk | P |
|---|---|---|---|---|
| Age (years) |  | 60.59 ± 12.10 | 60.60 ± 12.29 | 0.994 |
| Gender (%) | Female | 82 (35.3) | 75 (33.0) | 0.673 |
|  | Male | 150 (64.7) | 152 (67.0) |  |
| Grade (%) | G1+G2 | 128 (55.2) | 76 (33.5) | <0.001 |
|  | G3+G4 | 104 (44.8) | 151 (66.5) |  |
| Stage (%) | Stage I+II | 162 (69.8) | 102 (44.9) | <0.001 |
|  | Stage III+IV | 70 (30.2) | 125 (55.1) |  |

4B). These results indicated that the CSRNP family might impact the immune environment of ccRCC through the above-mentioned immunocytes. The immune infiltration profile is different in normal kidney tissues. CSRNP1 only positively regulated the infiltration of eight immunocytes and did not negatively regulate any, which was significantly different from its effects in ccRCC tissues. Meanwhile, CSRNP2 and CSRNP3 were both mostly positively associated with effector memory CD4 T cells, but not with type 2 T cells in tumor tissues (**Figure 4C**).

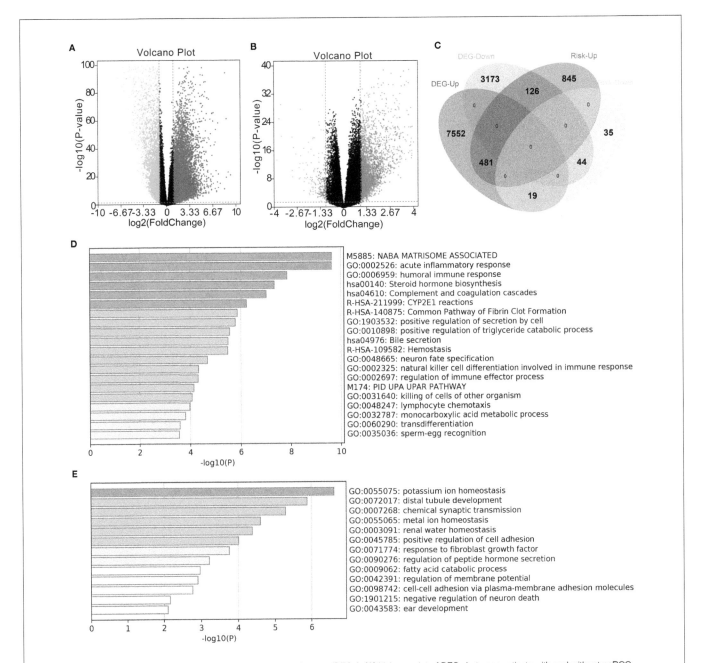

**FIGURE 3 |** Functional enrichment analysis of differentially expressed genes (DEGs). **(A)** Volcano plot of DEGs between patients with and without ccRCC.
**(B)** Volcano plot of DEGs between patients in the high- and low-risk groups. **(C)** Venn diagram merging DEGs from **(A, B)**. **(D, E)** Functional enrichment analysis of significantly **(D)** upregulated genes associated with both tumors and increased risk of tumors, and **(E)** downregulated genes associated with tumors and decreased risk of tumors.

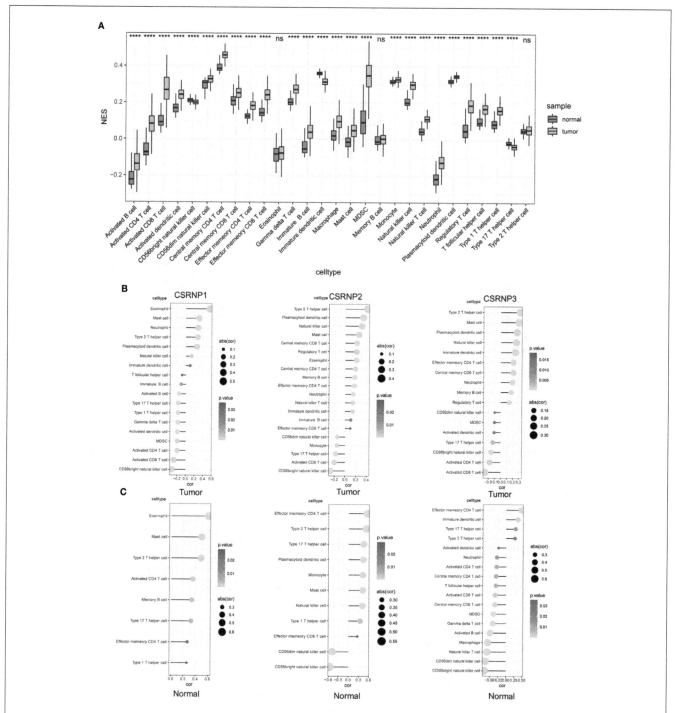

**FIGURE 4** | Correlations between CSRNP family and immune infiltration. **(A)** Normalized enrichment scores (NES) of 28 immunocytes between normal and tumor tissues. **(B, C)** Correlations between CSRNP family and significant infiltrated immunocytes in tumor **(B)** and normal **(C)** tissues.

## Genetic Alteration in *CSRNP*s

Genetic alterations play an important role in the regulation of gene expression. We found that the genetic alterations in *CSRNP1*, *CSRNP2*, and *CSRNP3* were approximately 11%, 0.2%, and 0.8%, respectively (**Figure 5A**). We then evaluated the prognostic values of *CSRNP*s in high- and low- mutant burden patients in all enrolled patients with ccRCC, and

found that both *CSRNP1* and *CSRNP3* act as protective factors in both high- and low-mutant burden patients (**Figures 5B, E, D, G**). Meanwhile, although we did not find a significant effect of *CSRNP2* on ccRCC OS in the entire group, we found that *CSRNP2* was a remarkable hazard factor in patients with a high-, but not with a low-mutant burden (**Figures 5C, F**).

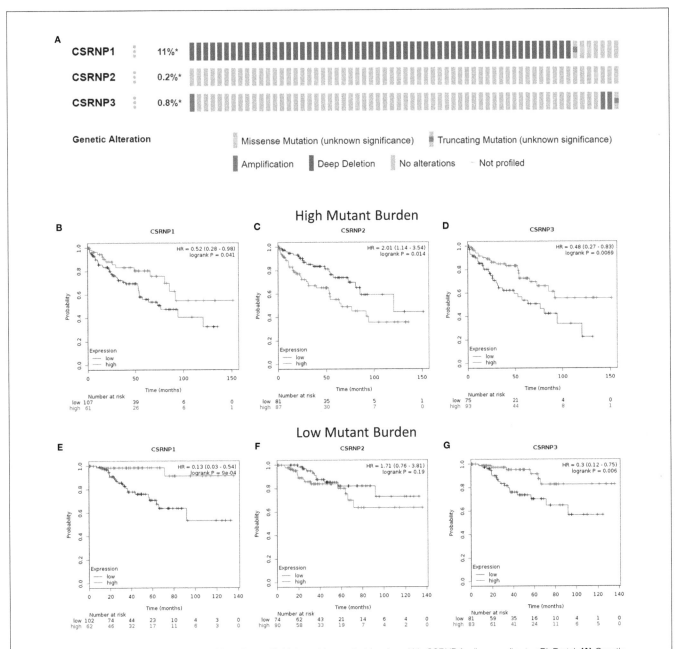

**FIGURE 5** | Genetic alterations and overall survival in patients with high- and low-mutant burden within CSRNP family according to cBioPortal. **(A)** Genetic alterations of *CSRNP* genes in patients from TCGA dataset (each rectangle represents one patient; not all patients were shown [n = 532]); **(B–G)** Overall survival of patients with high- **(B–D)** and low- **(E–G)** mutant burden within CSRNP family.

## DNA Methylation Sites Within *CSRNP*s

DNA methylation also plays a pivotal role in the regulation of gene expression and affects clinical outcomes. The DNA methylation sites of the *CSRNP* genes and the prognostic values of each CpG obtained from TCGA database were analyzed by MethSurv (**Figures 6A–C** and **Table 3**). We found that cg19538674 of CSRNP1, cg07772537 of CSRNP2, and cg07811002 of CSRNP3 were the most methylated sites (**Figures 6A–C**). However, cg03540589 (HR: 2.87, 95% CI: 1.571-5.243, *P* < 0.001), cg23618218 (HR: 2.037, 95% CI: 1.196-3.469, *P* = 0.009), and cg07811002 (HR: 0.588, 95% CI:

0.392-0.879, *P* = 0.010) of *CSRNP1*, *CSRNP2*, and *CSRNP3*, respectively, were the most powerful and DNA methylation locational risk factors. Overall, nine, ten, and two CpGs of *CSRNP1*, *CSRNP2*, and *CSRNP3*, respectively, indicated aberrant prognosis (**Figures 6A–C**).

## DISCUSSION

With the rapid development of bioinformatics tools for analyzing multiple databases with many clinical samples, outcomes, and

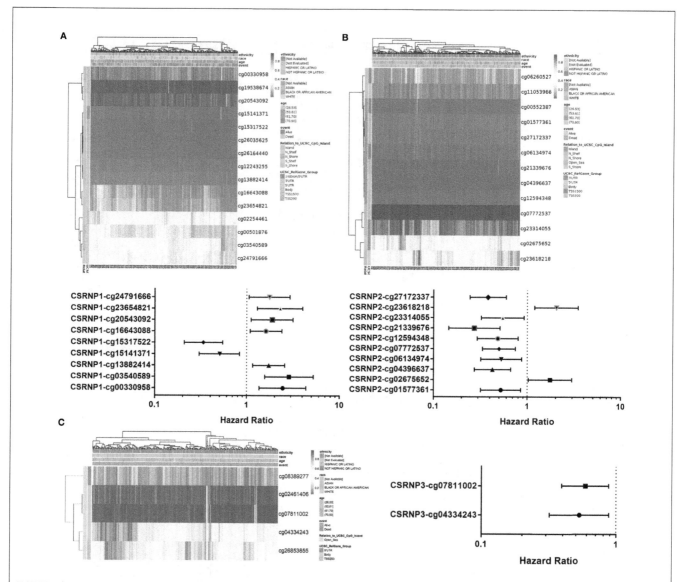

**FIGURE 6** | DNA methylation analysis of CSRNP family members using MethSurv. The DNA methylation clustered expression and forest plot of *CSRNP1* **(A)**, *CSRNP2* **(B)**, and *CSRNP3* **(C)**. Red to blue scale indicates high to low expression. Various colorful side boxes were used to characterize the ethnicity, race, age, event, and relation to UCSC_CpG_island and UCSC_refGene_Group.

different clinical features, prognoses can be predicted and specific cancers can be detected using biomarker molecules, especially some gene families. This study mainly explored the prognostic value and biology of *CSRNP* family genes in ccRCC using online bioinformatics tools.

*CSRNP1* has been considered as an immediate early gene (20) that binds the specific sequence AGAGTG and contains domains rich in cysteine and serine. The results of single, double, or triple gene knockouts *in vivo* indicated that the expression of *CSRNP1* could be highly induced by IL-2 in mouse T lymphocytes (6). In this study, we found that *CSRNP1* expression is positively associated with the infiltration of type 2 T helper cells in both normal and ccRCC tissues, confirming the previous findings. Noteworthy, in *Drosophila*, upregulated *CSRNP1* disturbs cell cycle progression by downregulating Cdk1 activity and

promoting apoptosis in a JNK-dependent manner (21). Besides, AXUD1 (CSRNP1) upregulates cytokine-increased MMP1 expression in the articular chondrocytes (22). These findings might facilitate our understanding of the role of CSRNP1 in the progression of various types of cancers. However, whether it affects the prognosis of patients with ccRCC requires further investigation. In this study, we found that CSRNP1 could be an important suppressive prognostic factor. Decreased mRNA expression of *CSRNP1* was associated with a poor prognosis in patients with ccRCC; whereas stage-specific expression profiles significantly differed. Moreover, in terms of potential genetic and epidemic alterations, CSRNP1 acts as a protective factor in patients with high- and low-mutant burdens. In addition, nine CpGs of *CSRNP1* were correlated with a significantly aberrant prognosis.

**TABLE 3 |** The significantly prognostic values of CpG in the CSRNP family.

| Gene-CpG | HR | 95% CI | P value |
|---|---|---|---|
| CSRNP1-Body-N_Shore-cg00330958 | 2.448 | 1.369-4.377 | 0.002525 |
| CSRNP1-5'UTR-N_Shore-cg03540589 | 2.87 | 1.571-5.243 | 0.000606 |
| CSRNP1-5'UTR-Island-cg13882414 | 1.732 | 1.167-2.571 | 0.006379 |
| CSRNP1-1stExon;5'UTR-Island-cg15141371 | 0.503 | 0.301-0.838 | 0.008363 |
| CSRNP1-TSS200-Island-cg15317522 | 0.335 | 0.208-0.542 | 8.07E-06 |
| CSRNP1-5'UTR-S_Shelf-cg16643088 | 1.615 | 1.092-2.388 | 0.016263 |
| CSRNP1-3'UTR-N_Shelf-cg20543092 | 1.88 | 1.118-3.161 | 0.017233 |
| CSRNP1-5'UTR-S_Shore-cg23654821 | 2.294 | 1.306-4.03 | 0.003876 |
| CSRNP1-5'UTR-N_Shelf-cg24791666 | 1.759 | 1.057-2.926 | 0.029723 |
| CSRNP2-TSS200-Island-cg01577361 | 0.523 | 0.32-0.854 | 0.009528 |
| CSRNP2-TSS1500-S_Shore-cg02675652 | 1.747 | 1.026-2.977 | 0.040103 |
| CSRNP2-5'UTR-Island-cg04396637 | 0.427 | 0.274-0.668 | 0.000188 |
| CSRNP2-TSS1500-Island-cg06134974 | 0.529 | 0.321-0.872 | 0.012577 |
| CSRNP2-Body-Open_Sea-cg07772537 | 0.501 | 0.335-0.748 | 0.000728 |
| CSRNP2-TSS200-Island-cg12594348 | 0.485 | 0.294-0.8 | 0.004652 |
| CSRNP2-TSS200-Island-cg21339676 | 0.273 | 0.146-0.512 | 5.18E-05 |
| CSRNP2-3'UTR-Open_Sea-cg23314055 | 0.548 | 0.325-0.922 | 0.023602 |
| CSRNP2-5'UTR-N_Shelf-cg23618218 | 2.037 | 1.196-3.469 | 0.008819 |
| CSRNP2-TSS200-Island-cg27172337 | 0.383 | 0.245-0.597 | 2.32E-05 |
| CSRNP3-Body-Open_Sea-cg04334243 | 0.53 | 0.318-0.882 | 0.014682 |
| CSRNP3-Body-Open_Sea-cg07811002 | 0.588 | 0.392-0.879 | 0.009772 |

CSRNP2 has been positively associated with many aberrant non-cancerous diseases, including obesity and type 2 diabetes mellitus (23). Moreover, Vargas et al. (24) reported that CSRNP2 acts as a potential drug repositioning candidate for the treatment of Alzheimer's disease. However, the present study found that CSRNP2 did not sufficiently correlated with the OS of patients with ccRCC to serve as an important prognostic factor, according to the GEPIA analysis results. Furthermore, CSRNP2 was a remarkable hazard factor for patients with a high-, but not with a low-, mutant burden. In addition, the DNA methylation sites of CSRNP2 showed significant hazard ratios, suggested that CSRNP2 might be a meaningful target gene for epigenetic therapy.

CSRNP3 was found to encode a transcriptional factor for muscle development in growing pigs (25), and was reported as a target gene to treat obesity and metabolic syndrome in an exome-wide mediated study (26). However, the role of CSRNP3 in cancer development requires further investigation. We found that mRNA expression of CSRNP3, like that of CSRNP1, was lower in ccRCC, and was associated with a poor prognosis. Moreover, CSRNP3 may be a protective factor in patients with high- and low-mutant burdens. In addition, two CpGs of CSRNP3 positively correlated with significantly aberrant prognosis, which might help clarify detailed biological functions.

The prognostic values of CSRNP genes were consistent with the above details. We constructed a novel risk score model based on the expression of the CSRNP family to improve the prediction of OS. We also classified all the samples into high- and low-risk groups according to the median cutoff value of the risk score. The expression profiles of the CSRNP family members were different between these groups, especially those of CSRNP1 and CSRNP3. The low-risk group had a better OS. Importantly, the AUC of the time-dependent ROC curve reached 0.69 over time. Moreover,

this signature was an independent predictor of prognosis among patients with ccRCC. Our model exhibited good diagnostic and predictive capacities, but further improvement is needed. The CSRNP family, particularly CSRNP1 and CSRNP3, was validated as a useful prognostic biomarker for patients with ccRCC.

Further investigation on functional enrichment analysis implied that the CSRNP family might function *via* immune-related biological pathways. We found that immunocyte infiltration was higher in tumor than in paracancerous tissues. The immune infiltration profile of the CSRNP family genes in ccRCC tumor tissues was different from that in normal tissues; natural killer cells and plasmacytoid dendritic cells showed positive correlations. It is known that natural killer cells destroy various cancer cells (27–29), including renal cell carcinoma (30). Plasmacytoid dendritic cell (pDC) infiltration predicts better survival in triple-negative breast cancer (31) and melanoma (32). In addition, effector memory CD4 T cells could be considered as a protective factor in HIV (33) and cytomegalovirus disease (34). Consistently, we found that CSRNP2 and CSRNP3 were both mostly positively associated with effector memory CD4 T cells in normal tissues. Taken together, the CSRNP family might play an important role in ccRCC immune infiltration and impact the immune environment of ccRCC through immunocyte infiltration.

There were some limitations to this study. The most important was that we generated conclusions mostly based on online integrative bioinformatics analysis tools; therefore, data from *in vitro* or *in vivo* experiments, and clinical validation are urgently needed. Limitations are also imposed by the retrospective design of the study and the small sample size. Therefore, we plan to cooperate with several urological centers to conduct a prospective study and maximize the sample size. We will also continue to conduct in-depth investigations into the occurrence and development of CSRNP family genes in ccRCC to support our conclusion that the CSRNP family could serve as a useful prognostic biomarker.

In conclusion, we comprehensively explored the prognostic value of the CSRNP family using online integrative bioinformatics analysis tools. The CSRNP family signature may serve as a prognostic biomarker to predict the OS of patients with ccRCC. The risk score model based on the CSRNP showed good diagnostic and independent predictive capacity. The association between the CSRNP family and immune infiltration might offer another clinical treatment option.

## AUTHOR CONTRIBUTIONS

GY designed the study. HZ and XQ performed the bioinformatics analyses and wrote the manuscript. All authors contributed to the article and approved the submitted version.

## SUPPLEMENTARY MATERIAL

**Supplementary Figure 1 |** Expression of CSRNPs in patients with different Fuhrman grade ccRCCs.

# REFERENCES

1. Dunnick NR. Renal cell carcinoma: staging and surveillance. *Abdominal Radiol (NY)* (2016) 41:1079–85. doi: 10.1007/s00261-016-0692-0

2. Siegel RL, Miller KD. Cancer statistics, 2020. *CA Cancer J Clin* (2020) 70:7–30. doi: 10.3322/caac.21590

3. Ferlay J, Soerjomataram I, Dikshit R, Eser S, Mathers C, Rebelo M, et al. Cancer incidence and mortality worldwide: sources, methods and major patterns in GLOBOCAN 2012. *Int J Cancer* (2015) 136:E359–86. doi: 10.1002/ijc.29210

4. Kroeger N, Seligson DB, Signoretti S, Yu H, Magyar CE, Huang J, et al. Poor prognosis and advanced clinicopathological features of clear cell renal cell carcinoma (ccRCC) are associated with cytoplasmic subcellular localisation of Hypoxia inducible factor-2alpha. *Eur J Cancer* (2014) 50:1531–40. doi: 10.1016/j.ejca.2014.01.031

5. Selvi I, Demirci U. The prognostic effect of immunoscore in patients with clear cell renal cell carcinoma: preliminary results. *Int Urol Nephrol* (2020) 52:21–34. doi: 10.1007/s11255-019-02285-0

6. Gingras S, Pelletier S, Boyd K, Ihle JN. Characterization of a family of novel cysteine- serine-rich nuclear proteins (CSRNP). *PLoS One* (2007) 2:e808–8. doi: 10.1371/journal.pone.0000808

7. Espina J, Feijóo CG, Solís C, Glavic A. csrnp1a is necessary for the development of primitive hematopoiesis progenitors in zebrafish. *PLoS One* (2013) 8:e53858. doi: 10.1371/journal.pone.0053858

8. Feijóo CG, Sarrazin AF, Allende ML, Glavic A. Cystein-serine-rich nuclear protein 1, Axud1/Csrnp1, is essential for cephalic neural progenitor proliferation and survival in zebrafish. *Dev Dyn* (2009) 238:2034–43. doi: 10.1002/dvdy.22006

9. Ishiguro H, Tsunoda T, Tanaka T, Fujii Y, Nakamura Y, Furukawa Y. Identification of AXUD1, a novel human gene induced by AXIN1 and its reduced expression in human carcinomas of the lung, liver, colon and kidney. *Oncogene* (2001) 20:5062–66. doi: 10.1038/sj.onc.1204603

10. Yang HL, Cho EY, Han KH, Kim H, Kim SJ. Characterization of a novel mouse brain gene (mbu-1) identified by digital differential display. *Gene* (2007) 395:144–50. doi: 10.1016/j.gene.2007.03.005

11. Kim B, Kang S, Kim SJ. Differential promoter methylation and histone modification contribute to the brain specific expression of the mouse Mbu-1 gene. *Mol Cells* (2012) 34:433–37. doi: 10.1007/s10059-012-0182-3

12. Tang Z, Li C, Kang B, Gao G, Li C, Zhang Z. GEPIA: a web server for cancer and normal gene expression profiling and interactive analyses. *Nucleic Acids Res* (2017) 45:W98–102. doi: 10.1093/nar/gkx247

13. Aguirre-Gamboa R, Gomez-Rueda H, Martínez-Ledesma E, Martínez-Torteya A, Chacolla-Huaringa R, Rodriguez-Barrientos A, et al. SurvExpress: an online biomarker validation tool and database for cancer gene expression data using survival analysis. *PLoS One* (2013) 8:e7425. doi: 10.1371/journal.pone.0074250

14. Zhou Y, Zhou B, Pache L, Chang M. Metascape provides a biologist-oriented resource for the analysis of systems-level datasets. *Nat Commun* (2019) 10:1523. doi: 10.1038/s41467-019-09234-6

15. Yoshihara K, Shahmoradgoli M, Martínez E, Vegesna R, Kim H, Torres-Garcia W, et al. Inferring tumour purity and stromal and immune cell admixture from expression data. *Nat Commun* (2013) 4:2612. doi: 10.1038/ncomms3612

16. Li Y, Gong Y, Ning X, Peng D, Liu L, He S, et al. Downregulation of CLDN7 due to promoter hypermethylation is associated with human clear cell renal cell carcinoma progression and poor prognosis. *J J Exp Clin Cancer Res* (2018) 37:276. doi: 10.1186/s13046-018-0924-y

17. Nam HY, Chandrashekar DS, Kundu A, Shelar S, Kho EY, Sonpavde G, et al. Integrative Epigenetic and Gene Expression Analysis of Renal Tumor Progression to Metastasis. *Mol Cancer Res MCR* (2019) 17:84–96. doi: 10.1158/1541-7786.MCR-17-0636

18. Gao J, Aksoy BA, Dogrusoz U, Dresdner G, Gross B, Sumer SO, et al. Integrative analysis of complex cancer genomics and clinical profiles using the cBioPortal. *Sci Signal* (2013) 6:pl. doi: 10.1126/scisignal.2004088

19. Modhukur V, Iljasenko T, Metsalu T, Lokk K, Laisk-Podar T, Vilo J. MethSurv: a web tool to perform multivariable survival analysis using DNA methylation data. *Epigenomics* (2018) 10:277–88. doi: 10.2217/epi-2017-0118

20. Hutton JJ, Jegga AG, Kong S, Gupta A, Ebert C, Williams S, et al. Microarray and comparative genomics-based identification of genes and gene regulatory regions of the mouse immune system. *BMC Genomics* (2004) 5:82. doi: 10.1186/1471-2164-5-82

21. Glavic A, Molnar C, Cotoras D, de Celis JF. Drosophila Axud1 is involved in the control of proliferation and displays pro-apoptotic activity. *Mech Dev* (2009) 126:184–97. doi: 10.1016/j.mod.2008.11.005

22. Macdonald CD, Falconer AMD, Chan CM, Wilkinson DJ, Skelton A, Reynard L, et al. Cytokine-induced cysteine- serine-rich nuclear protein-1 (CSRNP1) selectively contributes to MMP1 expression in human chondrocytes. *PLoS One* (2018) 13:e0207240. doi: 10.1371/journal.pone.0207240

23. Chen J, Meng Y, Zhou J, Zhuo M, Ling F, Zhang Y, et al. Identifying candidate genes for Type 2 Diabetes Mellitus and obesity through gene expression profiling in multiple tissues or cells. *J Diabetes Res* (2013) 2013:970435. doi: 10.1155/2013/970435

24. Vargas DM, De Bastiani MA, Zimmer ER, Klamt F. Alzheimer's disease master regulators analysis: search for potential molecular targets and drug repositioning candidates. *Alzheimers Res Ther* (2018) 10:59. doi: 10.1186/s13195-018-0394-7

25. Messad F, Louveau I, Koffi B, Gilbert H, Gondret F. Investigation of muscle transcriptomes using gradient boosting machine learning identifies molecular predictors of feed efficiency in growing pigs. *BMC Genomics* (2019) 20:659. doi: 10.1186/s12864-019-6010-9

26. Yamada Y, Sakuma J, Takeuchi I, Yasukochi Y, Kato K, Oguri M, et al. Identification of rs7350481 at chromosome 11q23.3 as a novel susceptibility locus for metabolic syndrome in Japanese individuals by an exome-wide association study. *Oncotarget* (2017) 8:39296–308. doi: 10.18632/oncotarget.16945

27. Jo H, Cha B, Kim H, Brito S, Kwak BM, Kim ST, et al. α-Pinene Enhances the Anticancer Activity of Natural Killer Cells via ERK/AKT Pathway. *Int J Mol Sci* (2021) 22:656. doi: 10.3390/ijms22020656

28. Zanker DJ, Owen KL, Baschuk N, Spurling AJ, Parker BS. Loss of type I IFN responsiveness impairs natural killer cell antitumor activity in breast cancer. *Cancer Immunol Immunother* (2021). doi: 10.1007/s00262-021-02857-z

29. Shi M, Li ZY, Zhang LM, Wu XY, Xiang SH, Wang YG, et al. Hsa_circ_0007456 regulates the natural killer cell-mediated cytotoxicity toward hepatocellular carcinoma via the miR-6852-3p/ICAM-1 axis. *Cell Death Dis* (2021) 12:94. doi: 10.1038/s41419-020-03334-8

30. Shaffer TM, Aalipour A, Schürch CM, Gambhir SS. PET Imaging of the Natural Killer Cell Activation Receptor NKp30. *J Nucl Med* (2020) 61:1348–54. doi: 10.2967/jnumed.119.233163

31. Oshi M, Newman S, Tokumaru Y, Yan L, Matsuyama R, Kalinski P, et al. Plasmacytoid Dendritic Cell (pDC) Infiltration Correlate with Tumor Infiltrating Lymphocytes, Cancer Immunity, and Better Survival in Triple Negative Breast Cancer (TNBC) More Strongly than Conventional Dendritic Cell (cDC). *Cancers (Basel)* (2020) 12:3342. doi: 10.3390/cancers12113342

32. Zhang W, Lim SM, Wang JH, Ramalingam S, Kim M, Jin JO. Monophosphoryl lipid A-induced activation of plasmacytoid dendritic cells enhances the anti-cancer effects of anti-PD-L1 antibodies. *Cancer Immunol Immunother* (2020) 70:689–700. doi: 10.1007/s00262-020-02715-4

33. Potter SJ, Lacabaratz C, Lambotte O, Perez-Patrigeon S, Vingert B, Sinet M, et al. Preserved central memory and activated effector memory CD4+ T-cell subsets in human immunodeficiency virus controllers: an ANRS EP36 study. *J Virol* (2007) 81:13904–15. doi: 10.1128/jvi.01401-07

34. Gamadia LE, Remmerswaal EB, Weel JF, Bemelman F, Van Lier RA, Ten Berge IJ. Primary immune responses to human CMV: a critical role for IFN-gamma-producing CD4+ T cells in protection against CMV disease. *Blood* (2003) 101(7):2686–92. doi: 10.1182/blood-2002-08-2502

# 3

# Identification of an m6A-Related lncRNA Signature for Predicting the Prognosis in Patients with Kidney Renal Clear Cell Carcinoma

*JunJie Yu[1], WeiPu Mao[1], Si Sun[1], Qiang Hu[1], Can Wang[1], ZhiPeng Xu[1], RuiJi Liu[1], SaiSai Chen[1], Bin Xu[2] and Ming Chen[2,3]\**

[1] *Medical College, Southeast University, Nanjing, China,* [2] *Department of Urology, Affiliated Zhongda Hospital of Southeast University, Nanjing, China,* [3] *Department of Urology, Affiliated Lishui People's Hospital of Southeast University, Nanjing, China*

**\*Correspondence:**
*Ming Chen*
*mingchenseu@126.com*

**Purpose:** This study aimed to construct an m6A-related long non-coding RNAs (lncRNAs) signature to accurately predict the prognosis of kidney clear cell carcinoma (KIRC) patients using data obtained from The Cancer Genome Atlas (TCGA) database.

**Methods:** The KIRC patient data were downloaded from TCGA database and m6A-related genes were obtained from published articles. Pearson correlation analysis was implemented to identify m6A-related lncRNAs. Univariate, Lasso, and multivariate Cox regression analyses were used to identifying prognostic risk-associated lncRNAs. Five lncRNAs were identified and used to construct a prognostic signature in training set. Kaplan–Meier curves and receiver operating characteristic (ROC) curves were applied to evaluate reliability and sensitivity of the signature in testing set and overall set, respectively. A prognostic nomogram was established to predict the probable 1-, 3-, and 5-year overall survival of KIRC patients quantitatively. GSEA was performed to explore the potential biological processes and cellular pathways. Besides, the lncRNA/miRNA/mRNA ceRNA network and PPI network were constructed based on weighted gene co-expression network analysis (WGCNA). Functional Enrichment Analysis was used to identify the biological functions of m6A-related lncRNAs.

**Results:** We constructed and verified an m6A-related lncRNAs prognostic signature of KIRC patients in TCGA database. We confirmed that the survival rates of KIRC patients with high-risk subgroup were significantly poorer than those with low-risk subgroup in the training set and testing set. ROC curves indicated that the prognostic signature had a reliable predictive capability in the training set (AUC = 0.802) and testing set (AUC = 0.725), respectively. Also, we established a prognostic nomogram with a high C-index and accomplished good prediction accuracy. The lncRNA/miRNA/mRNA ceRNA network and PPI network, as well as functional enrichment analysis provided us with new ways to search for potential biological functions.

**Conclusions:** We constructed an m6A-related lncRNAs prognostic signature which could accurately predict the prognosis of KIRC patients.

Keywords: prognostic signature, The Cancer Genome Atlas, long non-coding RNA, kidney renal clear cell carcinoma, M6A

## INTRODUCTION

Renal cell carcinoma (RCC) was the third most common malignant tumor of the urinary system worldwide (1), of which kidney renal clear cell carcinoma (KIRC) was the most frequent subtype (2). Despite the development of many targeted drugs and immunosuppressive drugs, radical nephrectomy was still the primary and most effective treatment method (3). Moreover, KIRC was insensitive to chemotherapy and radiotherapy and had a higher rate of recurrence and metastasis than other subtypes of RCC (3, 4). A better understanding of the molecular mechanisms of KIRC was crucial for the development of new therapeutic agents. It was urgent to identify an effective prognostic signature to predict the survival outcomes of KIRC patients.

DNA methylation and post-translational histone modifications were involved in the epigenetic regulation of cell development and differentiation (5). N6-methyladenosine (m6A) modification was the most abundant internal epistatic modification of mRNA and non-coding RNA (6) and was involved in many biological processes, including RNA splicing, export, and translation (7). The m6A modifications were regulated by m6A regulators, including methyltransferases complex ("writers"), signal transducers ("readers"), and demethylases ("erasers") (8). It has been reported that M6A was closely associated with a variety of tumors and was thought to be one of the drivers of tumorigenesis and progression. Cai et al. (9) reported that m6A Methyltransferase METTL3 promoted the growth of prostate cancer by regulating hedgehog pathway. Guo et al. (10) reported that RNA demethylases ALKBH5 prevented pancreatic cancer progression by post-transcriptional activation of PER1. Furthermore, m6A-regulated genes also played an essential role in the pathogenicity of KIRC. Zhuang et al. (11) reported that FTO suppressed KIRC progression through the FTO-PGC-1α signaling pathway. Gao et al. (12) reported that DMDRMR-mediated regulation of CDK4 promoted KIRC progression through m6A reader IGF2BP3.

Long non-coding RNAs (lncRNAs) were a class of RNAs that could not encode proteins and have been widely studied in recent years (13). lncRNAs were involved in various biological processes in eukaryotes, and their aberrant expressions were near related to tumor malignancy, including tumor proliferation, differentiation, apoptosis, drug resistance, and metastasis (14, 15). Nevertheless, whether m6A modification-related lncRNAs

could be involved in the progression of KIRC remained to be elucidated. Therefore, it was urgent to identify m6A-associated lncRNAs biomarkers for the early diagnosis and prognosis of patients with KIRC.

Here, based on the data of KIRC patients downloaded from The Cancer Genome Atlas (TCGA) database, we constructed an m6A-related lncRNAs prognostic signature by bioinformatic and statistical analysis to predict the prognostic outcomes of KIRC patients accurately. We found that the prognostic signature constructed with five m6A-associated lncRNAs had a high predictive ability. Moreover, a nomogram was constructed to predict the overall survival (OS) of KIRC patients quantitatively. Finally, a ceRNA network and PPI network were built to further explore the possible biological mechanisms of lncRNAs in preparation for identifying new biomarkers.

## METHODS

### Data Source and Preparation

As the flow chart of the study shown in **Figure S1**, we downloaded Transcriptome profiling data in fragment per kilobase method (FPKM) format of 530 KIRC patients from TCGA data portal (https://portal.gdc.cancer.gov/). Subsequently, these data were collated and annotated, and then collapsed into protein-coding genes and long non-coding RNAs employing the Ensembl human genome browser (http://asia.ensembl.org/info/data/index.html) using the Perl program (16). And 14,142 lncRNAs were identified. Then, the differential analysis of these lncRNAs was performed by the "limma" package in R 4.0.3 (logFC > 1 or<-1, p < 0.05), and 4,492 significantly differential lncRNAs were identified. In addition, 35 m6A-related genes were obtained from published articles (8, 17), and the expression matrixes were extracted from transcriptome profiling datasets, including regulators on writers [KIAA1429 (VIRMA), METTL3, METTL14, WTAP, RBM15, RBM15B, METTL16, ZC3H13, and PCIF1], readers [TRMT112, ZCCHC4, NUDT21 (CPSF5), CPSF6, CBLL1 (HAKAI), SETD2, HNRNPC, HNRNPG (RBMX), HNRNPA2B1, IGF2BP1, IGF2BP2, IGF2BP3, YTHDC1, YTHDF1, YTHDF2, YTHDF3, YTHDC2, SRSF3, SRSF10, XRN1, FMR1 (FMRP), NXF1, and PRRC2A], and erasers (FTO, ALKBH5, and ALKBH3). The differential analysis was also performed by the "limma" package in R software and 25 m6A-related genes were confirmed to be significantly different (p < 0.05, **Figure S2**). Then, Pearson correlation analysis between these lncRNAs and 25 m6A-related genes was performed, and 753 m6A-related lncRNAs were identified (cor > 0.5 or <-0.5, p < 0.05). The clinicopathological data were downloaded from the TCGA dataset, excluding those with survival time <30 days or unknown (n = 17), and those with

---

Abbreviations: KIRC, kidney renal clear cell carcinoma; TCGA, The Cancer Genome Atlas; lncRNA, long non-coding RNA; m6A: N6-methyladenosine; ROC, receiver operating characteristic; GO, Gene Ontology; KEGG, Kyoto Encyclopedia of Genes and Genomes; AUC, area under the curve; CI, Confidence intervals; OS, Overall survival; C-index, concordance index; HR, Hazard ratios; AJCC, American Joint Committee on Cancer.

unclear specific information including stage (n = 3), tumor grade (n = 3), and AJCC M stage (n = 3). Subsequently, we merged lncRNAs expression data with clinical data. Ultimately, a total of 505 cases were included in the study.

## Construction and Verification of an m6A-Related lncRNAs Prognostic Signature

To construct an effective prognostic prediction signature, we randomly classified the 505 cases into training set (253 samples) and testing set (252 samples) in a 1:1 ratio (**Table 1**). The training set was applied to construct a prognostic signature and to evaluate it in the testing set. The univariate Cox proportional hazards regression analysis was used to identify m6A-related lncRNAs, which were significantly linked with prognosis (p < 0.01) in the training set. Least absolute shrinkage and selection operator (LASSO) regression analysis was applied to eliminate those prognostic-related lncRNAs highly correlated with each other to avoid overfitting. Later, the multivariate Cox proportional hazards regression analysis was subjected to determine independent prognostic factors. Ultimately, we identified five prognostic risk-related lncRNAs to construct a prognostic risk score signature. The risk score of KIRC patients was calculated using the format $risk\ score = \sum_{i=1}^{n} coef(i)*lncRNA(i)\ expression$. The KIRC patients were classified into high-risk subgroup and low-risk subgroup based on median risk score as the cut-off value. The Kaplan–Meier survival curve was performed to compare the survival outcomes of the two groups. The receiver operating characteristic curves (ROC) and its area under the curve (AUC) values were utilized to evaluate the specificity and sensitivity of the signature by "ROC package" in R software.

## Establishment and Validation of a Prognostic Nomogram

To quantitatively predict the prognosis of KIRC patients, we constructed a prognostic nomogram based on risk score and traditional prognosis-related clinical variables, including age,

grade, AJCC T stage. Afterward, the concordance index (C-index) and calibration curves were used to evaluate the reliability and accuracy of the prognostic nomogram.

## Gene Set Enrichment Analysis (GSEA) and Weighted Gene Co-Expression Network Analysis (WGCNA)

GSEA software was performed to explore the potential biological processes and cellular pathways in the low- and high-risk subgroups in KIRC TCGA cohort. The expression profiles of mRNAs and lncRNAs of KIRC patients downloaded from the TCGA database were applied to construct gene co-expression networks using the "WGCNA package" implemented in R software. The construction process was the same as described previously (18). The FPKM method was used to standardize the data. The parameter settings of the dynamic tree cut method referred to previous literature.

## CeRNA Network Construction and PPI Analysis, As Well As Functional Enrichment Analysis

Previous literature has reported potential interactions between mRNAs, miRNAs, and lncRNAs, and to elucidate the regulatory role of m6A-related lncRNAs, we constructed a ceRNA network based on WGCNA and differentially expressed lncRNAs. The lncRNA and mRNAs modules with the highest correlation coefficient were selected. To further close the relationship with the clinical traits and increase the accuracy of prediction, the lncRNAs in the MEturquoise module were intersected with the differentially expressed lncRNAs in the KIRC dataset in the TCGA database, and 12 lncRNAs were finally selected as m6A-associated lncRNAs. The miRcode (http://www.mirco de.org/) database was utilized to predict miRNAs that interacted with 12 lncRNAs, identifying 161 pairs of interactions between 12 lncRNAs and 35 miRNAs. The relationship between miRNAs and target mRNAs was predicted by TargetScan (http://www.targe tscan.org/), miRDB (http://www.mirdb.org/miRDB/), and miRTarBase (http://mirtarbase.mbc.nctu.edu.tw),

---

**TABLE 1 |** Comparison of clinical characteristics of KIRC* patients in training set and testing set.

| Covariates | Type | Overall set | Training set | Testing set | P-value |
|---|---|---|---|---|---|
| age | <=60 | 258 (51.09%) | 122 (48.22%) | 136 (53.97%) | 0.2291 |
| | >60 | 247 (48.91%) | 131 (51.78%) | 116 (46.03%) | |
| gender | FEMALE | 173 (34.26%) | 90 (35.57%) | 83 (32.94%) | 0.5958 |
| | MALE | 332 (65.74%) | 163 (64.43%) | 169 (67.06%) | |
| grade | G1–2 | 228 (45.15%) | 119 (47.04%) | 109 (43.25%) | 0.6466 |
| | G3–4 | 272 (53.86%) | 132 (52.17%) | 140 (55.56%) | |
| | GX | 5 (0.99%) | 2 (0.79%) | 3 (1.19%) | |
| stage | Stage I–II | 306 (60.59%) | 157 (62.06%) | 149 (59.13%) | 0.5604 |
| | Stage III–IV | 199 (39.41%) | 96 (37.94%) | 103 (40.87%) | |
| T | T1–2 | 324 (64.16%) | 165 (65.22%) | 159 (63.1%) | 0.6859 |
| | T3–4 | 181 (35.84%) | 88 (34.78%) | 93 (36.9%) | |
| M | M0 | 404 (80%) | 203 (80.24%) | 201 (79.76%) | 0.9896 |
| | M1 | 77 (15.25%) | 38 (15.02%) | 39 (15.48%) | |
| | MX | 24 (4.75%) | 12 (4.74%) | 12 (4.76%) | |
| N | N0 | 228 (45.15%) | 120 (47.43%) | 108 (42.86%) | 0.0768 |
| | N1 | 15 (2.97%) | 11 (4.35%) | 4 (1.59%) | |
| | NX | 262 (51.88%) | 122 (48.22%) | 140 (55.56%) | |

*KIRC, kidney renal clear cell carcinoma.

and 149 mRNAs were identified. Cytoscape software was used to visualize the lncRNA/miRNA/mRNA ceRNA network. STRING (https://string-db.org/) was a website that could predict interactions between functional proteins (19, 20). Those 149 target mRNAs were applied to establish a PPI network. A medium confidence of >0.4 was considered significant. CytoHubba plugin of Cytoscape was used to extract hub genes from the PPI network. Subsequently, using the "clusterProfiler package" in R software, Gene Ontology (GO) enrichment analysis of the 149 targeted mRNA was used to identify molecular functions (MF), cellular components (CC), and biological processes (BP). The Kyoto Encyclopedia of Genes and Genomes (KEGG) was performed to search for potential signaling pathways.

## Cell Lines, Clinical Samples Collection, RNA Extraction, and Quantitative Real-Time Polymerase Chain Reaction (qRT-PCR)

The human KIRC cell lines,786-O, caki-1, and human kidney cell (HK-2 cell, proximal tubule epithelial cell) were originally purchased from cell repository of Shanghai Institute of Life Sciences, Chinese Academy of Sciences. RPMI 1640 medium, containing 10% fetal bovine serum (FBS), penicillin (25 U/ml), and streptomycin (25 mg/ml), was used to culture these KIRC cells at 37°C in a humidified 5% $CO_2$ environment. In addition, a total of 25 fresh samples from patients who underwent laparoscopic radical or partial nephrectomy for KIRC were collected in Southeast University Zhongda Hospital from 2019 to 2020, including tumor tissue and matched adjacent normal kidney tissue and stored at −80°C. All patients were diagnosed with KIRC and did not undergo any antitumor therapy before surgery. The research was authorized by the Medical Ethics Committee of the Southeast University Zhongda Hospital (ZDKYSB077), and each patient gave informed consent.

Total RNA was isolated from KIRC cells and clinical tissues using Total RNA Kit I (50) (OMEGAbiotec, China). Then cDNA was synthesized using the HiScript II Q RT SuperMix (R223-01) reagent kit (vazyme, Nanjing, China). Quantitative real-time PCR (qRT-PCR) was performed using the SYBR green PCR mix (vazyme, Nanjing, China) according to the manufacturer's instructions. The $2^{-\Delta\Delta CT}$ calculation method (21, 22), a relative quantification to calculate the proportion of transcripts in a sample, was applied to determine the relative expression levels of the five m6A-related lncRNAs in the prognostic signature. It described the expression levels of the target genes relative to the reference genes. The detailed calculation method of $\Delta\Delta CT$ was as follows: $\Delta\Delta CT=$ $(CT_{lncRNA} - CT_{GAPDH})$ sample− $(CT_{lncRNA} - CT_{GAPDH})$ control (The control group in this study was HK-2 cell or normal kidney tissue). GAPDH was employed as the endogenous control. The final results obtained from the $2^{-\Delta\Delta CT}$ calculation were the relative expression of the target genes. The primer sequences used in the present study were listed in **Table S1**.

## Statistical Analysis

The statistical analysis was performed in R software (version 4.0.2). The Perl programming language (Version 5.30.2) was used for data processing. Kaplan-Meier survival curve analysis with log-rank test was applied to analyze OS. Univariate, Lasso, and multivariate Cox regression analyses were used to evaluate prognostic significance. ROC curve analysis and its AUC value was used to evaluate the reliability and sensitivity of the prognostic signature. $P < 0.05$ was regarded as statistically significant.

# RESULTS

## Construction and Evaluation of an m6A-Related lncRNAs Prognostic Signature in Training Set

To construct a prognostic prediction signature for KIRC patients, we performed univariate Cox proportional hazards regression analysis of expression of the 753 m6A-related lncRNAs in the training set. Expression of 297 lncRNAs was shown to be significantly associated with the prognosis of KIRC patients. LASSO Cox analysis was applied to eliminate these prognostic-related lncRNAs highly correlated with each other to avoid overfitting, and 15 m6A-related lncRNAs were identified (**Figures 1A, B**). Subsequently, multivariate Cox proportional hazards regression analysis were adopted, and it generated the m6A-related lncRNAs prognostic signature which contained five m6A-related lncRNAs and coefficient of each (**Figure 1C**), using the formula as follows: risk score = 0.935053 * AC012170.2+ (−1.93775) * AC025580.3+0.416438 * AL157394.1+0.291862 * AP006621.2+(−0.35955) * AC124312.5. Also, forest plots of multivariate cox regression analysis displayed that AC012170.2, AL157394.1, and AP006621.2 were risk factors for Hazard Radio (HR) >1, whereas AC025580.3 and AC124312.5 were protective factors for HR <1 (**Figure 1D**).

To evaluate the reliability and sensitivity of the prognostic risk-related signature, the KIRC patients in the training dataset were assigned to low- and high-risk subgroups based on the median value of risk scores. Kaplan-Meier survival curves were performed and depicted that the survival outcomes of KIRC patients with high-risk subgroup were significantly worse than those with low-risk subgroup in the training set (p < 0.001) (**Figure 1E**). The 3-, 5-year survival rates were 60.7 and 46.2% for the high-risk subgroup and 90.6 and 86.5% for the low-risk subgroup, respectively. ROC curves showed that the AUC value for prognostic risk-related signature was 0.802 (**Figure 1F**). Moreover, the AUC value corresponding to 1, 3, 5 years of survival outcomes were 0.806, 0.785, and 0.814 (**Figure 1G**), which demonstrated that the prognostic risk-related signature harbored a promising ability to predict prognosis in the training set. In addition, scatter plot showed that high-risk score KIRC patients had worse survival times than low-risk score group; the risk Score distribution plot depicted that the high-risk subgroup had higher risk scores than the low-risk subgroup; furthermore, the heatmap showed significant differences in the expression profiles of five prognosis-related lncRNAs between the high-risk and low-risk subgroups (**Figure 1H**). Besides, the Kaplan-Meier survival curves were applied to evaluate prognostic roles of the five prognosis-related lncRNAs, and the results

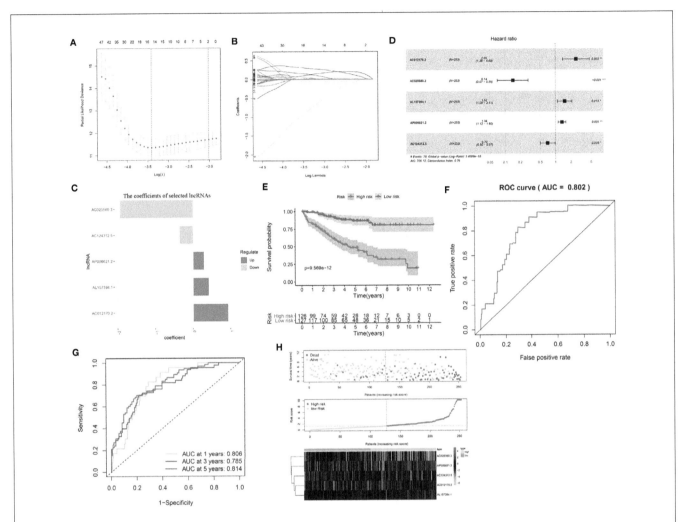

**FIGURE 1 |** Construction and evaluation of an m6A-related lncRNAs prognostic signature in Training set. **(A–C)** The least absolute shrinkage and selection operator (LASSO) Cox regression analysis was performed to avoid overfitting in training set after univariate Cox regression analysis. Lasso coefficient values and vertical dashed lines were calculated at the best log (lambda) value **(A, B)** and Lasso coefficient profiles of the prognostic-related lncRNAs were displayed **(C)**. **(D)** Forest plot of multivariate cox regression analysis for five prognostic-related lncRNAs. The Hazard Ratio (HR) value and its 95% confidence interval, as well as associated p-value, were showed. These HRs greater than 1 were risk factors, which indicated that high expression of these lncRNAs was unfavorable for prognosis, while HRs less than 1 were protective factors, which indicated that high expression of lncRNAs was favorable for prognosis. **(E)** Kaplan-Meier curves showed that the high-risk group had worse survival probability than the low-risk group in the training set. **(F)** Receiver operating characteristic (ROC) curves for the signature and its AUC value in training set. **(G)** ROC curves and their AUC value represented 1-, 3-, and 5-year predictions in training set. **(H)** Scatter plot showed the correlation between the survival status and risk score of KIRC patients; Risk score distribution plot showed the distribution of high-risk and low-risk KIRC patients; Heatmap of the five m6A-related lncRNA expression profiles showed the expression of risk lncRNAs in high-risk and low-risk group in training set. *p < 0.05; **p < 0.01; ***p < 0.001.

confirmed that higher expression of AC012170.2 (**Figure 2A**), AL157394.1 (**Figure 2D**), and AP006621.2 (**Figure 2E**) and lower expression of AC025580.3 (**Figure 2B**) and AC124312.5 (**Figure 2C**) were linked to poorer survival outcomes (p < 0.05). In summary, the prognostic risk-related signature we constructed had significant reliability and sensitivity in predicting the prognosis of KIRC patients.

## Validation of the m6A-Related lncRNAs Prognostic Signature in Testing Set

To further validate the predictive ability of the m6A-related lncRNAs prognostic signature, we calculated the risk scores in

both testing set and overall set using the same algorithm for KIRC patients, who were also divided into low- and high-risk subgroups. Kaplan-Meier survival curves displayed that the OS for KIRC patients were consistent with those in the testing set (**Figure 3A**) and overall set (**Figure 3B**) (p < 0.001). The 3-, 5-year survival rates were 67.9 and 46.8% for the high-risk subgroup and 82.1 and 70.7% in the low-risk subgroup in the testing set, and 64.8 and 46.4% for the high-risk subgroup and 86.2 and 78.4% in the low-risk subgroup in the overall set, respectively. ROC curves also indicated that the m6A-related lncRNAs prognostic signature had a reliable predictive capability in the testing set (AUC = 0.725; **Figure 3C**) and overall set

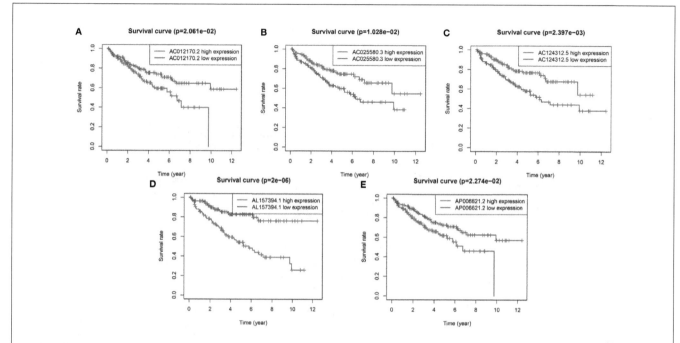

**FIGURE 2** | The Kaplan-Meier (K-M) survival curves of five m6A-related lncRNAs in the prognostic signature. **(A, D, E)** The K-M survival curves of AC012170.2, AL157394.1, and AP006621.2 showed high expression group had worse overall survival (OS) than the low expression group in the training set (p < 0.05). **(B, C)** The K-M survival curves of AC025580.3 and AC124312.5 showed high expression group had better OS than the low expression group in the training set (p < 0.05).

(AUC = 0.763; **Figure 3D**). Furthermore, the time-ROC curves and its AUC value also displayed that the prognostic signature had strong prognostic value for KIRC patients in testing set (1-year AUC = 0.726, 3-year AUC = 0.640, 5-year AUC = 0.677; **Figure 3E**) and overall set (1-year AUC = 0.765, 3-year AUC = 0.708, 5-year AUC = 0.741; **Figure 3F**). Besides, the scatter plot and risk score distribution plot also displayed the correlations between survival status and risk score of KIRC patients in high- and low-risk subgroup in the testing set (**Figure 3G**) and overall set (**Figure 3H**). Also, heatmaps showed that the expression profiles of the five prognosis-related lncRNAs were also consistent with those in the training set. These results indicated that the m6A-related lncRNAs prognostic signature had a robust and stable prognostic-predictive ability.

## Clinical Value and Application of the m6A-Related lncRNAs Prognostic Signature

To access the clinical value and application of the prognostic signature, the risk scores from prognostic signature and clinicopathological characteristics, including age, gender, grade, AJCC stage, TNM stage were integrated. As was shown in **Figure 4A**, the heatmap showed associations between the expression profiles of the five m6A-related lncRNAs and clinicopathological features in the low- and high-risk subgroup. We found that there were significant differences in age, grade, AJCC stage, and survival status between high- and low-risk subgroups (p < 0.05). In addition, forest plots showed the stable prognostic ability of the five m6A-related lncRNAs included in the prognostic risk model (**Figure 4B**). Multivariate ROC curve based on the risk score from prognostic

signature and clinicopathologic characteristics indicated that the AUC value for risk score was 0.802, which was higher than the AUC value of age (0.629), gender (0.484), Grade (0.708), AJCC stage (0.800), T stage (0.746), M stage (0.713), N stage (0.410) (**Figure 4C**). Furthermore, we compared the m6A-related lncRNAs prognostic signature (AUC = 0.765) with published prediction models [Sun et al. (2) AUC = 0.646; Wan et al. (23) AUC = 0.729; Xing et al. (24) AUC = 0.724] and found that our signature had higher prediction reliability and sensitivity than other published biomarkers (**Figure 4D**). Subsequently, the univariate (**Figure 4E**) and multivariate Cox regression analysis (**Figure 4F**) were performed and confirmed that risk score, age, grade were independent prognostic factors (p < 0.01). Overall, our results indicated that the prognostic risk score signature could be used independently and reliably to predict survival outcomes in patients with KIRC.

Finally, to develop a quantitative method to predict the prognosis of KIRC patients, we constructed a prognostic nomogram based on risk score and prognostic-related clinicopathological parameters to predict 1-, 3-, 5-year OS of KIRC patients (**Figure 4G**). The C-index value of this nomogram was 0.794. The calibration curve proved that the prognostic nomogram was reliable and accurate (**Figures 4H–J**).

## Stratification Analysis of the m6A-Related lncRNAs Prognostic Signature Based on Prognosis-Related Clinicopathological Features

To better evaluate the predictive ability of the m6A-related lncRNAs prognostic signature and to validate its ability to

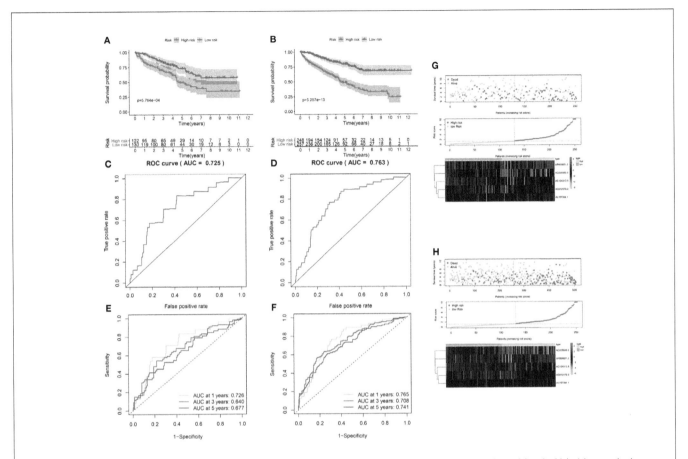

**FIGURE 3** | Validation of the prognostic signature for KIRC patients in testing set and overall set. Kaplan-Meier curves showed that the high-risk group had worse overall survival (OS) than the low-risk group in the testing set **(A)** and overall set **(B)**. Receiver operating characteristic (ROC) curves for the prognostic signature and its AUC value in the testing set **(C)** and overall set **(D)**. ROC curves and their AUC value represented 1-, 3-, and 5-year predictions in the testing set **(E)** and overall set **(F)**. Scatter dot plot showed the outcomes between the survival status and risk score of KIRC patients in high- and low-group; Risk score distribution plot showed the distribution of high-risk and low-risk KIRC patients; Heatmap of the five m6A-related lncRNA expression profiles showed the expression of risk lncRNAs in high-risk and low-risk group in the testing set **(G)** and overall set **(H)**, separately.

predict OS in high-and low-risk subgroups, we performed a stratified analysis based on clinicopathological features, including age (>60 years *vs.* ≤60 years), gender (FEMALE *vs.* MALE), AJCC grade (G1–2 *vs.* G3–4), stages (stage I–II *vs.* stage III–IV), AJCC T stage (T1–2 *vs.* T3–4). Kaplan-Meier survival analyses were performed and results showed that the high-risk subgroup had worse OS compared to the low-risk subgroup in different strata of clinical characteristics (p < 0.05; **Figures 5A–J**).

## GSEA of the High- and Low-Risk Subgroup in KIRC Patients Based on the m6A-Related lncRNAs Prognostic Signature

To investigate the potential biological processes and pathways involved in molecular heterogeneity, the GSEA was performed between the low- and high-risk subgroups in TCGA cohort. The results displayed that the altered genes in the high-risk subgroups belonged to pathways involving proteasome, cancer-muscle-contraction, glycosaminoglycan-biosynthesis-chondroitin-

sulfate, p53-signaling-pathway, complement-and-coagulation-cascades (**Figure 6A**). Besides, the GSEA analysis in the low-risk subgroups related to ERBB-signaling-pathway, tryptophan-metabolism, fatty-acid-metabolism, prostate-cancer, histidine-metabolism (**Figure 6B**). It indicated that activation of pathways in high- or low-risk subgroups could contribute to improving prognosis. As shown in **Figures 6C, D**, the top 10 KEGG signaling pathways in high- or low-risk subgroups were displayed and suggested enrichment scores in the high-risk subgroup were associated with proteasome, while valine-leucine-and-isoleucine-degradation in low-risk subgroup. These findings gave new insights into individualized treatment for different risk subgroups of patients with KIRC.

## Construction of a ceRNA Network and PPI Network Based on WGCNA and Functional Enrichment Analysis

To elaborate on how m6A-related lncRNAs regulate targeting mRNAs expression by sponging miRNAs in KIRC, we

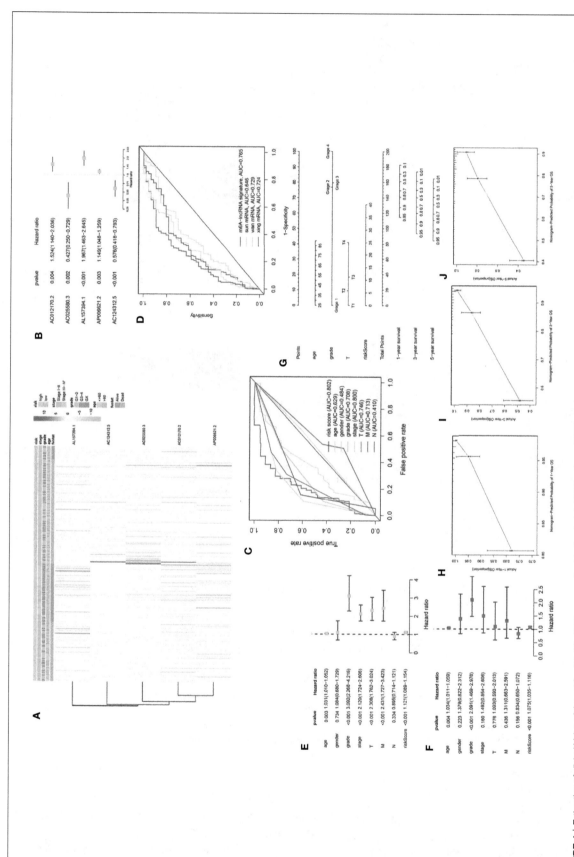

**FIGURE 4 |** Estimation of clinical Value of the m6A-related lncRNAs prognostic risk signature in KIRC patients. **(A)** The heatmap showed associations between the expression of the five m6A-related lncRNAs in the low- and high-risk group and clinicopathological features, including survival status (alive or dead), age (>60 y or <=60 y), AJCC stages (stages I–II or III–IV), and AJCC grade (1–2, 3–4, or NA) (all p < 0.05) in training set.
**(B)** The forest plots showed the prognostic ability of the five m6A-related lncRNAs in the prognostic risk model (p < 0.05). **(C)** The multivariate receiver operating characteristic (ROC) curve showed predictive accuracy of risk score was higher than other clinicopathological features. **(D)** Multivariate ROC curves showed the sensitivity and specificity of the prognostic risk signature were higher than other published biomarkers in predicting the prognosis of KIRC patients. **(E)** The univariate Cox regression analysis showed that risk score and clinicopathological features, included age, grade, AJCC stage, T and M stage were prognostic-related variables.
**(F)** The multivariate Cox regression analysis showed risk score, grade, age were independent prognostic factors. **(G)** Construction of a prognostic nomogram based on risk score and prognostic-related clinicopathological parameters to predict 1-, 3-, 5-year overall survival of KIRC patients. **(H–J)** The calibration curves of the nomogram displayed the concordance between predicted and observed 1-, 3-, and 5-year OS.

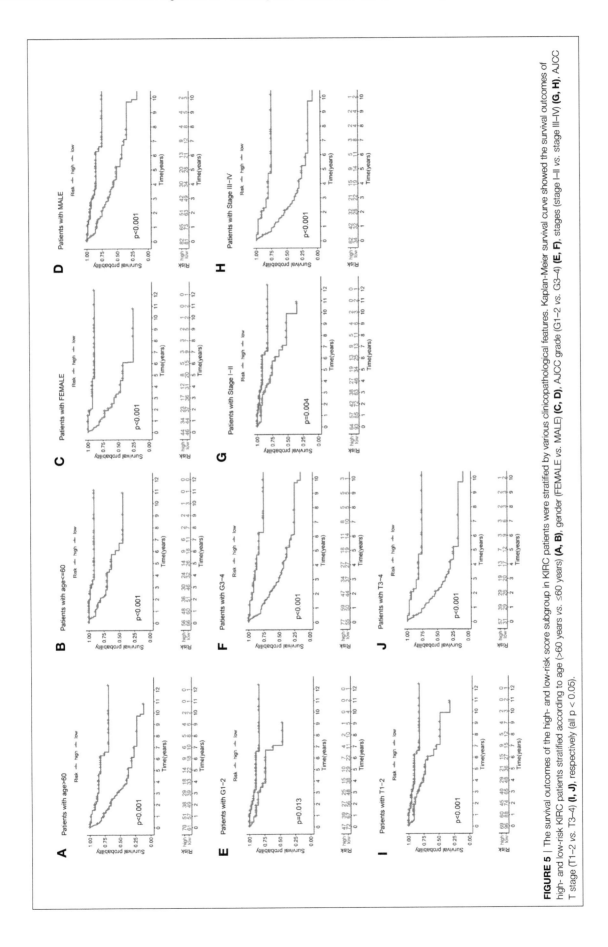

**FIGURE 5** | The survival outcomes of the high- and low-risk score subgroup in KIRC patients were stratified by various clinicopathological features. Kaplan-Meier survival curve showed the survival outcomes of high- and low-risk KIRC patients stratified according to age (>60 years vs. ≤60 years) **(A, B)**, gender (FEMALE vs. MALE) **(C, D)**, AJCC grade (G1–2 vs. G3–4) **(E, F)**, stages (stage I–II vs. stage III–IV) **(G, H)**, AJCC T stage (T1–2 vs. T3–4) **(I, J)**, respectively (all p < 0.05).

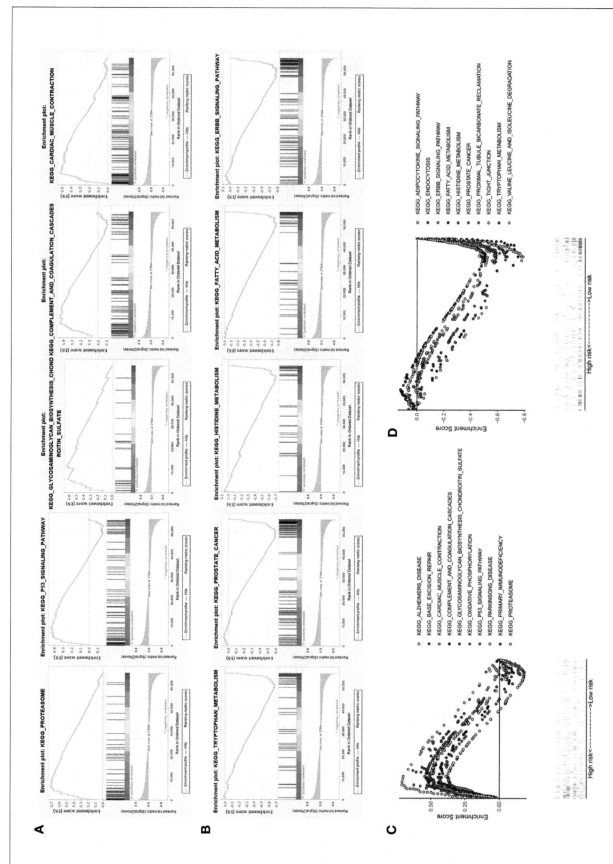

**FIGURE 6 |** Gene set enrichment analysis (GSEA) of the high- and low-risk subgroup in KIRC patients based on the prognostic signature. **(A)** GSEA showed that the top five tumor hallmarks were enriched in the high-risk group. **(B)** GSEA showed that the top five tumor hallmarks were enriched in the low-risk group. **(C)** The top 10 KEGG signaling pathways were enriched in the low-risk KIRC patients. **(D)** The top 10 KEGG signaling pathways in low-risk KIRC patients.

constructed a ceRNA network based on WGCNA and performed PPI analysis using the STRING database. WGCNA was performed to identify lncRNAs in modules associated with the clinical traits of KIRC and MEturquoise module was selected because of the highest correlation coefficient (**Figures 7A, B**). Likewise, these mRNAs in the MEgreen module were selected (**Figures 7C, D**). Then, we constructed a lncRNA-miRNA-mRNA ceRNA network that contained 12 lncRNAs, 35 miRNAs, and 149 mRNAs to investigate the potential biological function of m6A-related lncRNAs (**Figure 8A**). Subsequently, these 149 target mRNAs were applied to implement PPI analysis (**Figure 8B**). The connecting nodes of the top 30 target mRNAs were shown in PPI network, with VEGFA having the most interacting nodes (**Figure 8C**). Besides, we obtained the top 10 hub genes using CytoHubba plugin of Cytoscape software (**Figure 8D**). Ultimately, GO enrichment analysis and KEGG pathway analysis of 149 targeted mRNA

were implemented. We found that the top five GO terms for biological processes were T cell activation, leukocyte cell-cell adhesion, regulation of cell-cell adhesion, regulation of mononuclear cell proliferation, positive regulation of cell adhesion; The top five GO terms for cellular components were external side of plasma membrane, collagen-containing extracellular matrix, apical part of cell, basolateral plasma membrane, apical plasma membrane, and the top five GO terms for molecular functions were immune receptor activity, cytokine receptor activity, cytokine binding, cytokine activity, cytokine receptor binding (**Figure 8F**). The top five KEGG signaling pathways were cytokine-cytokine receptor interaction, cell adhesion molecules, human T-cell leukemia virus 1 infection, Epstein-Barr virus infection, viral protein interaction with cytokine and cytokine receptor (**Figure 8E**). These results provided us with new ways to search for potential functions of m6A-related lncRNAs in KIRC.

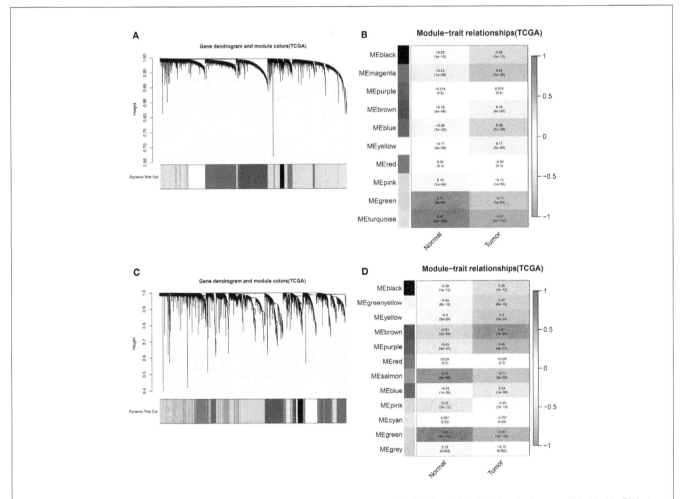

**FIGURE 7** | WGCNA was performed to identify modules associated with the clinical traits of KIRC. **(A)** Hierarchical clustering dendrogram of identified lncRNAs in modules of KIRC. **(B)** Heatmaps of the correlation between Eigengene of lncRNAs and clinical traits of KIRC were displayed. Each module with different colors contained the correlation and P-value, and MEturquoise module with the highest correlation coefficient was selected. **(C)** Hierarchical clustering dendrogram of identified mRNAs in modules of KIRC. **(D)** Heatmaps of the correlation between Eigengene of mRNAs and clinical traits of KIRC cancer were displayed. Each module with different colors contained the correlation and P-value, and MEgreen module with the highest correlation coefficient was selected.

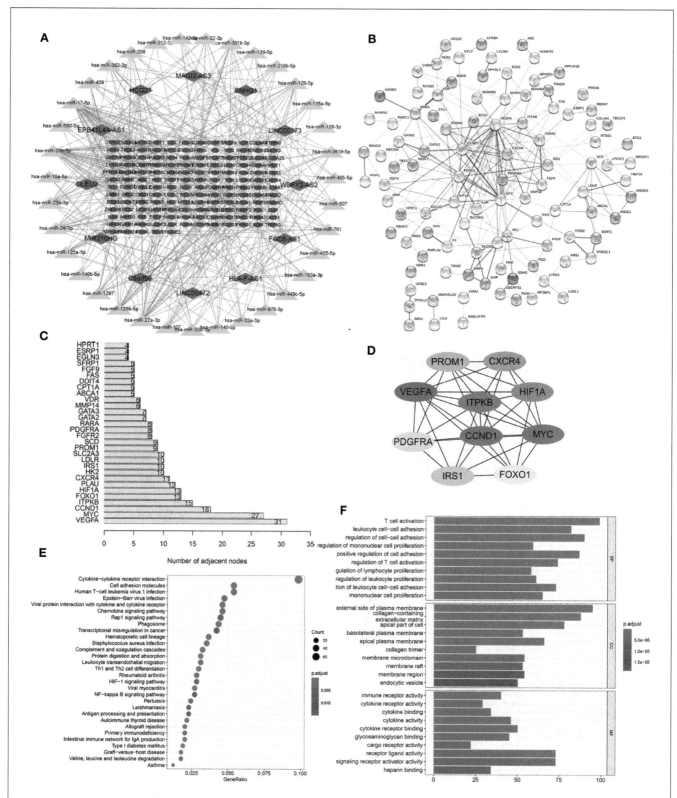

**FIGURE 8 |** Construction of a lncRNA-miRNA-mRNA ceRNA network and protein-protein interaction (PPI) network, as well as functional enrichment analysis. **(A)** The ceRNA network displayed 12 m6A-related lncRNAs and their sponged miRNAs and targeted mRNAs. **(B)** PPI network of target genes. **(C)** The bar chart showed the number of connecting nodes of target mRNAs in PPI network. **(D)** PPI network of the top 10 hub genes obtained from CytoHubba plugin of Cytoscape. **(E)** Bubble diagram of Kyoto Encyclopedia of Genes and Genomes (KEGG) pathway analysis revealed the enriched signaling pathways of targeted mRNAs. **(F)** Gene Ontology (GO) analysis of targeted mRNAs revealed the enriched biological processes, cell components, and molecular functions.

## Identification of Expression Levels of the Five m6A-Related lncRNAs in KIRC Cells and Clinical Tissue Samples

To further demonstrate the feasibility of the prognostic signature, we performed qRT-PCR assays in KIRC cells and clinical tissue samples to validate the expression levels of the five m6A-related lncRNAs. We first validated the expression level of the five lncRNAs in normal kidney cells (HK-2 cell) and two KIRC cell lines (786-O, caki-1). The results indicated that the expression level of AC012170.2, AL157394, AP006621.2, and AC025580.3 were significantly increased in KIRC cells compared with normal kidney cells, whereas AC124312.5 was downregulated in KIRC cell (**Figures 9A–E**). The same results were detected in tumor tissue and matched adjacent normal kidney tissue (**Figures 9F–J**). Collectively, these findings further validated the stability and reliability of the m6A-related lncRNAs prognostic signature.

## DISCUSSIONS

In our present study, we identified five prognostic-associated m6A-related lncRNAs (AC012170.2, AL157394.1, AP006621.2, AC025580.3, and AC124312.5) and constructed an m6A-related lncRNAs prognostic signature that could accurately predict the prognostic outcome of KIRC patients based on TCGA data. Firstly, the KIRC samples have been randomly divided into training set and testing set. Then, univariate Cox proportional hazards regression analysis was applied in the training set, and 297 lncRNAs were found to be associated with the prognosis significantly. Subsequently, LASSO Cox analysis and multivariate Cox proportional hazards regression analysis were

adopted. Five prognostic-associated m6A-related lncRNAs were identified as independent prognostic factors for KIRC patients used to construct the prognostic risk score model subsequently. To evaluate the predictive ability of the prognostic signature, we classified the KIRC patients into low- and high-risk subgroups based on the median value of risk scores. Subsequently, we performed Kaplan-Meier survival analysis and confirmed that the high-risk subgroup had a worse OS than low-risk subgroup in the training set, testing set, and overall set. It was consistent with the results of the ROC curves. Moreover, a prognostic nomogram was constructed to predict the OS of KIRC patients quantitatively. Finally, a lncRNA/miRNA/mRNA ceRNA network and a PPI network based on WGCNA were built further to explore the possible biological mechanisms of m6A-related lncRNAs. Besides, GO and KEGG enrichment analysis was performed to validate the main biological functions and downstream pathways of those m6A-related lncRNAs. Collectively, our results indicated that m6A-related lncRNAs prognostic signature had a robust and stable prognostic-predictive ability.

Several studies (2, 25) have reported that m6A-related gene models could predict the prognosis of KIRC patients well, but whether m6A-related lncRNAs prognostic signature could predict the prognosis of KIRC remained unknown. In the present study, we compared the m6A-related lncRNAs prognostic signature with published prediction models and found that our signature had reliable predictive reliability and sensitivity, superior to other published biomarkers. In addition, we developed a prognostic nomogram to accurately predict the prognosis of KIPC patients, which had a comparable predictive ability with the published literature (26, 27). Therefore, this could be a new and useful predictive tool for KIRC patients.

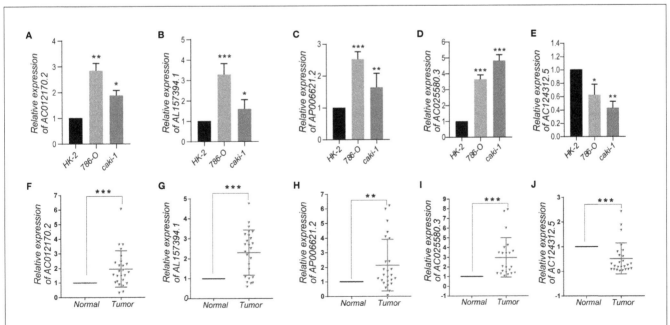

**FIGURE 9 | (A–E)** The expression levels of five m6A-related lncRNAs in the prognostic signature in normal kidney cell and KIRC cells. **(F–J)** The expression levels of five m6A-related lncRNAs in 25 paired KIRC and matched adjacent normal tissues were examined by qRT-PCR. *p < 0.05; **p < 0.01; ***p < 0.001.

Besides, to access the clinical value of the prognosis signature, we integrated risk scores and clinicopathological characteristics, and performed univariate and multivariate Cox regression analysis and stratification analysis. We found that risk score, age, grade were independent prognostic factors, which indicated that the m6A-lncRNAs prognostic signature could be used independently and reliably to predict OS in KIRC patients. Moreover, stratification analysis demonstrated that the high-risk subgroup had worse OS compared to the low-risk subgroup in different clinical characteristics. It also proved the reliability and usefulness of the prognostic signature.

Then, combined with the expression levels, we analyzed the five m6A-related lncRNAs in the prognostic signature. We found that AC012170.2, AL157394, AP006621.2 were upregulated in tumor tissues compared with normal tissues. Furthermore, AC012170.2, AL157394.1, and AP006621.2 were risk factors, which were upregulated in high-risk subgroup. The Kaplan-Meier survival curves showed that higher expression of AC012170.2, AL157394.1, and AP006621.2 were linked to poorer survival outcomes. These suggested that they might act as tumor suppressors in KIRC. On the contrary, AC124312.5 was downregulated in tumor tissues. Moreover, AC124312.5 were protective factors, which were upregulated in low-risk subgroup. And the lower expression of AC124312.5 was linked to poorer survival outcomes. These suggested that it might act as tumor promoters in KIRC. It gave us insight into their potential role in tumorigenesis and development for KIRC. Also, Xia et al. (28) reported the prognostic role of AP006621.2 and AC025580.3 in KIRC. However, the roles of the remaining three m6A-related lncRNAs in tumors have not been reported. Therefore, our next step will be to further verify its function and mechanism from *in vivo* and *in vitro* experiments.

Our study still had some limitations. Firstly, the dataset we used to construct and validate the m6A-related lncRNAs prognostic signature was obtained from TCGA. We failed to locate suitable external data from other public databases to evaluate the reliability of the model. Second, we only performed preliminary expression studies on these five m6A-related lncRNAs in the signature. However, further functional analysis and mechanistic studies were not carried out. Finally, we were not able to verify its specific biological functions and found the exact signaling pathways.

In conclusion, in the present study, we extracted data from public databases and analyzed the role of m6A-related lncRNAs in KIRC. We successfully constructed a prognostic risk signature based on five m6A-related lncRNAs and validated the reliability and sensitivity of the model. We also established a prognostic nomogram that could quantitatively predict the prognostic outcome of KIRC patients. Besides, the ceRNA network and PPI network were constructed and GO and KEGG functional enrichment analysis was performed, which provided us with new ways to search for potential functions of m6A-related lncRNAs in KIRC.

## AUTHOR CONTRIBUTIONS

JY and SS were responsible for study design, data acquisition and analysis, and manuscript writing. JY and WM performed bioinformatics and statistical analyses. QH, CW, ZX, SC, and RL were responsible for collecting clinical samples. JY and WM prepared the figures and tables for the manuscript. BX and MC were responsible for the integrity of the entire study and manuscript review. All authors contributed to the article and approved the submitted version.

## ACKNOWLEDGMENTS

The authors gratefully acknowledge the data generated by TCGA database used in this study.

## SUPPLEMENTARY MATERIAL

**Supplementary Figure 1 |** The flow chart of the study.

**Supplementary Figure 2 |** The heatmap was performed to visualize the differential expression of 35 N6-methyladenosine (m6A) related genes between 489 tumor tissues and 51 normal tissues in The Cancer Genome Atlas (TCGA) prostate cancer cohort. *p < 0.05; **p < 0.01; ***p < 0.001.

## REFERENCES

1. Miller KD, Nogueira L, Mariotto AB, Rowland JH, Yabroff KR, Alfano CM, et al. Cancer Treatment and Survivorship Statistics, 2019. *CA Cancer J Clin* (2019) 69(5):363–85. doi: 10.3322/caac.21565
2. Sun Z, Jing C, Xiao C, Li T, Wang Y. Prognostic Risk Signature Based on the Expression of Three m6A RNA Methylation Regulatory Genes in Kidney Renal Papillary Cell Carcinoma. *Aging (Albany NY)* (2020) 12(21):22078–94. doi: 10.18632/aging.104053
3. Escudier B, Porta C, Schmidinger M, Rioux LN, Bex A, Khoo V, et al. Renal Cell Carcinoma: ESMO Clinical Practice Guidelines for Diagnosis, Treatment and Follow-Up. *Ann Oncol* (2019) 30(5):706–20. doi: 10.1093/annonc/mdz056
4. Jonasch E, Gao J, Rathmell WK. Renal Cell Carcinoma. *BMJ* (2014) 349: g4797. doi: 10.1136/bmj.g4797
5. Jones PA. Functions of DNA Methylation: Islands, Start Sites, Gene Bodies and Beyond. *Nat Rev Genet* (2012) 13(7):484–92. doi: 10.1038/nrg3230
6. Liu N, Pan T. N6-Methyladenosine-Encoded Epitranscriptomics. *Nat Struct Mol Biol* (2016) 23(2):98–102. doi: 10.1038/nsmb.3162
7. Zhao BS, Roundtree IA, He C. Post-Transcriptional Gene Regulation by mRNA Modifications. *Nat Rev Mol Cell Biol* (2017) 18(1):31–42. doi: 10.1038/nrm.2016.132
8. Zaccara S, Ries RJ, Jaffrey SR. Reading, Writing and Erasing mRNA Methylation. *Nat Rev Mol Cell Biol* (2019) 20(10):608–24. doi: 10.1038/s41580-019-0168-5
9. Cai J, Yang F, Zhan H, Situ J, Li W, Mao Y, et al. RNA m (6)A Methyltransferase Mettl3 Promotes the Growth of Prostate Cancer by Regulating Hedgehog Pathway. *Onco Targets Ther* (2019) 12:9143–52. doi: 10.2147/OTT.S226796
10. Guo X, Li K, Jiang W, Hu Y, Xiao W, Huang Y, et al. RNA Demethylase ALKBH5 Prevents Pancreatic Cancer Progression by Posttranscriptional Activation of PER1 in an m6A-YTHDF2-Dependent Manner. *Mol Cancer* (2020) 19(1):91. doi: 10.1186/s12943-020-01158-w
11. Zhuang C, Zhuang C, Luo X, Huang X, Yao L, Li J, et al. N6-Methyladenosine Demethylase FTO Suppresses Clear Cell Renal Cell Carcinoma Through a Novel FTO-PGC-1α Signalling Axis. *J Cell Mol Med* (2019) 23(3):2163–73. doi: 10.1111/jcmm.14128

12. Gao S, Gu Y, Niu S, Wang Y, Duan L, Pan Y, et al. DMDRMR-Mediated Regulation of m6A-Modified CDK4 by m6A Reader IGF2BP3 Drives ccRCC Progression. *Cancer Res* (2020) 81(4):923–34. doi: 10.1158/0008-5472.CAN-20-1619

13. Mercer TR, Dinger ME, Mattick JS. Long Non-Coding RNAs: Insights Into Functions. *Nat Rev Genet* (2009) 10(3):155–9. doi: 10.1038/nrg2521

14. Hahne JC, Valeri N. Non-Coding RNAs and Resistance to Anticancer Drugs in Gastrointestinal Tumors. *Front Oncol* (2018) 8:226. doi: 10.3389/fonc.2018.00226

15. Müller V, Oliveira-Ferrer L, Steinbach B, Pantel K, Schwarzenbach H. Interplay of lncRNA H19/miR-675 and lncRNA NEAT1/miR-204 in Breast Cancer. *Mol Oncol* (2019) 13(5):1137–49. doi: 10.1002/1878-0261.12472

16. Yates AD, Achuthan P, Akanni W, Allen J, Allen J, Alvarez JJ, et al. Ensembl 2020. *Nucleic Acids Res* (2020) 48(D1):D682–8. doi: 10.1093/nar/gkz966

17. Sun T, Wu R, Ming L. The Role of m6A RNA Methylation in Cancer. *BioMed Pharmacother* (2019) 112:108613. doi: 10.1016/j.biopha.2019.108613

18. Langfelder P, Horvath S. WGCNA: An R Package for Weighted Correlation Network Analysis. *BMC Bioinformatics* (2008) 9:559. doi: 10.1186/1471-2105-9-559

19. von Mering C, Huynen M, Jaeggi D, Schmidt S, Bork P, Snel B. STRING: A Database of Predicted Functional Associations Between Proteins. *Nucleic Acids Res* (2003) 31(1):258–61. doi: 10.1093/nar/gkg034

20. Szklarczyk D, Morris JH, Cook H, Kuhn M, Wyder S, Simonovic M, et al. The STRING Database in 2017: Quality-Controlled Protein-Protein Association Networks, Made Broadly Accessible. *Nucleic Acids Res* (2017) 45(D1):D362–8. doi: 10.1093/nar/gkw937

21. Livak KJ, Schmittgen TD. Analysis of Relative Gene Expression Data Using Real-Time Quantitative PCR and the 2(-Delta Delta C(T)) Method. *Methods* (2001) 25(4):402–8. doi: 10.1006/meth.2001.1262

22. Mao W, Huang X, Wang L, Zhang Z, Liu M, Li Y, et al. Circular RNA hsa_circ_0068871 Regulates FGFR3 Expression and Activates STAT3 by Targeting miR-181a-5p to Promote Bladder Cancer Progression. *J Exp Clin Cancer Res* (2019) 38(1):169. doi: 10.1186/s13046-019-1136-9

23. Wan B, Liu B, Yu G, Huang Y, Lv C. Differentially Expressed Autophagy-Related Genes are Potential Prognostic and Diagnostic Biomarkers in Clear-Cell Renal Cell Carcinoma. *Aging (Albany NY)* (2019) 11(20):9025–42. doi: 10.18632/aging.102368

24. Xing Q, Ji C, Zhu B, Cong R, Wang Y. Identification of Small Molecule Drugs and Development of a Novel Autophagy-Related Prognostic Signature for Kidney Renal Clear Cell Carcinoma. *Cancer Med* (2020) 9(19):7034–51. doi: 10.1002/cam4.3367

25. Fang J, Hu M, Sun Y, Zhou S, Li H. Expression Profile Analysis of m6A RNA Methylation Regulators Indicates They are Immune Signature Associated and Can Predict Survival in Kidney Renal Cell Carcinoma. *DNA Cell Biol* (2020) 39(12):1–8. doi: 10.1089/dna.2020.5767

26. Schiavina R, Mari A, Bianchi L, Amparore D, Antonelli A, Artibani W, et al. Predicting Positive Surgical Margins in Partial Nephrectomy: A Prospective Multicentre Observational Study (the RECORd 2 Project). *Eur J Surg Oncol* (2020) 46(7):1353–9. doi: 10.1016/j.ejso.2020.01.022

27. Bianchi L, Schiavina R, Borghesi M, Chessa F, Casablanca C, Angiolini A, et al. Which Patients With Clinical Localized Renal Mass Would Achieve the Trifecta After Partial Nephrectomy? The Impact of Surgical Technique. *Minerva Urol Nefrol* (2020) 72(3):339–49. doi: 10.23736/S0393-2249.19.03485-4

28. Qi-Dong X, Yang X, Lu JL, Liu CQ, Sun JX, Li C, et al. Development and Validation of a Nine-Redox-Related Long Noncoding RNA Signature in Renal Clear Cell Carcinoma. *Oxid Med Cell Longev* (2020) 2020:6634247. doi: 10.1155/2020/6634247

# 4

# A Retrospective, Multicenter, Long-Term Follow-Up Analysis of the Prognostic Characteristics of Recurring Non-Metastatic Renal Cell Carcinoma after Partial or Radical Nephrectomy

Sung Han Kim[1], Boram Park[2], Eu Chang Hwang[3], Sung-Hoo Hong[4], Chang Wook Jeong[5], Cheol Kwak[5], Seok Soo Byun[6] and Jinsoo Chung[1*]

[1] Department of Urology, Urologic Cancer Center, Research Institute and Hospital of National Cancer Center, Goyang, South Korea,
[2] Statistics and Data Center, Research Institute for Future Medicine, Samsung Medical Center, Seoul, South Korea,
[3] Department of Urology, Chonnam National University Medical School, Gwangju, South Korea, [4] Department of Urology, Seoul St. Mary's Hospital, Seoul, South Korea, [5] Department of Urology, Seoul National University College of Medicine and Hospital, Seoul, South Korea, [6] Department of Urology, Seoul National University Bundang Hospital, Seongnam, South Korea

*Correspondence:
Jinsoo Chung
cjs5225@ncc.re.kr

This study aimed to compare the cancer-specific survival (CSS) and overall survival (OS) of nephrectomized patients with non-metastatic renal cell carcinoma (nmRCC) and local recurrence without distant metastasis (LR group), those with metastasis without local recurrence (MET group), and those with both local recurrence and metastasis (BOTH group). This retrospective multicenter study included 464 curatively nephrectomized patients with nmRCC and disease recurrence between 2000 and 2012; the follow-up period was until 2017. After adjusting for significant clinicopathological factors using Cox proportional hazard models, CSS and OS were compared between the MET (n = 50, 10.7%), BOTH (n = 95, 20.5%), and LR (n = 319, 68.8%) groups. The CSS and OS rates were 34.7 and 6.5% after a median follow-up of 43.9 months, respectively. After adjusting for significant prognostic factors of OS and CSS, the MET group had hazard ratios (HRs) of 0.51 and 0.57 for OS and CSS (p = 0.039 and 0.103), respectively, whereas the BOTH group had HRs of 0.51 and 0.60 for OS and CSS (p < 0.05), respectively; LR was taken as a reference. The 2-year OS and CSS rates from the date of nephrectomy and disease recurrence were 86.9% and 88.9% and 63.5% and 67.8%, respectively, for the LR group; 89.5% and 89.5% and 48.06% and 52.43%, respectively, for the MET group; and 96.8% and 96.8% and 86.6% and 82.6%, respectively, for the BOTH group. Only the LR and BOTH groups had significant differences in the 2-year OS and CSS rates (p < 0.05). In conclusion, our study showed that the LR group had worse survival prognoses than any other group in nephrectomized patients with nmRCC.

Keywords: prognosis, nephrectomy, metastasis, renal cell carcinoma, recurrence

# INTRODUCTION

Globally, the number of incidentally diagnosed localized non-metastatic renal cell carcinomas (nmRCCs) has increased due to improvements in diagnostic modalities (1). Given that the radical removal of primary RCC by partial or complete nephrectomy is the standard treatment for nmRCC, approximately 7–30% of surgically treated RCCs recur within 5 years (2), and another 20–40% of RCCs progress to metastasis after curative surgery, resulting in a poor 5-year overall survival (OS) of <20% (3–5). Both clinicians and researchers have attempted multiple times to overcome the diverse and unpredictable survival outcomes of local recurrence (LR) and distant metastasis in patients with nmRCC after nephrectomy, and various definitions of disease recurrence in multiple cohorts have shown different prognostic outcomes (4–7). Several predictive factors of OS and CSS, such as the interval between nephrectomy and LR or metastasis development, the characteristics of recurrent or metastatic tumors, and the different pathological and genetic backgrounds of primary tumors, have been suggested (5–7). However, some guidelines recommend a 5-year follow-up period, which is not adequate to manage RCC as it either presents with delayed LR or only as metastasis without LR (MET) in approximately 5–10% of patients, even after a 5-year disease-free period, due to its heterogenetic, intratumoral, and distinct histological characteristics (4–6). Therefore, researchers have put extensive efforts for several decades into finding significant predictive markers for LR and MET in RCC, after either radical or partial nephrectomy. Such markers can predict patients with a high risk of LR and MET after nephrectomy, even with clear resected margins.

This study aimed to assess the predisposing characteristics and survival prognoses of patients with LR and no metastasis (LR group), those with metastasis and no LR (MET group), and those with LR and metastasis (BOTH group). The data of 464 patients who underwent RCC nephrectomy with postoperative disease recurrence were collected retrospectively from six Korean institutions. The patients in this study either underwent nmRCC radical or partial nephrectomy with a follow-up period until the end of 2017. Survival prognosis analysis focused on the OS and cancer-specific survival (CSS) for all groups.

# MATERIALS AND METHODS

## Ethical Statement

This retrospective study was approved by the institutional review board of the National Cancer Center (approval number: NCC 2018–0045 and B1202/145-102), which waived the requirement for informed consent due to the retrospective nature of this study (8–10). All study procedures were performed in accordance with the tenets of the ethical guidelines and regulations of the Ethical Principles for Medical Research Involving Human Subjects of the World Medical Association Declaration of Helsinki.

## Patient Criteria and RCC Database

Data of the 4,246 enrolled patients with RCC were obtained from two multicenter RCC databases—the nmRCC (8) and mRCC (9) databases—that were obtained from the Multicenter Korean National Kidney Cancer (MKNKC) database. A total of 464 (10.9%) patients with RCC were selected for this study. All participants underwent curative partial or radical nephrectomy with or without lymphadenectomy between 2000 and 2012 and attended at least a follow-up period of 1 month until either local recurrence or distant metastasis was detected. Exclusion criteria were age <19 years (n = 12); histologically confirmed benign tumor (n = 73); postoperative disease recurrence within 1–3 months to exclude obscured synchronous metastasis at nephrectomy (n = 5); positive resection margins after partial/radical nephrectomy (n = 35); and a history of cytoreductive nephrectomy, incomplete medical records of survival outcomes, a history of previous cancers, and same patient visiting different hospitals (n = 73).

The parameters analyzed in this study were baseline anthropometric characteristics, including age, sex, and underlying diseases; preoperative baseline laboratory findings, including serum albumin, hemoglobin, and creatinine; intraoperative nephrectomy information; pathology results, including pTNM stage, histology, Fuhrman nuclear grade, sarcomatoid differentiation, lymphovascular invasion, necrosis, and capsule invasion; and survival outcomes, including all-cause and cancer-specific deaths. The surgical procedures of partial and radical nephrectomies were documented in a previous study (8–10); however, no specific standardized protocol was followed for surgical procedures during the collection of data for the RCC database. For the initial postoperative imaging follow-up, imaging intervals, that is, either 1- or 3-month intervals, were not standardized and were based on the preference of the urologist for the postoperative surveillance protocol established at the time.

## Patient Classification

Patients were categorized into the LR (n = 319, 68.8%), MET (n = 50, 10.7%), and BOTH (n = 95, 20.5%) groups. The LR group comprised nephrectomized patients with clear resection margins who were diagnosed with local recurrence at the renal fossa without distant metastasis throughout the postoperative 1–3-month imaging follow-up, whereas the MET group comprised only those with post-nephrectomy distant metastasis without LR around the renal fossa throughout the 1–3-month postoperative follow-up period. The BOTH group comprised nephrectomized patients diagnosed with only postoperative LRs in the operated renal fossa who later experienced disease progression in the distal metastatic organs. The BOTH group included four patients who were simultaneously diagnosed with local recurrence and distant metastasis.

## Statistical Analysis

Baseline characteristics are presented as frequencies (percentages) for categorical variables and as medians [interquartile range (IQR) or mean ± standard deviations (SD)] for continuous variables. Differences in distributions were compared among the three groups using a one-way analysis of variance or the Kruskal-Wallis test for continuous variables and Pearson's $\chi^2$ test or Fisher's exact test for categorical variables. A *post-hoc* analysis was performed to explore the clinicopathological factors that differed among the LR, MET, and BOTH groups. Given that we performed two analyses among the three groups, we set the significance cut-off at 0.05/2 for the *post-hoc* tests, taking multiple comparisons into consideration.

The survival indices OS and CSS were used to assess all-cause and RCC-related deaths, respectively. OS and CSS were compared among groups using the Cox proportional hazard models after adjusting for important covariates. A backward variable selection method with an elimination criterion of P > 0.05 was performed to complete the multivariable model. Survival curves were plotted using the survival probabilities of a multivariable model, and the survival rates of the three groups from 1 to 15 years were calculated using the Kaplan-Meier method. A two-sided p-value < 0.05 was considered statistically significant. Statistical analysis was performed using SAS 9.4 (SAS Institute Inc., Cary, NC, USA).

## Data Availability

The datasets generated and/or analyzed during the current study are available to be provided from the corresponding author upon reasonable request.

## RESULTS

Throughout the median follow-up of 43.9 (range, 19.0–76.1) months, the local recurrence, metastasis, and mortality rates following nephrectomy were 68.7, 31.3, and 41.2%, respectively,

including 161 (34.7%) and 30 (6.5%) RCC-related deaths and non-RCC-related deaths, respectively. Preoperative serum platelet and albumin levels, operative methods, and pathologic N stage were significantly different clinicopathological factors among the three groups (p < 0.05, **Table 1**). Moreover, baseline platelet levels and the nephrectomy method were significantly different between the LR and MET groups (**Supplementary Table 1A**), and the baseline albumin levels, pN1 stages, and intratumor necrosis characteristics were significantly different between the LR and BOTH groups (p < 0.05, **Supplementary Table 1B**).

**Supplementary Table 2** describes the analysis of the predictive clinicopathological factors of OS and CSS in each group. Multivariate analysis results (**Supplementary Table 2**) showed that the body mass index, hypertension, hemoglobin and albumin levels, pT3-4 and pN1 stageS, and Fuhrman nuclear grades 3–4 were significant risk factors of OS (p < 0.05), whereas body mass index, diabetes, hypertension, hemoglobin and albumin levels, pT3-4 and pN1 stageS, and Fuhrman nuclear grades 3–4 were the risk factors of CSS (p < 0.05). After adjusting for the significant risk factors of OS and CSS, the MET group had a significant hazard ratio (HR) of 0.51 (95% confidence interval [CI]: 0.27–0.97) for OS (p = 0.039) and an insignificant HR of 0.57 (CI: 0.29–1.12) for CSS (p = 0.103). The BOTH group had HRs of 0.51 (95% CI: 0.27–0.77) and 0.60 (95% CI: 0.39–0.92) for OS and CSS (p < 0.05), respectively, with the LR group (HR, 1.0) as a reference (**Table 2**).

**Table 3** describes the multivariate analyses of significant clinicopathological data within each group. Only capsular

**TABLE 1** | Baseline characteristics (N = 464).

| | | Total | LR group | MET group | BOTH group | p-value |
|---|---|---|---|---|---|---|
| Number | | 464 | 319 | 50 | 95 | |
| Follow-up duration | median (IQR) | 93.2 (48.4–127.7) | 93.2 (48.4–127.7) | 36.8 (13.8–100.9) | 93.2 (49.6–124.5) | |
| Age at operation | mean ± STD | 56.5 ± 11.6 | 56.5 ± 11.6 | 59.4 ± 9.9 | 56.7 ± 11 | 0.238 |
| Body mass index (kg/cm2) | mean ± STD | 23.9 ± 3 | 23.9 ± 3 | 24.5 ± 3.5 | 24 ± 2.9 | 0.481 |
| Diabetes | yes | 47 (14.7) | 47 (14.7) | 8 (16) | 13 (13.7) | 0.929 |
| Hypertension | yes | 109 (34.2) | 109 (34.2) | 24 (48.0) | 42 (44.2) | 0.059 |
| Hemoglobin | median (IQR) | 13.3 (11.4–14.6) | 13.3 (11.4–14.6) | 13.3 (11.6–14.6) | 13.8 (12.2–14.9) | 0.348 |
| Platelet | median (IQR) | 255.5 (212–318.5) | 255.5 (212–318.5) | 212 (181–261) | 251 (212–299) | 0.005 |
| Creatinine | median (IQR) | 1 (0.9–1.2) | 1 (0.9–1.2) | 1 (0.83–1.2) | 1 (0.9–1.16) | 0.916 |
| Albumin | median (IQR) | 4.1 (3.7–4.4) | 4.1 (3.7–4.4) | 4.2 (3.8–4.4) | 4.2 (3.9–4.5) | 0.034 |
| Nephrectomy | Open surgery | 328 (70.7) | 233 (73.0) | 23 (46.0) | 72 (75.8) | <.001 |
| | Laparoscopic | 127 (29.3) | 83 (26.0) | 26 (52.0) | 18 (19.0) | |
| Operative Extent | partial | 58(12.5) | 41 (12.9) | 7 (14.0) | 10 (10.5) | 0.994 |
| | radical | 196 (42.2) | 140 (43.9) | 23 (46.0) | 33 (34.7) | |
| pathologic T stage | T1 | 138 (43.3) | 138 (43.3) | 19 (38.0) | 31 (32.6) | 0.568 |
| | T2 | 57 (17.9) | 57 (17.9) | 10 (20.0) | 23 (24.2) | |
| | T3 | 111 (34.8) | 111 (34.8) | 19 (38.0) | 36 (37.9) | |
| | T4+Tx | 12 (3.8) | 12 (3.8) | 1 (2.0) | 2 (2.1) | |
| pathologic N stage | N0+Nx | 291 (91.2) | 291 (91.2) | 45 (90.0) | 92 (96.8) | 0.015 |
| | N1 | 27 (8.5) | 27 (8.5) | 4 (8.0) | 0 (0.0) | |
| Nuclear grade | grade 1-2 | 82 (25.7) | 82 (25.7) | 13 (26.0) | 20 (21.1) | 0.206 |
| | grade 3-4 | 147 (46.1) | 147 (46.1) | 31 (62.0) | 59 (62.1) | |
| Sarcomatoid differentiation | yes | 13 (4.1) | 13 (4.1) | 2 (4.0) | 8 (8.4) | 0.269 |
| Necrosis | yes | 43 (13.5) | 43 (13.5) | 8 (16.0) | 22 (23.2) | 0.075 |
| Lymphovascular invasion | yes | 39 (12.2) | 39 (12.2) | 10 (20.0) | 7 (7.4) | 0.084 |
| Capsular invasion | yes | 72 (22.6) | 72 (22.6) | 17 (34.0) | 22 (23.2) | 0.208 |
| Cause of death (n = 191) | RCC related | 117 (80.7) | 117 (80.7) | 11 (91.7) | 33 (97.1) | |
| | non-RCC-related | 28 (19.3) | 28 (19.3) | 1 (8.3) | 1 (2.9) | |

invasion was found to be a significant risk factor for both OS (HR: 8.97, CI: 1.83–44.09) and CSS (HR: 7.36, CI: 1.45–37.35) in the MET group (p < 0.05) in the subgroup analyses for selecting high-risk factors of OS and CSS. In the LR group, body mass index and preoperative hemoglobin and albumin levels were favorable risk factors of OS and CSS, whereas hypertension and pathologic T3-4 and N1 stages were unfavorable risk factors of both OS and CSS; a Fuhrman nuclear grade 3-4 was a risk factor of CSS only (p < 0.05). In the BOTH group, diabetes, lymphovascular invasion, and a Fuhrman nuclear grade 3-4 were significant factors of both OS and CSS (p < 0.05).

When the 2-year and 3-year survival rates from the nephrectomy date were analyzed in the three groups, the OS and CSS rates were 89.5% and 79.4% and 89.5% and 83.2%, respectively, for the MET group; 86.9% and 80.3% and 88.9% and 82.9%, respectively, for the LR group; and 96.8% and 93.2% and 96.8% and 93.2%, respectively, for the BOTH group (Table 4A). Only the LR and BOTH groups had significant differences in the 2- and 3-year OS and CSS rates (p < 0.05). Considering the starting date of disease recurrence, the 2-year and 3-year survival rates of OS and CSS rates were 48.1% and 48.1% and 52.4% and 52.4%, respectively, for the MET group; 63.5% and 57.3% and 67.8% and 61.8%, respectively, for the LR group; and 82.6% and 71.6% and 82.6% and 71.6%, respectively, for the BOTH group (Table 4B). Only the 2-year OS and CSS rats were significantly different between the LR and BOTH groups (p < 0.05).

**TABLE 2** | Univariable and multivariable Cox proportional hazard models for overall survival (OS) and cancer-specific survival (CSS) among three groups.

| Group | Metastasis | Recurrence | Total | Event (%) | Univariable model | | Multivariable model | |
|---|---|---|---|---|---|---|---|---|
| | | | | | HR (95% CI) | p-value | HR (95% CI) | p-value |
| **(1) Overall Survival (OS)** | | | | | | | | |
| LR group | no | yes | 319 | 145 (45.5) | 1 (ref) | (0.0187) | 1 (ref) | (0.0017) |
| MET group | yes | no | 50 | 12 (24.0) | 0.63 (0.35–1.15) | 0.1326 | 0.51 (0.27–0.97) | 0.0389 |
| Both group | yes | yes | 95 | 34 (35.8) | 0.61 (0.42–0.89) | 0.0104 | 0.51 (0.34–0.77) | 0.0015 |
| **(2) Cancer-Specific Survival (CSS)** | | | | | | | | |
| LR group | no | yes | 319 | 117 (36.7) | 1 (ref) | (0.2405) | 1 (ref) | (0.0302) |
| MET group | yes | no | 50 | 11 (22.0) | 0.73 (0.39–1.36) | 0.3147 | 0.57 (0.29–1.12) | 0.1026 |
| Both group | yes | yes | 95 | 33 (34.7) | 0.74 (0.50–1.10) | 0.1365 | 0.60 (0.39–0.92) | 0.0209 |

Adjusted for body mass index, hypertension, hemoglobin, albumin, pT stage, pN stage, and nuclear grade in OS multivariable model.
CI, confidence interval.

**TABLE 3** | Multivariable Cox proportional hazard model in each subgroup for overall survival (OS) and cancer-specific survival (CSS).

| | | | Overall survival (OS) | | Cancer-specific survival (CSS) | |
|---|---|---|---|---|---|---|
| | | | HR (95% CI) | p-value | HR (95% CI) | p-value |
| MET group | | | n = 50, event = 12 (24.0%) | | n = 50, event = 11 (22.0%) | |
| | Capsular invasion | yes | 8.97 (1.83–44.09) | 0.007 | 7.36 (1.45–37.35) | 0.016 |
| LR group | | | n = 304, event = 132 (43.4%) | | n = 319, event = 117 (36.7%) | |
| | Body mass index (kg/cm2) | | 0.89 (0.84–0.95) | <.001 | 0.87 (0.81–0.94) | <.001 |
| | Hypertension | yes | 2.07 (1.41–3.02) | <.001 | 2.78 (1.80–4.30) | <.001 |
| | Hemoglobin | female (≤12), male (≤13) | 1 (ref) | | 1 (ref) | |
| | | female (>12), male (>13) | 0.45 (0.30–0.68) | <.001 | 0.47 (0.30–0.74) | 0.001 |
| | Albumin | ≤3.0 | 1 (ref) | | 1 (ref) | |
| | | >3.0 | 0.21 (0.09–0.52) | <.001 | 0.20 (0.08–0.50) | 0.001 |
| | pathologic T stage | T1 | 1 (ref) | (<.001) | 1 (ref) | (<.001) |
| | | T2 | 1.30 (0.78–2.19) | 0.318 | 1.69 (0.92–3.08) | 0.089 |
| | | T3 | 1.98 (1.30–3.03) | 0.002 | 2.31 (1.42–3.76) | 0.001 |
| | | T4+Tx | 9.41 (4.02–22.02) | <.001 | 11.4 (4.66–27.86) | <.001 |
| | pathologic N stage | N0+Nx | 1 (ref) | | 1 (ref) | |
| | | N1 | 2.21 (1.18–4.13) | 0.014 | 2.63 (1.35–5.13) | 0.005 |
| | Nuclear grade | grade 1-2 | | | 1 (ref) | |
| | | grade 3-4 | | | 1.92 (1.09–3.38) | 0.024 |
| BOTH group | | | n = 95, event = 34 (35.8%) | | n = 95, event = 33 (34.7%) | |
| | Diabetes | yes | 2.69 (1.17–6.18) | 0.02 | 3.03 (1.30–7.07) | 0.011 |
| | Lymphovascular invasion | yes | 4.19 (1.41–12.46) | 0.01 | 4.01 (1.32–12.22) | 0.015 |
| | Nuclear grade | grade 1-2 | | | 1 (ref) | |
| | | grade 3-4 | | | 3.35 (1.11–10.08) | 0.032 |

CI, confidence interval.

**TABLE 4 |** Survival rate of 2 and 3 years according to three groups **(A)** from the date of nephrectomy and **(B)** from the date of local recurrence or metastasis.

| Group | N | Overall survival | | | | | | Cancer-specific survival | | | | | |
|---|---|---|---|---|---|---|---|---|---|---|---|---|---|
| | | 2 years | 95% CI | | 3 years | 95% CI | | 2 years | 95% CI | | 3 years | 95% CI | |
| | | survival rate | Lower | Upper | survival rate | Lower | Upper | survival rate | Lower | Upper | survival rate | Lower | Upper |
| **(A) Survival rates according to three groups from the date of nephrectomy** | | | | | | | | | | | | | |
| LR | 319 | 86.90% | 83.15% | 90.80% | 80.30% | 75.85% | 85.10% | 88.90% | 85.40% | 92.60% | 82.90% | 78.60% | 87.40% |
| MET | 50 | 89.50% | 80.20% | 99.90% | 79.40% | 66.60% | 94.60% | 89.50% | 80.17% | 99.90% | 83.20% | 71.61% | 96.60% |
| BOTH | 95 | 96.80% | 93.22% | 100.0% | 93.20% | 88.17% | 98.60% | 96.80% | 93.22% | 100.0% | 93.20% | 88.17% | 98.60% |
| **(B) Survival rates according to three groups from the date of local recurrence or metastasis** | | | | | | | | | | | | | |
| LR | 319 | 63.50% | 57.70% | 69.80% | 57.30% | 51.20% | 64.00% | 67.80% | 62.10% | 74.10% | 61.80% | 55.70% | 68.60% |
| MET | 50 | 48.06% | 29.20% | 79.00% | 48.06% | 29.20% | 79.00% | 52.43% | 32.90% | 83.60% | 52.43% | 32.90% | 83.60% |
| BOTH | 95 | 82.60% | 74.40% | 91.70% | 71.60% | 61.60% | 83.10% | 82.60% | 74.40% | 91.70% | 71.60% | 61.60% | 83.10% |

*CI, confidence interval.*

The OS and CSS curves adjusted for significant covariates showed significant differences among the three groups (p < 0.005, **Figure 1**). There was a significant difference in OS

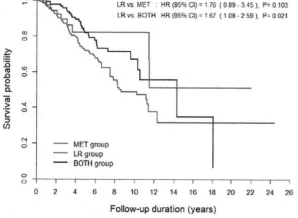

**FIGURE 1 |** Survival curves of the multivariable model for **(A)** overall survival and **(B)** cancer-specific survival among the three groups. CI, confidence interval.

between the LR group and each of the other two groups (*versus* MET, HR 1.96, and *versus* BOTH, HR 1.97) (p < 0.05, **Figure 1A**). However, only the BOTH group significantly differed in CSS from the LR group (LR *versus* BOTH, HR 1.67) (p = 0.021, **Figure 1B**).

**Supplementary Table 3** shows the extended long term-survival rates spanning up to 15 years postoperatively. A significant difference in both OS and CSS was observed between the LR and BOTH groups at 2–3 years postoperatively, whereas a significant difference in only OS was observed between the aforementioned groups at 4 and 9 years postoperatively (p < 0.05). There was a significant difference in both OSS and CSS between the MET and LR groups at 9, 10, and 11 years postoperatively, whereas there was a significant difference in only OS between the aforementioned groups at 8 years postoperatively. These differences remained in all groups until 15 years postoperatively (all, p < 0.05).

## DISCUSSION

Disease recurrence after curative nephrectomy in patients with nmRCC is challenging due to its rarity and unpredictability owing to the heterogenetic and pleomorphic pathophysiology of RCC, making large prospective studies, including randomized controlled trials, rare and inducing conflicting issues related to therapeutic and follow-up guidelines. These limitations allow retrospective multicenter studies comprising large study samples, such as in this study, to define significant independent disease recurrence predictive factors and characterize the prognostic survival of patients with nmRCC after nephrectomy (1–4, 11–14). This study selected a sufficient number of post-nephrectomized patients with recurrence and stratified them into LR, MET, and BOTH groups according to their recurrence patterns. Significant independent predictive and prognostic risk factors of OS and CSS were found, and some important characteristic findings regarding disease recurrence were obtained to improve postoperative surveillance and therapeutic strategic information.

The comparison of prognostic survival among the three groups demonstrated that both metastatic groups (HR < 1.0 for OS and CSS, **Table 2**) had significantly better OS and CSS than the LR group; however, there was an insignificant difference in CSS between the LR and MET groups (**Figures 1, 2**). Nevertheless, there were no significant differences in OS and CSS between both the MET and BOTH groups (p > 0.05, **Table 2**). Moreover, the 2- and 3-year OS and CSS rates supported the aforementioned unfavorable prognostic outcomes of the LR group, as well as the fact that the LR and BOTH groups had significantly different 2-year OS and CSS, regardless of the time from nephrectomy to disease recurrence (p < 0.05, **Table 4**). These results were unexpected and different from the general concepts of the survival of patients with RCC, which state that patients with mRCC had poorer survival outcomes than those with locally recurrent RCC (**Table 2**). This may be due to the distinguishing characteristics of this cohort compared to those in other studies (4, 5, 11–18). This study excluded patients who unsuccessfully underwent nephrectomy and have residual tumor cells at the renal fossa and those with obscured synchronous mRCCs who were at high risk of disease recurrence with suspicions of high tumor extents and aggressive tumor burdens. Moreover, this study includes a higher proportion of early stage patients with small tumor sizes (T1-staged RCC, 84.7%) and young patients (55.5 ± 12.4 years) compared to other studies. The characteristics of this cohort allowed us to focus on the primary tumor and disease progression, that is, either isolated local recurrence or distant metastasis, resulting in a lower number of patients in the MET (n = 50) and BOTH (n = 95) groups than in the LR group (n = 319) (3–5). The higher rate of early stage patients and small-sized

tumors and the lower rate of high stage patients and large-sized tumors in this study were due to the fact that the Korean National Cancer Screening Program performs testing twice at the age of 40 and 55 years, significantly affecting the survival outcomes of each group compared to previous studies (**Table 1**) (3–6, 11–18).

Another explanation for the differential survival outcomes among groups was the differential characteristics of the LR group, which included more advanced infiltrating diseases, poorer general conditions, and higher tumor burdens requiring more open surgery than the remaining two groups (**Tables 1, 3** and **Supplementary Table 1** and **Figure 1**). The higher baseline platelet levels and open surgery rate in the LR group than in the MET group and the more frequent nodal positivity and less necrotic primary lesions with lower albumin levels in the LR group than in the BOTH group supported the unfavorable prognoses of this group (p < 0.05, **Supplementary Table 1**) (14, 15, 19). Moreover, the therapeutic modalities of the LR and other groups were also important prognostic factors. This study did not discuss the therapeutic modalities of disease recurrence, but another Korean population-based study studying the therapeutic trends of disease recurrence (4.4%) after radical nephrectomy in 25,792 patients with nmRCCs between 2007 and 2013 showed significantly different OS rates between surgical methods (30.4 ± 18.7 months) and significantly different recurrence rates between targeted therapies (31 ± 22 months), other systemic therapies (25.4 ± 21.1 months), and radiation (24.1 ± 22.3 months) therapies. Therefore, it is possible to

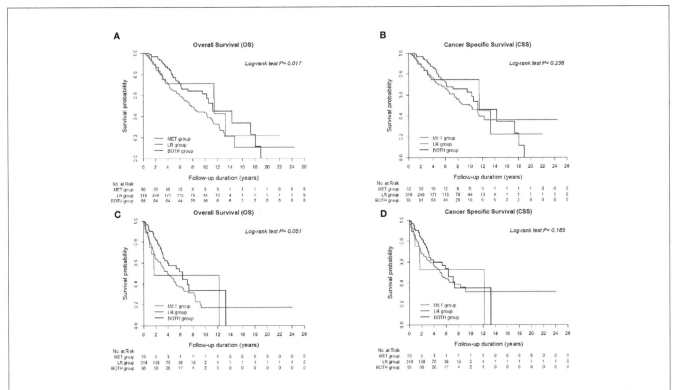

**FIGURE 2** | Kaplan-Meier curves between LR, BOTH, and MET groups for **(A)** Overall survival (OS) and **(B)** Cancer-specific survival (CSS) from the date of nephrectomy, and **(C)** OS and **(D)** CSS from the date of disease recurrence or metastasis.

identify patients at higher risk in the LR group who may need closer follow-ups and earlier consideration for various adjuvant therapeutic strategies including intervention measures according to recurrent sites compared to low-risk patients.

As for the predictive factors of OS and CSS in each group, this study found that baseline hypertension, pathologic T3-4, N1 staging, and Fuhrman nuclear grade 3-4 are significant unfavorable risk factors and that high body mass index and hemoglobin and albumin levels are significant favorable risk factors in the LR group (p < 0.05, **Table 3**) (16–18, 20). Capsular invasion in the MET group and diabetes, lymphovascular invasion, and high nuclear grade in the BOTH group were also important prognostic factors of poor OS and CSS (p < 0.05, **Table 4**) (4, 21, 22). These independent prognostic factors were clinically important to stratify high-risk patients with poor prognoses at recurrence diagnosis during follow-up. Moreover, the post-nephrectomized 2-year and 3-year follow-ups from the time of disease recurrence were important time points to compare the survival rates between groups (p < 0.05, **Table 4**). These data suggest that high-risk patients with diseased recurrence should be monitored more closely within 2 years, meaning that survival prognoses were determined within 2 years and that the more active and earlier administration of adjuvant therapies should be considered to improve survival outcomes. Therapeutic recommendations for LR lesions should be established according to the location, extent, and size of tumor in each recurrence as non-established guidelines, definitions, and recommendations for LR allow various therapies based on the discretion of clinicians, resulting in inconsistent prognostic results (1–5).

As for surgical or interventional LR measures, several studies have reported that diseases progressed in 40–60% of patients following therapeutic measures, even in a nephrectomized patient with nmRCC and an isolated LR, implying that survival improved following measures (11–14). Bruno et al. (11) reported a 2.9% overall LR (LR: 1.5% and BOTH: 1.4%) in 1165 pT1-4N0M0-staged nephrectomy patients during a median time of 16.9 months (range, 0.5 –103.6). Surgical intervention ensured a good OS and 3-year survival rates of 37.5 and 31%. Itano et al. (13) reported a disease recurrence rate of 2.9% (LR: 1.8%, and BOTH: 1.1%) in 1,737 pT1-3N0M0-staged radical nephrectomy patients. The disease control rate of surgical intervention was estimated at 60% of the OS rate. Margulis et al. (14) reported an LR rate of 1.8% during a median follow-up of 42 months in 2,945 pT1-3N0M0-staged nephrectomy patients. Surgical intervention ensured disease recurrence and overall mortality rates of 2.0% (27 distant metastases and 8 isolated LRs) and 1.8%, respectively. Therefore, further suggestions for effective surgical guidelines for LR and metastatic group indications should be discussed considering the association between metastases and other interventions and systemic therapy. Moreover, the surveillance of therapeutic strategies with close monitoring should also be considered within 2 years of recurrence until 4 years based on the type of metastasis (**Table 2** and **Supplementary Table 3**).

There is no consensus on preventive adjuvant systemic therapies and on when to apply adjuvant systemic therapies for disease recurrence after nephrectomy in patients with nmRCC because of contradicting results between previous clinical trials in this era of targeted therapy. The S-TRAC (sunitinib, positive), PROTECT (pazopanib), ARISER (girentuximab), and ATLAS (axitinib) trials showed contradicting results regarding the efficacy of adjuvant targeted therapies in a specified subset of nephrectomized patients with nmRCC (23, 24). In the upfront immune therapy era, several new ongoing trials showed that adjuvant immune-checkpoint inhibitors were efficient in nephrectomized patients with nmRCC (Keynote 564 trial, NCT03142334) (25), contradicting previous trials in the targeted therapy era. Immune checkpoint inhibitors potentiate systemic immune responses to the remnant cancer cells in secondary tumor sites after the complete removal of the primary kidney tumor (26). Some suggestions for future trials include investigating the effects of combining an immune-checkpoint inhibitor with targeted therapy and localized intervention for controlling disease recurrence and microtumor environments (26, 27).

Lastly, regarding the choice of surgical treatment, that is, radical or partial nephrectomy, and surgical technique, that is, open or laparoscopic surgery, survival was not influenced by nephrectomy itself, especially in early stage patients with confined nmRCC. Open and radical nephrectomy reportedly often showed poorer prognostic outcomes than other techniques and also disease recurrence because open nephrectomy was more suitable for patients with advanced stage tumors, as well as nodal infiltration, high intratumor burdens, poor preoperative characteristics and immunity, and a high likelihood of increased circulating cancer cells *via* the lymphovascular system intraoperatively, resulting in a higher probability of disease recurrence/progression after nephrectomy compared to other techniques (28–30). Selecting appropriate patients with nmRCC for nephrectomy is important to successfully remove all tumor cells to reduce disease recurrence.

This study had several inherent limitations due to its retrospective multicenter design, missing values, and missing information on postoperative prognoses, such as non-standardized surgical procedures, treatment modalities, specific locations, and disease recurrence criteria, and tumor burdens. However, only a few studies with large cohorts were available to characterize disease recurrence and predict prognostic factors after nephrectomy in patients with nmRCC. The findings from this study, along with several significant factors in each group, may help identify high-risk patients with nmRCC and better manage LR and MET with adequate follow-ups and therapeutic plans after nephrectomy. Future trials on postoperative preventive measures, on the determination of risk factors in patients with LR that can progress to distant metastasis and those who had the best survival outcomes, and on adjuvant therapy should be conducted.

This retrospective, multicenter, long-term follow-up nmRCC study showed that the LR group had worse survival prognoses than the remaining recurrent metastatic groups. The independent risk factors of survival in each group may indicate other high risk disease recurrence factors that may require adjuvant systemic therapies and local therapy to improve the prognosis of patients with nmRCC after either radical or partial nephrectomy. Further prospective cohort studies should be conducted to validate our findings and provide suggestions for LR and metastatic groups.

## AUTHOR CONTRIBUTIONS

SK: Conceptualization, data curation, investigation, methodology, project administration, supervision, and writing (original draft preparation). EH, S-HH, CJ, CK, and SB: Conceptualization, data curation, investigation, methodology, supervision, and writing (original draft preparation). BP: Conceptualization, data curation, formal analysis, investigation, methodology, project administration, supervision, and writing (original draft preparation). JC: Conceptualization, data curation, investigation, methodology, project administration, supervision, funding acquisition, and writing (original draft preparation). All authors contributed to the article and approved the submitted version.

## SUPPLEMENTARY MATERIAL

**Supplementary Table 1** | Comparison of baseline clinicopathological characteristics **(A)** between the LR and the MET and **(B)** between the LR and the BOTH groups

**Supplementary Table 2** | Univariable and multivariable Cox proportional hazard models between groups for overall survival (OS) and cancer-specific survival (CSS)

**Supplementary Table 3** | Survival rates for overall survival (OS) and cancer-specific survival (CSS) from 1 years to 15 years according to three groups

## REFERENCES

1. Kato M, Suzuki T, Suzuki Y, Terasawa Y, Sasano H, Arai Y. Natural History of Small Renal Cell Carcinoma: Evaluation of Growth Rate, Histological Grade, Cell Proliferation and Apoptosis. *J Urol* (2004) 172:863. doi: 10.1097/01.ju.0000136315.80057.99

2. Dabestani S, Marconi L, Kuusk T, Bex A. Follow-Up After Curative Treatment of Localised Renal Cell Carcinoma. *World J Urol* (2018) 36:1953–59. doi: 10.1007/s00345-018-2338-z

3. Patard JJ, Pignot G, Escudier B, Eisen T, Bex A, Sternberg C, et al. ICUD-EAU International Consultation on Kidney Cancer 2010: Treatment of Metastatic Disease. *Eur Urol* (2011) 60:684–90. doi: 10.1016/j.eururo.2011.06.017

4. Lee Z, Jegede OA, Haas NB, Pins MR, Messing EM, Manola J, et al. Local Recurrence Following Resection of Intermediate-High Risk Nonmetastatic Renal Cell Carcinoma: An Anatomical Classification and Analysis of the ASSURE (ECOG-ACRIN E2805) Adjuvant Trial. *J Urol* (2020) 203(4):684–9. doi: 10.1097/JU.0000000000000588

5. Frees SK, Kamal MM, Nestler S, Levien PM, Bidnur S, Brenner W, et al. Risk-Adjusted Proposal for >60 Months Follow Up After Surgical Treatment of Organ-Confined Renal Cell Carcinoma According to Life Expectancy. *Int J Urol* (2019) 26:385–90. doi: 10.1111/iju.13882

6. Beksac AT, Paulucci DJ, Blum KA, Yadav SS, Sfakianos JP, Badani KK. Heterogeneity in Renal Cell Carcinoma. *Urol Oncol* (2017) 35:507–15. doi: 10.1016/j.urolonc.2017.05.006

7. Guðmundsson E, Hellborg H, Lundstam S, Erikson S, Ljungberg B. Swedish Kidney Cancer Quality Register Group. Metastatic Potential in Renal Cell Carcinomas ≤7 Cm: Swedish Kidney Cancer Quality Register Data. *Eur Urol* (2011) 60:975–82. doi: 10.1016/j.eururo.2011.06.029

8. Byun SS, Hong SK, Lee S, Kook HR, Lee E, Kim HH, et al. The Establishment of KORCC (Korean Renal Cell Carcinoma) Database. *Investig Cli Urol* (2016) 57:50–7. doi: 10.4111/icu.2016.57.1.50

9. Kim JK, Kim SH, Song MK, Joo J, Seo SI, Kwak C, et al. Survival and Clinical Prognostic Factors in Metastatic non-Clear Cell Renal Cell Carcinoma Treated With Targeted Therapy: A Multi-Institutional, Retrospective Study Using the Korean Metastatic Renal Cell Carcinoma Registry. *Cancer Med* (2019) 8:3401–10. doi: 10.1002/cam4.2222

10. Kang HW, Seo SP, Kim WT, Yun SJ, Lee SC, Kim WJ, et al. Korean Renal Cell Carcinoma (KORCC) Group. Impact of Young Age at Diagnosis on Survival in Patients With Surgically Treated Renal Cell Carcinoma: A Multicenter Study. *J Korean Med Sci* (2016) 31:1976–82. doi: 10.3346/jkms.2016.31.12.1976

11. Schrodter S, Hakenberg OW, Manseck A, Leike S, Wirth MP. Outcome of Surgical Treatment of Isolated Local Recurrence After Radical Nephrectomy for Renal Cell Carcinoma. *J Urol* (2002) 167:1630–3. doi: 10.1016/S0022-5347(05)65167-1

12. Bruno JJ 2nd, Snyder ME, Motzer RJ, Russo P. Renal Cell Carcinoma Local Recurrences: Impact of Surgical Treatment and Concomitant Metastasis on Survival. *BJU Int* (2006) 97:933–8. doi: 10.1111/j.1464-410X.2006.06076.x

13. Itano NB, Blute ML, Spotts B, Zincke H. Outcome of Isolated Renal Cell Carcinoma Fossa Recurrence After Nephrectomy. *J Urol* (2000) 164:322–5. doi: 10.1016/S0022-5347(05)67350-8

14. Margulis V, McDonald M, Tamboli P, Swanson DA, Wood CG. Predictors of Oncological Outcome After Resection of Locally Recurrent Renal Cell Carcinoma. *J Urol* (2009) 181:2044–51. doi: 10.1016/j.juro.2009.01.043

15. Ito K, Seguchi K, Shimazaki H, Takahashi E, Tasaki S, Kuroda K, et al. Tumor Necrosis is a Strong Predictor for Recurrence in Patients With Pathological T1a Renal Cell Carcinoma. *Oncol Lett* (2015) 9:125–30. doi: 10.3892/ol.2014.2670

16. Zhang G, Wu Y, Zhang J, Fang Z, Liu Z, Xu Z, et al. Nomograms for Predicting Long-Term Overall Survival and Disease-Specific Survival of Patients With Clear Cell Renal Cell Carcinoma. *Onco Targets Ther* (2018) 11:5535–544. doi: 10.2147/OTT.S171881

17. Richards KA, Abel EJ. Surveillance Following Surgery for Nonmetastatic Renal Cell Carcinoma. *Curr Opin Urol* (2016) 26:432–8. doi: 10.1097/MOU.0000000000000308

18. Xia L, Hu G, Guzzo TJ. Prognostic Significance of Preoperative Anemia in Patients Undergoing Surgery for Renal Cell Carcinoma: A Meta-Analysis. *Anticancer Res* (2017) 37:3175–81. doi: 10.21873/anticanres.11677

19. Van Poppel H, Baert L. Nephrectomy for Metastatic Renal Cell Carcinoma and Surgery for Distant Metastases. *Acta Urologica Belgica* (1996) 64:11–7.

20. Xu Y, Zhang Y, Wang X, Kang J, Liu X. Prognostic Value of Performance Status in Metastatic Renal Cell Carcinoma Patients Receiving Tyrosine Kinase Inhibitors: A Systematic Review and Meta-Analysis. *BMC Cancer* (2019) 19:168. doi: 10.1186/s12885-019-5375-0

21. Bedke J, Heide J, Ribback S, Rausch S, de Martino M, Scharpf M, et al. Microvascular and Lymphovascular Tumour Invasion are Associated With Poor Prognosis and Metastatic Spread in Renal Cell Carcinoma: A Validation Study in Clinical Practice. *BJU Int* (2018) 121(1):84–92. doi: 10.1111/bju.13984

22. Rysz J, Franczyk B, Ławiński J, Olszewski R, Gluba-Brzózka A. The Role of Metabolic Factors in Renal Cancers. *Int J Mol Sci* (2020) 21(19):7246. doi: 10.3390/ijms21197246

23. Sharma T, Tajzler C, Kapoor A. Is There a Role for Adjuvant Therapy After Surgery in "High Risk for Recurrence" Kidney Cancer? An Update on Current Concepts. *Curr Oncol* (2018) 25:e444. doi: 10.3747/co.25.3865

24. Gross-Goupil M, Kwon TG, Eto M, Ye D, Miyake H, Seo SI, et al. Axitinib Versus Placebo as an Adjuvant Treatment of Renal Cell Carcinoma: Results From the Phase III, Randomized ATLAS Trial. *Ann Oncol* (2018) 29:2371–78. doi: 10.1093/annonc/mdy454

25. K. Choueiri T, I. Quinn D, Zhang T, Gurney, Doshi GK, Cobb PW, et al. Abstract CT162: Pembrolizumab Monotherapy for the Adjuvant Treatment of Renal Cell Carcinoma Post-Nephrectomy: Randomized, Double-Blind,

Phase III KEYNOTE-564 Study. *Cancer Res* (2019) 79(13):162. doi: 10.1158/1538-7445.AM2019-CT162

26. Pignot G, Loriot Y, Kamat AM, Shariat SF, Plimack ER. Effect of Immunotherapy on Local Treatment of Genitourinary Malignancies. *Eur Urol Oncol* (2019) 2:355–64. doi: 10.1016/j.euo.2019.01.002

27. Rieken M, Kluth LA, Fajkovic H, Capitanio U, Briganti A, Krabbe LM, et al. Predictors of Cancer-Specific Survival After Disease Recurrence in Patients With Renal Cell Carcinoma: The Effect of Time to Recurrence. *Clin Genitourin Cancer* (2018) 16:e903. doi: 10.1016/j.clgc.2018.03.003

28. Haga N, Onagi A, Koguchi T, Hoshi S, Ogawa S, Akaihata H, et al.

Perioperative Detection of Circulating Tumor Cells in Radical or Partial Nephrectomy for Renal Cell Carcinoma. *Ann Surg Oncol* (2020) 27:1272–81. doi: 10.1245/s10434-019-08127-8

29. Porta C, Bonomi L, Lillaz B, Klersy C, Imarisio I, Paglino C, et al. Immunological Stress in Kidney Cancer Patients Undergoing Either Open Nephrectomy or Nephron-Sparing Surgery: An Immunophenotypic Study of Lymphocyte Subpopulations and Circulating Dendritic Cells. *Oncol Rep* (2008) 20:1511–9.

30. Song T, Yin Y, Liao B, Zheng S, Wei Q. Capsular Invasion in Renal Cell Carcinoma: A Meta-Analysis. *Urol Oncol* (2013) 31:1321–6. doi: 10.1016/j.urolonc.2011.12.019

# 5

# TSPAN7 Exerts Anti-Tumor Effects in Bladder Cancer Through the PTEN/PI3K/AKT Pathway

Xi Yu[1†], Shenglan Li[2†], Mingrui Pang[1], Yang Du[1], Tao Xu[1], Tao Bai[3],
Kang Yang[1], Juncheng Hu[1], Shaoming Zhu[1], Lei Wang[1*] and Xiuheng Liu[1*]

[1] Department of Urology, Renmin Hospital of Wuhan University, Wuhan, China, [2] Department of Radiography, Renmin Hospital of Wuhan University, Wuhan, China, [3] Department of Urology, Wuhan No. 1 Hospital, Tongji Medical College, Huazhong University of Science and Technology, Wuhan, China

*Correspondence:
Lei Wang
Drwanglei@whu.edu.cn
Xiuheng Liu
drliuxh@hotmail.com

[†]These authors have contributed equally to this work

The tetraspanin protein superfamily participate in the dynamic regulation of cellular membrane compartments expressed in a variety of tumor types, which may alter the biological properties of cancer cells such as cell development, activation, growth and motility. The role of tetraspanin 7 (TSPAN7) has never been investigated in bladder cancer (BCa). In this study, we aimed to investigate the biological function of TSPAN7 and its therapeutic potential in human BCa. First, *via* reverse transcription and quantitative real-time PCR (qRT-PCR), we observed downregulation of TSPAN7 in BCa tissues samples and cell lines and found that this downregulation was associated with a relatively high tumor stage and tumor grade. Low expression of TSPAN7 was significantly correlated with a much poorer prognosis for BCa patients than was high expression. Immunohistochemistry (IHC) showed that low TSPAN7 expression was a high-risk predictor of BCa patient overall survival. Furthermore, the inhibitory effects of TSPAN7 on the proliferation and migration of BCa cell lines were detected by CCK-8, wound-healing, colony formation and transwell assays *in vitro*. Flow cytometry analysis revealed that TSPAN7 induced BCa cell lines apoptosis and cell cycle arrest. *In vivo*, tumor growth in nude mice bearing tumor xenografts could be obviously affected by overexpression of TSPAN7. Western blotting showed that overexpression of TSPAN7 activated Bax, cleaved caspase-3 and PTEN but inactivated Bcl-2, p-PI3K, and p-AKT to inhibit BCa cell growth *via* the PTEN/PI3K/AKT pathway. Taken together, our study will help identify a potential marker for BCa diagnosis and supply a target molecule for BCa treatment.

Keywords: cell cycle, apoptosis, PI3K/AKT, PTEN, bladder cancer, TSPAN7

## INTRODUCTION

Bladder cancer (BCa) is the most common malignancy of the urinary system, with more than 80,000 newly diagnosed cases and almost 18,000 deaths in the USA in 2019 (1). Approximately 70% of all diagnosed cases are non–muscle invasive bladder cancer (NMIBC), whereas the remaining cases are classified as muscle-invasive bladder cancer (MIBC). Despite advancements in the development of novel drugs and surgical treatments, approximately 50% of patients with BCa develop metastatic or recurrent disease within 2 years of diagnosis (2). Patients always require long-term follow-up with cystoscopy and computed tomography (CT) scans in case of relapse. As a result, the management costs of BCa seem to be considerably higher than other cancers (3). The overall survival of BCa patients remains very poor, thus, a better understanding of the molecular mechanisms of bladder carcinogenesis and elucidation of effective methods for predicting the prognosis of BCa are imperative.

Encoded by the TM4SF2 gene on XP114, tetraspanin 7 (TSPAN7) is a member of the tetraspanin protein superfamily of conserved membrane proteins (4–6). Most of the family members are cell-surface proteins that are characterized by the presence of four hydrophobic domains. TSPAN7 was first described as being strongly expressed in T-cell acute lymphoblastic leukemia (ALL) (7). Subsequently, TSPAN7 was found to be expressed in cancer of the stomach, pancreas, liver, esophagus, kidneys, and to be most strongly expressed in the brain (8–11). TSPAN7 mediates signal transduction events that play a role in the regulation of cell development, activation, growth, and motility (6, 12–14). In multiple myeloma (MM) patients, elevated TSPAN7 expression may be associated with better outcomes in up to 50% of patients (15). However, in lung cancer, TSPAN7 promotes migration and proliferation *via* epithelial-to-mesenchymal transition (16). Overall, TSPAN7 expression is associated with carcinogenesis, however, the precise role of TSPAN7 expression in BCa has not been defined.

Herein, by bioinformatics analysis of a dataset from The Cancer Genome Atlas (TCGA-BLCA), combined with fresh BCa and adjacent tissue samples studies, we identified that the downregulation of TSPAN7 expression plays an essential oncogenic role in BCa pathogenesis. In the current study, we first identified that the expression of TSPAN7 was significantly associated with tumor stage and grade in human BCa, and that low TSPAN7 expression was an independent predictive factor of overall survival (OS). Furthermore, overexpression of TSPAN7 exerted negative impacts on cell proliferation, colony formation, apoptosis, migration and invasion both *in vitro* and *in vivo via* the PTEN/PI3K/AKT signaling pathway. Thus, regulation of PTEN/PI3K/AKT signaling *via* TSPAN7 targeting may represent a new therapeutic approach for BCa treatment.

## MATERIALS AND METHODS

### Bioinformatics Analysis

The mRNA-read scount expression data for 427 bladder urothelial carcinoma patient samples (408 BCa and 19 normal bladder tissue samples) and clinical survival data for 412 patients were downloaded from TCGA-BLCA with "TCGAbiolinks" package in R language. An mRNA expression matrix was made with the raw counts of each RNA in each sample. The "Deseq2" package in R was used to calculate the differential expression of mRNAs between the bladder cancer tissues samples and paracancerous normal specimens. A fold change| >2 and p-value <0.05 were used as the threshold. A volcano plot for the

differentially expressed mRNAs was generated with "ggplot2" in R. Survival analysis was performed using these differentially expressed mRNAs with the "ggsurv" package in R with a p-value <0.05 used as the screening threshold. Then, the significant selected mRNAs were functionally analysed by Gene Ontology (GO) enrichment analysis and Kyoto Encyclopedia of Genes and Genomes (KEGG) pathway analysis with a p-value <0.05 set as the statistical threshold, the performing "clusterprofiler" R package was used to screen out significant enrichments in KEGG pathways and GO terms.

### Patients and Tissue Samples

Thirty-four pairs of fresh BCa and adjacent tissue specimens were obtained at the Department of Urology at Renmin Hospital of Wuhan University from March 2019 to December 2019. All specimens were collected by radical resection from patients without a prior history of BCa or adjuvant therapy and harvested after obtaining patients' written consent. BCa was defined by two pathologists. The tumor stage and grade of all patients were diagnosed according to the 2009 TNM staging system and 2004 World Health Organization grading system, respectively. All patients were under regular follow-up.

### Cell Lines and Cell Culture

The human bladder cancer cell lines 5637, T24, and EJ and human immortalized normal bladder epithelium cell line SV-HUC-1 were kindly provided by the Stem Cell Bank, Chinese Academy of Sciences (Shanghai, China). Identification of the cell lines was conducted at the China Centre for Type Culture Collection (Wuhan, China). 5637, T24, and EJ cells were maintained in RPMI-1640 medium (HyClone, China), and SV-HUC-1 cells were maintained in F-12K medium (HyClone, China) supplemented with 10% fetal bovine serum (FBS) (Gibco, Australia) and 1% penicillin G sodium/streptomycin sulfate. All the cells were grown in a humidified atmosphere consisting of 5% $CO_2$ and 95% air at 37°C

### Total RNA Isolation From Bladder Tissue Samples and BCa Cells

Total RNA was extracted from BCa cells and bladder tissue specimens using TRI Reagent (Cat. abs9331-100 ml, Absin, China) according to the manufacturer's instructions. The reverse transcription process was carried out with the RevertAid RT Reverse Transcription Kit (Cat. K1691, Thermo Scientific, China). Finally, the produced cDNA was stored at -20°C.

### Reverse Transcription and Quantitative Real-Time PCR

A total 20 μl-volume reaction system, which contained 1 μl cDNA, 1 μl of each primer, 10 μl NovoStart® SYBR qPCR SuperMix Plus (Cat.E096-01A, novoprotein, China), and 7 μl DNAse/RNAse-free water, was performed in triplicates. Fold enrichment was calculated with the 2−ΔΔCt method relative to the expression of GAPDH. The primer sequences were listed as follows: TSPAN7: 5`-CTCATCGGAACTGGCACCACTA-3`, 5`- CCTGAAA

TGCCAGCTACGAGCT-3`; GAPDH: 5`- GTCTCCTCTGA CTTCAACAGCG-3`, 5`- ACCACCCTGTTGCTGTAGCCAA-3`. All experiments were conducted in triplicate and repeated three times.

## Immunohistochemistry

For IHC, the procedures of dewaxing and rehydration were similar to those for HE staining. Then, the tissue sections were boiled in citrate buffer (pH 6.0) at 100°C for 15 min. A primary antibody (anti-TSPAN7, 1:50, 18695-1-AP, Proteintech) was added to the tissue sections after blocking with 3.0% hydrogen peroxide (H2O2) for 10 min at room temperature and incubated overnight at 4°C. A secondary antibody was added to the slides and incubated at room temperature for 30 min. Finally, the sections were incubated with DAB chromogen and then counterstained with hematoxylin.

Section assessment was completed by two experimental pathologists who were blinded to clinical outcomes. The scoring of TSPAN7 expression was defined as a score of 0, 1, 2, or 3 according to the staining intensity, and the overall staining score was summarized as low (0, 1) or high (2, 3).

## Transfections and Selection of BCa Cell Lines With Stable Overexpression of TSPAN7

The full sequence of TSPAN7 was inserted into a lentiviral vector to construct a TSPAN7-overexpression plasmid (Vigenebio, China). BCa cells ($1\times10^5$) were seeded in 6-well plates and grown to approximately 50% confluency. Then, the culture medium was removed, and fresh culture medium containing lentiviral particles carrying TSPAN7 cDNA or a negative control was added according to the manufacturer's instructions. The cells were cultured in an incubator at 37°C with 5% $CO_2$ for 18 h. Next, the culture medium was removed and replaced with fresh medium. After transfection for 72 h, culture medium containing an appropriate concentration of puromycin (Sigma, USA) was added to kill any nontransfected cells. The surviving cell clones were selected and expanded. The lentiviruses were designated pcDNA-TSPAN7. The empty vector was used as a negative control (pcDNA-vector). Western blot and qRT-PCR analyses were used to evaluate infection efficiency.

## Protein Extraction and Western Blot Analysis

Total cellular protein was extracted from BCa cells using a RIPA buffer solution. The samples were placed on ice for 30 min with discontinuous ultrasonic dispersion. The lysates were centrifuged at 12,000 rpm for 15 min at 4°C. The supernatant was harvested, and the protein concentration was detected with a bicinchoninic acid (BCA) assay using bovine serum albumin (BSA) as the standard. The extracted protein samples were denatured at 100°C for 10 min after 25% volume loading buffer was added. Finally, the protein samples were stored at -20°C. A total of 60 µg of protein from each sample was resolved by 8%–12% SDS-PAGE and transferred to PVDF membranes (Millipore, USA), which were blocked with 5% nonfat milk for at least 1 h at room temperature. The membranes were incubated with primary antibodies overnight at 4°C on a table concentrator, followed by secondary antibody incubation for 1 h at room temperature. Bands were detected with a corresponding protein development instrument and quantified with ImageJ software (W S Rasband, ImageJ, NIH).

## CCK-8-Based Cell Viability Assay

To assess cell proliferation, BCa cells were seeded at a density of $2\times10^3$ cells/well in 96-well plates and cultured for 24, 48, 72, or 96 h. At each end of the experiment, 10 µl of CCK-8 reagent (CK04, Dojindo, Japan) was added to each well, and the cells were further cultured for 1 h. Absorption values were measured at 450 nm. Cell growth curves were plotted according to the results of each experiment. All experiments were conducted in triplicate and repeated three times.

## Tumor Cell Colony Formation Assay

Tumor cell clonogenicity was assessed with a colony formation assay. Cells were seeded in 6-well plates at $1\times10^4$, $1\times10^3$, and $1\times10^2$ cells/well and grown for 10 days. Visible colonies (≥50 cells) were counted after 4% paraformaldehyde (PFA) fixation and 0.1% crystal violet staining. The experiment was repeated three times.

## Transwell Migration Assay

For transwell migration assays, we used a 24-well plate transwell chamber system (Corning, USA). In the upper chamber, $8\times10^4$ cells were suspended in 200 µl of serum-free medium, while 600 µl of 20% FBS medium was added to the lower chamber to induce cell migration. After 72 h, a cotton swab was used to remove any remaining cells in the upper chamber. The cells that migrated to the other side of the membrane were fixed in 4% PFA for 30 min and stained with 0.1% crystal violet for 4 hours. The stained chambers were left to dry and photographed. The experiment was repeated three times.

## Wound-Healing Assay

To assess cell motility, a wound-healing assay was used. Approximately $2–3\times10^6$ cells were plated in a 6-well plate. When the cells were 90%–95% confluent, the cell layer was carefully scratched with a sterile tip and washed with PBS three times. The cells were then incubated for 0 h, 12 h, 24 h, and 48 h, and images were acquired. The assays were repeated in triplicate.

## Cell Cycle and Apoptosis

BCa cells were harvested, centrifuged and then washed with cold PBS twice. For cell cycle analysis, cells were resuspended in 1× DNA Staining Solution containing propidium iodide and a permeabilization solution and incubated at 37°C for 30 min in the dark. The cell cycle distribution of each sample was analyzed by flow cytometry analysis. For cell apoptosis analysis, cells were stained with the Annexin-V FITC Apoptosis Detection Kit I (BD Biosciences, USA) according to the kit protocol and analyzed by flow cytometry analysis.

## TUNEL Assay

In brief, Prepare paraffin sections → dewaxing and hydration → cell transparency → add TUNEL reaction solution (TUNEL,

Roche Applied Science, Germany) → add Converter -POD→ react with substrate DAB to develop color → count and take photos with optical microscope.

## Xenograft Mouse Model

Specific pathogen-free (SPF) male BALB/c-nude mice (4 weeks old) were purchased from Beijing HFK Bioscience Co., Ltd. (Beijing, China). After a week of adaption at the laboratory animal facility of Renmin Hospital of Wuhan University, we randomly assigned mice to the control group and the test group. For a subcutaneous tumor growth assay, $1 \times 10^6$ pcDNA-TSPAN7 or pcDNA-NC T24 cells diluted in 0.2 ml of serum-free medium were subcutaneously injected into 5-week-old BALB/c-nude mice. After 5 weeks, the mice were sacrificed, all of the xenotransplanted tumors were dissected, and tumor weight and tumor size were measured with a Vernier caliper (tumor volume = length×width$^2$×0.5 mm$^3$). The tumors were fixed in 4% PFA and subsequently analyzed by IHC staining.

## Statistical Analysis

The 23.0 SPSS software package was used for all statistical analyses. The significance of differences was compared using the $\chi^2$ test and Student's t test. Overall survival was estimated by the Kaplan-Meier method, and differences in survival between two groups were analyzed by the log-rank test. For univariate and multivariate analyses, the Cox proportional hazards regression model was used. A two-sided P value < 0.05 was considered statistically significant.

## RESULTS

### Sixteen Key Marker Genes Were Selected by Bioinformatic Analysis

Through differential expression analysis of 19858 mRNAs between BCa and paracancerous normal specimens, 4943 significantly differentially expressed mRNAs including 2786 upregulated and 2157 downregulated mRNAs were obtained (**Figure 1A**). Herein, GAGE12D, CT45A5, GAGE2B, FGB, CT45A1, GAGE2D, GAGE1, and GAGE2A were upregulated with >10000-fold changes, and FAM180B, KCNB1, MYH11, PI16, MYOC, SYNM, GPR112, OSTN, MYH2, and GLP2R were downregulated with >40-fold changes in the BCa tissue samples compared to the normal bladder tissue samples. These differentially expressed RNAs were used to perform survival analysis exploring the effects of these mRNAs on the survival prognosis of BCa patients. Significantly (p-value <0.05), 596 mRNAs associated with a favorable or poor survival prognosis in bladder cancer were identified. The 596 mRNAs were

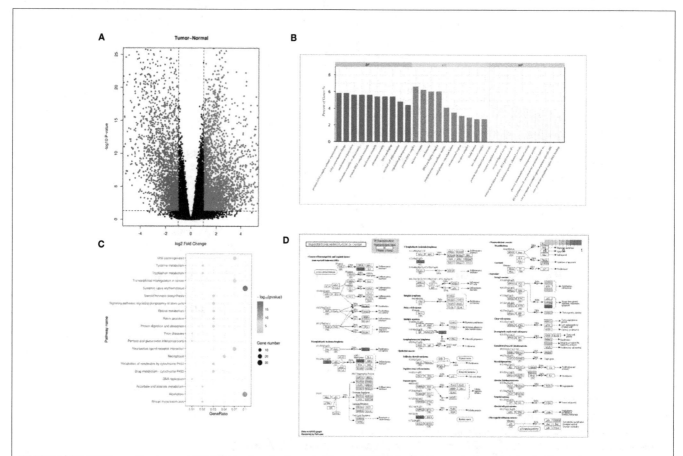

**FIGURE 1** | Differentially expressed genes in TCGA dataset, and pathway enrichment of TSPAN7. **(A)** Volcano plot visualizing the all differentially expressed genes in TCGA dataset, **(B)** GO enrichment, **(C)** KEGG pathway, and **(D)** Transcriptional misregulation in cancer.

functionally enriched in GO terms spanning the biological process (BP), molecular function (MF) and cellular component (CC) categories, and KEGG pathways, which showed relatively significant terms, such as DNA conformation changes, protein-DNA complex, receptor regulator activity and transcription factor activity (**Figures 1B–D**). Transcriptional misregulation in a cancer pathway was identified to be significant and found to involve 16 genes: HIST1H3D, HIST1H3B, HIST1H3F, HIST2H3D, CSF2, TLX3, HIST1H3A, HIST1H3E, IGFBP3, ETV7, WNT16, SLC45A3, GADD45A, ID2, TSPAN7, NFKBIZ, and IGF1.

## TSPAN7 Downregulation in BCa Tissue Specimens and Cell Lines

We first assessed TSPAN7 mRNA expression in BCa tissue samples compared to normal tissue samples (**Figures 2A, B**) and in cell lines (**Figure 2C**). qRT-PCR showed that TSPAN7 mRNA was significantly higher in the normal bladder tissue

specimens than in the BCa tissue specimens. The same result was found in Western blot (**Figures 2D, E**) of the BCa samples and cell lines. IHC staining results (**Figure 2F**) showed that the protein level of TSPAN7 was increased in normal bladder tissue specimens.

## Associations of TSPAN7 Expression With The Clinicopathological Features and Survival of Bladder Cancer Patients

As shown in **Table 1**, TSPAN7 expression was associated with tumor stage (p=0.01) and tumor grade (p=0.03) in BCa. However, no relationships were found between TSPAN7 expression and other clinical features, such as patient sex (p=0.68), age (p=0.41), tumor size (p=0.67), and tumor multiplicity (p=0.87), lymphnodes status (p=0.53). We then analyzed data from UCSC for patient overall survival and found that reduced TSPAN7 expression was significantly associated with poor overall survival (**Figure 3**).

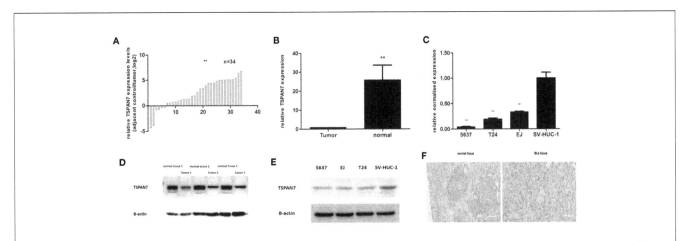

**FIGURE 2 |** TSPAN7 was downregulation in BCa patients and cell lines. **(A, B)** TSPAN7 mRNA expression in BCa tissue samples was lower than in normal tissue. **(C)** TSPAN7 mRNA was significantly downregulation in BCa cell lines (T24, 5637, EJ) compared with the normal bladder epithelial cell line (SV-HUC-1). **(D)** In Western blot, TSPAN7 showed a higher expression in normal tissue. **(E)** In Western blot, TSPAN7 showed a higher expression in normal bladder epithelial cell line. **(F)** Immunohistochemistry (IHC) showed the protein level of TSPAN7 was increased in normal bladder tissue. Scale bars, 100μm. **p<0.01.

**TABLE 1 |** Correlation between TSPAN7 expression and clinical features of patients.

| Variable | Groups | Total | Low | High | p |
|---|---|---|---|---|---|
| Gender | Male | 25 | 21 | 4 | 0.68 |
| | Female | 9 | 7 | 2 | |
| Age (years) | ≥60 | 22 | 19 | 3 | 0.41 |
| | <60 | 12 | 9 | 3 | |
| Tumor size (cm) | ≥ | 20 | 16 | 4 | 0.67 |
| | <3 | 14 | 12 | 2 | |
| Multiplicity of tumor | Single | 18 | 15 | 3 | 0.87 |
| | Multiple | 16 | 13 | 3 | |
| Tumor grade | PUNLMP, low grade | 8 | 3 | 5 | 0.01 |
| | High grade | 26 | 25 | 1 | |
| Tumor stage | Ta, T1 | 10 | 6 | 4 | 0.03 |
| | T2–T4 | 24 | 22 | 2 | |
| Lymphnodes | Negative | 26 | 22 | 4 | 0.53 |
| | Positive | 8 | 6 | 2 | |
| Distant metastasis | Absent | 34 | 28 | 6 | |
| | Present | 0 | | | |

## TSPAN7 Is Negatively Correlated With BCa Cell Proliferation, Viability, and Migration *In Vitro*

Our current data demonstrated that TSPAN7 expression was reduced in BCa tissue and cell lines and that TSPAN7 downregulation was associated with poor overall survival. We further assessed whether changes in TSPAN7 expression could affect BCa cell malignant behaviors. qRT-PCR (**Figure 4A**) and Western blot (**Figures 4B, C**) data confirmed that the expression of TSPAN7 was upregulated in pcDNA-TSPAN7 groups compared with pcDNA-vector groups. We then found that overexpression of TSPAN7 inhibited cell proliferation (**Figure 4D**). BCa cell colony formation assays showed that TSPAN7 overexpression reduced the number of BCa cell colonies (**Figure 4E**). Transwell invasion (**Figure 4F**) and wound-healing assays (**Figure 4G**) verified that TSPAN7 overexpression inhibited BCa cell invasion.

## Effects of TSPAN7 on BCa Cell Apoptosis *In Vitro*

Next, we determined the effects of TSPAN7 overexpression on BCa cell apoptosis. We found that the percentage of apoptotic cells was significantly higher in pcDNA-TSPAN7 groups than in pcDNA-vector groups (**Figure 5A**). Western blot data further showed that the expression of cleaved caspase-3 and Bax was upregulated, whereas that of Bcl-2 was downregulated in the pcDNA-TSPAN7 groups (**Figures 5B, C**).

## Effects of TSPAN7 on BCa Cell Cycle Arrest *In Vitro*

Moreover, TSPAN7 overexpression in 5637, EJ, and T24 cells increased the proportion of cells in the G1 phase compared to control expression (**Figure 6A**). Western blot data showed that CDK2 and cyclin E expression was downregulated in pcDNA-TSPAN7 groups compared to pcDNA-vector groups (**Figures 6B, C**). These findings suggested that TSPAN7 overexpression induced cell cycle arrest in the G1 phase of the cell cycle.

## TSPAN7 Inhibits Proliferation in BCa Cell Lines Through The PTEN/PI3K/AKT Pathway

Transactivation of PI3K/AKT can cause different biological activities, such as inflammation, immunity, cell growth, tumorigenesis, and apoptosis (17–19). In this study, we measured PI3K/AKT expression and activity in pcDNA-TSPAN7 and pcDNA-vector groups. We found that TSPAN7 overexpression in BCa cells downregulated the expression of p-PI3K and p-AKT, and upregulated the expression of PTEN, whereas pcDNA-vector did not impact these proteins (**Figures 7A, B**).

Then, we assessed whether the AKT agonist SC79 could reverse the effect of TSPAN7 overexpression on T24 cells. We also used PTEN inhibitor VO-Ohpic trihydrate to verify whether it caused the similar effect on pcDNA-vector T24 cells. The p-AKT levels in T24 cells were significantly elevated after SC79 treatment, and PTEN expression was markedly suppressed after VO-Ohpic trihydrate treatment (**Figures 7C, D**). Compared with no treatment, treatment of cells with SC79 or VO-Ohpic trihydrate dramatically produced opposite effects on the levels of these proteins. These findings indicated that SC79 partly reversed the inhibitory effect of TSPAN7 overexpression on T24 cells and that VO-Ohpic trihydrate showed an effect similar to that of TSPAN7 overexpression. To investigate the role of the PTEN/PI3K/AKT pathway in TSPAN7-mediated cell proliferation, migration and invasion, we performed rescue experiments also. In the presence of SC79, the proliferation, migration, and invasion of pcDNA-TSPAN7 T24 cells were clearly elevated. Similarly, inhibition of PTEN in T24 cells distinctly decreased cell growth, migration and invasion (**Figures 7E–G**). Altogether, these results confirmed that TSPAN7 inhibited the PTEN/PI3K/AKT pathway upstream of AKT and downregulated PTEN/PI3K/AKT pathway activation.

## Overexpression of TSPAN7 Suppresses BCa Cell Growth *In Vivo*

To confirm the inhibitory effects of TSPAN7 *in vivo*, we subcutaneously injected pcDNA-TSPAN7 or pcDNA-vector T24 cells into nude mice. We found significant differences in T24 cell xenograft formation, growth and weight between the two groups (**Figures 8A, B**). The size of tumor xenografts was larger in the pcDNA-vector T24 cell group than in the pcDNA-TSPAN7 groups. IHC showed that Ki67 expression was significantly downregulated in pcDNA-TSPAN7 T24 tumors compared to pcDNA-vector tumors (**Figure 8C**). Next, TUNEL staining validated that apoptotic cell numbers were increased in the pcDNA-TSPAN7 groups compared with the pcDNA-vector groups (**Figure 8D**). These results suggest that TSPAN7 suppresses tumor growth *in vivo*.

## DISCUSSION

In the present study, we showed that the expression of TSPAN7 in normal bladder tissue and cells was significantly higher than

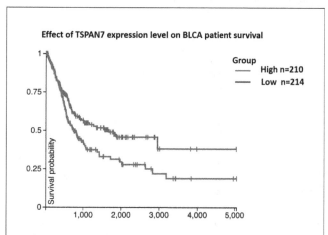

**FIGURE 3** | (**Table 1**) Association between TSPAN7 expression and clinicopathological features of human bladder cancer. (**Figure 3**) TSPAN7 expression was significantly associated with poor overall survival from UCSC.

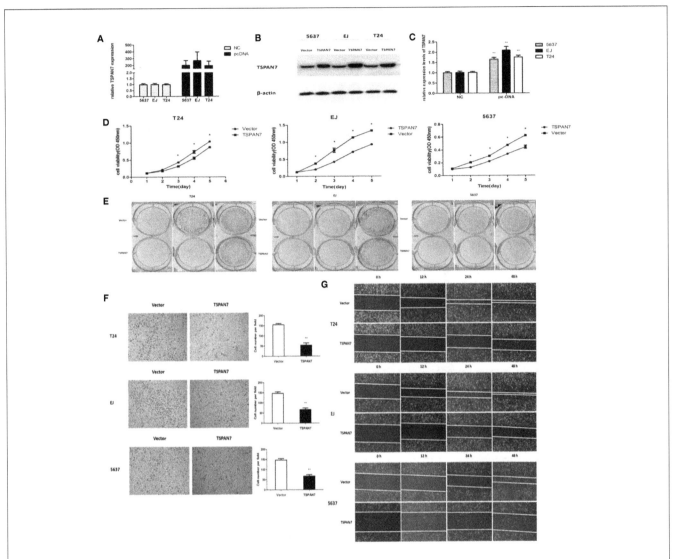

**FIGURE 4** | Overexpression of TSPAN7 repressed BCa cell proliferation and migration. **(A)** Verification of TSPAN7 overexpression efficacy at the mRNA level in T24, EJ, 5637 cells. **(B, C)** Verification of TSPAN7 overexpression efficacy at the protein level in T24, EJ, 5637 cells. CCK-8 assays **(D)** and colony formation assays **(E)** showed that TSPAN7 overexpression decreased the proliferation capacity. Transwell invasion **(F)** and wound-healing assays **(G)** showed that TSPAN7 overexpression attenuated cell migration ability *P < 0.05; **P < 0.01.

that in BCa tissue and cells. Furthermore, high expression of TSPAN7 was negatively correlated with a high T stage and tumor grade in BCa. The survival of patients with high expression of TSPAN7 was superior to that of those with low expression. Moreover, TSPAN7 overexpression inhibited BCa cell proliferation, cell cycle progression, invasion, and apoptosis.

TSPAN7 is a member of the transmembrane 4 superfamily, also called the tetraspanin family, which includes proteins characterized by four transmembrane domains, with one short and one large extracellular loop (20). Previous studies have found that in cerebellar granule cells, TSPAN7 promotes axonal branching, and the size of TSPAN7 clusters is increased by downregulation of IGSF3 expression, which might be at the center of a new signaling pathway controlling brain development (21). In oral tongue squamous cell carcinoma, differential methylation of TSPAN7 was found to be predictive of certain

clinical and epidemiologic parameters (22). There is also research suggesting that TSPAN7 plays an important role in the cytoskeletal organization required for the bone-resorbing function of osteoclasts by regulating signaling to Src, Pyk2, and microtubules (23). Lee SA disclosed a previously uncharacterized role for TSPAN7 in the regulation of the expression and functional activity of the dopamine D2 (DRD2) receptor, which was implicated in multiple neurologic and psychiatric disorders by postendocytic trafficking (24). In clear cell renal cell carcinoma (CCRCC), relatively high TSPAN7 expression in primary tumor cells is not associated with patient outcomes (25). However, increased TSPAN7 expression in CCRCC lung metastases is associated with prolonged metastasis-free survival (11). To the best of our knowledge, this is the first study to identify elevated TSPAN7 expression in BCa. Our study provides the first genetic evidence that TSPAN7 plays a critical role in BCa

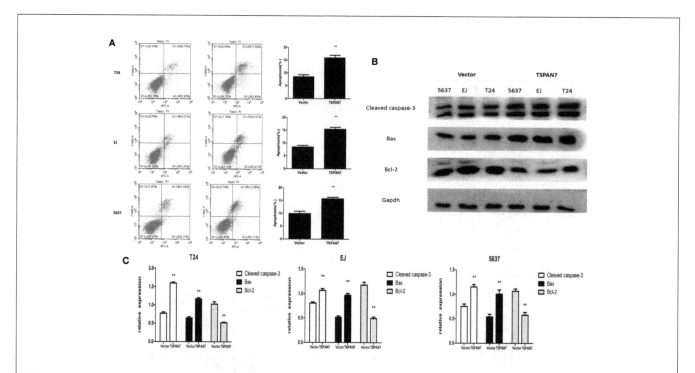

**FIGURE 5** | TSPAN7 overexpression promotes the apoptosis of BCa cell. **(A)** Quantitative flow cytometry measurements of apoptosis in T24, EJ, 5637 cells.
**(B, C)** TSPAN7 overexpression upregulated the expression of cleaved caspase-3 and Bax whereas that of Bcl-2 was downregulated. **p<0.01 vs. the control group.
All the above data are the mean ± SD from an average of three experiments.

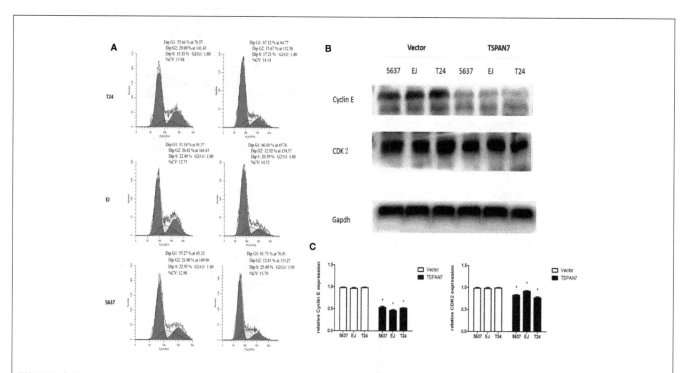

**FIGURE 6** | **(A)** TSPAN7 overexpression induced cell cycle arrest at the G1/S phase. **(B)** CDK2 and cyclin E expression was downregulated in pcDNA-TSPAN7
groups. **(C)** Densitometry analysis of western blots showed quantitation of Cyclin E and CDK2 levels. *p<0.05.

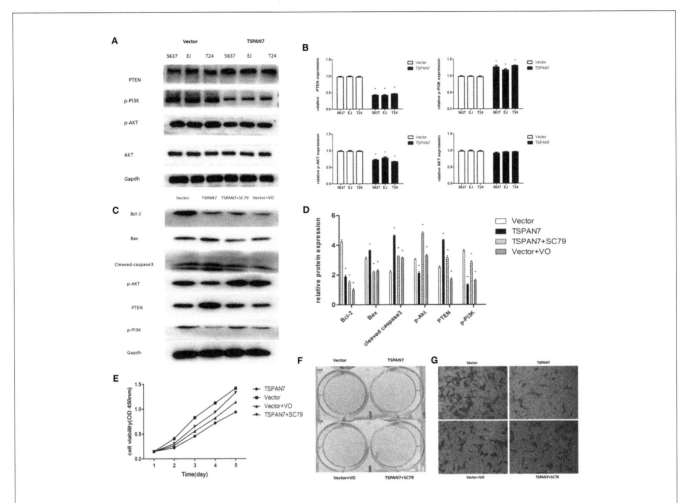

**FIGURE 7** | TSPAN7 inhibits proliferation in BCa cell lines *via* PTEN-PI3K/AKT pathways. **(A, B)** TSPAN7 overexpression in BCa cells downregulated the expression of p-PI3K and p-AKT, and upregulated the expression of PTEN. **(C, D)** In Western blot, AKT agonist SC79 could reverse the effect of TSPAN7 overexpression on T24 cells and PTEN inhibitor VO-Ohpic trihydrate caused the similar effect on pcDNA-vector T24 cells. **(E–G)** In the presence of SC79, the proliferation, migration and invasion of pcDNA-TSPAN7 T24 cells were clearly elevated and inhibition of PTEN in T24 cells distinctly decreased cell growth, migration and invasion. *P < 0.05 vs. the corresponding NC cells. All the above data are the mean ± SD from an average of three experiments.

tumorigenesis. Analyses of clinicopathological features showed that TSPAN7 was an independent prognostic factor of BCa that was significantly correlated with T stage and tumor grade, and low expression of TSPAN7 predicted a poor prognosis (OS) in BCa patients. According to our transcriptomic analysis, the mRNA expression of TSPAN7 was strongly downregulated in BCa tissue samples versus adjacent tissue samples, in accordance with the results from our TCGA database and qRT-PCR analyses. Consistent with the TCGA database analysis, the downregulation of TSPAN7 expression at both the transcriptional and translational levels in tumor specimens predicted high malignancy and a poor prognosis in BCa patients. Our results showed that overexpression of TSPAN7 inhibited BCa cell growth, migration and invasion *in vitro* and *in vivo*.

Furthermore, our findings revealed that overexpression of TSPAN7 could induce BCa cell apoptosis with caspase 3 cleavage and elevate the Bax/Bcl-2 ratio, indicating a potential role for TSPAN7 in facilitating apoptosis. The intrinsic apoptotic

pathway (mitochondria-dependent) activated in response to different stress conditions is mediated by intracellular signals that converge at the mitochondrial level (26). The Bcl-2 family regulates both proapoptotic and antiapoptotic pathways controlling MOMP alteration (27). Therefore, Bcl-2 family proteins serve as an "apoptotic switch" by mediating permeabilization of the mitochondrial membrane (28). The balance and interactions among Bcl-2 family members can determine whether a cell survives or undergoes apoptosis. While antiapoptotic proteins regulate apoptosis by blocking the mitochondrial release of cytochrome c, proapoptotic proteins act by promoting this release. Activation of the Bcl-2 family (Bax and Bak) neutralizes the antiapoptotic proteins Bcl-2 and Bcl-xL, leading to disruption of mitochondrial membrane outer membrane permeability (MOMP) so that proteins such as cytochrome-*c*, which plays a crucial role in activating mitochondrial-dependent death, are released into the cytosol (29). Then, cytochrome-c triggers the formation of apoptosomes, which recruit initiator pro-caspase-9 to the caspase recruitment

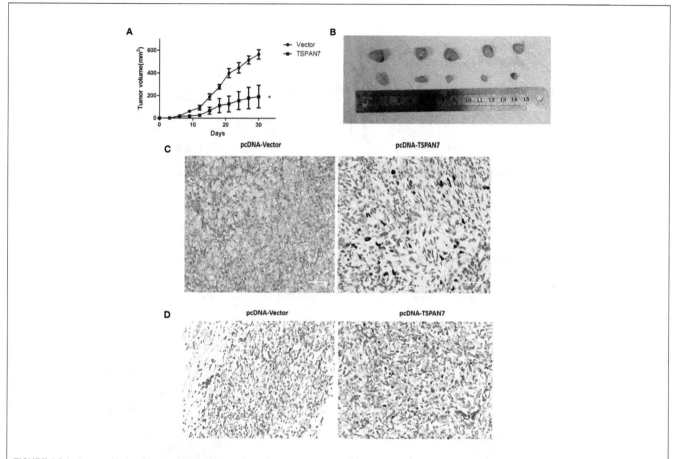

**FIGURE 8** | Anti-tumor effects of *in vivo*. **(A)** Mean tumor volume at each time point. **(B)** Morphology of the subcutaneous implanted tumor. **(C)** Immunohistochemistry (IHC) was performed to detect the protein of Ki67 in the tumor tissue. **(D)** A TUNEL assay was performed to detect the apoptotic cells in the tumor tissue. *P < 0.05 vs. the control. All the above data are the mean ± SD from an average of three experiments.

domain (CARD), resulting in autoactivation and proteolysis (30). Then, the process activates downstream executors, such as caspase-3, caspase-6 and caspase-7, for cleavage of cellular substrates, leading to apoptotic cell death (31).

Next, a series of gain-of-function assays was performed to elucidate the regulatory functions of TSPAN7 in BCa cells. Overexpression of TSPAN7 demonstrated a marked inhibitory effect on BCa cells by reducing proliferation, attenuating cell migration and inducing G1/S cell cycle arrest. Furthermore, Western blot analysis indicated that overexpression of TSPAN7 interfered with G0/G1 phase-related proteins, such as CCNA1/2, CCND1, and CDK2/4. Cancer often represents a pathological manifestation of uncontrolled cell division and cell cycle dysregulation. In mammalian cells, the G1-to-S phase transition requires the formation of cyclins D and E and activation of the cyclin D-CDK4/6 and cyclin E-CDK2 complexes (32). These proteins phosphorylate and inactivate Rb to release E2F, which mediates transcriptional activity. Then, the cell cycle will enter the S phase (33). The G2-to-M phase transition requires the activation of the cyclin B-CDK1 complex *via* the dephosphorylation of CDK1 (34). CDK2 promotes S phase initiation *via* the formation of functional cyclin A and cyclin E complexes (35). Upregulation of CDK2 expression can

be found in various solid tumors and is closely related to the development of tumors (36). In the present study, TSPAN7 was found to have a close relationship with CDK2, which binds to cyclin E to initiate the G1-to-S phase transition. This is accord with other studies (37, 38).

Phosphatase and tensin homolog (PTEN) is a tumor suppressor gene that was discovered in 1997 (39). It has been proven that the protein encoded by PTEN has protein phosphatase and lipid phosphatase activities, which can regulate a complex network dependent on phosphatase or nonphosphatase activity to affect cell biological functions (40–42). The frequent loss of heterozygosity, the inverse correlation between PTEN dose and tumorigenicity and the variety of PTEN regulatory mechanisms suggest that altering PTEN levels in cells may affect tumor progression, including that of thyroid, breast, and prostate cancer (41, 43–46). PTEN antagonizes growth factor-stimulated PI3K/AKT signaling by converting PIP3 to PIP2. PTEN dephosphorylates phosphatidylinositol 3,4,5-triphosphate (PIP3) and attenuates the activity of class I phosphatidylinositol 3-kinase (PI3K), which mediates survival factor signaling through PI3K effectors, such as AKT and mTOR (47). A previous study also indicated that PTEN is a tumor suppressor in the progression of cancers that functions by negatively regulating the PI3K/AKT signaling pathway (48). It has also been reported that, the activation of PI3K/AKT signaling, as a significant cancer-promoting pathway, blocks cellular apoptosis and accelerates cell proliferation *via* the activation of PTEN (49). Our present study was in accordance with the results of the aforementioned studies. We found elevated expression levels of PTEN and cleaved Caspase-3 but reduced expression levels of p-PI3K and p-AKT in the pcDNA-TSPAN7 group compared to the control group.

Finally, we established a xenograft tumor model using nude mice and demonstrated that TSPAN7 inhibited tumorigenesis *in vivo*.

In conclusion, we have shown, for the first time, the tumor-inhibiting effects of TSPAN7 on human BCa. TSPAN7 acts as a biomarker to predict the survival of BCa patients and the malignancy of tumors. TSPAN7 could be an oncogene that promotes apoptosis and inhibits tumor growth and cell cycle progression in BCa *via* the regulation of multiple key components of the PTEN/PI3K/AKT pathway. Specifically, it would be worthwhile to investigate whether restoring TSPAN7 expression can be a novel therapeutic strategy for BCa.

## AUTHOR CONTRIBUTIONS

XL and LW conceptualized the study. SL contributed to the data curation. MP conducted the formal analysis. XY, TX, and LW investigated the study. YD contributed to the methodology. KY and SZ conducted the project administration. TB and JH conducted the visualization. XY wrote the original draft. XY and SL wrote, reviewed, and edited the manuscript. All authors contributed to the article and approved the submitted version.

## REFERENCES

1. Siegel RL, Miller KD, Jemal A. Cancer statistics, 2020. *CA Cancer J Clin* (2020) 70(1):7–30. doi: 10.3322/caac.21590
2. Chen X, Zhang JX, Luo JH, Wu S, Yuan GJ, Ma NF, et al. CSTF2-Induced Shortening of the RAC1 3'UTR Promotes the Pathogenesis of Urothelial Carcinoma of the Bladder. *Cancer Res* (2018) 78(20):5848–62. doi: 10.1158/0008-5472.CAN-18-0822
3. Avritscher EB, Cooksley CD, Grossman HB, Sabichi AL, Hamblin L, Dinney CP, et al. Clinical model of lifetime cost of treating bladder cancer and associated complications. *Urology* (2006) 68(3):549–53. doi: 10.1016/j.urology.2006.03.062
4. Boucheix C, Rubinstein E. Tetraspanins. *Cell Mol Life Sci* (2001) 58(9):1189–205. doi: 10.1007/PL00000933
5. Ji G, Liang H, Wang F, Wang N, Fu S, Cui X. TSPAN12 Precedes Tumor Proliferation by Cell Cycle Control in Ovarian Cancer. *Mol Cells* (2019) 42 (7):557–67. doi: 10.14348/molcells.2019.0015
6. Boucheix C, Duc GH, Jasmin C, Rubinstein E. Tetraspanins and malignancy. *Expert Rev Mol Med* (2001) 2001:1–17. doi: 10.1017/S1462399401002381
7. Takagi S, Fujikawa K, Imai T, Fukuhara N, Fukudome K, Minegishi M, et al. Identification of a highly specific surface marker of T-cell acute lymphoblastic leukemia and neuroblastoma as a new member of the transmembrane 4 superfamily. *Int J Cancer* (1995) 61(5):706–15. doi: 10.1002/ijc.2910610519
8. Zemni R, Bienvenu T, Vinet MC, Sefiani A, Carrie A, Billuart P, et al. A new gene involved in X-linked mental retardation identified by analysis of an X;2 balanced translocation. *Nat Genet* (2000) 24(2):167–70. doi: 10.1038/72829
9. Hosokawa Y, Ueyama E, Morikawa Y, Maeda Y, Seto M, Senba E. Molecular cloning of a cDNA encoding mouse A15, a member of the transmembrane 4 superfamily, and its preferential expression in brain neurons. *Neurosci Res* (1999) 35(4):281–90. doi: 10.1016/s0168-0102(99)00093-0
10. Chakraborty S. In silico analysis identifies genes common between five primary gastrointestinal cancer sites with potential clinical applications. *Ann Gastroenterol* (2014) 27(3):231–6.
11. Wuttig D, Baier B, Fuessel S, Meinhardt M, Herr A, Hoefling C, et al. Gene signatures of pulmonary metastases of renal cell carcinoma reflect the disease-free interval and the number of metastases per patient. *Int J Cancer* (2009) 125 (2):474–82. doi: 10.1002/ijc.24353
12. Huang CI, Kohno N, Ogawa E, Adachi M, Taki T, Miyake M. Correlation of reduction in MRP-1/CD9 and KAI1/CD82 expression with recurrences in breast cancer patients. *Am J Pathol* (1998) 153(3):973–83. doi: 10.1016/s0002-9440(10)65639-8
13. Su JS, Arima K, Hasegawa M, Franco OE, Umeda Y, Yanagawa M, et al. Decreased expression of KAI1 metastasis suppressor gene is a recurrence predictor in primary pTa and pT1 urothelial bladder carcinoma. *Int J Urol* (2004) 11(2):74–82. doi: 10.1111/j.1442-2042.2004.00752.x

14. Sauer G, Windisch J, Kurzeder C, Heilmann V, Kreienberg R, Deissler H. Progression of cervical carcinomas is associated with down-regulation of CD9 but strong local re-expression at sites of transendothelial invasion. *Clin Cancer Res* (2003) 9(17):6426–31.
15. Cheong CM, Chow AW, Fitter S, Hewett DR, Martin SK, Williams SA, et al. Tetraspanin 7 (TSPAN7) expression is upregulated in multiple myeloma patients and inhibits myeloma tumour development in vivo. *Exp Cell Res* (2015) 332(1):24–38. doi: 10.1016/j.yexcr.2015.01.006
16. Wang X, Lin M, Zhao J, Zhu S, Xu M, Zhou X. TSPAN7 promotes the migration and proliferation of lung cancer cells via epithelial-to-mesenchymal transition. *Onco Targets Ther* (2018) 11:8815–22. doi: 10.2147/OTT.S167902
17. Xiang H, Xue W, Li Y, Zheng J, Ding C, Dou M, et al. CTRP6 attenuates renal ischemia-reperfusion injury through the activation of PI3K/Akt signaling pathway. *Clin Exp Pharmacol Physiol* (2020) 47(6):1030–40. doi: 10.1111/1440-1681.13274
18. Wang L, Yang M, Guo X, Yang Z, Liu S, Ji Y, et al. ERRalpha promotes gallbladder cancer development by enhancing the transcription of Nectin-4. *Cancer Sci* (2020) 111(5):1514–27. doi: 10.1111/cas.14344
19. Bu T, Wang C, Jin H, Meng Q, Huo X, Sun H, et al. Organic anion transporters and PI3K-AKT-mTOR pathway mediate the synergistic anticancer effect of pemetrexed and rhein. *J Cell Physiol* (2020) 235 (4):3309–19. doi: 10.1002/jcp.29218
20. Menager MM. TSPAN7, effector of actin nucleation required for dendritic cell-mediated transfer of HIV-1 to T cells. *Biochem Soc Trans* (2017) 45 (3):703–8. doi: 10.1042/BST20160439
21. Usardi A, Iyer K, Sigoillot SM, Dusonchet A, Selimi F. The immunoglobulin-like superfamily member IGSF3 is a developmentally regulated protein that controls neuronal morphogenesis. *Dev Neurobiol* (2017) 77(1):75–92. doi: 10.1002/dneu.22412
22. Krishnan NM, Dhas K, Nair J, Palve V, Bagwan J, Siddappa G, et al. A Minimal DNA Methylation Signature in Oral Tongue Squamous Cell Carcinoma Links Altered Methylation with Tumor Attributes. *Mol Cancer Res* (2016) 14(9):805–19. doi: 10.1158/1541-7786.MCR-15-0395
23. Kwon JO, Lee YD, Kim H, Kim MK, Song MK, Lee ZH, et al. Tetraspanin 7 regulates sealing zone formation and the bone-resorbing activity of osteoclasts. *Biochem Biophys Res Commun* (2016) 477(4):1078–84. doi: 10.1016/j.bbrc.2016.07.046
24. Lee SA, Suh Y, Lee S, Jeong J, Kim SJ, Kim SJ, et al. Functional expression of dopamine D2 receptor is regulated by tetraspanin 7-mediated postendocytic trafficking. *FASEB J* (2017) 31(6):2301–13. doi: 10.1096/fj.201600755RR
25. Wuttig D, Zastrow S, Fussel S, Toma MI, Meinhardt M, Kalman K, et al. CD31, EDNRB and TSPAN7 are promising prognostic markers in clear-cell renal cell carcinoma revealed by genome-wide expression analyses of primary tumors and metastases. *Int J Cancer* (2012) 131(5):E693–704. doi: 10.1002/ijc.27419

26. Green DR, Kroemer G. The pathophysiology of mitochondrial cell death. *Science* (2004) 305(5684):626–9. doi: 10.1126/science.1099320

27. Giam M, Huang DC, Bouillet P. BH3-only proteins and their roles in programmed cell death. *Oncogene* (2008) 27 Suppl 1:S128–36. doi: 10.1038/onc.2009.50

28. Adams JM, Cory S. The Bcl-2 apoptotic switch in cancer development and therapy. *Oncogene* (2007) 26(9):1324–37. doi: 10.1038/sj.onc.1210220

29. Danial NN, Korsmeyer SJ. Cell death: critical control points. *Cell* (2004) 116 (2):205–19. doi: 10.1016/s0092-8674(04)00046-7

30. Pistritto G, Trisciuoglio D, Ceci C, Garufi A, D'Orazi G. Apoptosis as anticancer mechanism: function and dysfunction of its modulators and targeted therapeutic strategies. *Aging (Albany NY)* (2016) 8(4):603–19. doi: 10.18632/aging.100934

31. Kuribayashi K, Mayes PA, El-Deiry WS. What are caspases 3 and 7 doing upstream of the mitochondria? *Cancer Biol Ther* (2006) 5(7):763–5. doi: 10.4161/cbt.5.7.3228

32. Ciemerych MA, Sicinski P. Cell cycle in mouse development. *Oncogene* (2005) 24(17):2877–98. doi: 10.1038/sj.onc.1208608

33. Leone G, DeGregori J, Jakoi L, Cook JG, Nevins JR. Collaborative role of E2F transcriptional activity and G1 cyclindependent kinase activity in the induction of S phase. *Proc Natl Acad Sci U S A* (1999) 96(12):6626–31. doi: 10.1073/pnas.96.12.6626

34. Seki A, Coppinger JA, Jang CY, Yates JR, Fang G. Bora and the kinase Aurora a cooperatively activate the kinase Plk1 and control mitotic entry. *Science* (2008) 320(5883):1655–8. doi: 10.1126/science.1157425

35. Huang Z, Wang L, Chen L, Zhang Y, Shi P. Induction of cell cycle arrest via the p21, p27-cyclin E,A/Cdk2 pathway in SMMC-7721 hepatoma cells by clioquinol. *Acta Pharm* (2015) 65(4):463–71. doi: 10.1515/acph-2015-0034

36. Asghar U, Witkiewicz AK, Turner NC, Knudsen ES. The history and future of targeting cyclin-dependent kinases in cancer therapy. *Nat Rev Drug Discov* (2015) 14(2):130–46. doi: 10.1038/nrd4504

37. Ferguson RL, Maller JL. Centrosomal localization of cyclin E-Cdk2 is required for initiation of DNA synthesis. *Curr Biol* (2010) 20(9):856–60. doi: 10.1016/j.cub.2010.03.028

38. Chae HD, Kim J, Shin DY. NF-Y binds to both G1- and G2-specific cyclin promoters; a possible role in linking CDK2/Cyclin A to CDK1/Cyclin B. *Bmb Rep* (2011) 44(8):553–7. doi: 10.5483/bmbrep.2011.44.8.553

39. Li J, Yen C, Liaw D, Podsypanina K, Bose S, Wang SI, et al. PTEN, a putative protein tyrosine phosphatase gene mutated in human brain, breast, and prostate cancer. *Science (New York NY)* (1997) 275(5308):1943–7. doi: 10.1126/science.275.5308.1943

40. Zhang L, Liu J, Lei S, Zhang J, Zhou W, Yu H. PTEN inhibits the invasion and metastasis of gastric cancer via downregulation of FAK expression. *Cell Signal* (2014) 26(5):1011–20. doi: 10.1016/j.cellsig.2014.01.025

41. Hopkins BD, Hodakoski C, Barrows D, Mense SM, Parsons RE. PTEN function: the long and the short of it. *Trends Biochem Sci* (2014) 39(4):183–90. doi: 10.1016/j.tibs.2014.02.006

42. Filbin MG, Dabral SK, Pazyra-Murphy MF, Ramkissoon S, Kung AL, Pak E, et al. Coordinate activation of Shh and PI3K signaling in PTEN-deficient glioblastoma: new therapeutic opportunities. *Nat Med* (2013) 19(11):1518–23. doi: 10.1038/nm.3328

43. Wang L, Hao S, Zhang S, Guo L, Hu C, Zhang G, et al. PTEN/PI3K/AKT protein expression is related to clinicopathological features and prognosis in breast cancer with axillary lymph node metastases. *Hum Pathol* (2017) 61:49–57. doi: 10.1016/j.humpath.2016.07.040

44. Ramírez-Moya J, Wert-Lamas L, Santisteban P. MicroRNA-146b promotes PI3K/AKT pathway hyperactivation and thyroid cancer progression by targeting PTEN. *Oncogene* (2018) 37(25):3369–83. doi: 10.1038/s41388-017-0088-9

45. Wise HM, Hermida MA, Leslie NR. Prostate cancer, PI3K, PTEN and prognosis. *Clin Sci (Lond Engl 1979)* (2017) 131(3):197–210. doi: 10.1042/CS20160026

46. Wang X, Jiang X. Post-translational regulation of PTEN. *Oncogene* (2008) 27 (41):5454–63. doi: 10.1038/onc.2008.242

47. Engelman JA, Luo J, Cantley LC. The evolution of phosphatidylinositol 3-kinases as regulators of growth and metabolism. *Nat Rev Genet* (2006) 7 (8):606–19. doi: 10.1038/nrg1879

48. Wang F, Li L, Chen Z, Zhu M, Gu Y. MicroRNA-214 acts as a potential oncogene in breast cancer by targeting the PTEN-PI3K/Akt signaling pathway. *Int J Mol Med* (2016) 37(5):1421–8. doi: 10.3892/ijmm.2016.2518

49. Gallardo A, Lerma E, Escuin D, Tibau A, Muñoz J, Ojeda B, et al. Increased signalling of EGFR and IGF1R, and deregulation of PTEN/PI3K/Akt pathway are related with trastuzumab resistance in HER2 breast carcinomas. *Br J Cancer* (2012) 106(8):1367–73. doi: 10.1038/bjc.2012.85

# 6

# Integrative Analysis of Methylation and Copy Number Variations of Prostate Adenocarcinoma Based on Weighted Gene Co-Expression Network Analysis

Yaxin Hou [1,2†], Junyi Hu [1,2†], Lijie Zhou [1,2], Lilong Liu [1,2], Ke Chen [1,2*] and Xiong Yang [1*]

[1] Department of Urology, Union Hospital, Tongji Medical College, Huazhong University of Science and Technology, Wuhan, China, [2] Shenzhen Huazhong University of Science and Technology Research Institute, Shenzhen, China

*Correspondence:
Ke Chen
shenke@hust.edu.cn
Xiong Yang
yangxiong1368@hust.edu.cn

†These authors have contributed equally to this work

Prostate adenocarcinoma (PRAD) is the most pervasive carcinoma diagnosed in men with over 170,000 new cases every year in the United States and is the second leading cause of death from cancer in men despite its indolent clinical course. Prostate-specific antigen testing, which is the most commonly used non-invasive diagnostic method for PRAD, has improved early detection rates in the past decade, but its effectiveness for monitoring disease progression and predicting prognosis is controversial. To identify novel biomarkers for these purposes, we carried out weighted gene co-expression network analysis of the top 10,000 variant genes in PRAD from The Cancer Genome Atlas in order to identify gene modules associated with clinical outcomes. Methylation and copy number variation analysis were performed to screen aberrantly expressed genes, and the Kaplan–Meier survival and gene set enrichment analyses were conducted to evaluate the prognostic value and potential mechanisms of the identified genes. Cyclin E2 (CCNE2), rhophilin Rho GTPase-binding protein (RHPN1), enhancer of zeste homolog 2 (EZH2), tonsoku-like DNA repair protein (TONSL), epoxide hydrolase 2 (EPHX2), fibromodulin (FMOD), and solute carrier family 7 member (SLC7A4) were identified as potential prognostic indicators and possible therapeutic targets as well. These findings can improve diagnosis and disease monitoring to achieve better clinical outcomes in PRAD.

Keywords: bioinformatics analysis, prostate adenocarcinoma, biomarker, prognosis, therapeutic target

## INTRODUCTION

Prostate adenocarcinoma (PRAD) is one of the most common neoplasms worldwide, ranking 4th among all cancer types in both sexes with an incidence of 7.1% (1). In the United States, PRAD is the most prevalent cancer in men and is estimated to have caused more than 30,000 deaths in 2020 (1, 2).

Cancer was previously considered as a genetic disease, but there is considerable evidence that epigenetic changes contribute to tumorigenesis and tumor progression (3–5). DNA methylation is the most widely studied epigenetic modification in both non-neoplastic and neoplastic diseases including PRAD (6). The methylation of CpG islands, which are often located in the gene promoter, results in transcriptional silencing (7). Recently, methylation of enhancer regions has also been shown to play an important role in regulating gene expression (8, 9). DNA methyltransferase 1 (DNMT1), DNMT3a, and DNMT3b are upregulated in PRAD tissue compared to normal benign prostatic hyperplastic tissue, and their expression is elevated in cancerous tissue with a higher Gleason score, suggesting a close association between epigenetic alterations and PRAD development and progression (10). Additionally, epigenetic marks are potential biomarkers for PRAD (11) and targets for next-generation drugs.

Copy number variations (CNVs) are the most common genetic alteration in cancers, and CNV burden is associated with the rates of recurrence and death in multiple neoplasms (12). E26 transformation-specific (*ETS*) genes, tumor protein 53 (*TP53*), phosphatase and tensin homolog (*PTEN*), and androgen receptor (*AR*) are the most frequently altered genes in primary prostate cancer, which leads to dysregulation of phosphoinositide 3-kinase (PI3K)/protein kinase B (AKT), RAS/RAF, and cell cycle

signaling pathways; moreover, alterations in *AR* and *TP53* have been linked to castration resistance (13, 14) and worse outcomes (15). Thus, CNVs have prognostic value in PRAD as they can reflect disease progression.

The development and progression of cancers involve gene–gene interactions within a gene co-expression network. In this study, we carried out weighted gene co-expression network analysis (WGCNA) (16) to identify genes associated with clinical outcomes in PRAD and can thus serve as biomarkers. We also investigated CNV and methylation status of genes in key module of the network and assessed their prognostic value for PRAD.

## MATERIALS AND METHODS
### Data Acquisition

The expression data matrix of The Cancer Genome Atlas (TCGA) PRAD database comprising 497 tumor and 52 normal tissue samples along with CNVs, DNA methylation, and clinical

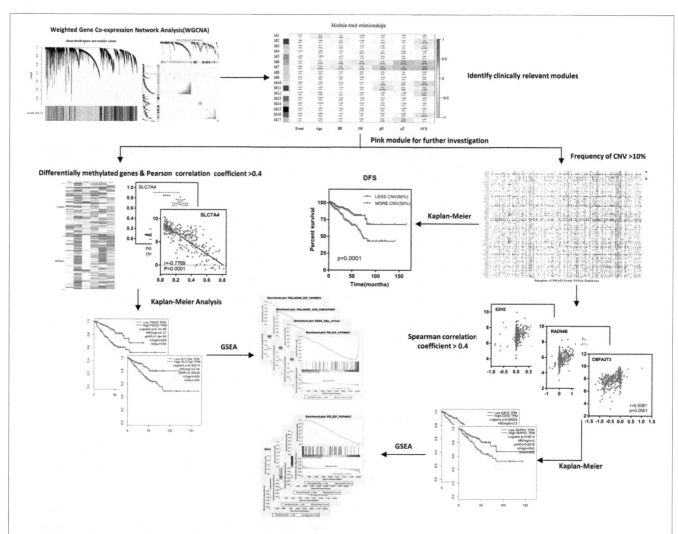

**FIGURE 1 |** Schematic diagram of the study. After identifying clinically relevant modules with WGCNA, the pink module (M7) was selected for further investigation including differentially methylated genes and frequency of CNVs, afterwards, the Kaplan–Meier survival analysis, and GSEA were used to obtain results and conclusions. WGCNA, weighted gene co-expression network analysis; DFS, disease-free survival; CNV, copy number variation; GSEA, Gene Set Enrichment Analysis.

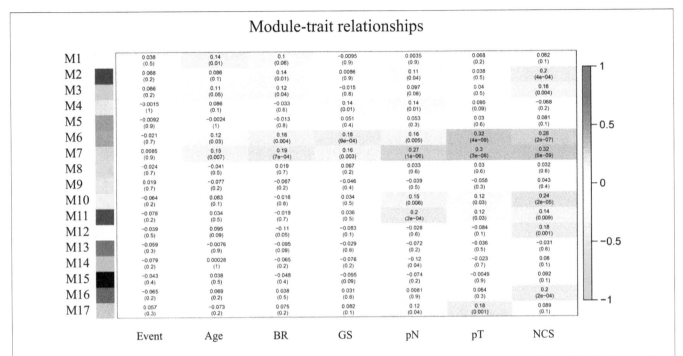

**FIGURE 2 |** Module–trait relationships. Each column corresponds to one trait, row to one module and every cell contains the correlation coefficient and *p*-value. The gray module represents genes not classified into any module. BR, biochemical recurrence. GS, Gleason score. pN, pathological N stage. pT, pathological T stage.

information was downloaded from the University of California at Santa Cruz (UCSC) Xena web server (https://xenabrowser.net/).

## Identification of Co-expression Module

Unlike ordinary clustering analysis, clustering criteria of WGCNA have biological significance, so the results obtained by this method have higher credibility. WGCNA clusters genes with similar expression patterns into a module and allows analysis of correlations between module and sample features. In this study, WGCNA was carried out to identify gene module closely related to clinical outcomes in PRAD. To minimize computational burden, the top 10,000 genes with the largest variance were selected. The topological overlap matrix (TOM) was performed to measure the correlation between genes and detection of module, which was able to identify not only the similarity of expression between gene A and gene C, but also the effect of gene A on gene C *via* gene B. A height of 220 in the sample cluster was used to detect outliers, with two outliers as filters. A power β of 8, minimal module size of 30, and branch merge cutoff height of 0.25 were used as the criteria for module construction.

## Copy Number Variation Analysis

The TCGA PRAD CNV profiles were originally measured using whole genome microarray at a TCGA genome characterization center, and GISTIC2 method was then conducted to acquire the estimated values to −2, −1, 0, 1, 2, respectively, representing homozygous deletion, single copy deletion, diploid normal copy, low-level copy number amplification, and high-level copy number amplification (17). The processed data was obtained from https://xenabrowser.net/. In addition, GISTIC2 was conducted to assess the possibility of CNV events in specific chromosomal regions. Genes with changes in frequency >10% were selected for further analysis. We calculated the Spearman correlation coefficient (*r*) between CNVs and gene expression levels, with *r* > 0.4 as the cutoff value, indicating the significant impact on gene expression of CNV.

## Methylation Analysis

The DNA methylation profiles of PRAD from TCGA were available at the University of California, Santa Cruz (UCSC) Xena browser (https://xenabrowser.net/), which were measured experimentally based on the Illumina Infinium HumanMethylation450 platform (Illumina, San Diego, CA, USA). DNA methylation values (β values, between 0 and 1) were recorded for every array probe in each sample by virtue of BeadStudio software (Illumina, San Diego, CA, USA), representing the ratio of the intensity of the methylated bead type to the combined locus intensity. The level of methylation evaluated by β values were derived from the Johns Hopkins University and University of Southern California TCGA genome characterization center.

## Gene Set Enrichment Analysis and Protein–Protein Interaction Network Analysis

Gene Set Enrichment Analysis (GSEA) (18) is a computational method used to determine whether a predefined set of genes can show significant differences between two biological

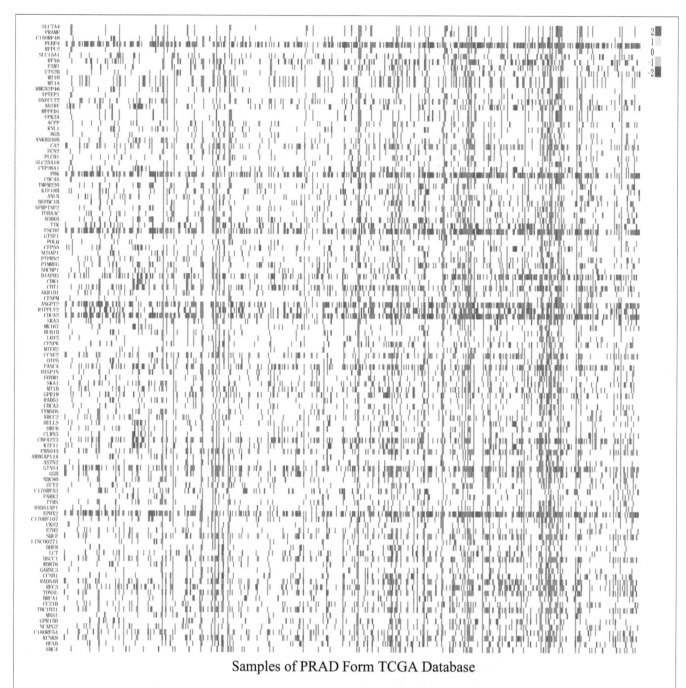

Samples of PRAD Form TCGA Database

**FIGURE 3 |** The level of gene copy number in PRAD samples. The estimated values –2, –1, 0, 1, 2, respectively representing homozygous deletion, single copy deletion, diploid normal copy, low-level copy number amplification, and high-level copy number amplification. The horizontal axis represents PRAD tumor samples in TCGA, whereas the vertical axis represents genes from M7 module with CNV > 10%.

statuses, which were performed by the GSEA software obtained from http://www.broad.mit.edu/gsea to assess the enrichment of identified genes with distinct CNVs and methylation levels in PRAD, with false discovery rate (FDR) < 25% and nominal $p$ < 0.05 as the cutoff values. Protein-protein interaction (PPI) network analysis of identified genes was completed by an online tool available at https://

string-db.org/ to assess possible interactions between their expression products.

## Survival and Statistical Analyses

The Kaplan–Meier survival analysis was performed with Prism 7.0 (GraphPad, La Jolla, CA, USA) and the online tool GEPIA (http://gepia.cancer-pku.cn/index.html) (19). Previous study by

**TABLE 1** | Gene copy number variation associated with PRAD clinicopathological staging.

| Gene | | pT | | p-value | | pN | | p-value |
|---|---|---|---|---|---|---|---|---|
| | | pT2 | pT3+pT4 | | | pN0 | pN1 | |
| **TMEM220** | | | | | | | | |
| −1 | 106 | 24 | 82 | | 96 | 71 | 25 | |
| 0 | 378 | 162 | 216 | <0.001 | 319 | 267 | 52 | 0.031 |
| **SQLE** | | | | | | | | |
| 0 | 334 | 153 | 181 | | 275 | 235 | 40 | |
| 1 | 150 | 33 | 117 | <0.001 | 140 | 103 | 37 | 0.003 |
| **RAD54B** | | | | | | | | |
| 0 | 330 | 153 | 177 | | 271 | 231 | 40 | |
| 1 | 154 | 33 | 121 | <0.001 | 144 | 107 | 37 | 0.006 |
| **HEXB** | | | | | | | | |
| −1 | 89 | 16 | 73 | | 82 | 61 | 21 | |
| 0 | 395 | 170 | 225 | <0.001 | 333 | 277 | 56 | 0.67 |
| **GINS4** | | | | | | | | |
| −1 | 160 | 47 | 113 | | 145 | 113 | 32 | |
| 0 | 324 | 139 | 185 | 0.004 | 270 | 225 | 45 | 0.177 |
| **FBXO43** | | | | | | | | |
| 0 | 325 | 152 | 173 | | 266 | 230 | 36 | |
| 1 | 159 | 34 | 125 | <0.001 | 149 | 108 | 41 | <0.001 |
| **EZH2** | | | | | | | | |
| 0 | 390 | 160 | 230 | | 332 | 270 | 62 | |
| 1 | 94 | 26 | 68 | 0.017 | 83 | 68 | 15 | 0.900 |
| **EPHX2** | | | | | | | | |
| −1 | 267 | 73 | 194 | | 235 | 184 | 51 | |
| 0 | 217 | 113 | 104 | <0.001 | 180 | 154 | 26 | 0.059 |
| **DSCC1** | | | | | | | | |
| 0 | 335 | 153 | 182 | | 276 | 235 | 41 | |
| 1 | 149 | 33 | 116 | <0.001 | 139 | 103 | 36 | 0.006 |
| **CCNE2** | | | | | | | | |
| 0 | 330 | 153 | 177 | | 271 | 232 | 39 | |
| 1 | 154 | 33 | 121 | <0.001 | 144 | 106 | 38 | 0.003 |
| **CBFA2T3** | | | | | | | | |
| −1 | 189 | 49 | 140 | | 169 | 131 | 38 | |
| 0 | 295 | 137 | 158 | <0.001 | 246 | 207 | 39 | 0.088 |
| **TBC1D31** | | | | | | | | |
| 0 | 334 | 153 | 181 | | 275 | 234 | 41 | |
| 1 | 150 | 33 | 117 | <0.001 | 140 | 104 | 36 | 0.007 |
| **TONSL** | | | | | | | | |
| 0 | 350 | 156 | 194 | | 290 | 246 | 44 | |
| 1 | 134 | 30 | 104 | <0.001 | 125 | 92 | 33 | 0.007 |
| **RHPN1** | | | | | | | | |
| 0 | 350 | 156 | 194 | | 290 | 246 | 44 | |
| 1 | 134 | 30 | 104 | <0.001 | 125 | 92 | 33 | 0.007 |

*"−1" for deletions and "1" for amplifications.*

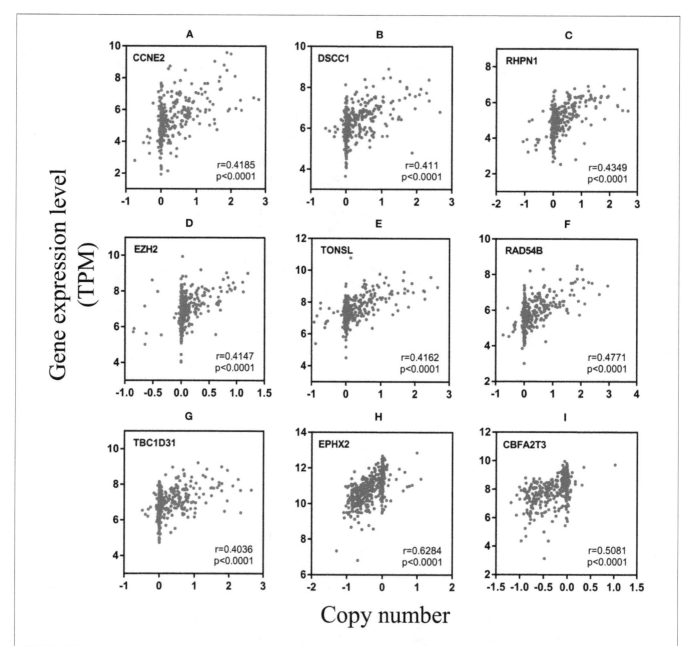

**FIGURE 4 |** The relevancy of copy number and expression level of nine genes with the Spearman correlation coefficient >0.4. **(A–G)** were mainly manifested as an increase in copy number (amplification) and positively correlated with the level of expression. **(H,I)** were mainly manifested as a loss of copy number (deletion) **(A)** CCNE2, **(B)** DSCC1, **(C)** RHPN1, **(D)** EZH2, **(E)** TONSL, **(F)** RAD54B, **(G)** TBC1D31, **(H)** EPHX2, and **(I)** CBFA2T3. TPM, transcripts per million.

Li et al. has established a prognostic model and verified with independent datasets after establishing a prognostic model (20); therefore, we downloaded the independent dataset GSE70769 (21) through the National Center for Biotechnology Information Search database (https://www.ncbi.nlm.nih.gov/) and analyzed the impact of the identified genes on the prognosis of prostate cancer patients. Multivariate analyses were carried out with the cox proportional hazards regression model. All data processing was performed using SPSS v22.0 software (SPSS Inc, Chicago, IL, USA) or R software (x64 3.5.1) (22).

The research process is illustrated in **Figure 1**.

## RESULTS

### Identification of Co-expression Module in PRAD

The top 10,000 genes with the largest variations in expression level relative to normal tissue were selected for WGCNA. We generated a module–trait association network with 7 clinicopathologic traits and 17 modules and calculated the

Pearson's correlation coefficients and *p*-values to evaluate the relationship between clinical traits and feature vectors of genes in the module. The module with highest correlation coefficient and module size >30 (pink module, M7, $p < 0.01$) was selected for further analysis (**Figure 2**).

## Copy Number Variation Analysis

After analyzing CNV profiles of TCGA PRAD data and combining the results with pink module (M7) from the WGCNA, we selected 111 genes with a variation frequency >10% and constructed a heatmap of the CN of genes in the PRAD samples (**Figure 3**), which allowed us to identify those with abnormal CN. Because our aim was to identify prognostic biomarkers for PRAD, we examined the pathologic stage associated with the CN variants. The 14 genes with the highest CNV and the corresponding clinicopathologic stage are shown in **Table 1**. Of these, nine genes with a Spearman correlation coefficient >0.4 were selected to evaluate the association between gene CN and expression level. Positive correlations were observed for the cyclin E2 (*CCNE2*), DNA replication and sister chromatid cohesion 1 (*DSCC1*), rhophilin Rho GTPase-binding protein (*RHPN1*), enhancer of zeste homolog 2 (*EZH2*), RAD54B, TBC1 domain family member 31 (*TBC1D31*), and tonsoku-like DNA repair protein (*TONSL*) genes ($p < 0.0001$), indicating the amplifications of CN events probably correlated with higher gene expression level. However, epoxide hydrolase 2 (*EPHX2*) and CBFA2/RUNX1 partner transcriptional co-repressor 3 (*CBFA2T3*) primarily showed deletions of CN events, which leading to the lower level of gene expression (**Figure 4**). To macro-evaluate the possibility of CNV events in specific chromosomal regions, the deletion and amplification plots based on G scores for CNV were demonstrated in **Supplementary Figure 2**. The higher G score of a region represents for the greater probability of CNV events in that region.

## The Kaplan–Meier Survival Analysis

We performed the Kaplan–Meier analysis to evaluate the relationship between CNV and disease-free survival (DFS). The survival curve indicated that CNV level was significantly associated with the prognosis of patients with PRAD, with lower CNV predicting longer DFS ($p = 0.0001$; **Figure 5**). We analyzed the relationship between CNV of the nine above-mentioned genes and patient prognosis and found that lower CNs of *CCNE2* [hazard ratio (HR) = 1.6; $p < 0.05$], *RHPN1* (HR = 2; $p < 0.05$), *EZH2* (HR = 2.2; $p < 0.001$), and *TONSL* (HR = 1.7; $p < 0.05$) were associated with better prognosis, whereas the opposite was true for *EPHX2* (HR = 0.47; $p < 0.001$) (**Figure 6**). A multivariate analysis of *CBFA2T3* CN suggested that it may be a protective factor in PRAD, whereas the Kaplan–Meier survival analysis suggested it was not statistically significant in the prognosis of patients with PRAD (**Figure 6I** and **Table 2**). The validation of identified biomarkers for prognosis value revealed the similar results as our former analysis, indicating the explicit prognostic significance of *CCNE2*, *SLC7A4*, *EZH2*, etc. (**Supplementary Figures 1B–H**).

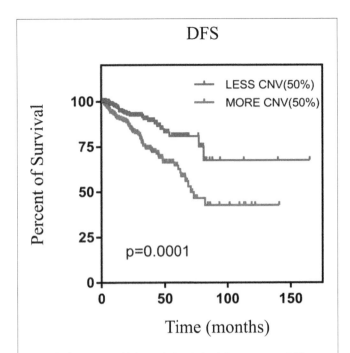

**FIGURE 5 |** The Kaplan–Meier survival analysis of nine genes. $p < 0.05$ was considered statistically different. DFS, disease-free survival; CNV, copy number variation.

## Gene Set Enrichment Analysis and PPI Network Analysis

To identify enriched gene sets in PRAD samples with high CNV and clarify the mechanisms of CNV in tumorigenesis, we performed GSEA to identify relevant biological pathways in the Kyoto Encyclopedia of Genes and Genomes (KEGG) database and Pathway Interaction Database (PID) using FDR < 25% and $p < 0.05$ as the criteria for significance. For *EZH2*, *TONSL*, and *CCNE2*, the GSEA curves revealed four enriched gene sets including "KEGG–cell cycle," "KEGG–P53 signaling pathway," "PID–ataxia–telangiectasia mutated (ATM) pathway," and "PID–E2F pathway," which are mainly related to cell cycle regulation, cell apoptosis, and DNA damage repair. Additionally, for *EPHX2*, two functional gene sets were enriched—namely, "Cell cycle pathway" and "PID–E2F pathway" (**Figure 7**). The PPI network analysis found that there was a co-expression between EZH2 and CCNE2, both of which play important roles in regulating cell cycle (**Supplementary Figure 1A**).

## Methylation Analysis

After establishing the co-expression module, the DNA methylation level of the genes was examined, and its correlation with gene expression level was evaluated with the Pearson's correlation coefficient. Differentially methylated genes with the Pearson's correlation coefficient >0.4 were identified, including fibromodulin (*FMOD*), transmembrane protein 220 (*TMEM220*), histone H2B type 1-H (*HIST1H2BH*), zinc finger 334 (*ZNF334*), RIC3 acetylcholine receptor chaperone (*RIC3*), and solute carrier family 7 member (*SLC7A4*); these genes were

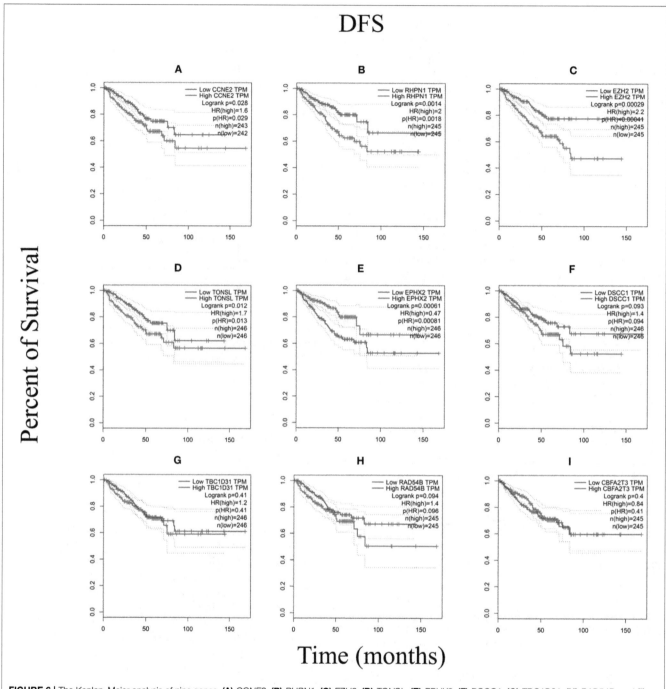

**FIGURE 6 |** The Kaplan–Meier analysis of nine genes. **(A)** *CCNE2*, **(B)** *RHPN1*, **(C)** *EZH2*, **(D)** *TONSL*, **(E)** *EPHX2*, **(F)** *DSCC1*, **(G)** *TBC1D31*, **(H)** *RAD54B*, and **(I)** *CBFA2T3*. $p < 0.05$ was considered statistically different. DFS, disease-free survival.

all hypermethylated in tumor samples ($n = 336$) compared to normal tissue ($n = 49$) (**Figures 8A, 9A**). There was a moderate inverse correlation between gene expression and methylation levels ($r > 0.4$, $p < 0.001$; **Figure 8B**).

The heatmap of DNA methylation revealed significantly higher levels in tumor tissue compared to normal tissue, especially for *SLC7A4*. The Kaplan–Meier survival curves showed an association between gene expression level and the prognosis of PRAD for *FMOD* [HR (high) = 0.37;

$p < 0.001$] and *SLC7A4* [HR (high) = 0.44; $p < 0.001$], with a higher level corresponding to better prognosis (**Figures 9B,E**), while others were not statistically significant (**Figures 9C,D,F,G**). The GSEA curves revealed four gene sets that were enriched, including "KEGG–cell cycle," "PID–E2F pathway," "Hallmark–E2F target," and "Hallmark–G2M checkpoint" (**Figures 9H–K**). These results indicate that *FMOD* and *SLC7A4* are significant genes related to the clinical outcome of PRAD.

## DISCUSSION

The number of new cases of PRAD in the United States has shown an increasing trend in the last 3 years, and PRAD is the second leading cause of death in men despite improvements in diagnostic methods and treatments (2, 23). Although magnetic resonance imaging and some biomarkers are used for the diagnosis of PRAD, the standard approach is tissue biopsy (24), which may only be performed at later stages of the disease when therapeutic options are limited.

Copy number variations occur in 4.8–9.5% of the human genome and play a critical role in tumor recurrence (25); and epigenetic modifications such as DNA methylation are potential biomarkers and targets for treatment in cancer (11). Given the increasing rates of PRAD, there is a need for new diagnostic and prognostic biomarkers with high specificity and sensitivity. In this study, we identified five novel genes with high CNV in PRAD by WGCNA (*CCNE2*, *RHPN1*, *EZH2*, *TONSL*, and *EPHX2*) along with two hypermethylated genes (*FMOD* and *SLC7A4*) that were significantly correlated with the prognosis of patients with PRAD and may thus be clinically useful biomarkers.

Cyclin E2 encodes cyclin E2, a regulatory subunit of cyclin-dependent kinase 2 (CDK2), which controls cell cycle entry from quiescence. Although the gene encoding the other subunit

**TABLE 2 |** Multivariate analysis of CBFA2T3 CNV and patient survival.

| Variable | Multivariate analysis | | |
|---|---|---|---|
| | HR | 95% CI | *p*-value |
| T stage (≥T3) | 2.361 | 1.175–4.743 | 0.016 |
| N stage | 1.363 | 0.494–3.726 | 0.557 |
| M stage | 1.254 | 0.713–2.196 | 0.457 |
| Gleason score (≥8) | 3.172 | 1.529–6.578 | 0.002 |
| PSA (≥10) | 1.486 | 0.869–2.432 | 0.119 |
| CBFA2T3 | 0.424 | 0.218–0.824 | 0.011 |

*HR estimated from Cox proportional hazard regression model; p < 0.05 was considered statistically significant.*
*DFS, disease-free survival; HR, hazard ratio.*

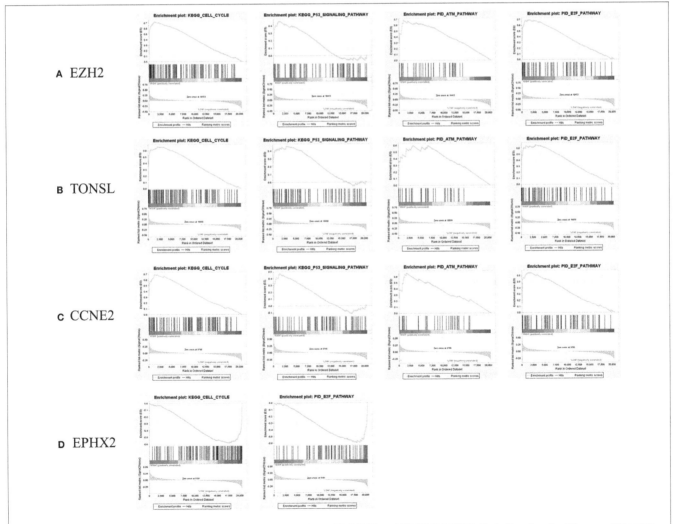

**FIGURE 7 |** Gene Set Enrichment Analysis (GSEA) curve. **(A)** *E2H2*, **(B)** *TONEL*, **(C)** *CCNE2*, and **(D)** *EPHX-2*. KEGG, Kyoto Encyclopedia of Genes and Genomes. ATM, ataxia telangiectasia-mutated.

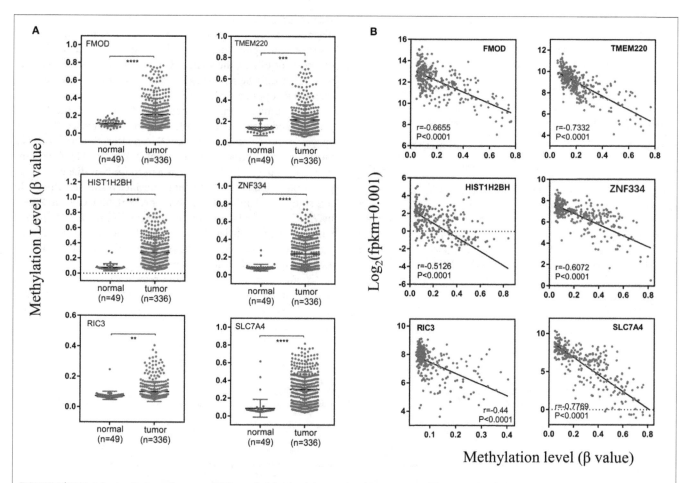

**FIGURE 8 |** Methylation levels of specific genes. **(A)** The methylation levels in normal and tumor groups, **(B)** the relationship between expression level and methylation level. The vertical axis of **(A)** and the horizontal axis of **(B)** indicate the DNA methylation level (β-value). And r represents the Pearson's correlation coefficient, the absolute value closer to 1 means the stronger the correlation. fpkm, fragments per kilobase million.

of CDK2, *CCNE1*, has been linked to poor prognosis in hepatocellular carcinoma (HCC), there is little known about the role of *CCNE2* in tumor progression (26). Cyclin E2 was shown to induce the G1-S transition in PC3 prostate cancer cells (27); our results suggest that it may have a similar function in PRAD, given that a lower *CCNE2* CN was associated with longer DFS in patients.

Rhophilin Rho GTPase-binding protein is a Rho GTPase-interacting protein that has not been previously reported in PRAD, but is known to modulate the glomerular filtration barrier and podocyte cytoskeletal architecture (28). The long non-coding RNA *RHPN1* antisense RNA 1 (RHPN1-AS1) was found to promote the progression of several tumors, including uveal melanoma, cervical cancer, and HCC (29–31). Our results provide the first demonstration that overexpression of *RHPN1* is associated with poor prognosis in PRAD.

Enhancer of zeste homolog 2, the catalytic subunit of the DNA methyltransferase polycomb repressive complex 2 (PRC2), is overexpressed in hormone-refractory metastatic PRAD and

may be correlated with disease progression and prognosis (32). Consistent with our findings, one study showed that an elevated level of *EZH2* was associated with over proliferation of tumor cells and worse prognosis and may have clinical utility for distinguishing indolent PRAD from aggressive disease with a fatal course (31). On the one hand, the utility of *EZH2* as a biomarker has been demonstrated in patients with intractable PRAD (33). On the other hand, EZH2 inhibitors have been linked to carcinogenesis and treatment resistance in clinical trials (34), though the detailed mechanisms underlying these effects remain to be determined.

Tonsoku-like DNA repair protein promotes homologous recombination during DNA repair in a complex with MMS22-like (MMS22L) (35). However, the role of TONSL in prostate cancer is unknown. We found that a high level of TONSL was associated with enrichment of genes related to the ATM and E2F pathways—which mediate DNA repair and negatively regulate the cell cycle—and decreased survival time in patients with PRAD. Thus, TONSL is a potential biomarker for the progression of PRAD.

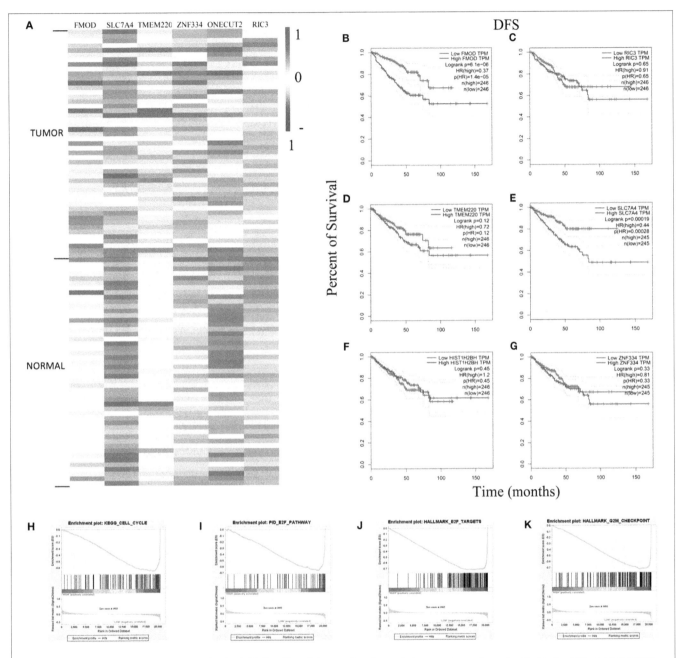

**FIGURE 9 |** Analysis of genes with high methylation level. **(A)** The differential expression of genes in tumor and normal samples. The Kaplan–Meier survival analysis curves in **(B–G)** demonstrated the relationship between DFS and expression level. **(H–K)** The GSEA curves of *FMOD* and *SLC7A4*. DFS, disease-free survival; GSEA, Gene Set Enrichment Analysis; HR, hazard ratio; TPM, transcripts per million.

Epoxide hydrolase 2 functions in arachidonic acid and androgen signaling (36–38) and has been linked to the biosynthesis and metabolism of cholesterol in the regulation of testosterone levels (39). *EPHX2* silencing induced apoptosis in PRAD cells and enhanced the antiproliferative effect of flutamide (40). In our study, decreased expression of *EPHX2* was associated with the enrichment of genes related to the cell cycle and E2F pathway while patients with an elevated level of *EPHX2* had better

prognosis, suggesting that EPHX2 has a protective role in PRAD.

Fibromodulin (encoded by *FMOD*) is thought to be involved in the inhibition of tumorigenesis and apoptosis in hematologic malignancies such as B-cell chronic lymphocytic leukemia and mantle cell lymphoma, like other proteoglycans (40). FMOD was shown to be overexpressed in PRAD cell lines and clinical specimens (41), which is supported by our findings. Our analysis revealed that higher expression of FMOD was associated with a better clinical outcome, highlighting its potential utility as a biomarker for monitoring disease progression.

Solute carrier family 7 member is a cationic amino acid transporter of unknown function; SLC7A4 expressed in the plasma membrane was insufficient to drive amino acid transport (42). Our results showed that *SLC7A4* methylation was higher in tumor specimens than in normal tissue, and that higher *SLC7A4* expression was associated with better clinical outcome. We speculate that SLC7A4 inhibits tumor formation in PRAD through regulation of the cell cycle. Thus, *SLC7A4* likely has clinical value for monitoring PRAD progression and predicting prognosis.

# CONCLUSION

In this study, we used WGCNA to identify seven genes that are potential prognostic biomarkers for PRAD based on CNV (*CCNE2*, *RHPN1*, *EZH2*, *TONSL*, and *EPHX2*) and DNA hypermethylation (*FMOD* and *SLC7A4*), all of which can serve as indicators of PRAD progression and potential therapeutic targets for the PRAD treatment as well. However, further experiments are needed to elucidate the precise roles and mechanisms

of these candidate biomarkers in PRAD and validate their clinical applicability.

# AUTHOR CONTRIBUTIONS

XY and KC: conception, design of study, and revising the manuscript. YH: drafting the manuscript. JH and LZ: analysis and interpretation of data. YH and LL: acquisition of data. All authors contributed to the article and approved the submitted version.

# SUPPLEMENTARY MATERIAL

**Supplementary Figure 1** | Protein–protein interaction (PPI) and validation of prognosis for identified biomarkers. **(A)** A co-expression between enhancer of zeste homolog 2 (EZH2) and Cyclin E2 (CCNE2), both of which play important roles in regulating cell cycle. **(B–H)** The prognostic value of identified genes in independent dataset GSE70769.

**Supplementary Figure 2** | The copy number variation (CNV) events in specific chromosomal regions. The higher G score represents for the greater probability of CNV events in that region. The previously identified genes were marked in the figure (*EZH2*: 7q36.1; *CCNE2*: 8q22.1; *RHPN1*: 8q24.3; *TONSL*: 8q24.3; *EPHX2*: 8p21.2-p21.1).

# REFERENCES

1. Bray F, Ferlay J, Soerjomataram I, Siegel RL, Torre LA, Jemal A. Global cancer statistics 2018: GLOBOCAN estimates of incidence and mortality worldwide for 36 cancers in 185 countries. *CA Cancer J Clin.* (2018) 68:394–424. doi: 10.3322/caac.21492
2. Siegel RL, Miller KD, Jemal A. Cancer statistics, (2020). *CA Cancer J Clin.* (2020) 70:7–30. doi: 10.3322/caac.21590
3. Jones PA, Baylin SB. The fundamental role of epigenetic events in cancer. *Nat Rev Genet.* (2002) 3:415–28. doi: 10.1038/nrg816
4. Berger SL, Kouzarides T, Shiekhattar R, Shilatifard A. An operational definition of epigenetics. *Genes Dev.* (2009) 23:781–3. doi: 10.1101/gad.1787609
5. Jones PA, Baylin SB. The epigenomics of cancer. *Cell.* (2007) 128:683–92. doi: 10.1016/j.cell.2007.01.029
6. Keil KP, Vezina CM. DNA methylation as a dynamic regulator of development and disease processes: spotlight on the prostate. *Epigenomics.* (2015) 7:413–25. doi: 10.2217/epi.15.8
7. Bogdanović O, Veenstra GJ. DNA methylation and methyl-CpG binding proteins: developmental requirements and function. *Chromosoma.* (2009) 118:549–65. doi: 10.1007/s00412-009-0221-9
8. King AD, Huang K, Rubbi L, Liu S, Wang CY, Wang Y, et al. Reversible regulation of promoter and enhancer histone landscape by DNA methylation in mouse embryonic stem cells. *Cell Rep.* (2016) 17:289–302. doi: 10.1016/j.celrep.2016.08.083
9. Benetatos L, Vartholomatos G. Enhancer DNA methylation in acute myeloid leukemia and myelodysplastic syndromes. *Cell Mol Life Sci.* (2018) 75:1999–2009. doi: 10.1007/s00018-018-2783-2
10. Gravina GL, Ranieri G, Muzi P, Marampon F, Mancini A, Di Pasquale B, et al. Increased levels of DNA methyltransferases are associated with the tumorigenic capacity of prostate cancer cells. *Oncol Rep.* (2013) 29:1189–95. doi: 10.3892/or.2012.2192
11. Valdés-Mora F, Clark SJ. Prostate cancer epigenetic biomarkers: next-generation technologies. *Oncogene.* (2015) 34:1609–18. doi: 10.1038/onc.2014.111
12. Hieronymus H, Murali R, Tin A, Yadav K, Abida W, Moller H, et al. Tumor copy number alteration burden is a pan-cancer prognostic factor associated with recurrence and death. *Elife.* (2018) 7:e37294. doi: 10.7554/eLife.37294.027

13. Robinson D, Van Allen EM, Wu YM, Schultz N, Lonigro RJ, Mosquera JM, et al. Integrative clinical genomics of advanced prostate cancer. *Cell.* (2015) 161:1215–28. doi: 10.1016/j.cell.2015.05.001
14. Taylor BS, Schultz N, Hieronymus H, Gopalan A, Xiao Y, Carver BS, et al. Integrative genomic profiling of human prostate cancer. *Cancer Cell.* (2010) 18:11–22. doi: 10.1016/j.ccr.2010.05.026
15. Hamid AA, Gray KP, Shaw G, MacConaill LE, Evan C, Bernard B, et al. Compound genomic alterations of TP53, PTEN, and RB1 tumor suppressors in localized and metastatic prostate cancer. *Eur Urol.* (2019) 76:89–97. doi: 10.1016/j.eururo.2018.11.045
16. Langfelder P, Horvath S. WGCNA: an R package for weighted correlation network analysis. *BMC Bioinform.* (2008) 9:559. doi: 10.1186/1471-2105-9-559
17. Mermel CH, Schumacher SE, Hill B, Meyerson ML, Beroukhim R, Getz G. GISTIC2.0 facilitates sensitive and confident localization of the targets of focal somatic copy-number alteration in human cancers. *Genome Biol.* (2011) 12:R41. doi: 10.1186/gb-2011-12-4-r41
18. Subramanian A, Kuehn H, Gould J, Tamayo P, Mesirov JP. GSEA-P: a desktop application for gene set enrichment analysis. *Bioinformatics.* (2007) 23:3251–3. doi: 10.1093/bioinformatics/btm369
19. Tang Z, Li C, Kang B, Gao G, Li C, Zhang Z. GEPIA: a web server for cancer and normal gene expression profiling and interactive analyses. *Nucleic Acids Res.* (2017) 45:W98–102. doi: 10.1093/nar/gkx247
20. Li R, Wang S, Cui Y, Qu H, Chater JM, Zhang L, et al. Extended application of genomic selection to screen multiomics data for prognostic signatures of prostate cancer. *Brief Bioinform.* (2020) bbaa197. doi: 10.1093/bib/bbaa197
21. Ross-Adams H, Lamb AD, Dunning MJ, Halim S, Lindberg J, Massie CM, et al. Integration of copy number and transcriptomics provides risk stratification in prostate cancer: A discovery and validation cohort study. *EBioMedicine.* (2015) 2:1133-44. doi: 10.1016/j.ebiom.2015.07.017
22. R Core Team. *R: A Language and Environment for Statistical Computing.* Vienna: R Foundation for Statistical Computing (2013).
23. Siegel RL, Miller KD, Jemal A. Cancer statistics, 2019. *CA Cancer J Clin.* (2019) 69:7–34. doi: 10.3322/caac.21551
24. Litwin MS, Tan HJ. The diagnosis and treatment of prostate cancer: a review. *JAMA.* (2017) 317:2532–42. doi: 10.1001/jama.2017.7248
25. Zarrei M, MacDonald JR, Merico D, Scherer SW. A copy number variation map of the human genome. *Nat Rev Genet.* (2015) 16:172–83. doi: 10.1038/nrg3871

26. Sonntag R, Giebeler N, Nevzorova YA, Bangen JM, Fahrenkamp D, Lambertz D, et al. Cyclin E1 and cyclin-dependent kinase 2 are critical for initiation, but not for progression of hepatocellular carcinoma. *Proc Natl Acad Sci USA.* (2018) 115:9282–7. doi: 10.1073/pnas.1807155115

27. Ye P, Shen L, Jiang W, Ye Y, Chen CT, Wu X, et al. Zn-driven discovery of a hydrothermal vent fungal metabolite clavatustide C, and an experimental study of the anti-cancer mechanism of clavatustide B. *Mar Drugs.* (2014) 12:3203–17. doi: 10.3390/md12063203

28. Lal MA, Andersson AC, Katayama K, Xiao Z, Nukui M, Hultenby K, et al. Rhophilin-1 is a key regulator of the podocyte cytoskeleton and is essential for glomerular filtration. *J Am Soc Nephrol.* (2015) 26:647–62. doi: 10.1681/ASN.2013111195

29. Lu L, Yu X, Zhang L, Ding X, Pan H, Wen X, et al. The long non-coding RNA RHPN1-AS1 promotes Uveal melanoma progression. *Int J Mol Sci.* (2017) 18:226. doi: 10.3390/ijms18010226

30. Duan H, Li X, Chen Y, Wang Y, Li Z. LncRNA RHPN1-AS1 promoted cell proliferation, invasion and migration in cervical cancer via the modulation of miR-299-3p/FGF2 axis. *Life Sci.* (2019) 239:116856. doi: 10.1016/j.lfs.2019.116856

31. Fen H, Hongmin Z, Wei W, Chao Y, Yang Y, Bei L, et al. RHPN1-AS1 drives the progression of hepatocellular carcinoma via regulating miR-596/IGF2BP2 axis. *Curr Pharm Des.* (2020) 25:4630–40. doi: 10.2174/1381612825666191105104549

32. Varambally S, Dhanasekaran SM, Zhou M, Barrette TR, Kumar-Sinha C, Sanda MG, et al. The polycomb group protein EZH2 is involved in progression of prostate cancer. *Nature.* (2002) 419:624–9. doi: 10.1038/nature01075

33. Xu K, Wu ZJ, Groner AC, He HH, Cai C, Lis RT, et al. EZH2 oncogenic activity in castration-resistant prostate cancer cells is Polycomb-independent. *Science.* (2012) 338:1465–9. doi: 10.1126/science.1227604

34. Comet I, Riising EM, Leblanc B, Helin K. Maintaining cell identity: PRC2-mediated regulation of transcription and cancer. *Nat Rev Cancer.* (2016) 16:803–10. doi: 10.1038/nrc.2016.83

35. Duro E, Lundin C, Ask K, Sanchez-Pulido L, MacArtney TJ, Toth R, et al. Identification of the MMS22L-TONSL complex that promotes homologous recombination. *Mol Cell.* (2010) 40:632–44. doi: 10.1016/j.molcel.2010.10.023

36. Newman JW, Morisseau C, Harris TR, Hammock BD. The soluble epoxide hydrolase encoded by EPXH2 is a bifunctional enzyme with novel lipid phosphate phosphatase activity. *Proc Natl Acad Sci USA.* (2003) 100:1558–63. doi: 10.1073/pnas.0437724100

37. Pinot F, Grant DF, Spearow JL, Parker AG, Hammock BD. Differential regulation of soluble epoxide hydrolase by clofibrate and sexual hormones in the liver and kidneys of mice. *Biochem Pharmacol.* (1995) 50:501–8. doi: 10.1016/0006-2952(95)00167-X

38. Tong M, Tai HH. Induction of NAD(+)-linked 15-hydroxyprostaglandin dehydrogenase expression by androgens in human prostate cancer cells. *Biochem Biophys Res Commun.* (2000) 276:77–81. doi: 10.1006/bbrc.2000.3437

39. Luria A, Morisseau C, Tsai HJ, Yang J, Inceoglu B, De Taeye et al. Alteration in plasma testosterone levels in male mice lacking soluble epoxide hydrolase. *Am J Physiol Endocrinol Metab.* (2009) 297:E375–83. doi: 10.1152/ajpendo.00131.2009

40. Vainio P, Gupta S, Ketola K, Mirtti T, Mpindi JP, Kohonen P, et al. Arachidonic acid pathway members PLA2G7, HPGD, EPHX2, and CYP4F8 identified as putative novel therapeutic targets in prostate cancer. *Am J Pathol.* (2011) 178:525–36. doi: 10.1016/j.ajpath.2010.10.002

41. Reyes N, Benedetti I, Bettin A, Rebollo J, Geliebter J. The small leucine rich proteoglycan fibromodulin is overexpressed in human prostate epithelial cancer cell lines in culture and human prostate cancer tissue. *Cancer Biomark.* (2016) 16:191–202. doi: 10.3233/CBM-150555

42. Wolf S, Janzen A, Vékony N, Martiné U, Strand D, Closs EI. Expression of solute carrier 7A4 (SLC7A4) in the plasma membrane is not sufficient to mediate amino acid transport activity. *Biochem J.* (2002) 364:767–75. doi: 10.1042/bj20020084

# 7

# Frontiers in Bladder Cancer Genomic Research

*Yi Li[1†], Lihui Sun[2†], Xiangyang Guo[1], Na Mo[3], Jinku Zhang[4,5*] and Chong Li[2,5,6,7*]*

[1] Department of Anesthesiology, Peking University Third Hospital, Beijing, China, [2] Core Facility for Protein Research, Institute of Biophysics, Chinese Academy of Sciences, Beijing, China, [3] Department of Pathology, Beijing Obstetrics and Gynecology Hospital, Capital Medical University, Beijing, China, [4] Department of Pathology, First Central Hospital of Baoding, Baoding, China, [5] Key Laboratory of Molecular Pathology and Early Diagnosis of Tumor in Hebei Province, First Central Hospital of Baoding, Baoding, China, [6] Department of Immunology, Beijing Jianlan Institute of Medicine, Beijing, China, [7] Department of Immunology, Beijing Zhongke Jianlan Biotechnology Co., Ltd., Beijing, China

*Correspondence:*
*Jinku Zhang*
*843561234@qq.com*
*Chong Li*
*lichong@moon.ibp.ac.cn*

[†]*These authors have contributed equally to this work*

Most of the etiology studies of bladder cancer focus on genetic changes, mainly including mutation and activation of oncogenes, mutation and inactivation of tumor suppressor genes, and rearrangement or heterozygous deletion of chromosomes. Moreover, bladder cancer is highly heterogeneous mainly due to abnormal changes in the genome and proteome of tumor cells. Surgery is the main treatment for bladder cancer, but because the recurrence rate is high after surgery and most of the muscle-invasive bladder cancer acquires distant metastasis. Therefore, there is a need to combine with chemotherapy to consolidate the treatment effect. However, there are differences in chemosensitivity among patients. In this article, we review the up-to-date genomic researches on bladder cancer occurrence, development, metastasis, and chemosensitivity in patients, in order to provide some theoretical support for the diagnosis and treatment strategy for bladder cancer.

Keywords: bladder cancer genomics, heterogeneity, epigenetics, oncogene sequencing method, precision treatment

## INTRODUCTION

Bladder cancer is the ninth most common malignant disease worldwide, with 549,393 new cases reported in 2018, and it ranks fourteenth in cancer mortality worldwide. Moreover, its incidence and mortality in males increased to the 6th and 9th place among cancers, respectively. Although men are more likely to develop bladder cancer, women often present with more advanced disease and have unfavorable prognosis. This disease can present as non-muscle-invasive bladder cancer (NMIBC), muscle-invasive bladder cancer (MIBC) and a metastatic form of the disease. The overall survival declines dramatically as the cancer progresses, especially when urothelial cells transition from noninvasive to invasive (1, 2). Each stage of the disease has different molecular drivers, and epigenetic dysregulation also plays an important role in the pathogenesis of bladder cancer (3). Furthermore, heterogeneity is a characteristic feature of bladder cancer, which exhibits a wide spectrum of clinical and pathologic features (4). In addition, chemotherapy is an important treatment method for bladder cancer, but chemotherapy has failed in a large proportion of patients with bladder cancer because of the gradual chemoresistance, which leads to the relapse and progression of tumors (5).

Recent advances in the next-generation sequencing technologies have significantly improved our understanding of the genomic landscape and the molecular underpinnings of bladder cancer (6).

This review will summarize the molecular mechanism of bladder cancer occurrence, development and metastasis, as well as the sensitivity towards chemotherapy in patients, in order to pave the way for diagnosis, monitoring, prognosis, and personalized care for bladder cancer. Meanwhile, the novel oncogene sequencing method and strategy will also be discussed.

## BLADDER CANCER GENOMICS

Carcinogenesis of cells is a very complicated process (7). At the genomic level, its cancerous mechanisms are mainly involved the following aspects: oncogene activation and overexpression; tumor suppressor gene mutations and deletions; loss of gene repair function; tandem duplication of nucleotide abnormalities in the genome, Microsatellite instability; dysfunction of signaling pathways; cell telomerase overexpression. In 2005, the United States launched the Oncology Genome Research Program (4), and hopes to find out all the oncogene in lung cancer, brain cancer, and ovarian cancer in the next 13 years in order to diagnose and treat these "terminally diseases". However, each tumor has its own unique genetic blueprint, even the cause of same tumor type is different between individuals. Scientists hope to use the "Tumor Genome Project" to establish global collaboration to unravel the secrets of all cancers and build a shared database. The successful implementation of this program is expected to truly benefit human health.

Bladder cancer genomics is a discipline based on the study of the bladder cancer genome to reveal the mechanism of bladder cancer development. Bladder cancer genomics can be divided into two aspects (8): to identify new mutation sites, genes and corresponding molecular signaling pathways related to bladder cancer, and to analyze the causes of tumorigenesis and development from the gene mutation spectrum.

### Bladder Cancer Genomics

Gene abnormalities can lead to cell cycle disorders, uncontrolled proliferation, and thus tumors. The genomic defects of bladder cancer are complicated, ranging from single DNA mutations to gene polymorphisms to whole or partial deletions of chromosomes.

The study has found that all human malignancies have somatic gene mutations (9). Activation of oncogenes and suppression of tumor suppressor genes are very common. Abnormal activation of oncogenes such as HER2 can facilitate tumor metastasis. Inactivation of *p53* and *p16* and other tumor suppressor genes involved in cell cycle regulation can inhibit apoptosis of tumor cells. Common mutations in bladder cancer include *TP53*, *PIK3CA*, *TSC1*, *FGFR3*, *HRAS*, and *HER2*. Moreover, common abnormal expression genes include *EGFR*, *Ki67*, *PD-L1*, *ERCC1*, and *BRCA1*. Shariat et al. found that the proportion of *p53* and *p16* abnormally expressed in bladder cancer patients were 56% and 54%, respectively. It was highly correlated with muscle-invasive bladder cancer which often indicates a poor prognosis (5). Soria et al. studied the expression of *HER2* in 354 bladder cancer patients and found

that *HER2* is highly expressed in more than 32% of patients. Higher expression of *HER2* indicates more aggressive tumor invasiveness (10). Hayashi et al. inhibited highly expressed *HER2* in bladder cancer cell lines and animal models with *HER2* inhibitor T-DM1 and found that T-DM1 has a more prominent inhibitory effect on bladder cancer cell growth than the trastuzumab. In addition, platinum-resistant bladder cancer cells with have higher levels of *HER2* expression. Interestingly, this group of cells is more sensitive to T-DM1, and cells treated with T-DM1 are more prone to apoptosis (11). The above studies indicate that the oncogene *HER2* plays an important role in the pathogenesis of bladder cancer. Inhibition of *HER2* expression and induction of apoptosis can significantly suppress the bladder cancer cell growth. *HER2* mutations are also present in bladder cancer. Tschui et al. studied both exon 19 and exon 20 of *HER2* gene in bladder cancer patients and found that mutations occur in exon 19 (12).

The cancer genome atlas (TCGA) analyzed DNA data from 131 patients with muscle-invasive bladder cancer and identified 32 mutant genes with high frequency. These mutations are mainly occurred in the cell cycle, chromatin regulation and kinase signaling pathways (13). Another comprehensive analysis of the full TCGA cohort of 412 MIBC cases was conducted in 2017. 58 significantly mutated genes (SMGs) were identified in the expanded cohort, in which 34 mutant genes were not identified in previous analysis and 7 mutant genes were identified in more than 10% of samples: *KMT2A* (11%), *SPTAN1* (12%), *ERBB2* (12%), *CREBBP* (12%), *FAT1* (12%), *ATM* (14%) and *KMT2C* (18%). Moreover, 158 genes that were epigenetically silenced were identified by analyzing DNA methylation and gene expression, for example, *SPATC1L* (silenced in 19%), nicotinate phosphoribosyltransferase (*NAPRT*) (13%), Poly(ADP-ribose) polymerase *PARP6* (26%) and latexin (*LXN*) (27%). However, the DNA hypermethylation in the promoter of other tumor suppressor genes were not found, such as *RB1*, *NF2*, *NF1*, *TSC2*, *TSC1*, *PTEN*, and *TP53* (14).

In addition to single DNA abnormality, bladder cancer genomic research also focuses on polymorphism sites. There are multiple gene polymorphisms in bladder cancer such as *ERCC1*, *XRCC1*, *GSTP1*, *CDA*, *GSTM1*, and *GSTT*. Different gene polymorphisms could predict chemotherapy sensitivity in bladder cancer. Xu et al. studied the efficacy of 41 patients at stage IV of muscle-invasive bladder cancer with different *ERCC1* genotypes after 2 to 6 cycles of platinum-based chemotherapy. The results suggest there is a discrepancy of short-term response to chemotherapy and median overall survival in patients with different ERCC1 genotype. Compared with C/T and T/T genotypes, patients with C/C genotype had a better short-term response to chemotherapy and median overall survival (15).

Studies have shown that there are changes in the PI3K, MAPK, Hedgehog, and Wnt pathways in the bladder cancer genome (16–18). Among them, the PI3K pathway is the most studied signaling pathway in bladder cancer. ERBB receptor family is the upstream promoter of the PI3K pathway. For example, ERBB1 (EGFR) can activate the PI3K pathway by activating RAS. Overexpression of EGFR, ERBB2 or ERBB3 is associated with tumor grade, stage, and prognosis in bladder cancer. Moreover, mutations in ERBB2 or ERBB3 have been found in some muscle-invasive bladder cancers (19). *PIK3CA* encodes the catalytic subunit p110α of PI3K, and its mutation occurs in 25% of non-muscle invasive bladder cancer (20). The above studies suggest that the mechanism of bladder cancer development and progression may be related to the PI3K signaling pathway.

## Genetics of Bladder Cancer Cell

Chromosomes are aggregates of genetic material, and chromosomal abnormalities are an important part of the genetic defects of bladder cancer. Based on genetic techniques such as genomic hybridization and loss of heterozygosity, it is found that bladder cancer has complex chromosome number and structural variation. Bartoletti et al. have shown that the partial or complete loss of genetic material at chromosome 9 can lead to the loss of tumor suppressor genes such as *p16* which often indicates the recurrence of low-grade bladder cancer. Abnormal numbers of chromosomes 3, 7, 13, and 17 have also occurred in bladder cancer (21). Among them, chromosome 3 polyploid and chromosome 7 aneuploidy may be related to the progression and malignancy of bladder cancer, and the aneuploidy of chromosome 17 often implies a high recurrence rate of bladder cancer (4, 22).

# HETEROGENEITY OF BLADDER CANCER GENOME

Tumor heterogeneity describes differences of genotype and phenotype between the same tumor type in different patients, and different sites in an individual, and even between the cancer cells within a tumor. For different individuals, tumor heterogeneity mainly depicts as differences in clinical characteristics such as pathological type, the degree of malignancy, invasion, and metastasis as well as gene mutation, and abnormal expression of proteins. For the same individual, tumor heterogeneity mainly exhibits as differences in gene expression profile and mutation at different sites of the same individual or between the cells of the same tumor, even between many subtypes of tumor cells in the tumor. Phenotypic and genomic (genetic) heterogeneity are two manifestations of tumor heterogeneity. Phenotypic heterogeneity is also the result of genomic heterogeneity to some extent (23). Therefore, the key to the study of tumor heterogeneity lies in genomic heterogeneity research.

According to the biological behavior of bladder cancer, it can be divided into muscle-invasive bladder cancer (MIBC) and non-muscle invasive bladder cancer (NMIBC). Studies have shown that there is a mutation of *Ha-ras/FGFR3* gene in NMIBC, and activation of the mouse *Ha-ras* gene can induce NMIBC, which is rare in MIBC. Inactivation of the *p53/Rb/PTEN* gene is more likely happen in MIBC. Activation of the *uroplakin II*-specific urothelial-specific promoter in transgenic mice demonstrated the expression of SV40T antigen in the urothelium which can

inactivate *p53* and *pRb*, thereby induces the invasion of tumor and metastasis of bladder cancer. Inactivation of *p53/Rb/PTEN* is less common in non-muscle invasive bladder cancer (24, 25). These findings suggest that the genomic heterogeneity (mutation and expression profile) between MIBC and NMIBC is likely to be significantly different in the biological behavior of the two bladder cancers.

Tumor heterogeneity can also exhibit as heterogeneity at the stage of tumor development. The infinite proliferation of cells is one of the main features of malignant tumors, and this characteristic requires *de novo* synthesis of telomeres by telomerase to prolong the loss of telomere ends in each round of DNA replication. Wu et al. performed whole genome and transcriptome sequencings of 97 bladder cancer patients and found that the telomere reverse transcriptase gene *TERT* is highly expressed in invasive and advanced bladder cancer patients as compared to the early and non-invasive bladder cancer patients. This group of patients has a higher mutation rate of the *TERT* promoter (26). This study showed a significant difference in the *TERT* promoter expression level and the mutation rate between early non-invasive and advanced invasive cancerous cells in bladder cancer.

Bladder cancer tumors have different biological characteristics of the tumor cells subsets, and there are certain differences in gene expression profiles among different cell subpopulations, which is well-described by the heterogeneity within the tumor. The most representative of intratumoral heterogeneity is the presence of a subset of tumor cells with different molecular markers in the bladder cancer. For instance, bladder cancer cells can be divided into common bladder cancer cells and bladder cancer stem cells, with a significant difference in genetic mutations at the latter. Li et al. extracted the single cell genomes of bladder cancer stem cells (BCSCs) and non-bladder cancer stem cells (non-BCSCs) for PCR amplification, and analyzed data from 20 cells. The single cell mutation rate of the *TERT* gene promoter C228T was found to be 50% higher in BCSCs and lower in non-BCSCs (27). There are two main hypotheses of the formation mechanism of malignant tumors heterogeneity in bladder cancer: clonal evolution hypothesis and cancer stem cell hypothesis (28, 29). The clonal evolution hypothesis was proposed by Nowell in 1976 which hypothesize that tumor cells originate from the first generation of single mutant cells. Thus, all tumor cell genomes are identical to the genome of the single cell, but complex factors such as mutations and environmental influences are involved in the proliferation and evolution process. Therefore, the subsequent formation of tumor cells is gradually varied in term of genotypes and phenotypes and eventually result in the tumor heterogeneity. Cancer stem cells are a research hot topic in molecular biology of tumor in recent years. The cancer stem cell hypothesis states that tumor cells are derived from cancer stem cells. Due to the multi-directional differentiation potential of tumor stem cells, various tumor cells proliferate and differentiate to produce subpopulation with different phenotypic functions and thus result in tumor heterogeneity. Kreso et al. found that the mutated genes of tumor cells in the same colorectal cancer case remained unchanged after continuous multiple implantations, but there were significant differences in phenotypes such as proliferative capacity and drug resistance (30). However, this hypothesis does not explain why there are differences in the genome of tumor cells of the same tumor type between different individuals.

Tumor heterogeneity is the result of genetic and environmental interactions. Although the current hypothesis does not completely reveal the cause of tumor heterogeneity, it offers research direction for tumor heterogeneity to some extent.

# EPIGENETIC AND BLADDER CANCER GENOME

## Telomerase Reverse Transcriptase

Telomerase is a ribonucleoprotein that is essential for the replication of most eukaryotic chromosome ends. In cancer cells, telomerase can be activated. In contrast, telomerase is epigenetically silenced and inactivated in normal cells (31). However, mutations of important genes can reverse telomerase silencings, such as tumor suppressor genes or mutations in the tumor suppressor pathway signaling molecules that may affect telomerase activity in human tumors (32). Telomerase consists of two subunits: telomerase RNA component (TERC) and telomerase reverse transcriptase tert (TERT) catalytic subunit. The TERT gene encodes a telomerase reverse transcriptase catalytic subunit and assembles into a ribonucleoprotein protease complex to maintain telomere length which plays an important role in the maintenance of tumor genome stability (33). In recent years, TERT promoter mutations have been found in malignant tumors such as melanoma (34) and glioma (35). Studies have shown that the TERT promoter mutation is highly correlated with the prognosis of transitional cell carcinoma and confirmed that the −124 C > T mutation (corresponding to C228T) is associated with high expression of TERT and telomerase activity (36).

Wu et al. found a coexistence relationship between the TERT promoter mutation point and the TC53/RB1 inert somatic mutation point. By determining the chromosomal instability index, it was found that the tumor chromosomal instability index of the TERT promoter mutation was significantly higher than that of the tumor without the TERT promoter mutation (26). TP53 is involved in the regulation of telomerase activity, maintenance of gene integrity, inert mutations, and its deletion is associated with chromosomal instability. These studies suggest that the coexistence of the two may have a synergistic effect on the chromosomal instability of bladder cancer (37).

Studies have found that the C228T mutation of the TERT promoter often occurs in BCSCs (27). Compared with non-BCSCs, C228T has a significantly higher mutation rate in BCSCs which is consistent with the phenomenon of high C228T expression in stem cells compared to normal somatic cells. Importantly, the TERT promoter C228T mutation can convert normal bladder stem cells (NBSCs) into tumor-initiating cells. This mutation is located at the promoter region and can lead to tumors formation which can be considered as tumor promoters.

It can be seen that the high mutation rate of TERT promoter in BCSCs is a new feature of bladder cancer, but the transformation of NBSCs mutation into BCSCs is complex and further research is needed.

Telomerase activity is observed in almost all human tumor types, thus monitoring the tumor's telomerase activity will greatly contribute to the diagnosis and screening of bladder cancer. Wu et al. screened for the presence of telomerase reverse transcriptase gene promoter somatic cell mutations by Sanger sequencing in 302 patients with different urological tumors. The result showed that 43% of genitourinary tumors had TERT promoter somatic mutations. This has determined high-frequency mutation hotspot of the telomerase reverse transcriptase gene promoter in clinical urogenital (26). In different types of urological organ tumors, the amplitude of somatic mutation of the TERT promoter was larger (0-63.7%). The urinary tract cancer has the highest mutation frequency among all, while the prostate cancer showed no mutation.

## Chromatin Remodeling

Chromatin remodeling is an important regulatory mechanism of epigenetics, which is characterized by changes in the nucleosome structure and its relative position to the DNA sequence, and alteration of the accessibility of gene promoter region sequences to further regulate gene expression. Chromatin remodeling works primarily through two pathways: ATP-dependent chromatin remodeling complex, the SWl/SNF complex; histone-modifying enzymes including histone methylation, acetylation, phosphorylation, and ubiquitination (38). Recent studies have found that chromatin remodeling related genes have high-frequency mutations in a variety of tumors including bladder cancer, kidney cancer, gastric cancer, ovarian clear cell carcinoma, breast cancer and glioblastoma (38). Mutations in chromatin remodeling-related genes can cause epigenetic changes in local histone modifications and chromatin conformation in cancer cells, leading to dysregulation of downstream signaling genes, changes in biological behavior such as cell proliferation and apoptosis, leading to tumor development (39).

Gui et al. performed full exon sequencing on 9 patients with transitional cell carcinoma and has found 8 frequently mutated chromatin remodeling genes in 59% of transitional cell bladder cancer: UTX, MLL-MLL3, CREBBP-EP300, NCOR1, ARID1A and CHD6 (40). UTX has a number of significantly enriched mutations including 11 nonsense mutations, 4 frameshift mutations, and 1 splice site change. One of these mutations was predicted to be able to truncate the JmjC domain, which is critical for the demethylase activity of the protein product. ARID1A has the same mutation pattern as UTX. In addition, mutations in the above genes have also been found in other malignant tumors such as ovarian cancer and renal cancer (41, 42). The study found that STAG2 is located on the X chromosome, encoding sister chromatid cohesion and segregation (SCCS) adhesion complex components, regulating the separation of sister chromosomes during cell division, and inactivation of STAG2 can cause weakening of chromosome binding and thus aneuploidy (43). Via gene sequencing and rigorous bioinformatics analysis, Guo et al. have found that

*STAG2*, *ESPL1* and *NIPBL* genes with frequent mutations in bladder cancer are involved in the SCCS process (44). The study further revealed that patients with mutant *STAG2* had a higher frequency of chromosomal aneuploidy by detecting copy number changes in the chromosome arm, and significantly worse in the prognosis of *STAG2* gene somatic cell mutation in bladder cancer patients compared with *STAG2* bladder cancer patients without the mutation. Collectively, in SCCS, other types of tumors only report rare or low-frequency mutations in oncogenes. Bladder cancer is a tumor type that is first known to have a high-frequency genetic damage gene in the SCCS process in which the genetic mutation rate is approximately 32%. The genetic changes affect the SCCS process which may involve the development of bladder cancer. Despite the detailed mechanism of *STAG2* leading to the pathogenesis of transitional cell carcinoma is still not known, the high-frequency recurrent mutant gene is indeed a new pathway associated with transitional cell carcinoma in the SCCS process of transitional cell bladder cancer (45).

## ONCOGENE SEQUENCING METHOD AND STRATEGY

The traditional sequencing method is Sanger sequencing. However, this method has the disadvantage of low sensitivity and it is difficult to obtain all genomic information, and high cost but low output which limits the application of Sanger sequencing in large-scale sequencing. High-throughput sequencing, the second-generation sequencing technology (also known as next-generation sequencing, deep sequencing) can simultaneously sequence a large number of genes, making it possible to accurately detect tumor and transcriptome abnormalities in tumor patients (46–48). This method can detect tumor genomic abnormalities including nucleotide substitution, insertion and deletion, copy number alteration and chromosome recombination, and improve the detection efficiency and resolution of the genome. As a next-generation sequencing technology, high-throughput sequencing has unparalleled advantages over the traditional sequencing methods. First, high-throughput sequencing can perform large-scale parallel sequencing of a large number of genes, resulting in a remarkable increase in gene detection efficiency. Second, high-throughput sequencing detects the number of occurrences of a certain gene in a sample can reflect the expression level of the gene to some extent. Finally, high-throughput sequencing is more economical than traditional large-scale gene sequencing.

### Whole Genome Sequencing

Whole genome sequencing is the sequencing of the entire genome of tumor tissue with the DNA sequence of the germ cells from the same patient (tumor cell mutation is not present in the germ cells) as a control can effectively identify the changes in all regions including nucleotide replacement, structural rearrangement, and copy number changes (49). Therefore, whole genome sequencing is the most comprehensive depiction

of the tumor genome, suitable for the study of tumor genome-wide association. However, whole genome sequencing requires the detection of a large number of sequences is redundant for studies that do not require the whole genome. In this case, shotgun sequencing based on the Sanger sequencing principle is more suitable for identifying somatic cell rearrangements and copy number changes in the genome.

Sanger sequencing is the gold standard for current gene sequencing. Wu et al. performed Sanger sequencing to sequence 302 different urinary tumor patients and found a high-frequency mutation hotspot of *TERT* promoter in urinary tumor patients wherein *TERT* promoter somatic mutation in 55.6% of bladder cancer (26). Guo et al. performed genome-wide sequencing of 99 tumors and corresponding peripheral blood samples from patients with transitional cell carcinoma by Sanger sequencing. SCCS-related gene mutations such as *STAG2* and *ESPL1* were confirmed from 11240 candidate somatic mutations. Moreover, mutant genes such as *FGFR3*, *TP53*, *PIK3CA*, and *RB1* are ubiquitous in malignant tumors (44). Second-generation sequencing invention has received extensive attention at the beginning compared to Sanger sequencing. Andrea et al. recruited 50 patients with muscle-invasive bladder cancer and performed whole-exome sequencing on germline and pretreatment tumor DNA. Then these patients were treated with neoadjuvant cisplatin-based chemotherapy and underwent surgery to evaluate the pathologic response. They identified *ERCC2*, one nucleotide excision repair gene, was only significantly mutated in responders compared with nonresponders (50). David et al. investigated the correlation of *ERCC2* with pathologic response to neoadjuvant cisplatin-based chemotherapy in an independent validation patient cohort, and they confirmed that *ERCC2* was indeed associated with response to chemotherapy (51). Desai et al. used the second-generation sequencing technology to map the mutations of primary and recurrent transitional cell bladder cancer. By comparing the differential expression of tumor-associated DNA damage response genes, they also found that especially *ERCC2* mutations indicate a better prognosis of chemoradiotherapy for transitional cell bladder cancer and a lower rate of recurrence and metastasis within 2 years (52).

### Exon Sequencing

Exon sequencing is a method of capturing whole genome exon DNA by using targeted sequence capture technology to enrich the construction of DNA library before performing high-throughput sequencing. It is characterized by sequencing of the open reading frame without sequencing the introns. Since exons account for only 2% of the entire genome, high-throughput sequencing of the targeted exon greatly reduces the amount of sequencing and achieves higher efficiency. Due to its deep sequencing of the coding region, it can be used to screen for mutations that Sanger sequencing could not. In addition, it is suitable for the study of single nucleotide polymorphism (SNP) and insertion-deletion (InDel) of the target gene. Longo et al. used targeted exon sequencing to detect 50 cases of patients with pTis-pT4b bladder cancer. Through the analysis of staged somatic mutations in patients with such high-risk bladder cancer, the mutated genes and mutation profiles were determined. In terms of single mutations, it was found that epigenetic and cell cycle-regulated genes have significantly higher mutation rates. PI3K/mTOR and cell cycle/DNA repair showed the highest mutation rate among the other assessed pathways. Moreover, *RB1* and *TP53* mutations were found to frequently coexist with *NF1* and *PIK3CA* mutations (53).

However, exon sequencing also has certain limitations. It is unable to sequence non-coding genes and thus fail to conduct a comprehensive study of intron-regulated genes associated with the target gene, and also impossible to identify copies.

## Single Cell Sequencing

In the past, genome sequencing was the extraction of DNA from many cells or a piece of tissue. It is inevitable that sequencing results are obtained from many cell genomes. However, tumors are heterogeneous and the genomic information of different subtypes is more or less different. Investigation of the total DNA information extracted from different cell populations will inevitably cause researchers to ignore the differences between cells to varying degrees and further bias the study of the target cell genome (54, 55). Single cell sequencing is the sequencing of genomes from a single cell. The process involves the isolation of single cells and extraction of DNA followed by single-cell genomic amplification and sequencing analysis. This will prevent the influence of other cell genomes on the sequencing results of the target cells and thus accurately measure the copy number of a single nuclear gene (56).

Bladder cancer is a solid tumor with significant heterogeneity, and the process of research needs to be careful to prevent bias resulted by other cells. In order to study *TERT* promoter mutations in the bladder cancer, Li et al. had isolated the single cells of BCSCs, non-BCSCs, NBBCs, and non-NBBCs and extracted their genomes for single-cell gene amplification and sequencing. The high-frequency mutation sites of C228T were found in the *TERT* promoters of BCSCs and non-BCSCs, and the effect of C228T mutation on bladder cancer and BCSCs was investigated (27). In order to study the genetic basis and origin of bladder cancer stem cells, Yang et al. had performed single-cell sequencing on 59 single cells including bladder cancer stem cells (BCSCs), bladder cancer non-stem cells (BCNSCs), bladder epithelial stem cells (BESCs), and normal bladder epithelial cells. It was found that BCSCs showed clonal homogeneity, and phylogenetic analysis indicated that BCSCs were derived from BESCs or BCNSCs. This study has confirmed that 21 abnormal key genes in BSCSs wherein 6 of which were not reported in bladder cancer in the past, which fully demonstrated the accuracy of single-cell sequencing (57). Faridani et al. demonstrated that microRNAs as the potential markers of different cell types and cell status by performing single-cell sequencing of the small-RNA transcriptome on human embryonic cells and tumor cells (58).

## Transcriptome Sequencing

The transcriptome sequencing is a technique to sequence the transcript RNA, which is a sequence of cDNA that is reverse transcribed from mRNA, total RNA or other RNAs (e.g., small RNAs) to obtain the sum of RNA in a state of the cell. It was found to be sensitive and effective for intron fusion including oncogene activation caused by in-frame fusion. Kekeeva et al. performed high-throughput transcriptome sequencing on bladder cancer patients and screened 4 fusion introns in bladder cancer from 819 suspected fusion introns such as *SEPT9/CYHR*, *IGF1R/TTC23*, *SYT8/TNNI2* and *CASZ1/DFFA* (59). Transcriptome sequencing can analyze gene expression profiles to reveal differentially expressed genes in tumors. Based on the transcriptome sequencing data, Zhang et al. confirmed the differential gene expressions of several bladder cancers through the comparison of bladder cancer and normal tissue transcriptome, in which *ELF3* and *MYBL2* are the tumor suppressors while *MEG3*, *APEX1*, and *EZH2* are the inducer of bladder cancer progression (60). In addition, transcriptome sequencing can also be applied to detect somatic mutations, but it is difficult to find a matching normal sample control which limits the application in this aspect. Liu et al. performed transcriptome sequencing of transitional cell carcinoma and identified 937 differentially expressed genes (61).

It is well known that miRNAs can form RNA silencing-inducing complexes to inhibit translation of target mRNAs which is an important mechanism for gene expression regulation. Studies have shown that miRNAs also play an important role in tumor pathogenesis (62). Therefore, transcriptome sequencing technology has broad application prospects in detecting the abnormal miRNA expression in tumors.

## BLADDER CANCER GENOMICS AND PRECISION TREATMENT

The traditional treatment strategy for bladder cancer is to formulate treatment plans according to grading and staging: early surgical treatment, middle and late stage surgery and perioperative radiotherapy and chemotherapy. However, the efficacy of treatment especially chemotherapy varies greatly in patients with the same type, grade, and stage of histology. It shows that there is still a considerable difference in the real situation of the patients with the same diagnosis. Since the differential sensitivity to chemotherapy in different patients, blind implementation of gold-standard chemotherapy is very likely to delay the treatment of chemotherapy-resistant patients. In response to the above problems, some researchers have proposed a strategy for precision medicine.

The essence of precise treatment of bladder cancer lies in the in-depth explanation of the molecular pathogenesis of bladder cancer. This is demonstrated on a more detailed molecular typing based on genome studies of bladder cancer. In addition, deletions of multiple tumor suppressor genes such as *CDKN2A* and *RB*, and amplification of oncogenes such as *E2F3*, *SOX4*, *EGFR*, and *CCND1* were also identified. By further analyzing the mRNA and protein expression levels of the gene, bladder cancer is classified into 4 types. Type I and type II have the characteristics of breast cancer-like cells namely in which *ERBB2* is highly expressed and estrogen receptor 2 (ESR2) pathway is activated. The difference is that type I mutations with fibroblast growth factor receptor 3 (FGFR3) and papillary histological phenotype III have similar characteristics of basal-like breast cancer cells, with the gene expression profile of squamous cells and stem cells, such as epidermal growth factor receptor (EGFR) and increased expression of keratin 5, 6A and 14 and the like. Type IV is between type II and type III (32). This gene expression-based typing provides a scientific basis for the new molecular typing of bladder cancer. However, the relationship between molecular typing and clinical efficacy and prognosis still needs further exploration.

Genomics research can explore the genes involved in disease recurrence, prognosis, and drug sensitivity to effectively predict and evaluate the efficacy of chemotherapy for bladder cancer. Choi et al. had classified bladder cancer into three types by clustering the gene expression profiles of 183 cases of bladder cancer (6). Among them, luminal- and basal-like cells are same as the type I and type III of the TCGA type. The difference is that bladder cancer caused by luminal-like cells with wild type p53 and its activation of the signaling pathway is divided into a new category, known as the p53-like type. Combined with clinical prognosis and efficacy analysis, the luminal type has the best prognosis and is sensitive to neoadjuvant chemotherapy while basal type has the worst prognosis, about 60% of patients are not sensitive to neoadjuvant chemotherapy. The prognosis of p53-like type is between the two aforementioned, but almost insensitive to neoadjuvant chemotherapy. Choi's research provides a promising reference for the development of chemotherapy for bladder cancer (63). Roland et al. used a single-sample genomic subtyping classifier (GSC) to predict four consensus subtypes: luminal, luminal-infiltrated, basal, and claudin-low. They validated the clinical impact of these consensus subtypes in independent neoadjuvant chemotherapy (NAC) and non-NAC datasets. Luminal tumors showed the best overall survival (OS) with and without NAC. Luminal-infiltrated tumors were associated with poor prognosis with and without NAC. Compared with surgery alone, basal tumors had the most improved OS with NAC. Claudin-low tumors had poor OS regardless of treatment regimen (64). Despite the current lacking of well-defined predictive genetic markers in bladder cancer, above studies provide a clear research direction for precise treatment.

In addition, bladder cancer genomics can reveal the molecular mechanisms involved in the development and progression of bladder cancer and provide new molecular targets for the treatment of bladder cancer. To date, targeted therapy has achieved outstanding results in a variety of cancer treatments, such as gefitinib targeted therapy in treating lung cancer. However, bladder cancer targeted therapy is still at the early stage of clinical research, thus targeted therapy is not the option in guideline treatment recommendations for bladder cancer. At the present, some high-frequency abnormalities of bladder cancer that have been discovered and identified by genomics may become potential therapeutic targets. This includes signaling pathways such as EGFR, P13K/mTOR, HER-2 and FGFR3. Notably, the Food and Drug Administration recently approved erdafitinib as a treatment for patients with advanced urothelial cancer (UC) with FGFR3/2

mutations, who progressed on platinum-based chemotherapy. Clinical trials showed the overall response rate of erdafitinib was 49% in patients with FGFR3 mutations (65, 66). Secondly, it is immunotherapy such as PD-1, and CTLA4. PD-1/PD-L1 immunotherapy can enhance the body's immune response to kill tumors and is effective for a variety of tumors including bladder cancer, lung cancer, stomach cancer, and kidney cancer. The US Food and Drug Administration (FDA) has approved this therapy for bladder cancer. Interestingly, bladder cancer has many tumor mutation burden (TMB). By analyzing the 443 bladder cancer samples from TCGA, single nucleotide polymorphism (SNP) and C>T were the most frequent mutation types, and significant differences in tumor immune microenvironment were observed between the low TMB group and the high TMB group, including Mast cells resting, NK cells resting, T cells CD4 memory activated and T cells CD8, which makes it sensitive to immunotherapy (67). However, some patients is resistant to PD-1/PD-L1 immunotherapy, partially because TGF-β in fibroblasts reduces anti-tumor immunity by inhibiting CD8+ T cell infiltration into the tumor parenchyma (68).Fortunately, a personalized neoantigen-based vaccine, NEO-PV-01, was designed by whole exome and RNA sequencing of each patient's formalin-fixed tumor and matched normal cells from blood, and it consisted of high-quality neoepitopes encoded by somatic mutations and selected using bioinformatics algorithms. The clinical trial showed NEO-PV-01 in combination with PD-1 blockade was a safe and effective treatment to patients with bladder cancer by inducing T cells to traffic to the tumor and mediate cell killing (69). The third is cell cycle regulatory molecules, such as Aurora kinase A and Polo-like kinase I (3). The fourth is the antibody-drug conjugate (ADC), for example, enfortumab vedotin comprises an anti nectin-4 monoclonal antibody, protease cleavable linker and monomethyl auristatin E (MMAE). Because nectin-4 is highly expressed in all metastatic UC tumors, once the bonded enfortumab vedotin is internalized, the microtubule-disrupting agent MMAE is released leading to apoptosis of the tumor cell. Clinical trials demonstrated enfortumab vedotin is a new therapeutic method in patients with platinum- and immune checkpoint inhibitor-refractory disease (70, 71).

## CONCLUSION AND PROSPECT

As shown **Table 1**, many genes are involved bladder cancer progression and metastasis, such as FGFR3, TP53, EGFR, HRAS and Ki67 (72–74), as well as HER2, TSC1, and ERCC1 which are the genes associated with bladder cancer. Among them, HER2 could be the potential therapeutic target, and ERCC1 is involved in the drug resistance of cisplatin and other chemotherapeutic drugs. Low expression of ERCC1 has a longer survival period. BRCA1 has DNA repair function and reduces the effect of chemotherapy drugs (12, 75, 76). However, the current molecular markers that predict the prognosis and chemotherapy efficacy of bladder cancer patients are still at premature stages. Genetic markers that can accurately predict the therapeutic effect of bladder cancer is yet to

**TABLE 1 |** Common gene alterations in bladder cancer.

| Gene Name | Function | Reference |
|---|---|---|
| *HER2* | Higher expression of *HER2* indicates more aggressive tumor invasiveness. | (10) |
| *ERCC1* | *ERCC1* is involved in the drug resistance of cisplatin and other chemotherapeutic drugs. Low expression of *ERCC1* has a longer survival period. | (13) |
| *EGFR,ERBB2,ERBB3* | Overexpression of *EGFR*, *ERBB2* or *ERBB3* is associated with tumor grade, stage, and prognosis in bladder cancer. | (19) |
| *PIK3CA* | Its mutation occurs in 25% of non-muscle invasive bladder cancer, associated with bladder cancer development and progression. | (20) |
| *p16* | The loss of tumor suppressor genes (*p16*) often indicates the recurrence of low-grade bladder cancer. | (21) |
| *p53,Rb,PTEN* | Inactivate *p53* and *pRb* induces the invasion of tumor and metastasis of bladder cancer. | (24, 25) |
| *TERT* | *TERT* is highly expressed in invasive and advanced bladder cancer patients as compared to the early and non-invasive bladder cancer patients. | (26) |
| *STAG2, ESPL1, NIPBL* | *STAG2, ESPL1* and *NIPBL* genes with frequent mutations in bladder cancer are involved in the sister chromatid cohesion and segregation process. | (44) |
| *ERCC2* | *ERCC2* mutations indicate a better prognosis of chemotherapy for bladder cancer and a lower rate of recurrence and metastasis within 2 years. | (50–52) |
| *ELF3, MYBL2* | Tumor suppressors. | (60) |
| *MEG3, APEX1, EZH2* | Inducer of bladder cancer progression. | (60) |
| *FGFR3* | The luminal-papillary subtype is characterized by *FGFR3* mutations, fusion with transforming acid coiled-coil containing protein 3 (*TACC3*), or amplification. | (65) |

found. In the future, intensive studies are needed to define the precise molecular characterization of bladder cancer (77). Genomics is an effective tool for studying the molecular pathology of bladder cancer. It is believed that with advances in sequencing technology, genomics may bring more help to the targeted therapy of bladder cancer (78).

# REFERENCES

1. Tran L, Xiao JF, Neeraj Agarwal N, Duex JE, Theodorescu D. Advances in Bladder Cancer Biology and Therapy. *Nat Rev Cancer* (2021) 21(2):104–21. doi: 10.1038/s41568-020-00313-1

2. Cao Y, Tian T, Li W, Xu H, Zhan C, Wu X, et al. Long non-Coding RNA in Bladder Cancer. *Clinica Chimica Acta* (2020) 503:113–21. doi: 10.1016/j.cca.2020.01.008

3. Porten SP. Epigenetic Alterations in Bladder Cancer. *Curr Urol Rep* (2018) 19 (12):102. doi: 10.1007/s11934-018-0861-5

4. Knowles MA, Hurst CD. Molecular Biology of Bladder Cancer: New Insights Into Pathogenesis and Clinical Diversity. *Nat Rev Cancer* (2015) 15(1):25–41. doi: 10.1038/nrc3817

5. Cai Z, Zhang F, Chen W, Zhang J, Li H. miRNAs: A Promising Target in the Chemoresistance of Bladder Cancer. *OncoTargets Ther* (2019) 12:11805–16. doi: 10.2147/OTT.S231489

6. Al-Ahmadie H, Netto GJ. Updates on the Genomics of Bladder Cancer and Novel Molecular Taxonomy. *Adv Anatomic Pathol* (2020) 27(1):36–43. doi: 10.1097/PAP.0000000000000252

7. Stratton MR. Exploring the Genomes of Cancer Cells: Progress and Promise. *Science* (2011) 331(6024):1553–8. doi: 10.1126/science.1204040

8. Garraway LA, Lander ES. Lessons From the Cancer Genome. *Cell* (2013) 153 (1):17–37. doi: 10.1016/j.cell.2013.03.002

9. Pleasance ED, Cheetham RK, Stephens PJ, McBride DJ, Humphray SJ, Greenman CD, et al. A Comprehensive Catalogue of Somatic Mutations From a Human Cancer Genome. *Nature* (2010) 463(7278):191–6. doi: 10.1038/nature08658

10. Soria F, Moschini M, Haitel A, Wirth GJ, Gust KM, Briganti A, et al. The Effect of HER2 Status on Oncological Outcomes of Patients With Invasive Bladder Cancer. *Urologic Oncol* (2016) 34(12):533.e531–533.e510. doi: 10.1016/j.urolonc.2016.07.006

11. Hayashi T, Seiler R, Oo HZ, Jäger W, Moskalev I, Awrey S, et al. Targeting HER2 With T-DM1, an Antibody Cytotoxic Drug Conjugate, is Effective in HER2 Over Expressing Bladder Cancer. *J Urol* (2015) 194(4):1120–31. doi: 10.1016/j.juro.2015.05.087

12. Tschui J, Vassella E, Bandi N, Baumgartner U, Genitsch V, Rotzer D, et al. Morphological and Molecular Characteristics of HER2 Amplified Urothelial Bladder Cancer. *Virchows Archiv an Int J Pathol* (2015) 466(6):703–10. doi: 10.1007/s00428-015-1729-4

13. Weinstein JN, Akbani R, Broom BM, Lerner SP, Creighton CJ, Kim J, et al. Comprehensive Molecular Characterization of Urothelial Bladder Carcinoma. *Nature* (2014) 507(7492):315–22. doi: 10.1038/nature12965

14. Robertson AG, Kim J, Al-Ahmadie H, Bellmunt J, Guo G, Cherniack AD, et al. Comprehensive Molecular Characterization of Muscle Invasive Bladder Cancer. *Cell* (2017) 171(3):540–556.e25. doi: 10.1016/j.cell.2017.09.007

15. Xu ZC, Cai HZ, Li X, Xu WZ, Xu T, Yu B, et al. ERCC1 C118T Polymorphism has Predictive Value for Platinum-Based Chemotherapy in Patients With Late-Stage Bladder Cancer. *Genet Mol Res GMR* (2016) 15(2):1–9. doi: 10.4238/gmr.15027801

16. Lee SJ, Lim JH, Choi YH, Kim WJ, Moon SK. Interleukin-28A Triggers Wound Healing Migration of Bladder Cancer Cells Via NF-kappaB-mediated MMP-9 Expression Inducing the MAPK Pathway. *Cell Signal* (2012) 24 (9):1734–42. doi: 10.1016/j.cellsig.2012.04.013

17. Lin J, Wang J, Greisinger AJ, Grossman HB, Forman MR, Dinney CP, et al. Energy Balance, the PI3K-AKT-mTOR Pathway Genes, and the Risk of Bladder Cancer. *Cancer Prev Res* (2010) 3(4):505–17. doi: 10.1158/1940-6207.CAPR-09-0263

18. Shin K, Lim A, Zhao C, Sahoo D, Pan Y, Spiekerkoetter E, et al. Hedgehog Signaling Restrains Bladder Cancer Progression by Eliciting Stromal Production of Urothelial Differentiation Factors. *Cancer Cell* (2014) 26 (4):521–33. doi: 10.1016/j.ccell.2014.09.001

19. Forster JA, Paul AB, Harnden P, Knowles MA. Expression of NRG1 and its Receptors in Human Bladder Cancer. *Br J Cancer* (2011) 104(7):1135–43. doi: 10.1038/bjc.2011.39

20. Sjodahl G, Lauss M, Gudjonsson S, Liedberg F, Halldén C, Chebil G, et al. A Systematic Study of Gene Mutations in Urothelial Carcinoma; Inactivating Mutations in TSC2 and PIK3R1. *PloS One* (2011) 6(4):e18583. doi: 10.1371/journal.pone.0018583

# AUTHOR CONTRIBUTIONS

JZ and CL designed and supervised the review. YL and LS searched literature and wrote the manuscript. XG and NM reviewed of the manuscript. All authors contributed to the article and approved the submitted version.

21. Bartoletti R, Cai T, Nesi G, Nesi G, Girardi LR, Baroni G, et al. Loss of P16 Expression and Chromosome 9p21 LOH in Predicting Outcome of Patients Affected by Superficial Bladder Cancer. *J Surg Res* (2007) 143(2):422–7. doi: 10.1016/j.jss.2007.01.012

22. Kruger S, Mess F, Bohle A, Feller AC. Numerical Aberrations of Chromosome 17 and the 9p21 Locus are Independent Predictors of Tumor Recurrence in non-Invasive Transitional Cell Carcinoma of the Urinary Bladder. *Int J Oncol* (2003) 23(1):41–8. doi: 10.3892/ijo.23.1.41

23. Almendro V, Marusyk A, Polyak K. Cellular Heterogeneity and Molecular Evolution in Cancer. *Annu Rev Pathol* (2013) 8:277–302. doi: 10.1146/annurev-pathol-020712-163923

24. Cordon-Cardo C. Molecular Alterations Associated With Bladder Cancer Initiation and Progression. *Scand J Urol Nephrol Supplementum* (2008) 218):154–65. doi: 10.1080/03008880802291915

25. Zhang ZT, Pak J, Huang HY, Shapiro E, Sun TT, Pellicer A, et al. Role of Ha-ras Activation in Superficial Papillary Pathway of Urothelial Tumor Formation. *Oncogene* (2001) 20(16):1973–80. doi: 10.1038/sj.onc.1204315

26. Wu S, Huang P, Li C, Huang Y, Li X, Wang Y, et al. Telomerase Reverse Transcriptase Gene Promoter Mutations Help Discern the Origin of Urogenital Tumors: A Genomic and Molecular Study. *Eur Urol* (2014) 65(2):274–7. doi: 10.1016/j.eururo.2013.10.038

27. Li C, Wu S, Wang H, Bi X, Yang Z, Du Y, et al. The C228T Mutation of TERT Promoter Frequently Occurs in Bladder Cancer Stem Cells and Contributes to Tumorigenesis of Bladder Cancer. *Oncotarget* (2015) 6(23):19542–51. doi: 10.18632/oncotarget.4295

28. Marusyk A, Polyak K. Tumor Heterogeneity: Causes and Consequences. *Biochim Biophys Acta* (2010) 1805(1):105–17. doi: 10.1016/j.bbcan.2009.11.002

29. Pietras A. Cancer Stem Cells in Tumor Heterogeneity. *Adv Cancer Res* (2011) 112:255–81. doi: 10.1016/B978-0-12-387688-1.00009-0

30. Kreso A, O'brien CA, Galen VP, Gan OI, Notta F, Brown AMK, et al. Variable Clonal Repopulation Dynamics Influence Chemotherapy Response in Colorectal Cancer. *Science* (2013) 339(6119):543–8. doi: 10.1126/science.1227670

31. Lingner J, Hughes TR, Shevchenko A, Mann M, Lundblad V, Cech TR, et al. Reverse Transcriptase Motifs in the Catalytic Subunit of Telomerase. *Science* (1997) 276(5312):561–7. doi: 10.1126/science.276.5312.561

32. Lin SY, Elledge SJ. Multiple Tumor Suppressor Pathways Negatively Regulate Telomerase. *Cell* (2003) 113(7):881–9. doi: 10.1016/S0092-8674(03)00430-6

33. Artandi SE, Depinho RA. Telomeres and Telomerase in Cancer. *Carcinogenesis* (2010) 31(1):9–18. doi: 10.1093/carcin/bgp268

34. Huang FW, Hodis E, Xu MJ, Kryukov GV, Chin L, Garraway LA. Highly Recurrent TERT Promoter Mutations in Human Melanoma. *Science* (2013) 339(6122):957–9. doi: 10.1126/science.1229259

35. Killela PJ, Reitman ZJ, Jiao Y, Bettegowda C, Agrawal N, Diaz LAJr, et al. TERT Promoter Mutations Occur Frequently in Gliomas and a Subset of Tumors Derived From Cells With Low Rates of Self-Renewal. *Proc Natl Acad Sci USA* (2013) 110(15):6021–6. doi: 10.1073/pnas.1303607110

36. Borah S, Xi L, Zaug AJ, Powell NM, Dancik GM, Cohen SB, et al. Cancer. TERT Promoter Mutations and Telomerase Reactivation in Urothelial Cancer. *Science* (2015) 347(6225):1006–10. doi: 10.1126/science.1260200

37. Veronese L, Tournilhac O, Callanan M, Prie N, Kwiatkowski F, Combes P, et al. Telomeres and Chromosomal Instability in Chronic Lymphocytic Leukemia. *Leukemia* (2013) 27(2):490–3. doi: 10.1038/leu.2012.194

38. Ho L, Crabtree GR. Chromatin Remodelling During Development. *Nature* (2010) 463(7280):474–84. doi: 10.1038/nature08911

39. Chi P, Allis CD, Wang GG. Covalent Histone Modifications–Miswritten, Misinterpreted and Mis-Erased in Human Cancers. *Nat Rev Cancer* (2010) 10(7):457–69. doi: 10.1038/nrc2876

40. Gui Y, Guo G, Huang Y, Hu X, Tang A, Gao S, et al. Frequent Mutations of Chromatin Remodeling Genes in Transitional Cell Carcinoma of the Bladder. *Nat Genet* (2011) 43(9):875–8. doi: 10.1038/ng.907

41. Wiegand KC, Shah SP, Al-Agha OM, Zhao Y, Tse K, Zeng T, et al. ARID1A Mutations in Endometriosis-Associated Ovarian Carcinomas. *New Engl J Med* (2010) 363(16):1532–43. doi: 10.1056/NEJMoa1008433

42. Dalgliesh GL, Furge K, Greenman C, Chen L, Bignell G, Butler A, et al. Systematic Sequencing of Renal Carcinoma Reveals Inactivation of Histone Modifying Genes. *Nature* (2010) 463(7279):360–3. doi: 10.1038/nature08672

43. Solomon DA, Kim T, Diaz-Martinez LA, Fair J, Elkahloun AG, Harris BT, et al. Mutational Inactivation of STAG2 Causes Aneuploidy in Human Cancer. *Science* (2011) 333(6045):1039–43. doi: 10.1126/science.1203619

44. Guo G, Sun X, Chen C, Wu S, Huang P, Li Z, et al. Whole-Genome and Whole-Exome Sequencing of Bladder Cancer Identifies Frequent Alterations in Genes Involved in Sister Chromatid Cohesion and Segregation. *Nat Genet* (2013) 45(12):1459–63. doi: 10.1038/ng.2798

45. Lawrence MS, Stojanov P, Polak P, Kryukov GV, Cibulskis K, Sivachenko A, et al. Mutational Heterogeneity in Cancer and the Search for New Cancer-Associated Genes. *Nature* (2013) 499(7457):214–8. doi: 10.1038/nature12213

46. Margulies M, Egholm M, Altman WE, Attiya S, Bader JS, Bemben LA, et al. Genome Sequencing in Microfabricated High-Density Picolitre Reactors. *Nature* (2005) 437(7057):376–80. doi: 10.1038/nature03959

47. Schuster SC. Next-Generation Sequencing Transforms Today's Biology. *Nat Methods* (2008) 5(1):16–8. doi: 10.1038/nmeth1156

48. Meyerson M, Gabriel S, Getz G. Advances in Understanding Cancer Genomes Through Second-Generation Sequencing. *Nat Rev Genet* (2010) 11(10):685–96. doi: 10.1038/nrg2841

49. Weir B, Zhao X, Meyerson M. Somatic Alterations in the Human Cancer Genome. *Cancer Cell* (2004) 6(5):433–8. doi: 10.1016/j.ccr.2004.11.004

50. Van Allen EM, Mouw KW, Kim P, Iyer G, Wagle N, Al-Ahmadie H, et al. Somatic ERCC2 Mutations Correlate With Cisplatin Sensitivity in Muscle-Invasive Urothelial Carcinoma. *Cancer Discovery* (2014) 4(10):1140–53. doi: 10.1158/2159-8290.CD-14-0623

51. David L, Plimack ER, Censits JH, Garraway LA, Bellmunt J, Allen EV, et al. Clinical Validation of Chemotherapy Response Biomarker ERCC2 in Muscle-invasive Urothelial Bladder Carcinoma. *JAMA Oncol* (2016) 2(8):1094–6. doi: 10.1001/jamaoncol.2016.1056

52. Desai NB, Scott SN, Zabor EC, Cha EK, Hreiki J, Sfakianos JP, et al. Genomic Characterization of Response to Chemoradiation in Urothelial Bladder Cancer. *Cancer* (2016) 122(23):3715–23. doi: 10.1002/cncr.30219

53. Longo T, Mcginley KF, Freedman JA, Etienne W, Wu Y, Sibley A, et al. Targeted Exome Sequencing of the Cancer Genome in Patients With Very High-Risk Bladder Cancer. *Eur Urol* (2016) 70(5):714–7. doi: 10.1016/j.eururo.2016.07.049

54. Navin N, Krasnitz A, Rodgers L, Cook K, Meth J, Kendall J, et al. Inferring Tumor Progression From Genomic Heterogeneity. *Genome Res* (2010) 20(1):68–80. doi: 10.1101/gr.099622.109

55. The biology of genomes. Single-Cell Sequencing Tackles Basic and Biomedical Questions. *Science* (2012) 336(6084):976–7. doi: 10.1126/science.336.6084.976

56. Navin N, Kendall J, Troge J, Andrews P, Rodgers L, McIndoo J, et al. Tumour Evolution Inferred by Single-Cell Sequencing. *Nature* (2011) 472(7341):90–4. doi: 10.1038/nature09807

57. Yang Z, Li C, Liu H, Liu H, Zhang X, Cai Z, et al. Single-Cell Sequencing Reveals Variants in ARID1A, GPRC5A and MLL2 Driving Self-renewal of Human Bladder Cancer Stem Cells. *Eur Urol* (2017) 71(1):8–12. doi: 10.1016/j.eururo.2016.06.025

58. Faridani OR, Abdullayev I, Hagemann-Jensen M, Schell JP, Lanner F, Sandberg R. Single-Cell Sequencing of the Small-RNA Transcriptome. *Nat Biotechnol* (2016) 34(12):1264–6. doi: 10.1038/nbt.3701

59. Kekeeva T, Tanas A, Kanygina A, Alexeev D, Shikeeva A, Zavalishina L, et al. Novel Fusion Transcripts in Bladder Cancer Identified by RNA-Seq. *Cancer Lett* (2016) 374(2):224–8. doi: 10.1016/j.canlet.2016.02.010

60. Zhang M, Li H, Zou D, Gao J. Ruguo Key Genes and Tumor Driving Factors Identification of Bladder Cancer Based on the RNA-seq Profile. *OncoTargets Ther* (2016) 9:2717–23. doi: 10.2147/OTT.S92529

61. Liu Y, Noon AP, Aguiar Cabeza E, Shen J, Kuk C, Ilczynski C, et al. Next-Generation RNA Sequencing of Archival Formalin-Fixed Paraffin-Embedded Urothelial Bladder Cancer. *Eur Urol* (2014) 66(6):982–6. doi: 10.1016/j.eururo.2014.07.045

62. Mendell JT, Olson EN. MicroRNAs in Stress Signaling and Human Disease. *Cell* (2012) 148(6):1172–87. doi: 10.1016/j.cell.2012.02.005

63. Kandoth C, Mclellan MD, Vandin F, Ye K, Niu B, Lu C, et al. Mutational Landscape and Significance Across 12 Major Cancer Types. *Nature* (2013) 502(7471):333–9. doi: 10.1038/nature12634

64. Seiler R, Ashab HAD, Erho N, van Rhijn BWG, Winters B, Douglas J, et al. Impact of Molecular Subtypes in Muscle-invasive Bladder Cancer on Predicting Response and Survival After Neoadjuvant Chemotherapy. *Eur Urol* (2017) 72(4):544–54. doi: 10.1016/j.eururo.2017.03.030

65. Casadei C, Dizman N, Schepisi G, Cursano MC, Basso U, Santini D, et al. Targeted Therapies for Advanced Bladder Cancer: New Strategies With FGFR Inhibitors. *Ther Adv Med Oncol* (2019) 11:1–14. doi: 10.1177/1758835919890285

66. Montazeri K, Bellmunt J. Erdafitinib for the Treatment of Metastatic Bladder Cancer. *Expert Rev Clin Pharmacol* (2020) 13(1):1–6. doi: 10.1080/17512433.2020.1702025

67. Lv J, Zhu Y, Ji A, Zhang Q, Liao G. Mining TCGA Database for Tumor Mutation Burden and Their Clinical Significance in Bladder Cancer. *Biosci Rep* (2020) 40(4):1–12. doi: 10.1042/BSR20194337

68. Mariathasan S, Turley SJ, Nickles D, Castiglioni A, Yuen K, Wang Y, et al. TGF-β Attenuates Tumour Response to PD-L1 Blockade by Contributing to Exclusion of T Cells. *Nature* (2018) 554(7693):544–8. doi: 10.1038/nature25501

69. Ott PA, Lieskovan SH, Bartosz Chmielowski B, Govindan R, Naing A, Bhardwaj N, et al. A Phase Ib Trial of Personalized Neoantigen Therapy Plus anti-PD-1 in Patients With Advanced Melanoma,non-Small Cell Lung Cancer, or Bladde Cancer. *Cell* (2020) 183(2):347–62.e24. doi: 10.1016/j.cell.2020.08.053

70. Alt M, Stecca C, Tobin S, Jiang DM, Sridhar SS. Enfortumab Vedotin in Urothelial Cancer. *Ther Adv Urol* (2020) 12:1–10. doi: 10.1177/1756287220980192

71. Park I, Lee JL. Systemic Treatment for Advanced Urothelial Cancer: An Update on Recent Clinical Trials and Current Treatment Options. *Korean J Internal Medcine* (2020) 35(4):834–53. doi: 10.3904/kjim.2020.204

72. Kompier LC, Lurkin I, Van Der Aa MN, van Rhijn BWG, van der Kwast TH, Zwarthoff EC. FGFR3, HRAS, KRAS, NRAS and PIK3CA Mutations in Bladder Cancer and Their Potential as Biomarkers for Surveillance and Therapy. *PloS One* (2010) 5(11):e13821. doi: 10.1371/journal.pone.0013821

73. Lopez-Beltran A, Luque RJ, Alvarez-Kindelan J, Quintero A, Merlo F, Carrasco JC, et al. Prognostic Factors in Stage T1 Grade 3 Bladder Cancer Survival: The Role of G1-S Modulators (p53, p21Waf1, P27kip1, Cyclin D1, and Cyclin D3) and Proliferation Index (Ki67-MIB1). *Eur Urol* (2004) 45 (5):606–12. doi: 10.1016/j.eururo.2003.11.011

74. Wang L, Feng C, Ding G, Ding Q, Zhou Z, Jiang H, et al. Ki67 and TP53 Expressions Predict Recurrence of non-Muscle-Invasive Bladder Cancer. *Tumour Biol J Int Soc Oncodevelop Biol Med* (2014) 35(4):2989–95. doi: 10.1007/s13277-013-1384-9

75. Klatte T, Seitz C, Rink M, Rouprêt M, Xylinas E, Karakiewicz P, et al. ERCC1 as a Prognostic and Predictive Biomarker for Urothelial Carcinoma of the Bladder Following Radical Cystectomy. *J Urol* (2015) 194(5):1456–62. doi: 10.1016/j.juro.2015.06.099

76. Font A, Taron M, Gago JL, Costa C, Sánchez JJ, Carrato C, et al. BRCA1 mRNA Expression and Outcome to Neoadjuvant Cisplatin-Based Chemotherapy in Bladder Cancer. *Ann Oncol Off J Eur Soc Med Oncol* (2011) 22(1):139–44. doi: 10.1093/annonc/mdq333

77. Iyer G, Al-Ahmadie H, Schultz N, Hanrahan AJ, Ostrovnaya I, Balar AV, et al. Prevalence and Co-Occurrence of Actionable Genomic Alterations in High-Grade Bladder Cancer. *J Clin Oncol Off J Am Soc Clin Oncol* (2013) 31 (25):3133–40. doi: 10.1200/JCO.2012.46.5740

78. Plimack ER, Dunbrack RL, Brennan TA, Andrake MD, Zhou Y, Serebriiskii IG, et al. Defects in DNA Repair Genes Predict Response to Neoadjuvant Cisplatin-Based Chemotherapy in Muscle-invasive Bladder Cancer. *Eur Urol* (2015) 68(6):959–67. doi: 10.1016/j.eururo.2015.07.009

# 8

# KIF15 Promotes Progression of Castration Resistant Prostate Cancer by Activating EGFR Signaling Pathway

Lin Gao[1†], Ru Zhao[1†], Junmei Liu[2], Wenbo Zhang[1], Feifei Sun[1], Qianshuo Yin[3], Xin Wang[1], Meng Wang[1], Tingting Feng[1], Yiming Qin[4], Wenjie Cai[1], Qianni Li[1], Hanchen Dong[1], Xueqing Chen[1], Xueting Xiong[5], Hui Liu[1,6], Jing Hu[1,6], Weiwen Chen[2] and Bo Han[1,6*]

[1] The Key Laboratory of Experimental Teratology, Ministry of Education and Department of Pathology, School of Basic Medical Sciences, Cheeloo College of Medicine, Shandong University, Jinan, China, [2] Department of Biochemistry and Molecular Biology, School of Basic Medical Sciences, Cheeloo College of Medicine, Shandong University, Jinan, China, [3] School of Basic Medical Sciences, Shandong University, Jinan, China, [4] College of Chemical Engineering and Materials Science, Shandong Normal University, Jinan, China, [5] Department of Molecular Genetics, University of Toronto, Toronto, ON, Canada, [6] Department of Pathology, Qilu Hospital, Cheeloo College of Medicine, Shandong University, Jinan, China

*Correspondence:
Bo Han
boh@sdu.edu.cn

†These authors have contributed equally to this work

Castration-resistant prostate cancer (CRPC) continues to be a major clinical problem and its underlying mechanisms are still not fully understood. The epidermal growth factor receptor (EGFR) activation is an important event that regulates mitogenic signaling. EGFR signaling plays an important role in the transition from androgen dependence to castration-resistant state in prostate cancer (PCa). Kinesin family member 15 (KIF15) has been suggested to be overexpressed in multiple malignancies. Here, we demonstrate that KIF15 expression is elevated in CRPC. We show that KIF15 contributes to CRPC progression by enhancing the EGFR signaling pathway, which includes complex network intermediates such as mitogen-activated protein kinase (MAPK) and phosphatidylinositol 3-kinase (PI3K)/AKT pathways. In CRPC tumors, increased expression of KIF15 is positively correlated with EGFR protein level. KIF15 binds to EGFR, and prevents EGFR proteins from degradation in a Cdc42-dependent manner. These findings highlight the key role of KIF15 in the development of CRPC and rationalize KIF15 as a potential therapeutic target.

Keywords: KIF15, EGFR, Cdc42, CRPC, protein stability

## INTRODUCTION

Prostate cancer (PCa) is the most commonly diagnosed cancer in men worldwide (1). Androgen deprivation treatment is the standard treatment for patients with advanced PCa (2). However, a more aggressive castration-resistant prostate cancer (CRPC) inevitably develops (3). Several novel therapeutic agents have been developed for CRPC, but the prognosis for patients with CRPC remains poor (4, 5). Therefore, the identification of novel therapeutic targets for CRPC is an urgent issue.

Epidermal growth factor receptor (EGFR), a member of the erbB family, regulates proliferation, differentiation, survival, and migration in multiple type of cells (6). EGFR plays an important role in the pathogenesis of PCa and in the CRPC progression (7–9). High levels of EGFR expression correlate with PCa progression (6, 7, 10, 11). EGFR usually acts at the plasma membrane or on vesicles belonging to the endosomal compartment (12); however, it can also localize to the nucleus and mitochondria (13). Epidermal growth factor (EGF) engagement activates the intrinsic kinase activity of EGFR which leads to the activation of several downstream intracellular signaling pathways, including the mitogen-activated protein kinase (MAPK) and phosphatidylinositol 3-kinase (PI3K)/AKT signaling (14, 15). These pathways can then mediate multiple physiological and pathological processes such as cell cycle progression and cell survival (16, 17). Constitutively activated MAPK and PI3K/AKT signaling occur in CRPC cells (18, 19), and they have been proposed as the important pathways in promoting PCa progression to CRPC (20).

Kinesins represent a superfamily of microtubule-dependent motor proteins that are involved in intracellular transport and mitosis (21). Kinesin family member 15 (KIF15) is an N-terminal and plus-end-directed motor that plays a critical role in the formation of bipolar spindles (22). It plays an important role in developing neuronal axons (23) and participates in the transport of macromolecules in several essential cellular processes, such as mitosis and meiosis (24). Recently, KIF15 was found to be overexpressed in several malignancies including pancreatic cancer, hepatocellular carcinoma, lung cancer, and breast cancer (25–28). Our previous study showed that KIF15 expression was elevated in enzalutamide resistant PCa, and promotes androgen receptor (AR) protein stabilization (29). KIF15 promotes cell proliferation in 22Rv1 and PC3 cells (29), which were CRPC cell lines, suggesting that KIF15 may correlate with CRPC progression. However, the function of KIF15 in CRPC cells has not been characterized.

In this study, we demonstrate that KIF15 expression is elevated in CRPC and KIF15 promotes CRPC progression. KIF15 inhibits degradation of EGFR protein in a cell division cycle 42 (Cdc42)-dependent manner, resulting in the activation of MAPK and PI3K/AKT signaling pathways. Therefore, our results highlight KIF15 as a potential novel therapeutic target for CRPC.

## MATERIALS AND METHODS

### Patients

A total of 49 PCa patients participated in our study. The tumor samples were obtained from Qilu Hospital of Shandong University (Jinan, China) between 2003 and 2015. The first group included 28 men with primary PCa who have undergone radical prostatectomy without receiving preoperative radiation or androgen deprivation treatment. The second group included 21 patients with CRPC treated by transurethral resection of the prostate to relieve symptomatic obstruction due to locally advanced disease. The initial treatment for patients was either observation or surgery. Development of CRPC was treated by flutamide or bicalutamide.

This study was conducted in accordance with the International Ethical Guidelines for Biomedical Research Involving Human Subjects. The study protocol was approved by the Institutional Review Board of Medicine School of Shandong University (ECSBMSSDU2019-1-021). The informed written consent was obtained from each patient.

### Immunohistochemistry

Immunohistochemistry (IHC) assays were performed as previously described using the PV9000 kit (Zsbio) (29). Slides were treated with antigen retrieval in EDTA (pH 8.0) in a pressure cooker for 10 minutes and then incubated with 3% $H_2O_2$ for 10 minutes at room temperature. Nonspecific antibody binding was blocked by subsequent incubation with goat serum (ZLI-9056; Zsbio) for 30 minutes at room temperature. Slides were then incubated overnight with anti-KIF15 (1:100, cat no. 55407-1-AP; Proteintech) or anti-EGFR (1:100, cat no. ab52894; Abcam) at 4°C. Tissues were analyzed by two independent pathologists (W.X.L. and H.B.) and KIF15 staining was scored semi-quantitatively based on cells with positive staining (0 = negative staining, 1 = weak staining, 2 = moderate staining, 3 = strong staining). For analysis, we combined both negative and weak KIF15 positive tumors into one group, and moderate and strong KIF15 positive tumors into the other. EGFR cell membrane-specific immunoreactivity was scored by estimating the percentage of positive tumor cells as previously described (7). score 0 (negative staining), no immunoreactive cell; score 1 (weak staining), positivity in 5% cancer cells; score 2 (moderate staining), positivity in 5–50% cancer cells; and score 3 (strong staining), positivity in 50% of cancer cells. Specimens were considered positive for EGFR expression (EGFR+) when the score was 2 or 3.

### Cell Culture and Reagents

LNCaP, C4-2B, and PC3 cells were purchased from American Type Culture Collection (ATCC) (Rockville, MD, USA) between 2015-2018, and cultured following ATCC's instructions except for the indicated treatment. Cells were authenticated by short tandem repeat analysis within the last 2 years. The cumulative culture length of the cells between thawing and use in this study was less than 15 passages. All of the newly revived cells were tested free of mycoplasma contamination by Hoechst 33258 staining (Beyotime, Jiangsu, China). EGF was obtained from Peprotech (NJ, USA), 20 ng/ml EGF was used for 20 minutes in this study.

### Western Blot

Western blot assays were performed as previously described (29). Primary antibodies used in Western blot assays are anti-KIF15 (2 μg/ml, cat no. H00056992-M01; Abnova), anti-EGFR (1:1000, cat no. 4267; Cell Signaling Technology), anti-Cdc42 (1:1000, cat no. ET1701-7; HUABIO), anti-MEK (1:1000, cat no. 4694; Cell Signaling Technology), anti-p-MEK (Ser217/221) (1:1000, cat no. 9154; Cell Signaling Technology), anti-ERK (1:1000, cat no. 4695; Cell Signaling Technology), anti-p-ERK (Thr202/Tyr204) (1:1000, cat no. 4370; Cell Signaling Technology), anti-AKT (1:1000, cat no. 4685; Cell Signaling Technology), anti-p-AKT

(Ser473) (1:1000, cat no. 4060; Cell Signaling Technology), anti-CDK2 (1:1000, cat no. CY5020; Abways), anti-CyclinD1 (1:1000, cat no. CY5404; Abways), anti-CyclinE1 (1:1000, cat no. CY5815; Abways), and anti-GAPDH (1:1000, cat no.ab181602; Abcam).

## Quantitative Real Time-PCR (qRT-PCR)

qRT-PCR was performed as previously described (30). The sequences of primers were as follows: KIF15 forward, 5'-CAAC CAAGTAATGAAGGTGATGCC-3'; KIF15 reverse, 5'-AAC GTGAAGGTCTTGGGCTC-3'; EGFR forward, 5'-AGGCA CGAGTAACAAGCTCAC-3'; EGFR reverse, 5'-ATGAGGA CATAACCAGCCACC-3'; GAPDH forward, 5'-GCACCGTC AAGGCTGAGAAC -3'; GAPDH reverse, 5'-TGGTGAAGAC GCCAGTGGA-3'. GAPDH was included as an endogenous control. The relative expression of indicated gene was calculated using the $2^{(-\Delta\Delta Ct)}$ method.

## Plasmids, siRNAs and Cell Transfection

KIF15 (Gene ID: 56992; vector: PcDNA3.1) cDNA expression vectors were designed and synthesized by Sangon Biotech (Shanghai, China). SiRNAs were purchased from GenePharma (Shanghai, China). The sequences of siRNAs were: siKIF15 #1: 5'-GGACAUAAAUUGCAAAUAC-3'; siKIF15 #2: 5'-GGAACA AAUGAGUGCUCUUTT-3'; siEGFR: 5'-GUAAUUAUGUG GUGACAGATT-3'. Cdc42-Q61L (Gene ID: 998; vector: PcDNA3.1) and Cdc42-T17N (Gene ID: 998; vector: PcDNA3.1) cDNA expression vectors were designed and synthesized by Biosune Biotech (Shanghai, China). Lipofectamine 3000 (Invitrogen, Carlsbad, CA) was used for transfection following the manufacturer's instruction. The effect of transfection efficiency was confirmed using qRT-PCR and Western blot assay. Lentiviral plasmids encoding shRNAs against control (NC; LV3-NC; 5'- GTTCTCCGAACGTGTCACGT -3') and KIF15 (shKIF15; LV3-shKIF15; 5'- GGAACAAATGAGTGCTCTT -3') were purchased from GenePharma (Shanghai, China). C4-2B cells with KIF15 knockdown were achieved by lentiviral approaches combined with puromycin selection as we reported (29).

## Cell Proliferation, Colony Formation, and Migration Assays

Cellular proliferation was measured by 3-(4,5-dimethylthiazol-2-yl)-5-(3-carboxymethoxyphenyl)-2-(4-sulfophenyl)-2H-tetrazolium inner salt (MTS) (Promega, Madison, WI, USA) and clonal formation assays. The transwell assay was used to measure the migration of PCa cells. Both assays were performed as previously described (30).

## Pulldown Assays

Rho GTPase pulldown assays were performed as previously described (31). GST-PAK-CRIB Rac/Cdc42 Isolation Kit was purchased from Kerafast (Boston, USA). The cells were lysed and centrifuged. The supernatant was transferred to new tubes containing agarose beads pre-coupled with PAK-CRIB and incubated with rotation at 4°C for 30 minutes. The beads were then washed, and the proteins bound on the beads were separated by SDS-PAGE. The amounts of active Cdc42 were determined by Western blot analysis with the corresponding antibodies.

## Tumor Xenografts

Five-week-old male nude mice were purchased from Weitonglihua Biotechnology (Beijing, China). To study the function of KIF15 in CRPC growth, a total of $6.0\times10^6$ C4-2B cells expressing a control shRNA (NC) or shKIF15 mixed with matrigel (1:1) were injected subcutaneously into the mice (n = 6/group). The mice were surgically castrated when the tumors reached 100-200 mm³. Tumor size was measured twice a week and the tumor volume was calculated with the formula: tumor volume = 0.5 × length × width². Tumor tissues were harvested and weighed after 4 weeks. All animal experiments were performed following a protocol approved by the Shandong University Animal Care Committee (Document No. LL-201602005).

## Bioinformatics Analysis

Datasets of GSE35988, GSE32269, GSE74367, and GSE2443 were downloaded from the GEO database (http://www.ncbi.nlm.nih.gov/geo). KIF15 expression in these datasets were analyzed in the groups between primary PCa and CRPC. The expressed genes of KIF15_High (top 2 KIF15 highest expression) and KIF15_Low (top 2 KIF15 lowest expression) obtained from GSE35988, GSE32269 and GSE2443 were subsequently analyzed for enrichment of biological themes using Gene Set Enrichment Analysis (GSEA) (http://software.broadinstitute.org/gsea/index.jsp).

## Statistical Analysis

Statistical analysis was carried out using GraphPad Prism 7 or SPSS 20.0 software. Statistical comparisons between groups were analyzed using two-sided Student's $t$ test. All experiments in vitro were performed in biological triplicate. All results are presented as the mean and the standard error of the mean. $P < 0.05$ was considered statistically significant. *, $P <0.05$; **, $P < 0.01$; ***, $P <0.001$; ****, $P < <0.0001$.

## RESULTS

### KIF15 Expression Is Elevated in CRPC

Our previous study showed that KIF15 promotes cell proliferation in androgen dependent cell line LNCaP and CRPC cell lines, including C4-2B, 22Rv1, and PC3 (29), these results suggest that KIF15 may correlate with CRPC progression. To investigate the clinicopathological significance of KIF15 expression in CRPC patients, we first analyzed the level of KIF15 using published datasets. As shown in **Figure 1A**, KIF15 expression was significantly upregulated in CRPC compared to primary PCa tissues in GSE32269 (32) ($P < 0.0001$), GSE35988 (33) ($P < 0.0001$) and GSE74367 (34) ($P < 0.0001$) datasets. Furthermore, KIF15 expression is elevated in androgen-independent than androgen-dependent PCa in GSE2443 (35) (**Figure 1B**, $P < 0.05$). In GSE35988 and GSE32269 datasets, PCa samples were divided into either the KIF15 high expression group (50% cut off) or KIF15 low expression group. Patients with high KIF15 expression were tightly clustered apart from

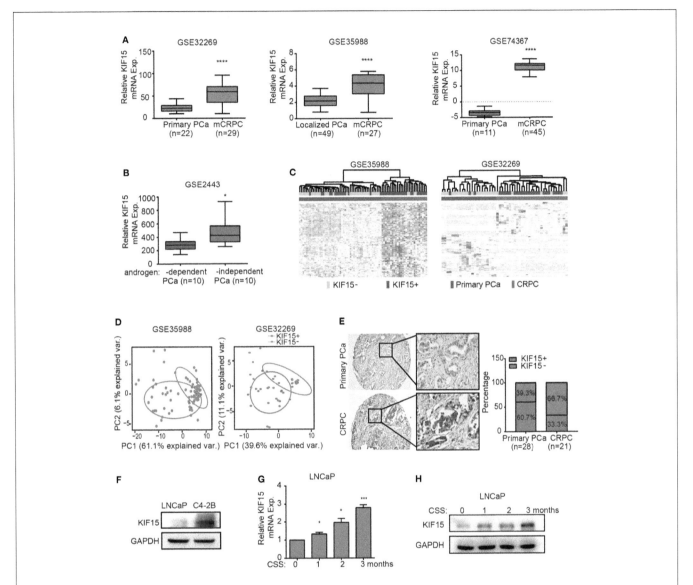

FIGURE 1 | KIF15 is overexpressed in CRPC. (A) Expression of KIF15 in primary PCa and CRPC tissues taken from publicly available datasets of GSE32269 (left), GSE35988 (middle) and GSE74367 (right). KIF15 expression was analyzed in a) 22 samples with primary PCa from hormone-naive patients, and 29 samples with CRPC (GSE32269); b) 49 samples with localized PCa, and 27 samples with metastatic CRPC (GSE35988); c) 11 samples with primary PCa tumor and 45 samples with CRPC metastases from 32 patients (GSE74367). The statistical analysis was based on Student's $t$ test. ****$P$ <0.0001. (B) KIF15 expression in androgen-dependent and independent PCa. KIF15 expression was analyzed in 10 samples with androgen-dependent primary PCa and 10 samples with androgen-independent primary PCa (GSE2443). The statistical analysis was based on Student's $t$ test. *$P$ <0.05. (C) Unsupervised clustering analyses of GSE35988 (left) and GSE32269 (right) datasets based on differentially expressed genes of primary PCa and CRPC tissues. Patients statue are shown in the annotation column. Patients were categorized according to KIF15 expression or PCa risk assessment. Green: patients with low KIF15 expression (50% cutoff; KIF15-); Purple: patients with high KIF15 expression (50% cutoff; KIF15 +); Blue: patients with primary PCa (Primary PCa); Red: patients with CRPC. (D) PCA analysis of unique CRPC-upregulated gene expression pattern between KIF15+ (high KIF15 expression, 50% cutoff) and KIF15- (low KIF15 expression, 50% cutoff) of PCa patients from GSE35988 and GSE32269 datasets. CRPC-upregulated genes were obtained from the top100 high expressed genes in CRPC compared with primary PCa in each dataset. Each point represents a patient. (E) The percentage of KIF15 expression distributed in PCa cases in Qilu Hospital with primary PCa or CRPC. Left panel: representative IHC images for KIF15 expression. Right panel: the percentage of KIF15 expression distributed in 49 PCa cases in Qilu Hospital with primary PCa or CRPC. (F) KIF15 levels in LNCaP and C4-2B cells analyzed by Western blot assay. LNCaP and C4-2B cells were harvested and whole lysates were subjected to Western blot. (G, H) Levels of KIF15 mRNA (G) and protein (H) in LNCaP cells with prolonged androgen-deprivation treatment. qRT-PCR and Western blot analysis were performed to detect KIF15 expression in LNCaP cells after androgen-deprived treatment in charcoal-stripped medium for the indicated time periods. CSS, Charcoal stripped fetal bovine serum; Exp., Expression; *$P$ < 0.05; ***$P$ < 0.001 vs. 0 month.

ones with low KIF15 expression and were congruent with CRPC subgroup (**Figure 1C**). As shown in **Figure 1D**, principal component analysis (PCA) demonstrated that PCa patients with high KIF15 expression displayed an expression pattern of

CRPC-upregulated genes distinct from PCa patients with low KIF15 expression. To confirm our findings, we then analyzed KIF15 expression in clinical specimens from primary PCa and CRPC cases from Qilu Hospital of Shandong University. As shown in **Figure 1E**, KIF15 is mainly expressed in the cytoplasm of tumor cells and its expression was significantly higher in CRPC samples than in primary PCa samples. Remarkably, among primary PCa cases, 17 (60.7%) showed negative or weak staining (7 cases: negative; 10 cases: weak), and only 11 (39.3%) had moderate or strong staining for KIF15 (6 cases: moderate; 5 cases: strong). However, 7 (33.3%) were negative or weak (2 cases: negative; 5 cases: weak), whereas 14 (66.7%) CRPC cases showed moderate or strong expression (6 cases: moderate; 8 cases: strong). Overall, CRPC specimens showed significantly stronger expression of KIF15 than primary PCa samples (**Figure 1E**, *P* = 0.034). Next, we evaluated the KIF15 expression in androgen-dependent LNCaP and CRPC cell lines of C4-2B. As shown in **Figure 1F**, KIF15 was dramatically upregulated in C4-2B. Notably, prolonged androgen deprivation for 3 months in LNCaP cells continuously enhanced KIF15 expression at both mRNA and protein levels (**Figures 1G, H**). These results indicate that enhanced KIF15 expression is highly correlated in CRPC.

## KIF15 Promotes CRPC Progression *In Vitro* and *In Vivo*

To determine whether KIF15 serves a functional role in CRPC progression, we overexpressed its expression in LNCaP cells and suppressed its expression in C4-2B cells with or without androgen depletion. We found that KIF15 greatly enhanced LNCaP cell proliferation under androgen depletion (charcoal stripped fetal bovine serum, CSS) than androgen-repletion conditions (fetal bovine serum, FBS; CSS *vs.* FBS; 1.8 folds *vs.* 1.4 folds) (**Figures 2A, B** and **Supplementary Figure S1A**). SiRNAs against KIF15 significantly reduced the total cell numbers of C4-2B under FBS as well as CSS conditions relative to their control counterparts (**Figures 2C, D** and **Supplementary Figure S1A**). Furthermore, siRNA knockdown of KIF15 in PC3 cells, an AR-negative CRPC cells (20), significantly inhibited cell proliferation (**Figure 2E**). Due to higher efficiency of transfection, siKIF15#2 was chosen for KIF15 knockdown in following experiments. As shown in **Supplementary Figures S1B–D**, KIF15 promoted cells

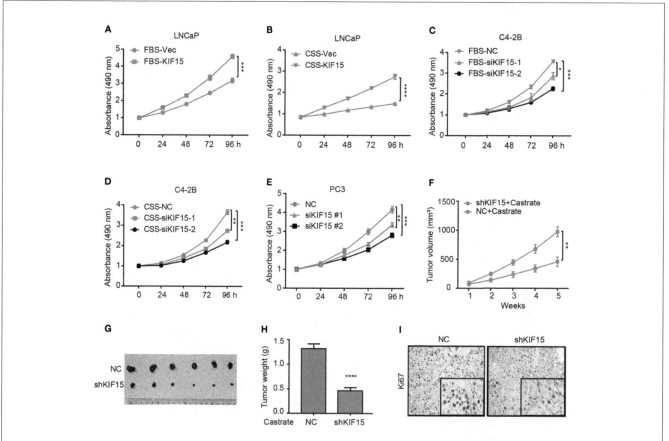

**FIGURE 2 |** KIF15 promotes CRPC *in vitro* and *in vivo*. **(A, B)** Cell proliferation of LNCaP cells with FBS or CSS treatment assessed by MTS assays. LNCaP cells were cultured in FBS medium **(A)** or CSS medium for 48 hours **(B)**, these cells were transfected with corresponding siRNA and subjected to MTS assays. Vec, vector. ***P <0.001; ****P <0.0001. **(C, D)** Cell proliferation of C4-2B cells with FBS or CSS treatment assessed by MTS assays. C4-2B cells were cultured in FBS medium **(C)** or CSS medium for 48 hours **(D)**, these cells were transfected with corresponding siRNA and subjected to MTS assays. NC, negative control; *P <0.05; **P < 0.01; ***P <0.001. **(E)** Cell proliferation of PC3 cells assessed by MTS assays. PC3 cells were transiently transfected with corresponding siRNA, the cells were subjected to MTS assays. **P < 0.01; ***P <0.001. **(F–H)** Xenograft tumor growth after KIF15 depletion. C4-2B cells with stable KIF15 knockdown or its control were injected subcutaneously into nude mice (6 mice per group). Tumor size was measured twice every week **(F)**. At the endpoint, tumors isolated from euthanized mice were photographed **(G)** and weighed **(H)**. **P < 0.01; ****P <0.0001. **(I)** Representative images of Ki67 IHC staining of xenograft tumor derived from C4-2B NC/shKIF15 cells.

migration and clone formation in both LNCaP and C4-2B cells. In addition, cell cycle distribution analysis demonstrated that silencing KIF15 could lead to a significant number of C4-2B and PC3 cells to accumulate in the G1 phase (**Supplementary Figure S1E**). Furthermore, KIF15 depletion of C4-2B xenografts in castrated nude mice resulted in delayed tumor progression; the mean tumor volume 463.5 ± 79.92 mm$^3$ in C4-2B shKIF15 xenografts while it was 979 ± 84.57 mm$^3$ in the control group ($P = 0.001$) (the weight of tumors; shKIF15 *vs.* control; 0.4633 ± 0.06312 g *vs.* 1.313 ± 0.09698 g; $P < 0.0001$) (**Figures 2F–H**). Moreover, the Ki67 percentage score of tumor cells in the shKIF15 group was relatively low when compared to cells in the NC group (**Figure 2I**). Collectively, our data suggested that KIF15 is required for the proliferation of CRPC cells.

## KIF15 Regulates EGFR Signaling in CRPC Cells

EGFR signaling plays an important role in the progression of PCa and the transformation to CRPC (7). We firstly utilized multiple public datasets to characterize the relationship between EGFR and KIF15 in CRPC progression. As shown in **Figure 3A**, GSEA was performed using microarray datasets from GEO database (GSE35988) and revealed that genes positively related to EGFR were enriched in the KIF15_High samples (NES = 2.32; $P < 0.0001$; FDR q< 0.0001). Additionally, genes down-regulated after treatment with EGFR inhibitor were enriched in the KIF15_High samples, which were analyzed by GSEA using GSE32269 (NES = 2.79; $P < 0.0001$; FDR q< 0.0001) as well as in GSE2443 (NES = 2.57; $P < 0.0001$; FDR q< 0.0001) microarray data (**Figure 3B** and **Supplementary Figure S2A**). These results suggested that EGFR pathway was positively related with KIF15 high expression in PCa. Importantly, 6 out of 28 (21.4%) primary PCa cases from Qilu Hospital showed KIF15+/EGFR+ by IHC staining (moderate or strong staining for both KIF15 and EGFR). Accordingly, 15 out of 28 (53.6%) cases were KIF15-/EGFR- by IHC staining (negative or weak staining for both KIF15 and EGFR). By contrast, only 5 (17.9%) cases demonstrated KIF15+/EGFR- (moderate or strong staining for KIF15 whereas negative or weak staining for EGFR) and 2 (7.1%) cases demonstrated KIF15-/EGFR+ (negative or weak staining for KIF15 and moderate or strong staining for EGFR). Among CRPC cases, IHC staining showed that 13 (61.9%) cases were KIF15+/EGFR+, 5 (23.8%) cases with KIF15-/EGFR-. By contrast, only 1 (4.8%) case was KIF15+/EGFR- and 2 (9.5%) cases were KIF15-/EGFR+ (**Figures 3C, D**). A positive correlation of KIF15 and EGFR expression was observed in primary PCa cases ($P = 0.0299$, $r = 0.462$) and CRPC cases ($P = 0.0055$, $r = 0.671$) (**Figure 3E**). Overall, these data suggest that high protein levels of KIF15 correlated with increased EGFR protein levels in prostate tumor samples. In addition, EGFR protein expression was significantly downregulated in C4-2B xenografts with KIF15 depletion as shown in **Figures 3F, G**. Then, we monitored EGFR expression after KIF15 overexpression in LNCaP cells, and KIF15 depletion in C4-2B and PC3 cells. As shown in **Figure 3H** and **Supplementary Figure S2B**, KIF15 overexpression enhanced EGFR protein

levels in LNCaP cells, while KIF15 depletion reduced EGFR protein levels in C4-2B and PC3 cells. These effects were more significantly in CSS condition in these cells. However, EGFR mRNA levels were not altered even though these cells showed marked increases or reductions in KIF15 expression (**Figures 3I, J** and **Supplementary Figure S2C**). Together, our results suggest that KIF15 may regulate EGFR protein levels, especially in the androgen deprivation condition.

To examine how KIF15 regulates EGFR signaling, we tested the key molecules in MAPK and PI3K-AKT signaling pathways which were reported as downstream of EGFR (19, 36). As shown in **Figure 4A**, KIF15 overexpression significantly increased p-MEK, p-ERK, and p-AKT protein levels in LNCaP cells, while KIF15 knockdown reduced p-MEK, p-ERK and p-AKT levels in C4-2B and PC3 cells. However, these effects of KIF15 were more significant with EGF treatment in the corresponding cells (**Figures 4B, C**). Since KIF15-depleted cells showed attenuation in MAPK and AKT activity and accumulation at the G1 phase, we examined the expression of cell cycle regulatory proteins (37) in these PCa cell lines. As shown in **Figure 4D**, KIF15 knockdown significantly reduced CyclinD1, CyclinE1, and CDK2 protein levels in both C4-2B and PC3 cells, while KIF15 overexpression increased their levels in LNCaP cells. Importantly, EGFR depletion reversed KIF15 overexpression-induced activation of MEK, ERK, and AKT, and cell proliferation in LNCaP cells (**Figures 4E, F** and **Supplementary Figure S2D**). These data demonstrated that KIF15 promotes CRPC progression by activating EGFR signaling pathway.

## KIF15 Inhibits Degradation of EGFR in CRPC Cells

To explore the mechanism by which KIF15 modulates EGFR protein level, we performed co-immunoprecipitation (co-IP) assays in both C4-2B and PC3 cells. As shown in **Figure 5A**, KIF15 binds to EGFR in these two cell lines. Since KIF15 regulated EGFR expression at protein levels but not at mRNA levels, we tested whether KIF15 affects EGFR protein degradation in PCa cells. C4-2B, PC3, and LNCaP cells were treated with cycloheximide (CHX) to block *de novo* protein synthesis, and EGFR protein level was analyzed by Western blot. The results showed that knockdown of KIF15 remarkably accelerates the degradation of EGFR proteins in comparison to the control cells, and KIF15 overexpression inhibited EGFR protein degradation (**Figure 5B**). These data suggest that KIF15 can stabilize the EGFR protein. It has been previously reported that Cdc42, a member of Rho GTPase family protein and a key regulator of the actin cytoskeleton, plays an important role in the process of internalization and degradation of receptors (38). Cdc42 activity is controlled by exchanging between the inactive GDP-bound form (Cdc42$^{GDP}$) and active GTP-bound form (Cdc42$^{GTP}$) (39). Unlike Ras, which is activated primarily by point mutations that impair its GTPase activity in human cancers, Cdc42 is activated by changes in upstream regulators. Hirsch et al. showed that EGFR protein degradation is correlated with activation of Cdc42 (40). To demonstrate the potential mechanism of KIF15 silencing-induced EGFR degradation, we tested Cdc42 activity by pulldown assays in C4-2B and PC3 cells transfected with

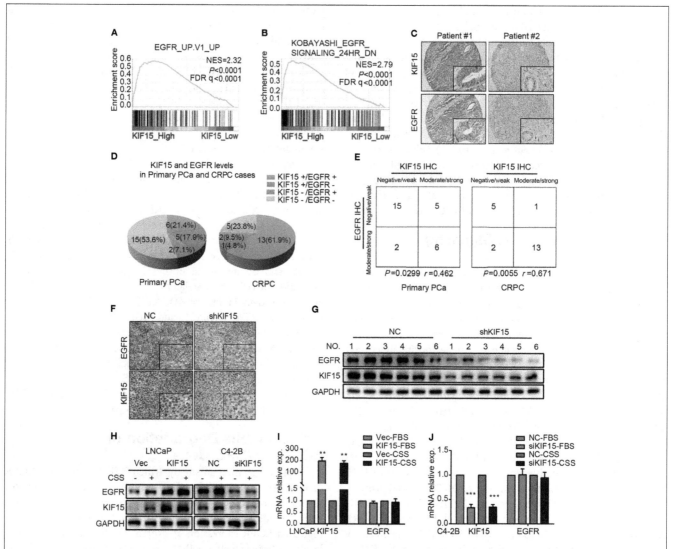

**FIGURE 3** | KIF15 promotes EGFR expression in PCa. **(A)** GSEA analysis of EGFR signatures (genes upregulated upon EGFR elevated) from a microarray dataset (GSE35988) that profiled CRPC cases with KIF15_High (the highest 2 samples) or KIF15_Low (the lowest 2 samples) expression. NES = 2.32; P < 0.0001, FDR q < 0.0001. **(B)** GSEA analysis of EGFR signatures (down-regulated after treatment with EGFR inhibitor) from a microarray dataset (GSE32269) that profiled CRPC cases with KIF15_High (the highest 2 samples) or KIF15_Low (the lowest 2 samples) expression. NES = 2.79; P < 0.0001, FDR q < 0.0001. **(C, D)** Representative IHC images **(C)** and quantitative analysis **(D)** for EGFR and KIF15 expression in PCa cases in Qilu Hospital. KIF15-, negative and weak KIF15 positive tumors examined by IHC staining; KIF15+, moderate and strong KIF15 positive tumors examined by IHC staining; EGFR-, negative and weak EGFR positive tumors examined by IHC staining; EGFR+, moderate and strong EGFR positive tumors examined by IHC staining. **(E)** Contingency table for KIF15 expression and EGFR status by IHC in primary PCa cases and CRPC cases in Qilu Hospital. **(F, G)** EGFR protein expression in C4-2B xenograft examined by IHC staining **(F)** and Western blot **(G)**. **(H)** EGFR protein expression in LNCaP cells (left) and C4-2B (right) cells. These cells were cultured and passaged in CSS medium or FBS medium for 1 month, and then they were transfected with corresponding expression plasmids for 48 hours or siRNA for 72 hours. Then cells were collected, lysed for Western blot assay. **(I, J)** The relative mRNA expression of KIF15 and EGFR in LNCaP **(I)** and C4-2B **(J)** cells with indicated treatment. LNCaP **(I)** and C4-2B **(J)** cells with indicated treatment as **(H)** were transfected with expression plasmids or siRNAs for 48 hours. The total RNA was extracted, and the mRNA levels of KIF15 and EGFR were determined by qRT-PCR. **P < 0.01; ***P < 0.001.

siRNA against KIF15 and in LNCaP cells transfected with KIF15 expression plasmids. As shown in **Figures 5C, D**, Cdc42 activity was significantly attenuated in KIF15-depleted C4-2B and PC3 cells, and enhanced in LNCaP cells with KIF15 overexpression. Furthermore, Cdc42 knockdown reversed KIF15 overexpression-induced EGFR protein upregulation in LNCaP cells (**Figure 5E**). Cdc42-Q61L was a form of Cdc42-active mutant (41), and Cdc42-T17N was a form of Cdc42-

inactive mutant (42, 43). EGFR protein level was elevated when Cdc42-Q61L but not Cdc42-T17N plasmids were transfected into the KIF15-depleted C4-2B and PC3 cells (**Figures 5F, G**). Our data supports that KIF15 inhibits degradation of EGFR in a Cdc42-dependent manner.

Together, KIF15 stabilizes EGFR in a Cdc42-dependent manner and activates EGFR signaling pathways to promote CRPC progression. A schematic diagram was shown in **Figure 6**.

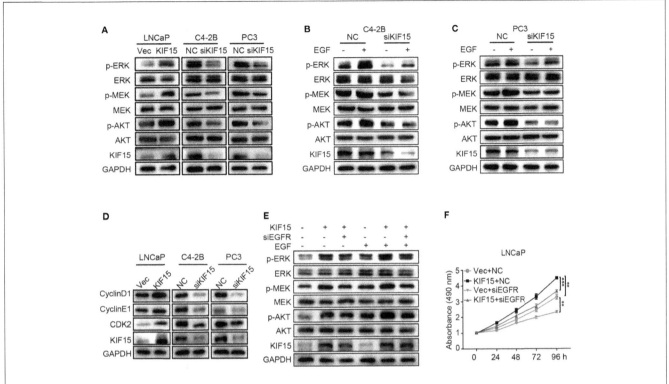

FIGURE 4 | KIF15 activates EGFR signaling in CRPC cells. **(A-C)** Expression of the key molecules in MAPK and PI3K-AKT signaling pathways determined by Western blot in KIF15-overexpressed or depleted PCa cells with or without 20 ng/ml EGF treatment for 20 minutes. **(D)** The expression of cell cycle-related proteins, CyclinD1, CyclinE1, and CDK2 determined by Western blot in the indicated PCa cells with KIF15 overexpression or depletion. **(E)** Expression of the key molecules in MAPK and PI3K-AKT signaling pathways determined by Western blot in KIF15 overexpressed and EGFR depleted LNCaP cells with or without 20 ng/ml EGF treatment for 20 minutes. **(F)** Cell proliferation of LNCaP cells assessed by MTS assays. LNCaP cells were transiently transfected with the indicated expression plasmids and/or siRNA, and cell proliferation was assessed by MTS assays. **P < 0.01; ***P <0.001.

## DISCUSSION

Our studies reveal a novel role of KIF15 that promotes CRPC by activating EGFR signaling pathway in both AR-positive and AR-negative cells. We show that KIF15 is elevated in CRPC cells, and that there is a positive correlation between KIF15 expression and EGFR protein expression levels. Upregulation of EGFR by KIF15 is mediated via a transcription-independent mechanism that involves inhibiting EGFR protein degradation. KIF15 overexpression induced the activation of ERK, MEK, and AKT, which are important molecules downstream of EGFR signaling. Our results indicate that, at least in part, KIF15 promotes CRPC cell proliferation via EGFR-dependent signaling, which highlights a novel and prominent role of KIF15 in contributing to CRPC progression. In addition, our previous studies showed that KIF15 promotes PCa progression by increasing AR protein levels (29). These new findings reveal the extensive role of KIF15 in the progression of CRPC especially in these AR-negative cells.

Although PCa is initially androgen sensitive and responds to androgen deprivation therapies, adaptive survival pathways culminate and CRPC inevitably develops. Multiple mechanisms contribute to the progression to CRPC, including both AR-dependent (44) and AR-independent pathways (45). Although AR is an important driver of CRPC progression (44), the PI3K–AKT–mTOR pathway, Src signaling pathway and growth factor

pathways, which are AR-independent pathways, also play a crucial role in CRPC (7, 18, 46, 47). Thus, novel therapies beside AR inhibition occupy an increasingly important role in the treatment of CRPC (5). Our previous studies showed that KIF15 promotes AR protein stabilization by enhancing the interaction between USP14 and AR in C4-2B enzalutamide resistant cells and 22Rv1 cells (29), suggesting that KIF15 may promote enzalutamide resistance via the AR pathway. In the current study, we focus on the role of KIF15 in CRPC progression and found that KIF15 could enhance the EGFR signaling pathway in both AR positive and negative cells.

Our new findings in this study that KIF15 activates EGFR signaling demonstrates that KIF15 may expedite CRPC progression by multiple pathways including AR-dependent and independent pathways. Multiple studies have highlighted the key role of AR signaling pathway in CRPC. Reactivation of AR signaling is sufficient and necessary to trigger the CRPC phenotype (48, 49). Therefore, although activation of AR and EGFR by KIF15 may simultaneously exist in AR positive CRPC cells, activation of EGFR signaling might act as a collaborative pathway. However, in AR negative CRPC cells, KIF15 may promote tumor cell proliferation through activating EGFR signaling pathway. One limitation of this study is how PTEN status affects KIF15-EGFR axis. LNCaP and C4-2B cells are PTEN-null and exhibit constitutively activated PI3K, whereas

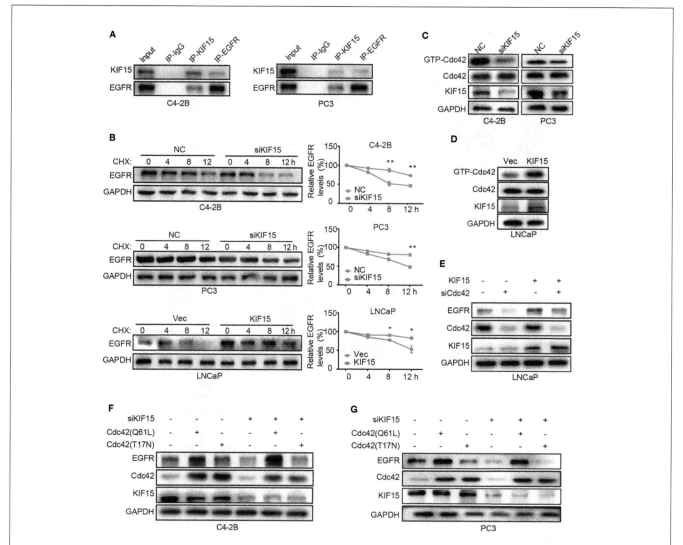

**FIGURE 5 |** KIF15 forms a protein complex with EGFR and inhibits EGFR degradation through Cdc42 in CRPC cells. **(A)** Co-IP assays performed to detect the interaction between KIF15 and EGFR in C4-2B and PC3 cells. Protein lysis was collected from C4-2B and PC3 cells to perform co-IP with control IgG or KIF15 or EGFR antibody, followed by Western blot with indicated antibodies. **(B)** EGFR protein levels determined by immunoblotting. C4-2B (top), PC3 (middle), and LNCaP (bottom) cells were transfected with KIF15 siRNA or KIF15 expression plasmids as indicated. At 24 hours post transfection, cells were then treated with 10 μg/ml CHX and collected at 0, 4, 8, and 12 hours. Western blot assays were performed to analyze EGFR protein levels. $*P < 0.05$; $**P < 0.01$. **(C, D)** GTP-Cdc42 levels analyzed by Western blot in C4-2B, PC3 **(C)**, and LNCaP **(D)** cells with the indicated treatment. C4-2B, PC3, and LNCaP cells were transfected with KIF15 siRNA or KIF15 expression plasmids as indicated. Rho GTPase pulldown assays were performed, and activated Cdc42 (GTP-Cdc42) was measured by Western blot assay. **(E–G)** EGFR protein expression in LNCaP **(E)**, C4-2B **(F)**, and PC3 **(G)** cells with the indicated treatment. LNCaP cells were transfected with KIF15 expression plasmids and siRNA against Cdc42 **(E)**, while C4-2B **(F)**, and PC3 **(G)** cells were transfected with siRNA against KIF15 and Cdc42(T17N) or Cdc42(Q61L) expression plasmids for 48 hours, then were harvested and lysed for Western blot assay.

22Rv1 cells express wild-type PTEN. In the current study, we found that KIF15 could affect EGFR protein expression both in LNCaP, C4-2B as well as in 22Rv1 (**Supplementary Figure S2E**) cells. These data suggested that PTEN status might not affect KIF15-EGFR axis in PCa cells.

Our study showed that AR-induced gene KIF15 is highly expressed in CRPC, which is consistent with the previous study (50). KIF15 expression pattern in PCa is similar with that of COBLL1, an AR-induced gene, which is highly induced in androgen-deprived cells (51). Our explanation of the mechanisms is as follows: 1) Androgen deprivation may result in reactivation of

AR. In this setting, AR is high-sensitive to low androgen. Hypersensitive AR activity is correlated with upregulation of AR-binding genes. As another possibility for inducing AR-binding genes in CRPC cells, previous studies have reported the reprogramming of AR downstream genes (52, 53). 2) Some key genes related with PCa progression are upregulated in androgen-deprived condition, including OCT1 (50), ANCCA (54), and B7-H3 (55). These genes have been reported to regulate KIF15 expression in solid tumors (25, 50, 56) as well as in androgen-deprived condition. 3) Androgen deprivation is associated with pro-inflammatory in PCa (57), and KIF15 has been reported to be

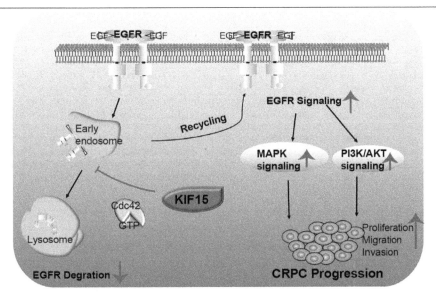

FIGURE 6 | A putative model illustrating the role of KIF15 in up-regulation of EGFR signaling to promote CRPC. EGFR is ubiquitinated by EGF stimulation and sorted to the endosome, resulting in its degradation in lysosomes. KIF15 blocks EGFR from undergoing lysosomal degradation by activating Cdc42 and increases EGFR recycling back to the cell membrane. The MAPK/ERK and PI3K/AKT signaling pathways are activated, both of which can promote the proliferation and invasion of CRPC cells.

upregulated in inflammatory microenvironment (58). Overall, KIF15 may be an important AR-induced gene in the transition from hormone sensitive PCa to CRPC cells.

Di Lorenzo et al. and Jathal et al. have revealed that high EGFR protein correlates with PCa progression and CRPC state (7, 11). There are many mechanisms of EGFR to promote CRPC. The first is the "cross-talk" between EGFR and AR pathways in CRPC cells (59). EGFR enhances AR stability and transcriptional function, and may contribute to AR activity in CRPC (60, 61). Combining the results from our previous studies that KIF15 promotes AR protein stabilization, our new findings in this study suggest that KIF15 may regulate AR not only directly but also in an EGFR-dependent way. The second mechanism involves MAPK and PI3K/AKT pathways activation by EGFR to sustain the growth, survival, invasion and metastasis of CRPC (6). EGFR-stimulated ERK activation is required for the induction and maintenance of the increased expression of Cyclin D1, and ensures G1 phase progression in the cell-cycle (6). As one of the chromokinesin family members, KIF15 is well known for its role in regulating mitotic spindle microtubules to promote cell mitosis (22). Therefore, KIF15 may expedite the cell cycle by accelerating mitosis and by activating ERK to accelerate entrance into the S phase in interphase. Together, our results demonstrate that KIF15 can utilize multiple pathways to expedite CRPC progression.

The degradation of EGFR is regulated by multiple factors. After EGFR binds to ligands, it undergoes dimerization, autophosphorylation, and internalization. Phosphorylated EGFR is ubiquitinated and degraded in lysosomes or recycled back to the cell surface (38, 62). Our findings show that function of KIF15 reduces EGFR degradation by activating Cdc42 in PCa cells. Cdc42 is a ras-related GTP-binding protein that serves as a molecular switch in cells and directs a wide range of cellular processes and signaling activities. Activated Cdc42, through an

interaction with its target/effector, inhibits the binding of c-Cbl (E3 ubiquitination ligase of EGFR) (63) to EGFR and thus prevents c-Cbl from catalyzing receptor ubiquitination. KIF15 promotes EGFR protein stabilization by activating Cdc42, whose mode of action is different from STAP-2, δ-Catenin, and UCHL1 inhibition of EGFR lysosomal degradation by competitive inhibition c-Cbl–mediated ubiquitination or abrogation of EGFR ubiquitination (64–66). These findings also posed additional questions if KIF15 can modulate other proteins in addition to EGFR in a Cdc42-dependent manner to promote CRPC. These implications warrant further investigations.

In conclusion, we further explored the functional role of KIF15 in CRPC and investigated the potential mechanisms of KIF15 in EGFR-mediated development of CRPC. Our findings uncovered that KIF15 inhibition may be considered as a potential novel strategy in CRPC patients.

## AUTHOR CONTRIBUTIONS

LG and RZ contributed to the conception and design of the study as well as data acquisition and interpretation. LG drafted the manuscript. JL, WZ, XW, FS, HL and JH extracted the information from the databases. TF, MW, QL, HD, QY, YQ, WJC and XC contributed to development of methodology. XX, WWC, and BH reviewed the manuscript critically. BH supervised and designed the study. All authors contributed to the article and approved the submitted version.

## SUPPLEMENTARY MATERIAL

Supplementary Figure 1 | KIF15 promotes proliferation and migration of prostate cancer cells in vitro. (A) Western blot analysis of KIF15 protein levels in indicated PCa cells. LNCaP and C4-2B cells were cultured in FBS (RPMI-1640 supplemented with 10% fetal bovine serum) medium or CSS (phenol red-free RPMI-1640 supplemented with 10% charcoal-stripped fetal bovine serum) medium for 48 hours. These cells were transfected with KIF15 expression plasmid for 48 hours (LNCaP cells) or corresponding siRNA for 72 hours (C4-2B cells), then were collected and lysed for Western blot assay. Vec, empty vector; NC, negative control. **(B)** Migration ability of indicated cells determined by transwell assays. Left panel: representative images of cell migration. Right panel: quantitative results of migration assays from triplicate experiments. *$P$ <0.05, **$P$ < 0.01. **(C, D)** Cell proliferation determined by colony formation assays. Data shown are means ± SEM of triplicate wells and are representative of at least three replicate experiments. Comparisons between groups were analyzed using t-tests (two-sided). *$P$ <0.05, **$P$ < 0.01. **(E)** Effects of KIF15 on the cell cycle determined by flow cytometry. Percentage of cells in G1, S and G2 phases are shown. C4-2B and PC3 cells were transfected with corresponding siRNA for 48 hours, then were harvested, and stained with propidium iodide dye for flow cytometric analysis of cell cycle distribution.

**Supplementary Figure 2 |** Relationship between KIF15 and EGFR level in prostate cancer cells. **(A)** GSEA analysis of EGFR signatures (down-regulated after treatment with EGFR inhibitor) from a microarray dataset (GSE2443) that profiled with KIF15_High (the highest 2 samples) or KIF15_Low (the lowest 2 samples) expression. NES = 2.57; $P$ < 0.0001, FDR q < 0.0001. **(B, C)** The protein **(B)** and mRNA **(C)** expression of EGFR determined by Western blot and qRT-PCR analysis after KIF15 transient knockdown in PC3 cells. PC3 cells were transfected with corresponding siRNA for 72 hours, then were harvested and lysed for Western blot assay **(B)**. PC3 cells were transfected with corresponding siRNA for 48 hours. The total RNA was extracted, and the mRNA levels of KIF15 and EGFR were then determined by qRT-PCR **(C)**. *$P$ <0.05, **$P$ < 0.01, ***$P$ <0.001. **(D)** EGFR and KIF15 protein expression levels examined by Western blot in LNCaP cells. LNCaP cells were transiently transfected with the indicated expression plasmids and/or siRNA for 48 hours. The cells were then harvested and lysed for Western blot assay. **(E)** EGFR and KIF15 protein expression levels examined by Western blot after KIF15 siRNA knockdown in 22Rv1 cells. 22Rv1 cells were transiently transfected with corresponding siRNA for 72 hours. The cells were then harvested and lysed for Western blot assay.

# REFERENCES

1. Balk SP. Androgen Receptor Functions in Prostate Cancer Development and Progression. *Asian J Androl* (2014) 16(4):561–4. doi: 10.4103/1008-682X.126396
2. Scher HI, Fizazi K, Saad F, Taplin ME, Sternberg CN, Miller K, et al. Increased Survival With Enzalutamide in Prostate Cancer After Chemotherapy. *N Engl J Med* (2012) 367(13):1187–97. doi: 10.1056/NEJMoa1207506
3. Chen X, Li Q, Liu X, Liu C, Liu R, Rycaj K, et al. Defining a Population of Stem-Like Human Prostate Cancer Cells That Can Generate and Propagate Castration-Resistant Prostate Cancer. *Clin Cancer Res* (2016) 22(17):4505–16. doi: 10.1158/1078-0432.CCR-15-2956
4. Kregel S, Kiriluk KJ, Rosen AM, Cai Y, Reyes EE, Otto KB, et al. Sox2 is an Androgen Receptor-Repressed Gene That Promotes Castration-Resistant Prostate Cancer. *PloS One* (2013) 8(1):e53701. doi: 10.1371/journal.pone.0053701
5. Huang Y, Jiang X, Liang X, Jiang G. Molecular and Cellular Mechanisms of Castration Resistant Prostate Cancer (Review). *Oncol Lett* (2018) 15(5):6063–76. doi: 10.3892/ol.2018.8123
6. Thamilselvan V, Menon M, Stein GS, Valeriote F, Thamilselvan S. Combination of Carmustine and Selenite Inhibits EGFR Mediated Growth Signaling in Androgen-Independent Prostate Cancer Cells. *J Cell Biochem* (2017) 118(12):4331–40. doi: 10.1002/jcb.26086
7. Di Lorenzo G, Tortora G, D'Armiento FP, De Rosa G, Staibano S, Autorino R, et al. Expression of Epidermal Growth Factor Receptor Correlates With Disease Relapse and Progression to Androgen-Independence in Human Prostate Cancer. *Clin Cancer Res* (2002) 8(11):3438–44. doi: 10.3816/cgc.2003.n.013
8. Liao Y, Guo Z, Xia X, Liu Y, Huang C, Jiang L, et al. Inhibition of EGFR Signaling With Spautin-1 Represents a Novel Therapeutics for Prostate Cancer. *J Exp Clin Cancer Res* (2019) 38(1):157. doi: 10.1186/s13046-019-1165-4
9. Shah RB, Ghosh D, Elder JT. Epidermal Growth Factor Receptor (ErbB1) Expression in Prostate Cancer Progression: Correlation With Androgen Independence. *Prostate* (2006) 66(13):1437–44. doi: 10.1002/pros.20460
10. Hernes E, Fossa SD, Berner A, Otnes B, Nesland JM. Expression of the Epidermal Growth Factor Receptor Family in Prostate Carcinoma Before and During Androgen-Independence. *Br J Cancer* (2004) 90(2):449–54. doi: 10.1038/sj.bjc.6601536
11. Jathal MK, Steele TM, Siddiqui S, Mooso BA, D'Abronzo LS, Drake CM, et al. Dacomitinib, But Not Lapatinib, Suppressed Progression in Castration-Resistant Prostate Cancer Models by Preventing HER2 Increase. *Br J Cancer* (2019) 121(3):237–48. doi: 10.1038/s41416-019-0496-4
12. Tzouvelekis A, Ntolios P, Karameris A, Vilaras G, Boglou P, Koulelidis A, et al. Increased Expression of Epidermal Growth Factor Receptor (EGF-R) in Patients With Different Forms of Lung Fibrosis. *BioMed Res Int* (2013) 2013:654354. doi: 10.1155/2013/654354
13. Sigismund S, Avanzato D, Lanzetti L. Emerging Functions of the EGFR in Cancer. *Mol Oncol* (2018) 12(1):3–20. doi: 10.1002/1878-0261.12155
14. Wee P, Wang Z. Epidermal Growth Factor Receptor Cell Proliferation Signaling Pathways. *Cancers (Basel)* (2017) 9(5):52. doi: 10.3390/cancers9050052
15. Yang Y, Goldstein BG, Nakagawa H, Katz JP. Kruppel-Like Factor 5 Activates MEK/ERK Signaling *via* EGFR in Primary Squamous Epithelial Cells. *FASEB J* (2007) 21(2):543–50. doi: 10.1096/fj.06-6694com
16. Parida S, Pal I, Parekh A, Thakur B, Bharti R, Das S, et al. GW627368X Inhibits Proliferation and Induces Apoptosis in Cervical Cancer by Interfering With EP4/EGFR Interactive Signaling. *Cell Death Dis* (2016) 7:e2154. doi: 10.1038/cddis.2016.61
17. Sathya S, Sudhagar S, Sarathkumar B, Lakshmi BS. EGFR Inhibition by Pentacyclic Triterpenes Exhibit Cell Cycle and Growth Arrest in Breast Cancer Cells. *Life Sci* (2014) 95(1):53–62. doi: 10.1016/j.lfs.2013.11.019
18. Chen H, Zhou L, Wu X, Li R, Wen J, Sha J, et al. The PI3K/AKT Pathway in the Pathogenesis of Prostate Cancer. *Front Biosci (Landmark Ed)* (2016) 21:1084–91. doi: 10.2741/4443
19. Kumar R, Srinivasan S, Pahari P, Rohr J, Damodaran C. Activating Stress-Activated Protein Kinase-Mediated Cell Death and Inhibiting Epidermal Growth Factor Receptor Signaling: A Promising Therapeutic Strategy for Prostate Cancer. *Mol Cancer Ther* (2010) 9(9):2488–96. doi: 10.1158/1535-7163.MCT-10-0180
20. Wu W, Yang Q, Fung KM, Humphreys MR, Brame LS, Cao A, et al. Linking Gamma-Aminobutyric Acid A Receptor to Epidermal Growth Factor Receptor Pathways Activation in Human Prostate Cancer. *Mol Cell Endocrinol* (2014) 383(1-2):69–79. doi: 10.1016/j.mce.2013.11.017
21. Hirokawa N, Noda Y, Tanaka Y, Niwa S. Kinesin Superfamily Motor Proteins and Intracellular Transport. *Nat Rev Mol Cell Biol* (2009) 10(10):682–96. doi: 10.1038/nrm2774
22. Drechsler H, McAinsh AD. Kinesin-12 Motors Cooperate to Suppress Microtubule Catastrophes and Drive the Formation of Parallel Microtubule Bundles. *Proc Natl Acad Sci U S A* (2016) 113(12):E1635–44. doi: 10.1073/pnas.1516370113
23. Liu M, Nadar VC, Kozielski F, Kozlowska M, Yu W, Baas PW. Kinesin-12, a Mitotic Microtubule-Associated Motor Protein, Impacts Axonal Growth, Navigation, and Branching. *J Neurosci* (2010) 30(44):14896–906. doi: 10.1523/jneurosci.3739-10.2010
24. Zhao H, Bo Q, Wu Z, Liu Q, Li Y, Zhang N, et al. KIF15 Promotes Bladder Cancer Proliferation *via* the MEK-ERK Signaling Pathway. *Cancer Manag Res* (2019) 11:1857–68. doi: 10.2147/CMAR.S191681
25. Li Q, Qiu J, Yang H, Sun G, Hu Y, Zhu D, et al. Kinesin Family Member 15 Promotes Cancer Stem Cell Phenotype and Malignancy *via* Reactive Oxygen Species Imbalance in Hepatocellular Carcinoma. *Cancer Lett* (2020) 482:112–25. doi: 10.1016/j.canlet.2019.11.008
26. Qiao Y, Chen J, Ma C, Liu Y, Li P, Wang Y, et al. Increased KIF15 Expression Predicts a Poor Prognosis in Patients With Lung Adenocarcinoma. *Cell Physiol Biochem* (2018) 51(1):1–10. doi: 10.1159/000495155
27. Wang J, Guo X, Xie C, Jiang J. KIF15 Promotes Pancreatic Cancer Proliferation *via* the MEK-ERK Signalling Pathway. *Br J Cancer* (2017) 117(2):245–55. doi: 10.1038/bjc.2017.165

28. Zou JX, Duan Z, Wang J, Sokolov A, Xu J, Chen CZ, et al. Kinesin Family Deregulation Coordinated by Bromodomain Protein ANCCA and Histone Methyltransferase MLL for Breast Cancer Cell Growth, Survival, and Tamoxifen Resistance. *Mol Cancer Res* (2014) 12(4):539–49. doi: 10.1158/1541-7786.Mcr-13-0459

29. Gao L, Zhang W, Zhang J, Liu J, Sun F, Liu H, et al. KIF15-Mediated Stabilization of AR and AR-V7 Contributes to Enzalutamide Resistance in Prostate Cancer. *Cancer Res* (2021) 81(4):1026–39. doi: 10.1158/0008-5472

30. Liu H, Wu Z, Zhou H, Cai W, Li X, Hu J, et al. The SOX4/miR-17-92/RB1 Axis Promotes Prostate Cancer Progression. *Neoplasia* (2019) 21(8):765–76. doi: 10.1016/j.neo.2019.05.007

31. Kim JC, Crary B, Chang YC, Kwon-Chung KJ, Kim KJ. Cryptococcus Neoformans Activates RhoGTPase Proteins Followed by Protein Kinase C, Focal Adhesion Kinase, and Ezrin to Promote Traversal Across the Blood-Brain Barrier. *J Biol Chem* (2012) 287(43):36147–57. doi: 10.1074/jbc.M112.389676

32. Cai C, Wang H, He HH, Chen S, He L, Ma F, et al. ERG Induces Androgen Receptor-Mediated Regulation of SOX9 in Prostate Cancer. *J Clin Invest* (2013) 123(3):1109–22. doi: 10.1172/JCI66666

33. Grasso CS, Wu YM, Robinson DR, Cao X, Dhanasekaran SM, Khan AP, et al. The Mutational Landscape of Lethal Castration-Resistant Prostate Cancer. *Nature* (2012) 487(7406):239–43. doi: 10.1038/nature11125

34. Roudier MP, Winters BR, Coleman I, Lam HM, Zhang X, Coleman R, et al. Characterizing the Molecular Features of ERG-Positive Tumors in Primary and Castration Resistant Prostate Cancer. *Prostate* (2016) 76(9):810–22. doi: 10.1002/pros.23171

35. Best CJ, Gillespie JW, Yi Y, Chandramouli GV, Perlmutter MA, Gathright Y, et al. Molecular Alterations in Primary Prostate Cancer After Androgen Ablation Therapy. *Clin Cancer Res* (2005) 11(19 Pt 1):6823–34. doi: 10.1158/1078-0432.CCR-05-0585

36. Liu F, Shangli Z, Hu Z. CAV2 Promotes the Growth of Renal Cell Carcinoma Through the EGFR/PI3K/Akt Pathway. *Onco Targets Ther* (2018) 11:6209–16. doi: 10.2147/OTT.S172803

37. Singh RK, Lokeshwar BL. The IL-8-Regulated Chemokine Receptor CXCR7 Stimulates EGFR Signaling to Promote Prostate Cancer Growth. *Cancer Res* (2011) 71(9):3268–77. doi: 10.1158/0008-5472.CAN-10-2769

38. Min P, Zhao S, Liu L, Zhang Y, Ma Y, Zhao X, et al. MICAL-L2 Potentiates Cdc42-Dependent EGFR Stability and Promotes Gastric Cancer Cell Migration. *J Cell Mol Med* (2019) 23(6):4475–88. doi: 10.1111/jcmm.14353

39. Zhu GF, Xu YW, Li J, Niu HL, Ma WX, Xu J, et al. Mir20a/106a-WTX Axis Regulates RhoGDIa/CDC42 Signaling and Colon Cancer Progression. *Nat Commun* (2019) 10(1):112. doi: 10.1038/s41467-018-07998-x

40. Hirsch D, Shen Y, Wu WJ. Growth and Motility Inhibition of Breast Cancer Cells by Epidermal Growth Factor Receptor Degradation is Correlated With Inactivation of Cdc42. *Cancer Res* (2006) 66: (7):3523–30. doi: 10.1158/0008-5472.Can-05-1547

41. Nalbant P. Activation of Endogenous Cdc42 Visualized in Living Cells. *Science* (2004) 305(5690):1615–9. doi: 10.1126/science.1100367

42. Djiane A, Riou J, Umbhauer M, Boucaut J, Shi D. Role of Frizzled 7 in the Regulation of Convergent Extension Movements During Gastrulation in Xenopus Laevis. *Development* (2000) 127(14):3091–100. doi: 10.1242/dev.127.14.3091

43. Su W, Cheng CY. Cdc42 is Involved in NC1 Peptide-Regulated BTB Dynamics Through Actin and Microtubule Cytoskeletal Reorganization. *FASEB J* (2019) 33(12):14461–78. doi: 10.1096/fj.201900991R

44. Chandrasekar T, Yang JC, Gao AC, Evans CP. Mechanisms of Resistance in Castration-Resistant Prostate Cancer (CRPC). *Transl Androl Urol* (2015) 4(3):365–80. doi: 10.3978/j.issn.2223-4683.2015.05.02

45. Ferraldeschi R, Nava Rodrigues D, Riisnaes R, Miranda S, Figueiredo I, Rescigno P, et al. PTEN Protein Loss and Clinical Outcome From Castration-Resistant Prostate Cancer Treated With Abiraterone Acetate. *Eur Urol* (2015) 67(4):795–802. doi: 10.1016/j.eururo.2014.10.027

46. Kokal M, Mirzakhani K, Pungsrinont T, Baniahmad A. Mechanisms of Androgen Receptor Agonist- and Antagonist-Mediated Cellular Senescence in Prostate Cancer. *Cancers (Basel)* (2020) 12(7):1833. doi: 10.3390/cancers12071833

47. Spreafico A, Chi KN, Sridhar SS, Smith DC, Carducci MA, Kavsak P, et al. A Randomized Phase II Study of Cediranib Alone Versus Cediranib in Combination With Dasatinib in Docetaxel Resistant, Castration Resistant Prostate Cancer Patients. *Invest New Drugs* (2014) 32(5):1005–16. doi: 10.1007/s10637-014-0106-5

48. Huang Y, Jiang X, Liang X, Jiang G. Molecular and Cellular Mechanisms of Castration Resistant Prostate Cancer. *Oncol Lett* (2018) 15(5):6063–76. doi: 10.3892/ol.2018.8123

49. Coutinho I, Day TK, Tilley WD, Selth LA. Androgen Receptor Signaling in Castration-Resistant Prostate Cancer: A Lesson in Persistence. *Endocr Relat Cancer* (2016) 23(12):T179–t97. doi: 10.1530/erc-16-0422

50. Yamamoto S, Takayama KI, Obinata D, Fujiwara K, Ashikari D, Takahashi S, et al. Identification of New Octamer Transcription Factor 1-Target Genes Upregulated in Castration-Resistant Prostate Cancer. *Cancer Sci* (2019) 110(11):3476–85. doi: 10.1111/cas.14183

51. Takayama KI, Suzuki T, Fujimura T, Takahashi S, Inoue S. COBLL1 Modulates Cell Morphology and Facilitates Androgen Receptor Genomic Binding in Advanced Prostate Cancer. *Proc Natl Acad Sci U S A* (2018) 115(19):4975–80. doi: 10.1073/pnas.1721957115

52. Wang Q, Li W, Zhang Y, Yuan X, Xu K, Yu J, et al. Androgen Receptor Regulates a Distinct Transcription Program in Androgen-Independent Prostate Cancer. *Cell* (2009) 138(2):245–56. doi: 10.1016/j.cell.2009.04.056

53. Jin HJ, Zhao JC, Wu L, Kim J, Yu J. Cooperativity and Equilibrium With FOXA1 Define the Androgen Receptor Transcriptional Program. *Nat Commun* (2014) 5:3972. doi: 10.1038/ncomms4972

54. Zou JX, Guo L, Revenko AS, Tepper CG, Gemo AT, Kung HJ, et al. Androgen-Induced Coactivator ANCCA Mediates Specific Androgen Receptor Signaling in Prostate Cancer. *Cancer Res* (2009) 69(8):3339–46. doi: 10.1158/0008-5472.Can-08-3440

55. Benzon B, Zhao SG, Haffner MC, Takhar M, Erho N, Yousefi K, et al. Correlation of B7-H3 With Androgen Receptor, Immune Pathways and Poor Outcome in Prostate Cancer: An Expression-Based Analysis. *Prostate Cancer Prostatic Dis* (2017) 20(1):28–35. doi: 10.1038/pcan.2016.49

56. Ma Y, Zhan S, Lu H, Wang R, Xu Y, Zhang G, et al. B7-H3 Regulates KIF15-Activated ERK1/2 Pathway and Contributes to Radioresistance in Colorectal Cancer. *Cell Death Dis* (2020) 11(10):824. doi: 10.1038/s41419-020-03041-4

57. Mangiola S, Stuchbery R, McCoy P, Chow K, Kurganovs N, Kerger M, et al. Androgen Deprivation Therapy Promotes an Obesity-Like Microenvironment in Periprostatic Fat. *Endocr Connect* (2019) 8(5):547–58. doi: 10.1530/ec-19-0029

58. Kitagawa A, Masuda T, Takahashi J, Tobo T, Noda M, Kuroda Y, et al. KIF15 Expression in Tumor-Associated Monocytes Is a Prognostic Biomarker in Hepatocellular Carcinoma. *Cancer Genomics Proteomics* (2020) 17(2):141–9. doi: 10.21873/cgp.20174

59. Traish AM, Morgentaler A. Epidermal Growth Factor Receptor Expression Escapes Androgen Regulation in Prostate Cancer: A Potential Molecular Switch for Tumour Growth. *Br J Cancer* (2009) 101(12):1949–56. doi: 10.1038/sj.bjc.6605376

60. Mellinghoff IK, Tran C, Sawyers CL. Growth Inhibitory Effects of the Dual ErbB1/ErbB2 Tyrosine Kinase Inhibitor PKI-166 on Human Prostate Cancer Xenografts. *Cancer Res* (2002) 62(18):5254–9. doi: 10.1016/s1359-6349(07)71012-1

61. Gregory CW, Fei X, Ponguta LA, He B, Bill HM, French FS, et al. Epidermal Growth Factor Increases Coactivation of the Androgen Receptor in Recurrent Prostate Cancer. *J Biol Chem* (2004) 279(8):7119–30. doi: 10.1074/jbc.M307649200

62. Zhang B, Zhang Y, Jiang X, Su H, Wang Q, Wudu M, et al. JMJD8 Promotes Malignant Progression of Lung Cancer by Maintaining EGFR Stability and EGFR/PI3K/AKT Pathway Activation. *J Cancer* (2021) 12(4):976–87. doi: 10.7150/jca.50234

63. Wu WJ, Tu S, Cerione RA. Activated Cdc42 Sequesters C-Cbl and Prevents EGF Receptor Degradation. *Cell* (2003) 114(6):715–25. doi: 10.1016/s0092-8674(03)00688-3

64. Kitai Y, Iwakami M, Saitoh K, Togi S, Isayama S, Sekine Y, et al. STAP-2 Protein Promotes Prostate Cancer Growth by Enhancing Epidermal Growth Factor Receptor Stabilization. *J Biol Chem* (2017) 292(47):19392–9. doi: 10.1074/jbc.M117.802884

65. Shrestha N, Shrestha H, Ryu T, Kim H, Simkhada S, Cho YC, et al. Delta-Catenin Increases the Stability of EGFR by Decreasing C-Cbl Interaction and Enhances EGFR/Erk1/2 Signaling in Prostate Cancer. *Mol Cells* (2018) 41(4):320–30. doi: 10.14348/molcells.2018.2292

66. Bi HL, Zhang XL, Zhang YL, Xie X, Xia YL, Du J, et al. The Deubiquitinase UCHL1 Regulates Cardiac Hypertrophy by Stabilizing Epidermal Growth Factor Receptor. *Sci Adv* (2020) 6(16):eaax4826. doi: 10.1126/sciadv.aax4826

# 9

# Clinical Utility of $^{18}$F-PSMA-1007 Positron Emission Tomography/Magnetic Resonance Imaging in Prostate Cancer

*Ao Liu[1†], Miao Zhang[2†], Hai Huang[1], Chuanjie Zhang[1], Xiaohao Ruan[1], Wenhao Lin[1], Biao Li[2\*], Lu Chen[1\*] and Danfeng Xu[1\*]*

[1] Department of Urinary Surgery, Ruijin Hospital, Shanghai Jiaotong University School of Medicine, Shanghai, China,
[2] Department of Nuclear Medicine, Ruijin Hospital, Shanghai Jiaotong University School of Medicine, Shanghai, China

**\*Correspondence:**
Lu Chen
cl12063@rjh.com.cn
Biao Li
lb10363@rjh.com.cn
Danfeng Xu
xdf12036@rjh.com.cn

†These authors have contributed equally to this work

**Purpose:** This study aimed to evaluate the clinical utility of $^{18}$F-PSMA-1007 positron emission tomography (PSMA PET)/magnetic resonance imaging (MRI) imaging in patients with suspected or defined prostate cancer.

**Methods:** In the pilot study, we retrospectively investigated 62 patients who underwent PSMA-PET/MRI for suspected or defined PCa between June 2019 and June 2020. Patients were grouped into three subgroups: (1) suspected PCa without histological evidence, (2) primary PCa, (3) biochemical recurrent prostate cancer (BRPCa). Two nuclear physicians independently interpreted the results of PSMA-PET/MRI. Management strategies before PSMA-PET/MRI were retrospectively reported, and the management strategy was re-evaluated for each patient considering the PSMA-PET/MRI result. The changes in strategies were recorded. Besides, the correlation between prostate specific antigen (PSA) level and management changes was also accessed by Fisher exact test, and two-side $p < 0.05$ was assumed as statistical significance.

**Results:** There were 28 patients in the suspected PCa group (group 1), 12 in the primary PCa group (group 2), and 22 in the BRPCa group (group 3). Overall, the intended decisions were changed in 26 (41.9%) of 62 patients after PSMA-PET/MRI, including 11/28 (39.3%) in suspected PCa group, 1/12 (8.4%) in primary PCa group, and 14/24 (63.6%) in BCR group. In group 1, the main impact on subsequent management included decreased active surveillance (from 20 to 9) and increased prostate biopsy (from 8 to 19). PSA levels were not significantly associated with management changes in suspected PCa patients ($p = 0.865$). In group 2, the main impact on subsequent management included decreased radical surgery (from 8 to 7), and multimodal therapy appearance ($n = 1$). Only in the category of PSA levels of $\geq 20$ ng/ml, the management of primary PCa was changed. In group 3, the main impact on subsequent management included decreased salvage radiotherapy (from 5 to 2), increased systemic therapy (from 6 to 7), and increased multimodal therapy (from 11 to 13). The highest proportion of management changes occurred in BCR patients with 0.5≤PSA<1 ng/ml.

**Conclusion:** From our preliminary experience, PSMA-PET/MRI may be a valued tool for defining PCa lesions and changing management. The biggest impact of management intent was in patients with BRPCa, especially in patients with 0.5≤PSA<1 ng/ml. However, further studies are needed to confirm our pilot findings.

**Keywords: prostate specific membrane antigen, positron emission tomography, magnetic resonance imaging, prostate cancer, management**

# INTRODUCTION

Prostate cancer (PCa) is the most frequent malignancy in men in the western world (1). In China, though lower incidence rate, significantly increased incidence and mortality of PCa are worth to rise our guard (2). Multi-parametric magnetic resonance imaging (mpMRI) is a standard imaging technique in the field of PCa, and confirmed its value in improving the detection of clinically significant PCa (csPCa) and guiding prostate biopsy (3). However, missed diagnoses of PCa and unnecessary biopsies are still unavoidable (4). For primary PCa, localized or locally advanced PCa is mainly treated with radical prostatectomy (RP), while metastatic PCa require systemic treatment *via* androgen deprivation therapy (ADT) or chemotherapy. Nevertheless, exact local and whole-body staging in a single investigation remains a challenge with conventional imaging techniques. Additionally, after primary treatment, increasing serum PSA levels greater than 0.2 ng/ml, confirmed by two consecutive measurements, can be defined as biochemical recurrence (BCR). In patients with recurrent disease, accurate evaluation of recurrence location and whole-body tumor burden are essential in patient-specific therapy planning. However, conventional imaging modalities including CT, bone scan, MRI, and more recently choline-PET/CT are all typically negative at low PSA values (5).

To solve this challenging issue, a new molecular imaging technique named prostate specific membrane antigen (PSMA) PET was introduced into clinical practice. This new PET tracer relies on the highly specific expression of PSMA by PCa cells. PSMA is a transmembrane type II glycoprotein, overexpressed in PCa cells, and increased with higher grades, metastasis development, and disease recurrence (6). A series of studies have indicated the priority of this new technique over conventional imaging in the field of primary staging and recurrence location (7). MRI provides much better soft tissue contrast and shows a higher sensitivity in detecting bone metastases in PCa. A combined approach with PSMA PET and mpMRI is capable of acquiring PET and MR data simultaneously or sequentially in a single examination. A potential added value of PSMA PET/MRI can be expected in prostate cancer. Recent studies suggested that PSMA-PET/MRI can provide superior detection efficacy as well as a considerable impact on decision-making (8). Sangwon Han et al. reviewed all studies assessing the impact of PSMA PE/CT and PET/MRI in patients with PCa, and found the proportion of management changes was 54% (9).

To our knowledge, the impact of PSMA PET/MRI on the management has not been determined in patients with defined PCa. Moreover, its impact regarding changes in decision-making for patients suspected of PCa has not been assessed. It is important to evaluate the role of PSMA PET/MRI in management changes for wide acceptance of this new technology by referring physicians in clinical practice.

We initially performed simultaneous [18]F-PSMA-1007 PET/MRI in patients with suspected PCa, primary PCa, and BRPCa patients, and investigated its impact on decision-making. Besides, we explored the potential association between PSA levels and management change.

# MATERIAL AND METHODS

## Patients and Methods

Patients were retrospectively identified and grouped into three subgroups: group 1 comprised patients with suspected PCa (PSA level >4 ng/ml, and/or digital rectal examination abnormality, and/or positive imaging); group 2 included men undergoing primary staging for primary PCa; group 3 comprised patients undergoing imaging for BCR with PSA levels greater than 0.2 ng/ml. Other inclusion criteria: age between 18 to 85 years, ability to understand study procedures, and volunteering to participate in this study. Exclusion criteria were acute prostatitis, the presence of any other concomitant cancers, PSA values less than 0.2 ng/ml, and transurethral resection of prostate (TURP) history. The study was approved by the Ethics Committee of Shanghai Ruijin Hospital (Approved No. 2019-18), and written informed consent was obtained from all patients.

Patient-related clinical information was collected by a urologist with more than 3 years' experience. Serum PSA levels were recorded closest to the scan. Two records of PSA value for each BRPCa patient within a 12-mo period before the scan were applied to calculate PSA doubling time (PSADT). A questionnaire was adapted from Roach et al. (10) to record management plans before and after PSMA PET/MRI. Management strategies were decided by a multidisciplinary meeting (MDM) consisting of urologists, pathologists, radiologists, and nuclear medicine physicians. All patients underwent a simultaneous [18]F-FDG PET and mpMRI before PSMA-PET/MRI examination. The initial management strategy was retrospectively decided by MDM discussion according to simultaneous [18]F-FDG PET and mpMRI results. After PSMA-PET/MRI examination, each pre-planned strategy was modified according to the PSMA-PET/MRI result, and revised managements from MDM discussion were recorded. The impact of PSMA PET/MRI on management was measured as the proportion of patients whose treatment was changed from a previous plan.

## Imaging Protocol and Interpretation

[18]F-PSMA-1007 was produced as described by Cardinale et al. (11). Each patient received an intravenous injection of [18]F-PSMA-1007 with a median dose of 263 MBq (range 164-353 MBq), then a PET/MRI examination was performed from the vertex to mid-thighs after 60 min of tracer uptake time using an integrated PET/MRI system (Biograph mMR, Siemens Healthcare). All [18]F-PSMA-1007 PET/MRI images were analyzed independently with dedicated software (Syngovia version VB 10, Siemens Healthcare). In line with published literature, any focal uptake of [18]F-PSMA-1007 ligand higher than the surrounding background without correspondence to physiologic uptake was considered positive. Two experienced nuclear medicine physicians (M.Z., B.L.) interpreted the [18]F-PSMA-1007 PET/MRI images, and disagreements were resolved by consensus.

## Management Decision Review

Based on the NCCN guidelines strictly, both the initial management plan and the revised management plan were made by MDM discussion (two urologist, one pathologist, one radiologist, and two nuclear medicine physicians), and all disagreements were resolved by consensus. For patients with suspected PCa, management decisions were categorized as active surveillance (AS) and prostate biopsy. A prostate biopsy was suggested for patients with elevated PSA levels (more than 4 ng/ml), or digital rectal examination abnormality, or positive imaging. For defined PCa patients, management decisions were categorized as active surveillance (AS), surgery (radical prostatectomy with or without pelvic lymph nodes dissection), salvage radiotherapy (sRT), systemic therapy (anti-androgen therapy or chemotherapy), and multimodal therapy (more than one type of the therapies mentioned above). Radical prostatectomy (RP) was a standard therapy for primary localized or locally advanced PCa. Systemic therapy was considered when patients with positive lymph nodes (LNs) out of pelvic and/or distant metastases in patients with primary PCa. For BRPCa patients, when the imaging was negative, AS, sRT, or ADT were selected according to clinical treatment history or doctor's experience. Systemic therapy or multimodal therapy was considered when imaging was positive. Additionally, simultaneous integrated boost intensity-modulated RT (SIB-IMRT) was considered when imaging was positive in the prostate bed or pelvic LNs. Stereotactic body radiotherapy (SBRT) is also considered as an option in oligometastatic patients.

## Statistical Analysis

All the demographic and clinical data were assessed by descriptive analysis. For continuous variables, medians and interquartile range (IQR) were reported. For categorical variables, counts

and percentages were calculated. PSADT was calculated according to the method described by Khan et al. (12). All analysis was assessed using SPSS software (version 22.0.0, IBM Corp., Armonk, NY, USA) and R 3.6.2 framework. Relationships between clinical variables and positive rates or management change accessed by Fisher's exact test, and two-side $p < 0.05$ was assumed as statistical significance.

# RESULTS

## Patient Characteristics

From June 2019 to June 2020, 62 consecutive patients who underwent PSMA-PET/MRI were retrospectively identified. The basic information of patients was summarized in **Table 1**. There were 28 patients in group 1 with median age of 63.5 years (IQR 60.5–68.0 years), and median PSA level of 9.8 ng/ml (IQR 6.5–13.1). Fifteen (53.6%) patients in group 1 had received a prostate biopsy in the past. There were 12 patients in group 2 with median age of 68.5 years (IQR 64.5–73.8 years), and median PSA level of 29.9 ng/ml (IQR 7.0–100.7). Four patients in group 2 had distant metastasis. Moreover, five patients in group 2 were receiving ADT at PET/MRI. There are 22 patients in group 3 with median age of

**TABLE 1** | Basic characteristics of patients.

| Clinical variable | Suspected PCa (n = 28) | Primary PCa (n = 12) | BRPCa (n = 22) |
|---|---|---|---|
| Mean age, years, (IQR) | 63.5 (60.5–68.0) | 68.5 (64.5–75.8) | 70.5 (63.0–75.8) |
| Median PSA, ng/ml, (IQR) | 9.8 (6.5–13.1) | 29.9 (7.0–100.7) | 2.0 (0.9–4.7) |
| Median PSAdt, months, (IQR) | / | / | 2.1 (1.5–5.6) |
| ISUP group, n (%) | / | | |
| 2 | | 5 (41.7) | 5 (22.7) |
| 3 | | 1 (8.3) | 6 (27.3) |
| 4 | | 1 (8.3) | 2 (9.1) |
| 5 | | 4 (33.3) | 5 (4.5) |
| NA | | 1 (8.3) | 4 (18.1) |
| Tumor stage, n (%) | / | | |
| T2 | | 6 (50.0) | 7 (31.8) |
| T3 | | 1 (8.3) | 11 (50.0) |
| T4 | | 5 (41.7) | 3 (13.6) |
| NA | | 0 | 1 (4.5) |
| Nodal stage, n (%) | / | | |
| N0 | | 7 (58.3) | 16 (72.7) |
| N1 | | 5 (41.7) | 5 (22.7) |
| NA | | 0 | 1 (4.5) |
| Metastasis stage | / | | |
| M0 | | 8 (66.7) | 17 (77.3) |
| M1 | | 4 (33.3) | 4 (18.2) |
| NA | | 0 | 1 (4.5) |
| Previous management, n (%) | | | |
| Prostate biopsy | 15 (53.6) | 12 (100) | 22 (100) |
| Curative therapy | 0 | 0 | 17 (77.3) |
| ADT history, n (%) | 0 | 0 | 17 (77.3) |
| Ongoing ADT, n (%) | 0 | 4 (33.3) | 13 (59.1) |

*Note. PCa, prostate cancer; BRPCa, biochemical recurrence prostate cancer; PSA, prostate specific antigen; ADT, androgen deprivation therapy; PSADT, prostate specific antigen doubling time.*

70.5 years (IQR 63.0–75.8 years), and median PSA level of 2.0 ng/ml (IQR 0.94–4.67). In 17 (77.3%) of 22 patients, the initial treatment was curative therapy, and in 5 (22.7%) of 22 patients, the initial treatment was ADT. There were 15 patients in group 3 were receiving ADT at PET/MRI, and 19 patients had ADT history. Management change details and follow-up information were presented in **Table 2**. A rose diagram shows the distribution of managements before PSMA PET/MRI, after PSMA PET/MRI, and implemented management in **Figure 1**. The management changes of each patient were detailed in **Supplementary Figure 1**.

## Changes in Suspected Prostate Cancer

[18]F-PSMA-1007 PET/MRI was positive in 17 (60.7%) patients and negative in 11 (39.3%) patients. [18]F-PSMA-1007 PET/MRI resulted in a change of management in 11 (39.3%) patients. Before PSMA, 8 patients planned to perform prostate biopsy, and 20 patients planned to undergo AS. After [18]F-PSMA-1007 PET/MRI, we suggested 19 patients perform prostate biopsy, and 9 patients to perform AS. In 27 suspected PCa patients with PSA data before PSMA PET/MRI, the positive rates were 0, 73, and 75% with PSA levels of <4 ng/ml, 4 ≤ PSA < 10 ng/ml, and PSA ≥ 10 ng/ml, respectively. The proportions of management changes were 0, 55, and 42% with PSA <4 ng/ml, 4 ≤ PSA < 10 ng/ml, and PSA ≥ 10 ng/ml, respectively (**Figure 2**). There was a significant association between PSA groups and PSMA positivity (p = 0.027). Higher PSA levels were not associated with decision-making changes (p = 0.865). A patient who shifted treatment was exemplified in **Figure 3**.

Follow-up is available for a median of 5.5 months (range 4–15 months) in 28 suspected patients. Details of management implementation were given in **Figure 1** and **Table 2**. There were 13 patients underwent biopsy (one patient have RP directly), 14 patients insisted on active surveillance, and one patient without pathological evidence underwent ADT directly, and was followed with decreased PSA level. Finally, seven patients were confirmed as PCa, six patients were negative for PCa. For the three positive patients who insisted on active surveillance, one patient had increased PSA (up to 13.8 ng/ml), one patient was lost, and one patient had stable PSA (19.2 ng/ml). For the 11 patients with negative PSMA PET/MRI, all of them selected AS, and no PCa was found till the last follow-up date. The follow-up PSA evolution and pathology evolution were detailed in **Table 2**.

## Changes in Primary Prostate Cancer

[18]F-PSMA-1007 PET/MRI was positive in all primary patients and resulted in a change of management in 1 (8.3%) patient. One patient shifted management from RP with PLND to multimodal therapy because of the detection of oligometastatic lesions. As shown in **Figure 2**, No management changes occurred in patients with PSA less than 20 ng/ml. Only in the category of PSA levels of ≥20 ng/ml, the management of primary PCa was changed (14% of patients).

Follow-up is available for a median of 9 months (range 4–15 months) in 12 primary PCa patients. Details of management implementation and follow-up PSA evolution were given in **Figure 1** and **Table 2**. PSMA PET/MRI identified localized or locally advanced PCa in seven patients, and PCa with distant metastases in five patients. In the seven patients without metastases, five patients underwent RP and the majority was

**TABLE 2 |** Management before and after [18]F-PSMA-1007 PET/MRI in patients with suspected PCa, primary PCa, and BRPCa.

| Management blinded to PSMA | Revised management plan | Implemented management | Follow-up PSA or pathological evolution |
|---|---|---|---|
| **Patients with suspected PCa (n = 28)** | | | |
| AS (20) | AS (9) | AS (9) | 8↓and 1→ |
| | Prostate biopsy (11) | AS (2) | 1↑and 1NA |
| | | Prostate biopsy (8) | 4 pos and 4 neg |
| | | RP (1) | 1 pos |
| Prostate biopsy (8) | Prostate biopsy (8) | AS (3) | 3→ |
| | | Prostate biopsy (4) | 2 pos and 2 neg |
| | | Systemic therapy (1) | 1↓ |
| **Primary PCa patients (n =12)** | | | |
| Surgery (8) | Surgery (7) | Surgery (5) | 4↓↓and 1↓ |
| | | Systemic therapy (2) | 1↓↓and 1↓ |
| | Multimodal therapy (1) | Systemic therapy (1) | 1↓ |
| Systemic therapy (4) | Systemic therapy (4) | AS (1) | 1↓ |
| | | Systemic therapy (3) | 3↓ |
| **BRPCa patients (n = 22)** | | | |
| sRT (5) | sRT (2) | Systemic therapy (2) | 2↓↓ |
| | Multimodal therapy (3) | Multimodal therapy (3) | 3↓↓ |
| Systemic therapy (6) | Systemic therapy (6) | Systemic therapy (5) | 2↑and 2↓and 1→ |
| | | Multimodal therapy (1) | 1→ |
| Multimodal therapy (11) | Systemic therapy (1) | Systemic therapy (1) | 1↓↓ |
| | Multimodal therapy (10) | Systemic therapy (1) | 1↑ |
| | (all with minor change) | Multimodal therapy (9) | 5↓↓and 2↓and 2↑ |

PCa, prostate cancer; BRPCa, biochemical recurrence prostate cancer; AS, Active surveillance; RP, Radical prostatectomy; sRT, salvage radiotherapy.
PSA evolution, ↑ (increased PSA level); ↓ (measurable decreased PSA level); ↓↓(indosable PSA level);→ (stable PSA level); NA (not available).
Pathological evolution : pos (positive pathology); neg (negative pathology).

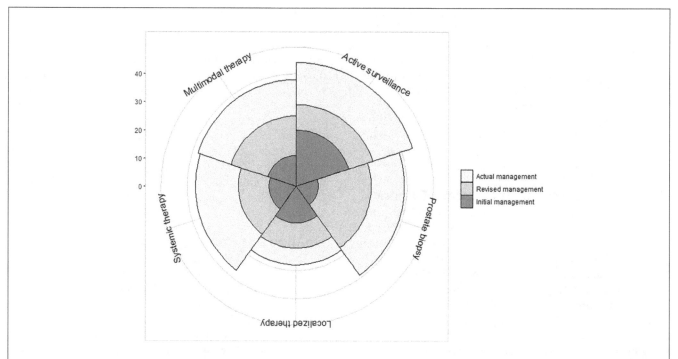

**FIGURE 1** | Rose diagram shows the distribution of managements before 18F-PSMA-1007 PET/MRI (initial management), after 18F-PSMA-1007 PET/MRI (revised management), and implemented management (actual management). Management decisions were categorized as active surveillance, prostate biopsy, localized therapy (surgery and salvageable pelvic radiotherapy), systemic therapy (anti-androgen therapy or chemotherapy), and multimodal therapy (more than one therapy type).

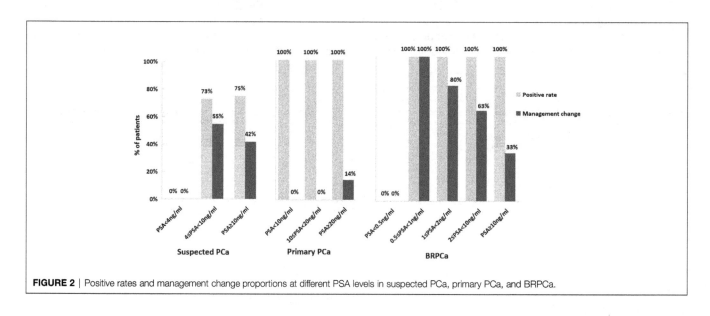

**FIGURE 2** | Positive rates and management change proportions at different PSA levels in suspected PCa, primary PCa, and BRPCa.

followed with undetectable PSA level (defined as <0.008 ng/ml), one patient with advanced PCa was planned to underwent neoadjuvant complete androgen blockade (CAB) for 3 to 6 months, and one patient with life expectancy <5 years also received CAB therapy. In the five patients with distant metastases, four patients with systemic therapy was followed with decreased PSA level, one patient was treated with Chinese traditional medicine and was followed with decreased PSA level.

## Changes in Biochemical Recurrent Prostate Cancer

In the BRPCa group, [18]F-PSMA-1007 PET/MRI was positive in 20 (90.9%) of 22 patients. Fourteen (63.6%) of 22 patients changed management plans after the examination. In three patients with positive finding beyond pelvis, the initial pelvic radiotherapy was changed into multimodal therapy. One patient in the multimodal group shifted to systemic therapy, and the

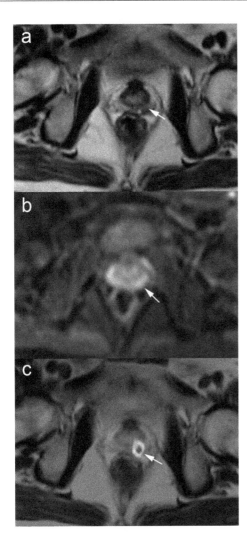

FIGURE 3 | A patient treated with management change in suspected PCa. Images from a 59-year-old male with a PSA level of 7.07 ng/ml. No tumor detection within the prostate is achievable with T2-weighted or DWI sequence alone (A, B), but fused PET/MRI demonstrates tumor involvement of the left lobe (C, white arrow). The management plan was shifted from active surveillance to biopsy. The subsequent prostate biopsy confirmed Gleason 4 + 3 prostate cancer in the ipsilateral lobe.

other 10 patients in multimodal therapy also had minor management changes (the combination of therapy types changed, or the same treatment types with more or less aggressive/extended approach), as exemplified in **Figure 4**. Finally, the number of patients of sRT decreased from 5 to 2, systemic therapy increased from 6 to 7, and multimodal therapy increased from 11 to 13. No patients with PSA values less than 0.5 ng/ml had positive imaging, and all patients with PSA values of ≥0.5 ng/ml had at least one positive lesion. Management change rate ranged from 0 to 100% for the several categories of PSA levels. The highest proportion of management change occurred in patients with $0.5 \leq$ PSA $< 1$ ng/ml (**Figure 2**). Higher PSA levels were significantly associated with positive results (p = 0.004). There was no significant association between

PSA and management change (p = 1.000). We also explored the relation between PSADT and positive rates or proportions of management change, though only 16 patients had sufficient information. From patients with PSADT levels of ≤3 months to >3 months, the positive rate decreased from 90.9 to 80.0% and the proportion of management change decreased from 63.6 to 40.0%. PSADT categories were not significantly associated with positive rates (p = 1.000) or proportions of management change (p = 0.596).

Follow-up is available for a median of 9 months (range 4–15 months) in 22 BRPCa patients. Details of management implementation were given in **Figure 1** and **Table 2**. Two patients with negative [18]F-PSMA-1007 PET/MRI results selected combined androgen blockade (CAB) therapy, as there was ongoing concern about regional recurrent disease due to a continuing rise in PSA, and finally achieved undetectable PSA level. In the 20 patients with positive PSMA-PET/MRI imaging, 7 patients underwent CAB therapy or ADT plus abiraterone therapy, and 13 patients underwent multimodal therapy. The majority of patients with multi-modal treatment received ADT and sRT except one patient who received salvage PLND combined with CAB therapy. The follow-up PSA evolution was detailed in **Table 2**.

## Management Plans Remained After [18]F-PSMA-1007 Positron Emission Tomography/Magnetic Resonance Imaging

Concerning the patients whose treatment plans were not revised after [18]F-PSMA-1007 PET/MRI, group 1 included 17/28 patients, group 2 included 11/12 patients, and group 3 included 8/22 patients. In the suspected PCa group, nine patients with negative PSMA results remained AS, and eight patients met the criteria of biopsy and were suggested to perform prostate biopsy. In group 2, surgery was already planned in seven patients with localized PCa, and subsequent PSMA PET/MRI confirmed localized disease. Four patients with multiple metastases were unfit for focal treatment after the initial evaluation and then confirmed by the PSMA PET/MRI. In group 3, there were six patients with multiple metastasis remained systemic therapy, and two patients with both negative conventional imaging and PSMA-PET/MRI remained sRT. The plans that were not altered are presented in detail in **Table 3**.

## DISCUSSION

Accurate detection of tumor existence, tumor staging as well as the recurrent lesions is crucial for patients before initiation of any kind of management. PET/MRI has emerged as a promising molecular imaging technique being explored in the field of prostate cancer (9). Despite a relatively small sample size, we reports that [18]F-PSMA-1007 PET/MRI could change the clinical decision-making in 39.3% of suspected PCa patients, 8.4% of primary PCa patients, and 63.6% of BRPCa patients. Our results

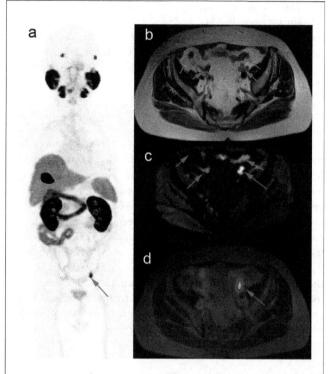

**FIGURE 4 |** A patient treated with management change in BRPCa. Images from 79-year-old male after radical prostatectomy (June 2018, Gleason score 4 + 4), following with combined androgen blockade therapy, and with PSA values rising to 0.375 ng/ml (August 2019). T2-weighted and DWI images show multiple suspicious nodes in the pelvis **(B, C)**. However, maximum-intensity projection of $^{18}$F-PSMA-1007 PET and fused PET/MRI images show intense tracer-associated uptake in only two lymph nodes **(A, D**, red arrow). Management plan was revised from androgen deprivation therapy combined with external beam radiotherapy to salvage pelvic lymph nodes dissection in combination with external beam radiotherapy.

**TABLE 3 |** Management plans that were not altered after $^{18}$F-PSMA-1007 PET/MRI.

| Patient types | Management plan | Reasons |
|---|---|---|
| Suspected PCa (17) | Prostate biopsy (8) AS (9) | Negative PSMA results (9); PSA >4 ng/ml and/or abnormal nodes in prostate and/or positive imaging (8). |
| Primary PCa (11) | Systemic therapy (4) Surgery (7) | Polymetastasis was seen on conventional imaging, PSMA detected more lesions but without influence on management (4); PSMA confirmed localized PCa (7). |
| BRPCa (8) | sRT (2) Systemic therapy (6) | BCR patients with negative imaging (2) CRPC patients with polymetastasis (6). |

*PCa, prostate cancer; BRPCa, biochemical recurrence prostate cancer; CRPC, castration resistant prostate cancer; EBRT, external beam radiotherapy; PLND, pelvic lymph nodes dissection; sRT, salvageable radiotherapy.*

indicate that the biggest impact caused by $^{18}$F-PSMA-1007 PET/MRI on decision-making occurred in the BRPCa group, especially in patients with 0.5 ≤ PSA <1 ng/ml. A review of the literature shows that 27 studies also reported the impact of PSMA-PET on management in patients with primary PCa or

BRPCa, but only one looked at primary PCa patients was based on PSMA-PET/MRI (**Supplementary Table 1**). To our knowledge, this is the first study to explore the impact of simultaneous $^{18}$F-PSMA-1007 PET/MRI on clinical management in suspected PCa, primary PCa, and BRPCa patients. Totally, we conducted a real-life clinical utility of $^{18}$F-PSMA-1007 PET/MRI in PCa field and it has been shown to be promising and useful tools in the clinical decision making of PCa patients, especially for BRPCa patients.

## Changes in Suspected Prostate Cancer

In recent years, several small-scale reports have successively confirmed the application of PSMA-PET in suspected PCa. Especially, PSMA-PET guided prostate biopsy may be a valuable alternative to improve the detection rate of clinically significant prostate cancer (csPCa). Le-Le Zhang et al. included 60 patients with suspected PCa, 25 patients with positive results underwent PSMA-PET guided target biopsy. Finally, PCa and csPCa were detected in 21/60 (35.0%) and 20/60 (33.3%) patients, respectively (13). Chen Liu et al. investigated 31 suspected PCa patients with prior negative biopsy. All patients underwent PSMA PET-ultrasound fusion image-guided biopsy. Imaging was positive in 18 patients, and csPCa was detected in 12 of 31 patients (38.7%) (14). Lopci et al. prospectively observed 45 patients suspicious for prostate cancer. The cohort comprised men with equivocal mpMRI and at least one negative biopsy. Twenty-five patients (55.5%) with positive results underwent PSMA-PET guided prostate biopsy, and the detection rate of prostate cancer was 44% (15). In our study, 13/17 patients with positive results underwent biopsy (including one patient who underwent RP directly). Finally, seven (53.8%) and six (46.2%) patients were confirmed as PCa and csPCa (Gleason score 7 or greater), respectively. Compared with Lopci et al., we included three patients with positive MRI and only 15 of 23 (53.6%) patients had negative biopsy history, which may partly explain the high positive rates of imaging and pathology. After $^{18}$F-PSMA-1007 PET/MRI, there was an increase in the use of prostate biopsy and a decrease in the use of AS. Our results indicate that PSMA PET/MRI may improve the detection rate of PCa and avoid unnecessary biopsy.

## Changes in Primary Prostate Cancer

Many published data confirmed the performance of PSMA PET regarding the detection of lymph node and distant metastases in staging before surgery. The treatment modification was due to the high sensitivity of the PSMA-PET for small distant metastatic spread. Kulkarni et al. prospectively investigated 50 patients with high-risk PCa. Of the 50 patients, 12 (24%) had management changed after PSMA PET/CT imaging (16). Hofman et al. designed a randomized phase 3 study, and recruited men with high-risk PCa in Australia, the result provided compelling evidence that PSMA-PET/CT conferred management change in 41/148 (28%) patients (17). In our study, PSMA-PET/MRI changed the clinical strategy in 8.3% of the patients with primary PCa, which was lower than Hofman's and Kulkarni's study. On the one hand, the number of the patient was quietly limited in this subgroup. On the other hand, we analyzed all primary PCa patients, rather than focused on high-risk PCa, as high-risk PCa is more likely to develop metastasis. This may underestimate the impact on management change. In our study, only one patient with PSA >20 ng/ml changed management after imaging, no management change happened in patients with PSA <20 ng/ml. However, Kulkarni et al. demonstrated that patients with PSA <20 ng/ml had more frequent management changes than PSA >20 ng/ml, which was contrary to ours. The relationship between PSA and management change in primary PCa is still inconclusive.

## Changes in Biochemical Recurrent Prostate Cancer

Our study found that the biggest impact of management intent was in patients with BRPCa, with a 63.6% intended management change noted. We found that PSMA-PET/MRI detected no site of uptake in patients with PSA levels less than 0.5 ng/ml, whereas published literature described detection rates in the order of 45–60% (18). All patients with PSA levels of more than 0.5 ng/ml had positive images, suggested the great performance of $^{18}$F-PSMA-1007 PET/MRI. A meta-analysis showed the pooled detection rate of $^{18}$F-labeled PSMA PET/CT was 49% for PSA <0.5 ng/ml and 86% for PSA ≥0.5 ng/ml (19). There are two possible explanations for the different positive rates between meta-analysis and our reports. On the one hand, our patient number is too limited. On the other hand, the detection rates of PSMA PET in BRPCa patients influenced by many heterogeneous factors, such as received ADT before PSMA-PET, types of tracer ($^{68}$Ga or $^{18}$F labeled), scan model (PET/MRI or PET/CT), or have undergone either RP and RT history. The impact of PSMA PET on the management in BRPCa patients has been widely evaluated. Overall management impact has been reported in the range from 51 to 76% (9, 20). In the present study, management change occurred in 63.6% BRPCa patients, which was comparable with other published studies. Moreover, the concomitant administration of ADT in patients, PET positivity, PSA levels, and PSADT had recently been reported as the most common heterogeneous source of management change. Our result suggested that management changes occurred mostly in patients with 0.5 ≤ PSA <1 ng/ml. For patients with PSA >1 ng/ml, there is a decreased trend of the proportion of management change in BRPCa patients. One possible explanation for the trend may be the advantage of PSMA-PET/MRI over conventional imaging is not obvious at a high recurrent PSA level, and the proportion of management change decreased. This finding was consistent with the EAU guideline, which suggested PSMA PET in BRPCa patients with lower recurrent PSA levels.

Previous studies on this new technology have mostly been based on $^{68}$Ga-PSMA-11 PET/CT, while studies focusing on $^{18}$F-PSMA-1007 PET/MRI were less numerous. Compared with $^{68}$Ga-labeled radiotracers, $^{18}$F-PSMA-1007 has a longer half-life, is easily available, and has significant hepatobiliary clearance (21). Therefore, $^{18}$F-PSMA-1007 PET/MRI may have advantages in detecting local recurrence and easily popularize in clinical practice. Our study evaluated changes between the intended management plan and the revised plan after PSMA PET/MRI, then indicated the clinical value of PSMA PET/MRI. However, a prior study suggested that the implanted management was quite different from the revised treatment plan (22). Studies evaluated the impact of this new technology on actual management is also necessary. Additionally, a cost-effectiveness analysis has to be addressed in a dedicated evaluation before clinical recommendation. Moreover, whether the treatment decision based on PSMA-PET/MRI is beneficial for longer or better survival have yet to be concluded. A multicenter phase III trial (SPPORT trial) in patients with BCR showed freedom-from-progression rate increased from 71.7% in patients who received prostate bed radiation alone to 89.1% in patients who received prostate bed radiation, pelvic lymph node radiation and short-term ADT (23). Such changes in practice could mean that PSMA-PET may add survival benefit when extra-pelvic oligometastatic lesions are detected which may benefit from targeted radiation (24). Further studies are warranted to elucidate whether the change of management will directly translate into survival benefit.

Some limitations of the present study should be noted. Firstly, the patient number is lower than previous studies, with a median patient number of 117 patients (range 15–431) per study, which affects the confidence of our results. However, we report a 41.9% of management change, which is comparable to previous studies (**Supplementary Figures 2-3**). This limitation can be explained by that only preliminary results from our institution are presented, and will disappear once our future larger prospective study is completed (ChiCTR2000036425). For the same reason, to date, no long-term follow-up is available. Secondly, the lack of histological validation is a common limitation in imaging studies. Only a part of patients in suspected and primary PCa groups have pathological confirmation. We were unable to report confirmed pathological data in the BRPCa patients of PSMA-positive lesions due to ethical reasons. Certainly, our study was also limited by the retrospective nature. Finally, our patient cohort was heterogeneous. For one thing, we included patients of suspected PCa, primary PCa, and BRPCa. For another, types of initial treatments in BRPCa patients were also different (including curative and palliative therapy). Nonetheless, this showed a real-life situation that physicians always preferred to apply new imaging technology into different types of patients, and then the best appropriate indications were identified.

## CONCLUSION

From our preliminary experience, PSMA-PET/MRI altered intended decision-making in 39.3% of patients with suspected PCa, 8.3% of patients with primarily diagnosed PCa, and 63.6% patients with BRPCa respectively. The biggest impact of management intent was in patients with BRPCa, especially in patients with 0.5 ≤ PSA <1 ng/ml. This result indicated that PSMA-PET/MRI could be a valued tool for defining lesions in the PCa field and making a personalized clinical decision. However, further larger studies are needed to confirm our pilot findings.

## AUTHOR CONTRIBUTIONS

DX had full access to all the data in the study and takes responsibility for the integrity of the data and the accuracy of the data analysis. DX and AL conceptualized and designed the study. MZ and HH acquired the data. HH and LC analyzed and interpreted the data. AL and LC drafted the manuscript. BL and DX critically revised the manuscript for important intellectual content. WL and XR peformed the statistical analysis. DX and BL obtained the funding. CZ provided administrative, technical, or material support. AL and XR supervised the study. All authors contributed to the article and approved the submitted version.

## SUPPLEMENTARY MATERIAL

**Supplementary Figure 1 |** Details of managements before $^{18}$F-PSMA-1007 PET/MRI, after $^{18}$F-PSMA-1007 PET/MRI, and implemented managements based on per patient. AS, active surveillance; RP, radical prostatectomy; sRT, salvage radiotherapy.

**Supplementary Figure 2 |** Summarize related literatures, regarding the positive rate and management impact of PSMA-PET in PCa patients. Our results were in line with previous studies.

**Supplementary Figure 3 |** Point diagram describes the positive rate and management impact of PSMA-PET in PCa patients at per study level.

## REFERENCES

1. Siegel RL, Miller KD, Jemal A. Cancer statistics, 2019. *CA: Cancer J Clin* (2019) 69:7–34. doi: 10.3322/caac.21551
2. Chen W, Zheng R, Baade PD, Zhang S, Zeng H, Bray F, et al. Cancer statistics in China, 2015. *CA: Cancer J Clin* (2016) 66:115–32. doi: 10.3322/caac.21338
3. Kasivisvanathan V, Rannikko AS, Borghi M, Panebianco V, Mynderse LA, Vaarala MH, et al. MRI-Targeted or Standard Biopsy for Prostate-Cancer Diagnosis. *N Engl J Med* (2018) 378:1767–77. doi: 10.1056/NEJMoa1801993
4. Stabile A, Giganti F, Rosenkrantz AB, Taneja SS, Villeirs G, Gill S, et al. Multiparametric MRI for prostate cancer diagnosis: current status and future directions. *Nat Rev Urol* (2020) 17:41–61. doi: 10.1038/s41585-019-0212-4
5. Zacho HD, Nielsen JB, Afshar-Oromieh A, Haberkorn U, deSouza N, De Paepe K, et al. Prospective comparison of (68)Ga-PSMA PET/CT, (18)F-sodium fluoride PET/CT and diffusion weighted-MRI at for the detection of bone metastases in biochemically recurrent prostate cancer. *Eur J Nucl Med Mol Imaging* (2018) 45:1884–97. doi: 10.1007/s00259-018-4058-4
6. Perner S, Hofer MD, Kim R, Shah RB, Li H, Moller P, et al. Prostate-specific membrane antigen expression as a predictor of prostate cancer progression. *Hum Pathol* (2007) 38:696–701. doi: 10.1016/j.humpath.2006.11.012
7. Pernthaler B, Kulnik R, Gstettner C, Salamon S, Aigner RM, Kvaternik H. A Prospective Head-to-Head Comparison of 18F-Fluciclovine With 68Ga-PSMA-11 in Biochemical Recurrence of Prostate Cancer in PET/CT. *Clin Nucl Med* (2019) 44:e566–e73. doi: 10.1097/rlu.0000000000002703
8. Grubmuller B, Baltzer P, Hartenbach S, D'Andrea D, Helbich TH, Haug AR, et al. PSMA Ligand PET/MRI for Primary Prostate Cancer: Staging Performance and Clinical Impact. *Clin Cancer Res* (2018) 24:6300–7. doi: 10.1158/1078-0432.CCR-18-0768
9. Han S, Woo S, Kim YJ, Suh CH. Impact of 68Ga-PSMA PET on the Management of Patients with Prostate Cancer: A Systematic Review and Meta-analysis. *Eur Urol* (2018) 74:179–90. doi: 10.1016/j.eururo.2018.03.030
10. Roach PJ, Francis R, Emmett L, Hsiao E, Kneebone A, Hruby G, et al. The impact of68Ga-PSMA PET/CT on management intent in prostate cancer: Results of an australian prospective multicenter study. *J Nucl Med* (2018) 59:82–8. doi: 10.2967/jnumed.117.197160
11. Giesel FL, Hadaschik B, Cardinale J, Radtke J, Vinsensia M, Lehnert W, et al. F-18 labelled PSMA-1007: biodistribution, radiation dosimetry and histopathological validation of tumor lesions in prostate cancer patients. *Eur J Nucl Med Mol Imaging* (2017) 44:678–88. doi: 10.1007/s00259-016-3573-4
12. Khan MA, Carter HB, Epstein JI, Miller MC, Landis P, Walsh PW, et al. Can prostate specific antigen derivatives and pathological parameters predict significant change in expectant management criteria for prostate cancer? *J Urol* (2003) 170:2274–8. doi: 10.1097/01.ju.0000097124.21878.6b
13. Zhang LL, Li WC, Xu Z, Jiang N, Zang SM, Xu LW, et al. (68)Ga-PSMA PET/CT targeted biopsy for the diagnosis of clinically significant prostate cancer compared with transrectal ultrasound guided biopsy: a prospective randomized single-centre study. *Eur J Nucl Med Mol Imaging* (2020). doi: 10.1007/s00259-020-04863-2
14. Liu C, Liu T, Zhang Z, Zhang N, Du P, Yang Y, et al. (68)Ga-PSMA PET/CT Combined with PET/Ultrasound-Guided Prostate Biopsy Can Diagnose Clinically Significant Prostate Cancer in Men with Previous Negative Biopsy Results. *J Nucl Med* (2020) 61:1314–9. doi: 10.2967/jnumed.119.235333

15. Lopci E, Saita A, Lazzeri M, Lughezzani G, Colombo P, Buffi NM, et al. (68)Ga-PSMA Positron Emission Tomography/Computerized Tomography for Primary Diagnosis of Prostate Cancer in Men with Contraindications to or Negative Multiparametric Magnetic Resonance Imaging: A Prospective Observational Study. *J Urol* (2018) 200:95–103. doi: 10.1016/j.juro.2018.01.079
16. Kulkarni M, Hughes S, Mallia A, Gibson V, Young J, Aggarwal A, et al. The management impact of (68)gallium-tris(hydroxypyridinone) prostate-specific membrane antigen ((68)Ga-THP-PSMA) PET-CT imaging for high-risk and biochemically recurrent prostate cancer. *Eur J Nucl Med Mol Imaging* (2020) 47:674–86. doi: 10.1007/s00259-019-04643-7
17. Hofman MS, Lawrentschuk N, Francis RJ, Tang C, Vela I, Thomas P, et al. Prostate-specific membrane antigen PET-CT in patients with high-risk prostate cancer before curative-intent surgery or radiotherapy (proPSMA): a prospective, randomised, multicentre study. *Lancet* (2020) 395:1208–16. doi: 10.1016/s0140-6736(20)30314-7
18. Wang R, Shen G, Yang R, Ma X, Tian R. (68)Ga-PSMA PET/MRI for the diagnosis of primary and biochemically recurrent prostate cancer: A meta-analysis. *Eur J Radiol* (2020) 130:109131. doi: 10.1016/j.ejrad.2020.109131
19. Treglia G, Annunziata S, Pizzuto DA, Giovanella L, Prior JO. Detection Rate of (18)F-Labeled PSMA PET/CT in Biochemical Recurrent Prostate Cancer: A Systematic Review and a Meta-Analysis. *Cancers* (2019) 11(5):710. doi: 10.3390/cancers11050710
20. Hoffmann MA, Wieler HJ, Baues C, Kuntz NJ, Richardsen I, Schreckenberger M. The Impact of 68Ga-PSMA PET/CT and PET/MRI on the Management of Prostate Cancer. *Urology* (2019) 130:1–12. doi: 10.1016/j.urology.2019.04.004
21. Freitag MT, Kesch C, Cardinale J, Flechsig P, Floca R, Eiber M, et al. Simultaneous whole-body (18)F-PSMA-1007-PET/MRI with integrated high-resolution multiparametric imaging of the prostatic fossa for comprehensive oncological staging of patients with prostate cancer: a pilot study. *Eur J Nucl Med Mol Imaging* (2018) 45:340–7. doi: 10.1007/s00259-017-3854-6
22. Calais J, Fendler WP, Eiber M, Gartmann J, Chu FI, Nickols NG, et al. Impact of (68)Ga-PSMA-11 PET/CT on the Management of Prostate Cancer Patients with Biochemical Recurrence. *J Nucl Med* (2018) 59:434–41. doi: 10.2967/jnumed.117.202945
23. Pollack A, Karrison TG, Balogh AG, Low D, Bruner DW, Wefel JS, et al. Short Term Androgen Deprivation Therapy Without or With Pelvic Lymph Node Treatment Added to Prostate Bed Only Salvage Radiotherapy: The NRG Oncology/RTOG 0534 SPPORT Trial. *Int J Radiat Oncol Biol Phys* (2018) 102:1605–. doi: 10.1016/j.ijrobp.2018.08.052
24. Jadvar H. Oligometastatic Prostate Cancer: Molecular Imaging and Clinical Management Implications in the Era of Precision Oncology. *J Nucl Med* (2018) 59:1338–9. doi: 10.2967/jnumed.118.213470
25. Bianchi L, Schiavina R, Borghesi M, Ceci F, Angiolini A, Chessa F, et al. How does (68) Ga-prostate-specific membrane antigen positron emission tomography/computed tomography impact the management of patients with prostate cancer recurrence after surgery? *Int J Urol* (2019) 26:804–11. doi: 10.1111/iju.14012
26. Rousseau E, Wilson D, Lacroix-Poisson F, Krauze A, Chi K, Gleave M, et al. A Prospective Study on (18)F-DCFPyL PSMA PET/CT Imaging in Biochemical

Recurrence of Prostate Cancer. *J Nucl Med* (2019) 60:1587–93. doi: 10.2967/jnumed.119.226381

27. Schmidt-Hegemann NS, Eze C, Li M, Rogowski P, Schaefer C, Stief C, et al. Impact of (68)Ga-PSMA PET/CT on the Radiotherapeutic Approach to Prostate Cancer in Comparison to CT: A Retrospective Analysis. *J Nucl Med* (2019) 60:963–70. doi: 10.2967/jnumed.118.220855

28. Müller J, Ferraro DA, Muehlematter UJ, Garcia Schüler HI, Kedzia S, Eberli D, et al. Clinical impact of (68)Ga-PSMA-11 PET on patient management and outcome, including all patients referred for an increase in PSA level during the first year after its clinical introduction. (2019) 46:889–900. doi: 10.1007/s00259-018-4203-0

29. Mattiolli AB, Santos A, Vicente A, Queiroz M, Bastos D, Herchenhorn D, et al. Impact of 68GA-PSMA PET / CT on treatment of patients with recurrent / metastatic high risk prostate cancer - a multicenter study. *Int Braz J Urol* (2018) 44:892–9. doi: 10.1590/s1677-5538.ibju.2017.0632

30. Farolfi A, Ceci F. (68)Ga-PSMA-11 PET/CT in prostate cancer patients with biochemical recurrence after radical prostatectomy and PSA <0.5 ng/ml. Efficacy and impact on treatment strategy. *Eur J Nucl Med Mol Imaging* (2019) 46:11–9. doi: 10.1007/s00259-018-4066-4

31. Roach PJ, Francis R, Emmett L, Hsiao E, Kneebone A, Hruby G, et al. The Impact of (68)Ga-PSMA PET/CT on Management Intent in Prostate Cancer: Results of an Australian Prospective Multicenter Study. *J Nucl Med* (2018) 59:82–8. doi: 10.2967/jnumed.117.197160

32. Hope TA, Aggarwal R, Chee B, Tao D, Greene KL, Cooperberg MR, et al. Impact of (68)Ga-PSMA-11 PET on Management in Patients with Biochemically Recurrent Prostate Cancer. *J Nucl Med* (2017) 58:1956–61. doi: 10.2967/jnumed.117.192476

33. Habl G, Sauter K, Schiller K, Dewes S, Maurer T, Eiber M, et al. (68) Ga-PSMA-PET for radiation treatment planning in prostate cancer recurrences after surgery: Individualized medicine or new standard in salvage treatment. *Prostate* (2017) 77:920–7. doi: 10.1002/pros.23347

34. Albisinni S, Artigas C, Aoun F, Biaou I, Grosman J, Gil T, et al. Clinical impact of (68) Ga-prostate-specific membrane antigen (PSMA) positron emission tomography/computed tomography (PET/CT) in patients with prostate cancer with rising prostate-specific antigen after treatment with curative intent: preliminary analysis of a multidisciplinary approach. *BJU Int* (2017) 120:197–203. doi: 10.1111/bju.13739

35. van Leeuwen PJ, Stricker P, Hruby G, Kneebone A, Ting F. (68) Ga-PSMA has a high detection rate of prostate cancer recurrence outside the prostatic fossa in patients being considered for salvage radiation treatment. *BJU Int* (2016) 117:732–9. doi: 10.1111/bju.13397

36. Fendler WP, Ferdinandus J, Czernin J, Eiber M, Flavell RR, Behr SC, et al. Impact of (68)Ga-PSMA-11 PET on the Management of Recurrent Prostate Cancer in a Prospective Single-Arm Clinical Trial. *J Nucl Med* (2020) 61:1793–9. doi: 10.2967/jnumed.120.242180

37. Grubmüller B, Baltzer P, D'Andrea D, Korn S, Haug AR, Hacker M, et al. (68) Ga-PSMA 11 ligand PET imaging in patients with biochemical recurrence after radical prostatectomy - diagnostic performance and impact on therapeutic decision-making. *Eur J Nucl Med Mol Imaging* (2018) 45:235–42. doi: 10.1007/s00259-017-3858-2

38. Shakespeare TP. Effect of prostate-specific membrane antigen positron emission tomography on the decision-making of radiation oncologists. *Radiat Oncol* (2015) 10:233. doi: 10.1186/s13014-015-0548-8

39. Bluemel C, Linke F, Herrmann K, Simunovic I, Eiber M, Kestler C, et al. Impact of (68)Ga-PSMA PET/CT on salvage radiotherapy planning in patients with prostate cancer and persisting PSA values or biochemical relapse after prostatectomy. *EJNMMI Res* (2016) 6:78. doi: 10.1186/s13550-016-0233-4

40. Sterzing F, Kratochwil C, Fiedler H. 68)Ga-PSMA-11 PET/CT: a new technique with high potential for the radiotherapeutic management of prostate cancer patients. (68)Ga-PSMA-11 PET/CT: a new technique with high potential for the radiotherapeutic management of prostate cancer patients. *Eur J Nucl Med Mol Imaging* (2016) 43:34–41. doi: 10.1007/s00259-015-3188-1

41. Rousseau C, Le Thiec M, Ferrer L, Rusu D, Rauscher A, Maucherat B, et al. Preliminary results of a (68) Ga-PSMA PET/CT prospective study in prostate cancer patients with occult recurrence: Diagnostic performance and impact on therapeutic decision-making. *Prostate* (2019) 79:1514–22. doi: 10.1002/pros.23869

42. Dewes S, Schiller K, Sauter K, Eiber M, Maurer T, Schwaiger M, et al. Integration of (68)Ga-PSMA-PET imaging in planning of primary definitive radiotherapy in prostate cancer: a retrospective study. *Radiat Oncol* (2016) 11:73. doi: 10.1186/s13014-016-0646-2

43. Gauthé M, Belissant O, Girard A, Zhang Yin J, Ohnona J, Cottereau AS, et al. [PET/CT and biochemical recurrence of prostate adenocarcinoma: Added value of (68)Ga-PSMA-11 when (18)F-fluorocholine is non-contributive]. *Progres en Urol J l'Assoc Fr d'urol la Soc Fr d'urol* (2017) 27:474–81. doi: 10.1016/j.purol.2017.04.004

44. Henkenberens C, Derlin T, Bengel FM, Ross TL, Wester HJ, Hueper K, et al. Patterns of relapse as determined by (68)Ga-PSMA ligand PET/CT after radical prostatectomy : Importance for tailoring and individualizing treatment. *Strahlentherapie und Onkol Organ der Dtsch Rontgengesellschaft [et al]* (2018) 194:303–10. doi: 10.1007/s00066-017-1231-9

45. Song H, Harrison C, Duan H, Guja K, Hatami N, Franc BL, et al. Prospective Evaluation of (18)F-DCFPyL PET/CT in Biochemically Recurrent Prostate Cancer in an Academic Center: A Focus on Disease Localization and Changes in Management. *J Nucl Med* (2020) 61:546–51. doi: 10.2967/jnumed.119.231654

46. Zacho HD, Nielsen JB, Dettmann K, Haberkorn U, Langkilde NC, Jensen JB, et al. 68Ga-PSMA PET/CT in Patients With Biochemical Recurrence of Prostate Cancer: A Prospective, 2-Center Study. *Clin Nucl Med* (2018) 43:579–85. doi: 10.1097/rlu.0000000000002169

47. Mena E, Lindenberg ML, Shih JH, Adler S, Harmon S, Bergvall E, et al. Clinical impact of PSMA-based (18)F-DCFBC PET/CT imaging in patients with biochemically recurrent prostate cancer after primary local therapy. *Eur J Nucl Med Mol Imaging* (2018) 45:4–11. doi: 10.1007/s00259-017-3818-x

# 10

# Genome-Wide Analyses of Prognostic and Therapeutic Alternative Splicing Signatures in Bladder Urothelial Carcinoma

*Zhongru Fan, Zhe Zhang\*, Chiyuan Piao, Zhuona Liu, Zeshu Wang and Chuize Kong\**

*Department of Urology, The First Affiliated Hospital of China Medical University, China Medical University, Shenyang, China*

**\*Correspondence:**
*Zhe Zhang*
*zhangzhe@cmu1h.com*
*Chuize Kong*
*kongchuize_cmu@sina.cn*

**Background:** Alternative splicing (AS) is an indispensable post-transcriptional modification applied during the maturation of mRNA, and AS defects have been associated with many cancers. This study was designed to thoroughly analyze AS events in bladder urothelial carcinoma (BLCA) at the genome-wide level.

**Methods:** We adopted a gap analysis to screen for significant differential AS events (DASEs) associated with BLCA. DASEs with prognostic value for OS and the disease-free interval (DFI) were identified by Cox analysis. In addition, a differential AS network and AS clusters were identified using unsupervised cluster analysis. We examined differences in the sensitivity to chemotherapy and immunotherapy between BLCA patients with high and low overall survival (OS) risk.

**Results:** An extensive number of DASEs (296) were found to be clinically relevant in BLCA. A prognosis model was established based prognostic value of OS and DFI. CUGBP elav-like family member 2 (CELF2) was identified as a hub splicing factor for AS networks. We also identified AS clusters associated with OS using unsupervised cluster analysis, and we predicted that the effects of cisplatin and gemcitabine chemotherapy would be different between high- and low-risk groups based on OS prognosis.

**Conclusion:** We completed a comprehensive analysis of AS events in BLCA at the genome-wide level. The present findings revealed that DASEs and splicing factors tended to impact BLCA patient survival and sensitivity to chemotherapy drugs, which may provide novel prospects for BLCA therapies.

Keywords: alternative splicing (AS), bladder urothelial carcinoma (BLCA), prognosis signature, regulatory network, splicing factor, immuno/chemotherapies

## INTRODUCTION

Bladder urothelial carcinoma (BLCA) is a common genitourinary malignancy, with an estimated 430,000 cases diagnosed annually worldwide, associated with 165,000 deaths (1). Some effective methods used for diagnosis and treatment include intravesical Bacillus Calmette and Guérin, which is used to treat intermediate- and high-risk, non-muscle-invasive bladder cancer; and immunotherapy with checkpoint inhibition, targeted therapies, and antibody–drug conjugates, which are used to treat muscle-invasive and advanced diseases. These treatments have been developed due to the profound understanding of the molecular biology and genetics underlying BLCA (2). However, studies are continuously necessary to continue probing unexploited mechanisms for the treatment of BLCA. One study identified over 4,632 survival-associated alternative splicing (AS) events (SASEs) in BLCA and indicated that the overall incidence of SASEs correlated strongly with survival (3), which indicated that AS might be a noteworthy regulatory mechanism in BLCA.

The AS process represents a critical post-transcriptional modification that allows for a single gene to produce diverse mRNA and protein isoforms, contributing to the rich proteome in somatic cells (4). Aberrations in splicing events and their regulators, which are known as splicing factors (SFs), can lead to the development and progression of cancer (5). The identified correlations between AS and some cancers, such as prostate, lung, gastric, and breast cancers, have suggested that AS may serve as a cancer hallmark and treatment target (6–9). Researchers have long recognized that AS events are relevant to bladder cancer (10). Recently, studies have expanded the exploration of the SF–AS regulatory pathway in tumor biology and function in BLCA. For example, polypyrimidine tract-binding protein 1 (PTBP1) directly regulates the splicing of pyruvate kinase isozyme M2 (PKM2) and MEIS2-L, and these two splicing events induce cell proliferation and lymph node metastasis, respectively (11). Similarly, non-POU domain-containing octamer-binding protein (NONO) can mediate a series of oncogenic expression events by regulating the SET domain and mariner transposase fusion gene (SETMAR) (12). The AS–SF network appears to play a strong regulatory role in BLCA. Therefore, the in-depth analysis of AS in BLCA at the whole-genome level may be clinically relevant.

Bioinformatics analyses examining AS in recent years have commonly been based on SASEs, which has allowed for the construction of prognostic models with good performance. To determine intrinsic discrepancies between tumor and normal tissues, gap analysis is crucial for oncology research. Differential AS events (DASEs) describe discrepancies in the splice sites between a pair of samples, which is vital to understanding AS and its regulatory mechanisms. Thus, we aimed to explore DASEs in BLCA.

In this study, we systematically analyzed DASEs using data obtained from The Cancer Genome Atlas (TCGA) SpliceSeq database and prognosis biomarkers associated with BLCA. We conducted survival analyses and established an overall survival (OS) and DFI prognosis model for BLCA. Based on our results, we explored differences in the sensitivity to immunotherapy and chemotherapy among BLCA patients with high or low OS risk. In addition, we performed an unsupervised cluster analysis and constructed a differential AS network, in which we defined three sample clusters and identified eight key SFs associated with 186 DASEs.

**Abbreviations:** AS, alternative splicing; BLCA, bladder urothelial carcinoma; CELF2, CUGBP Elav-Like Family Member 2; DASE, differential alternative splicing event; DFI, disease-free interval; MBNL1, muscleblind-like 1; OS, overall survival.

## MATERIALS AND METHODS

### Data Gathering and Processing

TCGA SpliceSeq (https://bioinformatics.mdanderson.org/TCGASpliceSeq/) is a database for studying the splicing patterns identified among TCGA RNA sequencing (RNAseq) data. The percent spliced in (PSI) value, which is an intuitive ratio ranging from 1 to 0, can be utilized to quantify AS events and categorize seven AS types: alternate acceptor site (AA), alternate donor site (AD), alternate promoter (AP), alternate terminator (AT), exon skip (ES), mutually exclusive exons (ME), and retained intron (RI) (**Figure 1A**) (13). Following the standards of "the percentage of samples with PSI = 100%", we screened the splicing patterns of protein-encoding genes among BLCA patients. The upsetR package was used to draw an upsetR plot to describe the quantity of genes alternatively spliced. We also obtained RNAseq data for BLCA patients from TCGA (using the Genomic Data Commons data portal at https://portal.gdc.cancer.gov/). Clinical data, including survival, age, sex, and cancer stage, were obtained from UCSC Xena (http://xena.ucsc.edu/). The inclusion criteria for BLCA patient samples included date regarding survival time and survival state and OS > 30 days. We included 425 cancer-related samples (including 406 tumor tissues and 19 normal adjacent tissues) in our study, based on the integration of AS data, expression profiles, and other clinical information (**Table 1**). All statistical analysis in the context were performed using R (version: 3.6.2).

### Differential Splicing Event Analysis

We compared tumor samples with adjacent normal tissue samples to identify DASEs with an average PSI > 0.05. The Wilcoxon rank-sum test was performed to evaluate the significance of DASEs between samples, and the Benjamini–Hochberg method was used to correct for multiple testing. We then defined DASEs with adjusted P-values < 0.05 and |log$_2$ (fold change)| > 1 as significant. To detect commonly occurring AS events, the following quality control rules were defined: first, the percentage of samples with PSI = 100% were included, and, second, the average PSI > 0.05. This allowed for the exclusion of rare AS events. We used pheatmap R package to draw a heatmap of top 20 DASEs and ggpubr package to draw a box plot of top 3 DASEs in order to show overall condition of DASEs in BLCA. Therefore, the model established here can be applied to non-special and larger sample populations. In addition, we also analyzed the differential expression of protein-encoding genes between tumor tissues and normal adjacent tissues using the edgeR package (standardized by calcNormFactors [expr, method = "TMM"] in edgeR). Differentially expressed genes (DEGs) were corrected by the Benjamini–Hochberg method by defining significant DEGs as those with P-values < 0.05 and |log$_2$ (fold change)| > 1. To further understand the regulatory role played by AS-associated genes in BLCA, we submitted the identified DASE-related genes to the STRING database (www.string-db.org/) to generate a protein–protein interaction (PPI) network. The "multiple proteins" column was selected.

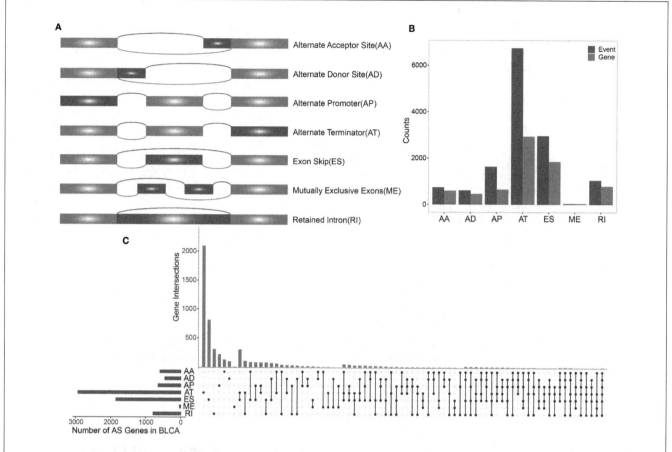

**FIGURE 1** | **(A)** Schematic diagram of AS. **(B)** Histogram of overall AS events and the number of genes involved. **(C)** The UpSetR plot showing the relationships between overall AS event-related genes across different types.

## Survival Analysis

First, we used a survival R package to perform a univariate Cox regression analysis to identify correlations between DASEs and survival in BLCA (including OS and DFI; samples with OS and DFI values greater than 30 days were retained for analysis). Second, the top 10 survival-related DASEs in BLCA were included in the stepwise Cox regression analysis, and a prognostic risk score was determined based on a linear combination of the AS PSI multiplied by the corresponding regression coefficient (b), which was used to represent the correlation weight. This regression coefficient was calculated from the multivariate Cox proportional hazard regression model, and the risk score formula was as follows:

$$\text{Risk Score} = \text{PSI of } AS_1 \times b_{AS1} + \text{PSI of } AS_2 \times b_{AS2} + \ldots$$
$$+ \text{PSI of } AS_{10} \times b_{AS10}$$

$$\text{Risk Score}_{OS} = \text{PSI of } AS_{3412\_PTGER3\_AT} \times 1.937$$
$$+ \text{PSI of } AS_{46432\_CIRBP\_RI} \times -1.890$$
$$+ \text{PSI of } AS_{30219\_CCNDBP1\_AA} \times -3.301$$

$$\text{Risk Score}_{DFI} = \text{PSI of } AS_{84100\_C8orf34\_AT} \times -5.738$$
$$+ \text{PSI of } AS_{82597\_TNKS\_AT} \times -6.495$$
$$+ \text{PSI of } AS_{63304\_FANCD2\_AT} \times 6.383$$
$$+ \text{PSI of } AS_{48124\_TPM4\_AP} \times 1.028$$
$$+ \text{PSI of } AS_{84681\_COX6C\_AT} \times -2.798$$

Based on the results of the stepwise Cox regression analysis, prognostic AS events in BLCA were identified, and corresponding OS and DFI prognostic models were constructed. We used the survminer R package to draw a Kaplan–Meier curve, which shows the top 10 individual DASEs and survival times to determine whether the prognosis models were able to distinguish favorable or poor patient prognoses. We calculated the area under the receiver operating characteristic (ROC) curve (AUC) using a survivalROC R package to further evaluate the OS and DFI prognosis models over a 5-year survival period.

## The Construction of an Alternative Splicing Network

The SF is a key regulator of AS. In the tumor microenvironment, a limited number of SFs can regulate multiple AS events. First, we

**TABLE 1 |** Clinical features of bladder urothelial carcinoma.

| Clinical Features | | Patient | Percent (%) |
|---|---|---|---|
| OS | Alive | 229 | 56.40 |
| | Dead | 177 | 43.60 |
| OS Time | ≤ 5 years | 358 | 88.18 |
| | > 5 years | 47 | 11.58 |
| | Missing Value | 1 | 0.24 |
| DFI | Disease-Free | 155 | 38.18 |
| | Recurrence | 31 | 7.64 |
| | Missing Value | 220 | 54.18 |
| DFI time | ≤ 5 years | 160 | 39.41 |
| | > 5 years | 26 | 6.40 |
| | Missing Value | 220 | 54.19 |
| Sex | Female | 105 | 25.86 |
| | Male | 301 | 74.14 |
| Age | ≤ 60 | 107 | 26.35 |
| | > 60 | 299 | 73.65 |
| T | T0 | 1 | 0.24 |
| | T1 | 3 | 0.74 |
| | T2 | 119 | 29.31 |
| | T3 | 192 | 47.29 |
| | T4 | 58 | 14.29 |
| | Missing Value | 33 | 8.13 |
| N | N0 | 235 | 57.88 |
| | N1 | 46 | 11.33 |
| | N2 | 75 | 18.47 |
| | N3 | 8 | 1.97 |
| | Missing Value | 42 | 10.35 |
| M | M0 | 196 | 48.28 |
| | M1 | 11 | 2.71 |
| | Missing Value | 199 | 49.01 |
| Stage | I | 2 | 0.49 |
| | II | 130 | 32.02 |
| | III | 138 | 33.99 |
| | IV | 134 | 33.01 |
| | Missing Value | 2 | 0.49 |
| **Total** | | **406** | **100** |

OS, overall survival; DFI, disease-free survival; T, tumor; N, node; M, metastasis.

collated a list of human SFs from a human SF database (14, 15). Second, we extracted SF-related gene expression profile data for BLCA, analyzed the identified SFs with an edgeR package, and corrected them using the Benjamin–Hochberg method. SFs with P-values < 0.05 and |log$_2$ (fold change)| > 1 were defined as differential expressing SFs. Third, the Spearman test was used to analyze the potential regulatory correlations between the expression of various SFs and the occurrence of DASEs, in which correlations with P-values < 0.05 and |R| > 0.4 were deemed significant. The regulatory network of AS events and SFs in BLCA was constructed by using Cytoscape (version:3.6.0). Finally, we adopted the ClueGO plug-in for Cytoscape to analyze the gene ontology (GO) and functional enrichment of the related genes in the network, and we identified significantly related GO terms (P-value < 0.05). In addition, univariate Cox regression analysis and survival analysis were employed to identify the impacts of identified SFs on survival.

## Identification of Alternative Splicing Clusters Associated With Prognosis and Molecular Subtypes

AS events vary greatly at the individual level. We applied an unsupervised consensus method performed by ConsensusClusterPlus R package to

identify AS clusters for BLCA (related parameters: distance = "Euclidean"; clusterAlg = "km"). We analyzed the relationships between AS clusters and survival time and further examined relevant clinical information (including age, sex, T, N, M, and stage) to identify associations between clinical information and AS clusters.

## Predictions for Immunotherapy and Chemotherapy

Based on the data obtained from the publicly available pharmacogenomics database, The Genomics of Drug Sensitivity in Cancer (GDSC at https://www.cancerrxgene.org/) (16), we predicted the chemotherapeutic response of each sample. During this process, the pRRophetic R package was used to generate forecasts, in which the minimal inhibitory concentration (IC$_{50}$) value of the sample was estimated by ridge regression, and the prediction accuracy was evaluated based on a ten-fold cross-validation of the GDSC training set (pRRopheticPredict [test matrix = Data; drug = Drug; tissue type = "allSolidTumors"; batchCorrect = "eb"; remove Low Varying Genes = 0.2], all other parameters were set to default). We selected two commonly used chemicals (cisplatin and gemcitabine) to individually predict the IC$_{50}$ values of each BLCA sample, and we calculated the differences in chemotherapeutic responses between the two drugs for the high- and low-risk groups, categorized by the AS-based OS prognosis using the Wilcoxon rank-sum test (P-values < 0.05). We also utilized the submap algorithm of TIDE (http://tide.dfci.harvard. edu/) and GenePattern (https://cloud.genepattern.org/gp) to predict discrepancies in the clinical responses to immune checkpoint blockades among BLCA patients who were at either high or low risk, according to the AS-based OS prognoses. On the TIDE, we chose "others" in the column "Cancer type" and "no" in the column of "Previous immunotherapy." Fisher's exact test was used to verify the relevance between OS-grouping and the immunotherapy response. On GenePattern, a submap was used for analysis and Bonferroni's *post hoc* test was used to correct P-values. The overall framework of this study is shown in **Figure 2**.

## RESULTS

### Overview of Alternative Splicing Events in BLCA

A synthetic analysis of AS profiles in human BLCA was employed. A total of 13,747 AS events associated with 5,174 genes were identified. In detail, we detected 736 instances of the AA splice type, involving 598 genes; 609 instances of the AD splice type, involving 459 genes; 1,629 instances of the AP splice type, involving 651 genes; 6,739 instances of the AT splice type,

involving 2,937 genes; 2,957 instances of the ES splice type, involving 1,855 genes; 38 instances of the ME splice type, involving 38 genes; and 1,039 instances of the RI splice type, involving 791 genes, as shown in **Figures 1A, B**. The AT splice type was the most common type identified (> 49%), and ES was the second most frequent type (> 21%), whereas ME was the rarest type. A given gene could be associated with multiple types of AS events, with some genes associated with up to five or six variable splicing types (**Figure 1C**). The information of 425 included samples is shown in **Supplementary Table S1**.

### Identification of Differential Alternative Splicing Events

We identified 296 DASEs by comparing the BLCA group with the control group, associated with 272 genes (**Figure 3A**). To investigate the relationship between DEGs and DASEs, 4,752 DEGs were identified in BLCA compared with the control group (2,679 upregulated genes and 2,073 downregulated genes) Representative DASE are shown as heat plot (**Figure 3B**) and box plot (**Figure 3C**).The results of all and selected DASEs and DEGs were offered as **Supplementary Table S2-S5**.

### The Construction of the PPI Network

We performed a PPI network analysis of differentially AS-related genes in BLCA and identified several hub genes based on the

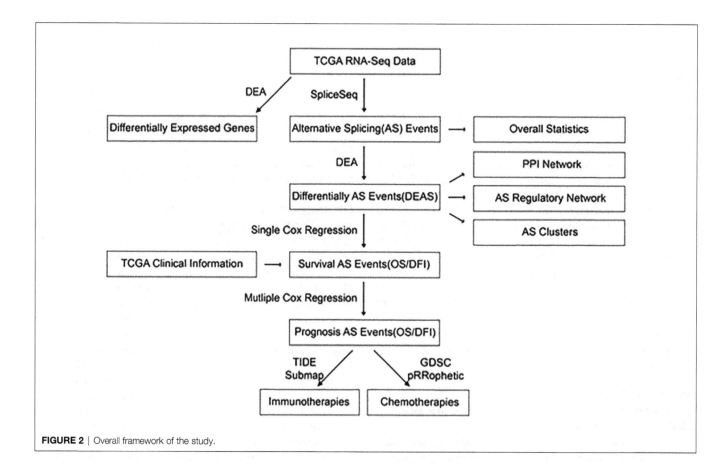

**FIGURE 2** | Overall framework of the study.

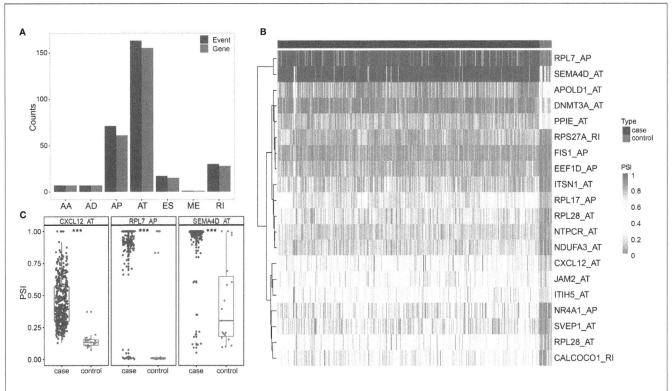

**FIGURE 3 | (A)** Histogram of DASE distribution in BLCA. **(B)** Heat map of the top 20 differentially AS events in BLCA. **(C)** Box plot of variable shear events among the top three alternative splice events in BLCA. *** represents p values < 0.0001.

number of collected genes. We identified 186 nodes and 392 edges in the PPI network, including the hub nodes *UBA52* (degree = 35), *RPS27A* (degree = 32), *PSMC5* (degree = 16), *RPL7* (degree = 15), and *PKM* (degree = 15) (**Figure 4**). The GO analysis of proteins in the network was shown in **Supplementary Table S6**.

## The Construction of a Prognostic Alternative Splicing Event Model

To probe the prognostic value of AS events in BLCA patients, we first adopted a univariate Cox regression analysis to evaluate the influence of AS events on the prognoses of BLCA patients. We detected 87 OS-related and 12 DFI-related AS events among the identified DASEs in BLCA. Both groups of AS events were most commonly associated with the AT and AP types (21 APs and 33 ATs in the OS group, accounting for > 62%; all DFIs were either AP or AT types, with 3 APs and 9 ATs). We also identified events that were related to both OS and DFI (total two), and plotted a forest map (**Figure 5C**).

Next, we attempted to identify independent prognostic factors associated with BLCA patients. We selected the top 10 OS- and DFI-related AS events in BLCA as candidate factors and utilized a stepwise Cox regression analysis to select independent prognostic-related AS events to establish various prognostic models (the top four event-related survival curves are shown in **Figures 5A, B**; the remaining six curves are shown in **Supplementary Figure S1**). Three independent prognostic factors were associated with OS, and five independent prognostic factors were associated with DFI

(**Figure 5D**). In the light of the median risk scores calculated for the OS and DFI prognostic models, BLCA patients were separated into a low-risk group and a high-risk group. Both the OS and DFI prognostic models showed the significant ability to differentiate survival among BLCA patients, and the DFI model showed better performance (OS: p = 1.03505e−05, AUC = 0.6767398; DFI: p = 0.0003621185, AUC = 0.8965976; see **Figures 5E, F**). The detailed parameters of clusters are submitted as "**Data Sheet File for clustering**".

## The Construction of an Alternative Splicing Network Based on Gap Analysis

Considering the notable differences in AS events in BLCA, we further analyzed the relationships between AS events and SFs. First, we investigated the differentially expressed SFs in BLCA, and we distinguished eight differential SFs: *CELF2*, *MBNL1*, *NOVA1*, *PTBP2*, *KHDRBS2*, *ELAVL2*, *ELAVL3*, and *ELAVL4*. Of these, *ELAV2*, *ELAVL3*, and *ELAVL4* were upregulated in BLCA, and *CELF2*, *MBNL1*, *NOVA1*, *PTBP2*, and *KHDRBS2* were downregulated (**Figure 6A**). Then we evaluated the correlations between DASEs and differentially expressed SFs, and we chose highly correlated pairs (|R| > 0.4 and P-value < 0.05) to generate a differential AS network. Among these SFs, *CELF2* is a pivotal splicing factor in the network, associated with 37 different AS events but is also negatively correlated with 26 different AS events. The *MBNL1* and *NOVA1* SFs also tended to be negatively correlated with most AS events (**Figure 6B**). In addition, we analyzed the GO-based functional enrichment of genes in the AS

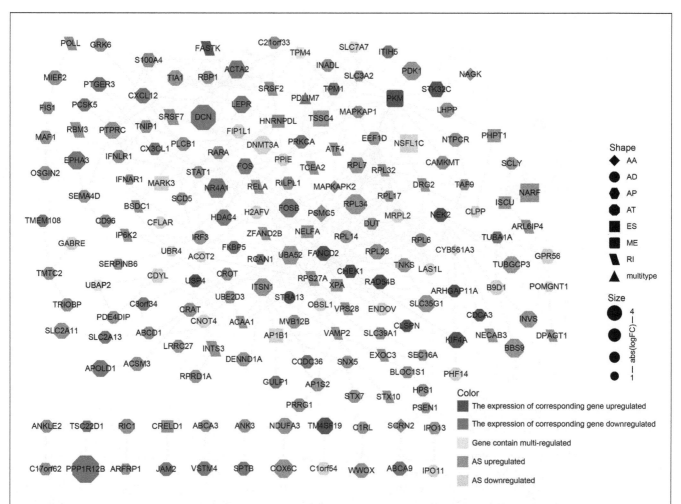

**FIGURE 4** | PPI network constructed by different alternative splicing-related genes in BLCA. The dots represent alternatively spliced genes, whereas the edges represent the relationships between the proteins corresponding to those genes. The shapes of the dots represent the AS types; the color of the dots represents the changes in gene expression. The size of the node represents |log2 (fold change)|.

network for BLCA, and a total of six GO terms were significantly enriched (**Figure 6C**). Ultimately, to evaluate the "performance" of these differential SFs, we performed a survival analysis and found that *NOVA1* was associated with survival-related ability, as were *ELAV4* and *ELAV3* (**Figure 7**).

## Prognosis-Associated Alternative Splicing Clusters

We performed an unsupervised analysis of all selected samples based on the AS events in BLCA to further identify different AS patterns. According to a consensus cluster plus analysis, using a consensus value range from 0 (white, samples never gathered together) to 1 (dark blue, samples always gathered together), three groups of samples were categorized, as follows: C1 (n = 116, 28.57%), C2 (n = 125, 30.79%) and C3 (n = 165, 40.64%) (**Figure 8A**).

Subsequently, we conducted a survival analysis of BLCA samples to appraise the relevance of the identified clusters for OS/DFI prognosis. The results showed that AS clusters were associated with different OS survival modes (P = 0.0003680077, see **Figure 8B**) but not with different DFI survival modes (P = 0.4414947, see **Figure 8C**).

We further analyzed related information for BLCA samples, such as OS (alive or dead), DFI (disease-free or recurrence), survival time (OS/DFI > 5 years or ≤ 5 years), age (age > 60 or ≤ 60), sex (female or male), T, N, M, stage, and the presence of *TP53*, *KRAS*, *BRAF*, and other common cancer-driving genetic mutations. Some of this information was not randomly distributed. For example, discrepancies in the OS, T, N, and stage values were identified among the AS clusters associated with BLCA (Chi-square test, P-values < 0.05). Among these, the driving gene *TP53* was mutated in 192 samples (accounting for > 47%), but no significant difference was observed for the *TP53* distribution across the AS clusters (Chi-square test, P-values > 0.05; **Figure 8D**). Therefore, we were also able to identify molecular subtypes associated with prognoses through AS events.

## Sensitivity Differences to Immunotherapy and Chemotherapy Between the High- and Low-Risk Groups

First, we analyzed the response to immunotherapy in BLCA and used the TIDE algorithm to predict the response to

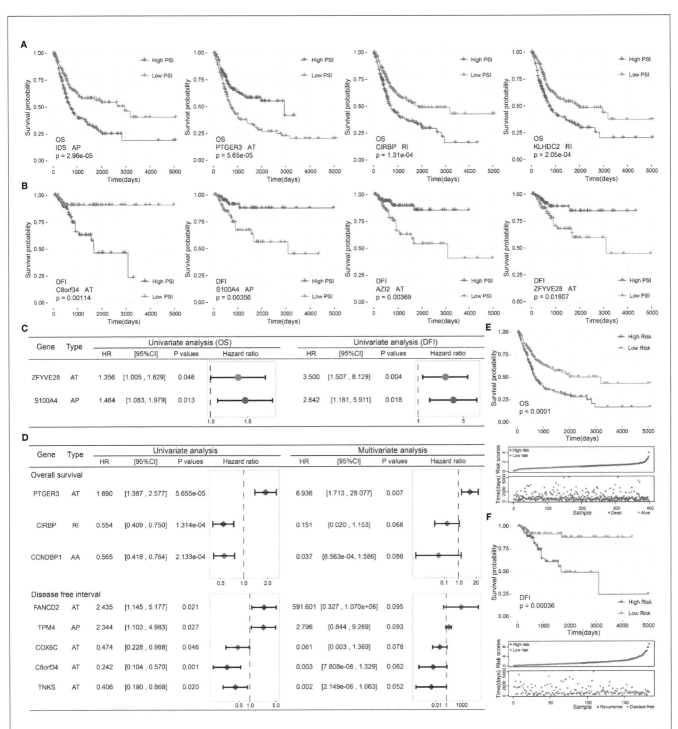

FIGURE 5 | **(A)** Kaplan–Meier curve of the four AS events associated with OS. **(B)** Kaplan–Meier curve of the top four AS events associated with DFI. **(C)** Comparison of AS events associated with OS and DFI in univariate Cox regression analysis of BLCA. **(D)** Comparison of univariate Cox analysis and stepwise Cox analysis of AS events associated with OS and DFI prognoses. **(E, F)**: Kaplan–Meier plot, risk score plot, and survival state plot of OS and DFI prognostic models for BLCA.

immunotherapy. Notable differences in the responses to immunotherapy were observed between the high-risk group (19.10%, 38/199) and the low-risk group (57.58%, 114/198) (using Fishers exact test, p = 1.674e−15, and the Chi-square test, p = 7.065e−15). In addition to the TIDE prediction, we also compared the expression profiles of BLCA patients with high and

low risk for OS using a submap algorithm, and we compared these outcomes with another data set derived from melanoma patients who were responsive to immunotherapy (17). We found that although no significant responses to immunotherapy were identified after correction *via* the Benjamini–Hochberg method in patients with high and low risk for OS, anti-programmed cell

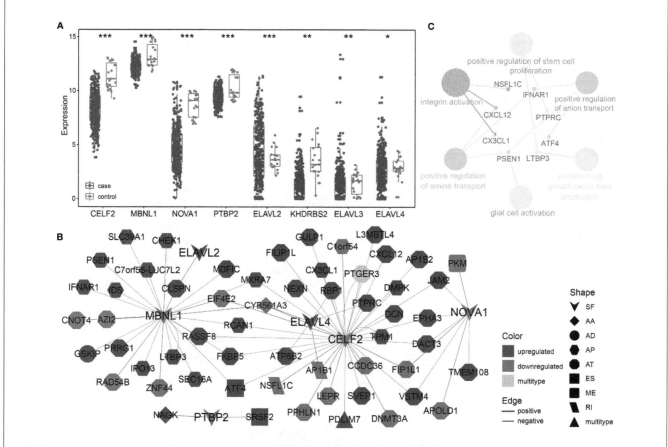

**FIGURE 6 | (A)** Box plot of differentially expressed SFs in BLCA. **(B)** Different AS networks in BLCA. **(C)** Gene-rich GO terms in different AS networks in BLCA. *
represents p values< 0.05, ** represents p values < 0.01, *** represents p values< 0.001.

death protein 1 (PD-1) and cytotoxic T-lymphocyte-associated protein (CTLA4) therapy appears to be effective in the high-risk group without correction (PD-1 P = 0.04995005; CTLA4 P = 0.03496503; see **Figure 9A**).

Next, we considered the discrepancies in the responses to chemotherapy among BLCA patients and attempted to assess the differences in the responses to two chemicals (cisplatin and gemcitabine) between patients with high and low risk for OS. Thus, we trained a prediction model using the R package "pRRophetic" on the GDSC cell line dataset, using a ridge regression. We appraised its prediction accuracy through a ten-fold cross-validation. Based on the prediction model for these two chemicals, we estimated the $IC_{50}$ values for each sample in the BLCA group. For these two chemicals, we observed significant differences in the $IC_{50}$ values for cisplatin and gemcitabine in patients with high and low risk for OS associated with BLCA (cisplatin P = 1.918960e–07; gemcitabine P = 1.303591e–03; see **Figure 9B**).

## DISCUSSION

Changes in AS events can have significant effects on oncogenesis and tumor progression (18). For example, the SF SF3B3 is upregulated and contributes to tumorigenesis by regulating *EZH2* pre-mRNA

splicing, representing a key prognostic factor and therapeutic target in clear cell renal cell carcinoma (19). Similarly, many recent studies have shown that DASEs regulated by differentially expressed SFs have effects on tumorigenesis, the epithelial–mesenchymal transition, and lymphatic metastasis (12, 20–24). Therefore, analyses of DASEs can be meaningful in an oncogenic context. Alternative splicing is widely present in metazoans. The genes regulated by AS typically differ from DEGs, emphasizing a different biological process. **Figure 4** shows that DEGs can be differentially spliced, as can many non-DEGs, indicating that differential AS is a widespread regulatory mechanism that can act to supplement DEGs. We therefore aimed to emphasize the study of DASEs, rather than DEGs. To achieve this goal, we set the "percentage of samples with PSI value = 100%" and the average PSI > 0.05, which ensured that the incorporated DASEs occurred in all samples, making our analyses and models applicable to most cases. As for the gathering of DEGs, we used conventional methods with edge R package, and this can be regarded "another system" compared with the methods of gathering DASEs.

Given the potential importance of AS events in tumor biology, attention has been paid to the clinical relevance of AS events in cancer. Previous research based on TCGA datasets revealed the prognostic value of AS events in BLCA (3). Guo et al. reported that single-nucleotide polymorphisms can influence specific splicing events and are associated with BLCA risk scores (25). We also examined the

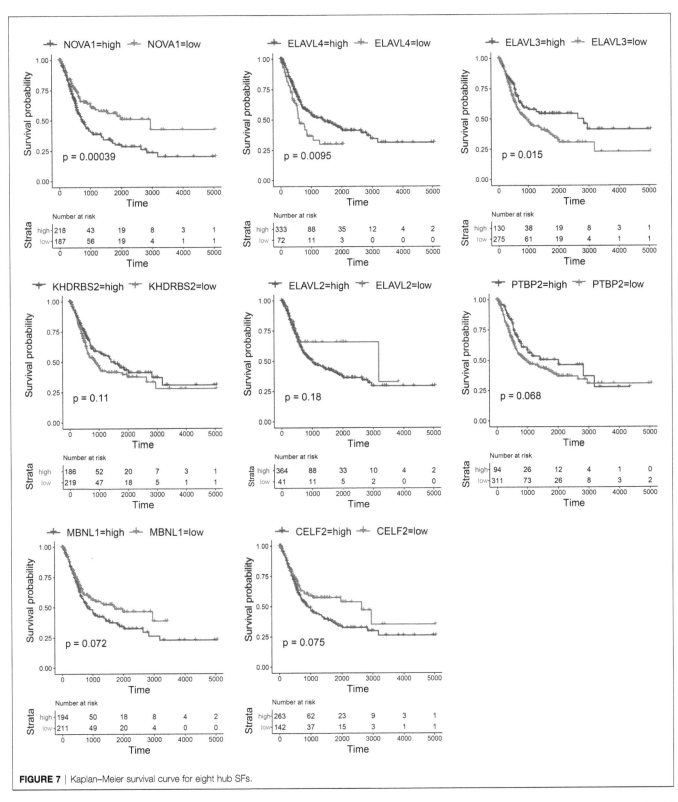

**FIGURE 7** | Kaplan–Meier survival curve for eight hub SFs.

profile and clinical relevance of AS events in BLCA by performing a pan-cancer analysis (26). Recently, some AS bioinformatics analyses reported the good performance of AS events in predicting prognosis (27–29). However, these studies have been based on SASEs, which explains their good prognosis-predicting performance. According to

other studies (30, 31), the analysis of DASEs or cancer-specific AS events can also show significant results. In this study, we performed systematic analyses to determine the prognostic value of DASEs in BLCA. The results of univariate Cox regression analysis showed a strong correlation between DASEs and survival, suggesting that

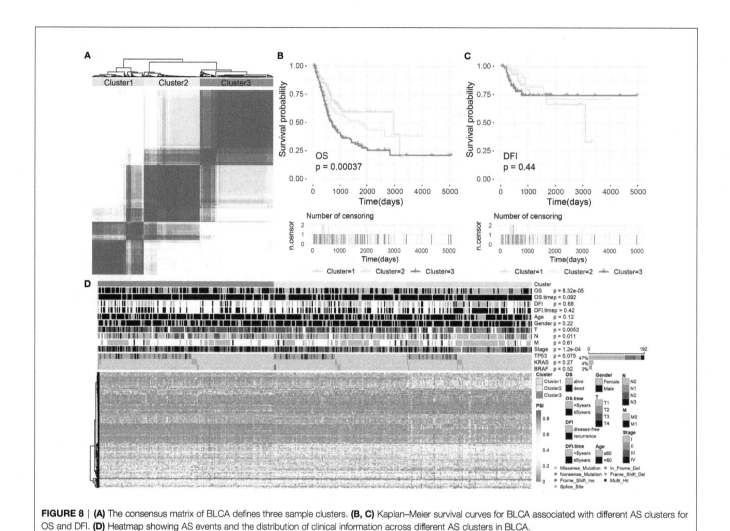

FIGURE 8 | (A) The consensus matrix of BLCA defines three sample clusters. (B, C) Kaplan–Meier survival curves for BLCA associated with different AS clusters for OS and DFI. (D) Heatmap showing AS events and the distribution of clinical information across different AS clusters in BLCA.

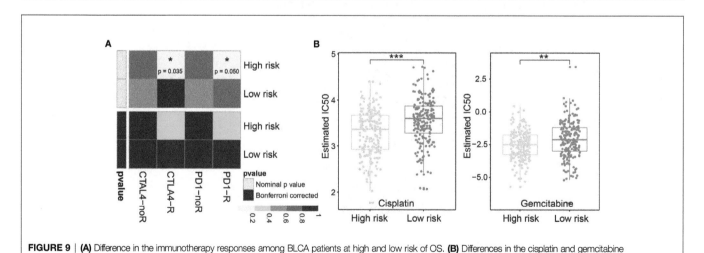

FIGURE 9 | (A) Difference in the immunotherapy responses among BLCA patients at high and low risk of OS. (B) Differences in the cisplatin and gemcitabine chemotherapy responses among patients with BLCA at high and low risk of OS. * represents p values< 0.05, ** represents p values < 0.01, *** represents p values< 0.001.

several DASEs events affect survival. The top 10 events identified in OS and DFI showed strong correlations with survival time. In the stepwise Cox regression analysis, independent prognostic AS events were identified in association with both OS and DFI. For the constructed prognostic model, however, the AUC value of OS was unfortunately not higher than 0.7, suggesting an insignificant result.

AS is regulated by a complex network and anomalous AS events and their associated regulatory factors should be investigated. Based on the differential AS genes, we constructed a PPI network to display how differential protein variants interact in BLCA (**Figure 4**). The plot offers a glimpse into changes in AS gene expression, AS types, and PPI. However, only a minority of the genes in the network have been identified as being alternatively spliced. For example, PKM exon 9 is skipped more frequently in BLCA (11). Although this network may be forward-looking, the available evidence to support the authenticity of this model is currently insufficient.

SFs are a series of RNA-binding proteins that can shear pre-RNA, and studying AS is vital. According to the network, eight SFs and numerous predictive pathways were associated with DASEs in BLCA. Little mechanism-based research exists for these eight SFs (CELF2, MBNL1, NOVA1, PTBP2, KHDRBS2, ELAVL2, ELAVL3, and ELAVL4) in BLCA; thus, further studies remain necessary. CELF2, an RNA-binding protein, can modulate RNA stability and translation by attaching to UG-rich sequence elements of introns, which can promote apoptosis and autophagy and regulate alternative polyadenylation (32–37). In this analysis, CELF2 was identified as a hub SF within the network; it was expressed at remarkably low levels and played a regulatory role for 37 DASEs. In addition, MBNL1 was the second most important SF. CELF2 and MBNL1 share some downstream genes and were both expressed at low levels, which agrees with the results of a recent research on the reciprocal regulatory roles of CELF2 and other SF (38). Most intensive studies have suggested that AS is regulated in a combinatorial manner by several SFs, which can be either synergistic or antagonistic (39). The cross-regulatory roles of SFs may have multifaceted effects for shaping cellular functions. Thus, further research referencing our AS network may be of great value. In the survival analysis, the SFs associated with DASEs did not present strong survival-related abilities. However, an increased potential population of downstream factors increases the functional complexity. These SFs were obtained by gap analysis, instead of survival analysis, which may explain why only NOVA1 appears to be a survival-related SF (**Figure 7**).

We did not identify any optimal prognostic AS clusters after conducting various classifications. BLCA has diverse biological specificity, suggesting that an increase in the number of clustering groups should be beneficial. According to the prognostic value of DASEs, we separated the sample into three groups of clusters related to prognoses in the case of OS while we failed to make the clustering relate to prognoses in the case of DFI. After overall consideration, we chose to retain this triple classification scheme.

AS events can also affect tumor immunity and sensitivity to chemotherapy drugs (40). To explore the immunotherapy response, the TIDE algorithm was used to determine significant differences in immunotherapy responses among the AS clusters (the

responses were better in the low-risk group). Although the TIDE algorithm is the most effective method for predicting the immunotherapy response in melanoma (41), it may not be valid in other tumors. We have found that the TIDE algorithm appears to be useful for cervical squamous cell carcinoma (42) and BLCA. Predicting the response to immune checkpoint blockade therapy can be difficult, and only a small portion of patients obtain benefits from therapy; however, no currently available alternative methods can predict the response to immunotherapy. In this situation, any attempts to predict the immunotherapy response may be useful. We were able to identify differences in the immunotherapy response between groups according to OS. We then used a submap algorithm to predict whether differences could be identified in response to anti-PD-1 and anti-CTAL-4 between the low- and high-risk groups. Although no significant differences were detected after correction, the high-risk group showed promise for the response to anti-PD-1 and anti-CTAL-4 treatment without correction. In the prediction to chemotherapy response, cisplatin and gemcitabine showed significant differences between patients with high and low BLCA risks. We tested two clustering mechanisms, including AS clustering (dividing samples into three groups) and high/low-risk of OS grouping (mentioned in section 3.6), and found that risk grouping provided better predictive results.

Within this limited study, we systematically analyzed AS events, associated SFs, prognostic signatures, and sensitivity to immunotherapy and chemotherapy in BLCA. Further verification of these findings remains necessary through subsequent studies of DASEs and SFs, both *in vivo* and *in vitro*, and examining AS signatures in various population cohort studies is worth pursuing.

## CONCLUSION

Overall, we performed a novel study of the AS regulatory networks that may be involved in the oncogenesis of BLCA. In addition, an AS-based prognostic model was established, and the low-risk group showed greater sensitivity to immuno- and chemotherapy.

## AUTHOR CONTRIBUTIONS

CK, ZZ, and ZF designed the research study. ZF performed all the bioinformatics analyses described here. ZF wrote and edited the manuscript. CK and ZZ reviewed the article and made modification suggestions. CK and ZZ supervised the project. CP, ZL, and ZW offered advice. All authors contributed to the article and approved the submitted version.

## REFERENCES

1. Torre LA, Bray F, Siegel RL, Ferlay J, Lortet-Tieulent J, Jemal A. Global Cancer Statistics. *CA Cancer J Clin* (2015) 65:87–108. doi: 10.3322/caac.21262

2. Lenis AT, Lec PM, Chamie K, Mshs MD. Bladder Cancer: A Review. *JAMA* (2020) 324:1980–91. doi: 10.1001/jama.2020.17598

3. He RQ, Zhou XG, Yi QY, Deng CW, Gao JM, Chen G, et al. Prognostic Signature of Alternative Splicing Events in Bladder Urothelial Carcinoma Based on Spliceseq Data from 317 Cases. *Cell Physiol Biochem* (2018) 48:1355–68. doi: 10.1159/000492094

4. Baralle FE, Giudice J. Alternative Splicing as a Regulator of Development and Tissue Identity. *Nat Rev Mol Cell Biol* (2017) 18:437–51. doi: 10.1038/nrm.2017.27

5. David CJ, Manley JL. Alternative Pre-mRNA Splicing Regulation in Cancer: Pathways and Programs Unhinged. *Genes Dev* (2010) 24:2343–64. doi: 10.1101/gad.1973010

6. Coomer AO, Black F, Greystoke A, Munkley J, Elliott DJ. Alternative Splicing in Lung Cancer. *Biochim Biophys Acta Gene Regul Mech* (2019) 1862:194388. doi: 10.1016/j.bbagrm.2019.05.006

7. Li Y, Yuan Y. Alternative RNA Splicing and Gastric Cancer. *Mutat Res* (2017) 773:263–73. doi: 10.1016/j.mrrev.2016.07.011

8. Paschalis A, Sharp A, Welti JC, Neeb A, Raj GV, Luo J, et al. Alternative Splicing in Prostate Cancer. *Nat Rev Clin Oncol* (2018) 15:663–75. doi: 10.1038/s41571-018-0085-0

9. Yang Q, Zhao J, Zhang W, Chen D, Wang Y. Aberrant Alternative Splicing in Breast Cancer. *J Mol Cell Biol* (2019) 11:920–9. doi: 10.1093/jmcb/mjz033

10. Thompson TE, Rogan PK, Risinger JI, Taylor JA. Splice Variants but not Mutations of DNA Polymerase Beta are Common in Bladder Cancer. *Cancer Res* (2002) 62:3251–6.

11. Xie RH, Chen X, Chen ZY, Huang M, Dong W, Gu P. Polypyrimidine Tract Binding Protein 1 Promotes Lymphatic Metastasis and Proliferation of Bladder Cancer via Alternative Splicing of MEIS2 and PKM. *Cancer Lett* (2019) 449:31–44. doi: 10.1016/j.canlet.2019.01.041

12. Xie RH, Chen X, Cheng L, Huang M, Zhou QH, Zhang JT, et al. NONO Inhibits Lymphatic Metastasis of Bladder Cancer via Alternative Splicing of SETMAR. *Mol Ther* (2021) 29: (1):291–307. doi: 10.1016/j.ymthe.2020.08.018

13. Schafer S, Miao K, Benson CC, Heinig M, Cook SA, Hubner N. Alternative Splicing Signatures in RNA-seq Data: Percent Spliced in (PSI). *Curr Protoc Hum Genet* (2015) 87:11.16.1–11.16.14. doi: 10.1002/0471142905.hg1116s87

14. Giulietti M, Piva F, D'Antonio M, D'Onorio De Meo P, Paoletti D, Castrignanò T, et al. SpliceAid-F: A Database of Human Splicing Factors and Their RNA-Binding Sites. *Nucleic Acids Res* (2013) 41:D125–31. doi: 10.1093/nar/gks997

15. Piva F, Giulietti M, Burini AB, Principato G. SpliceAid 2: A Database of Human Splicing Factors Expression Data and RNA Target Motifs. *Hum Mutat* (2012) 33:81–5. doi: 10.1002/humu.21609

16. Yang W, Soares J, Greninger P, Edelman EJ, Lightfoot H, Forbes S, et al. Genomics of Drug Sensitivity in Cancer (GDSC): A Resource for Therapeutic Biomarker Discovery in Cancer Cells. *Nucleic Acids Res* (2013) 41:D955–61. doi: 10.1093/nar/gks1111

17. Roh WJ, Chen PL, Reuben A, Spencer CN, Prieto PA, Miller JP. Integrated Molecular Analysis of Tumor Biopsies on Sequential CTLA-4 and PD-1 Blockade Reveals Markers of Response and Resistance. *Sci Transl Med* (2017) 9:eaah3560. doi: 10.1126/scitranslmed.aah3560

18. Chang HL, Lin JC. SRSF1 and RBM4 Differentially Modulate the Oncogenic Effect of HIF-1α in Lung Cancer Cells Through Alternative Splicing Mechanism. *Biochim Biophys Acta Mol Cell Res* (2019) 1866:118550. doi: 10.1016/j.bbamcr.2019.11855

19. Chen K, Xiao H, Zeng J, Yu G, Zhou H, Huang C, et al. Alternative Splicing of EZH2 pre-mRNA by SF3B3 Contributes to the Tumorigenic Potential of Renal Cancer. *Clin Cancer Res* (2017) 23:3428–41. doi: 10.1158/1078-0432.Ccr-16-2020

20. Yu LL, Kim JC, Jiang L, Feng BB, Ying Y, Ji KY, et al. MTR4 Drives Liver Tumorigenesis by Promoting Cancer Metabolic Switch Through Alternative Splicing. *Nat Commun* (2020) 11:708. doi: 10.1158/1078-0432.CCR-16-2020

21. Hu XH, Harvey SE, Zheng R, Lyu JY, Grzeskowiak CL, Powell E, et al. The RNA-Binding Protein AKAP8 Suppresses Tumor Metastasis by Antagonizing EMT-Associated Alternative Splicing. *Nat Commun* (2020) 11:486. doi: 10.1038/s41467-020-14304-1

22. Sznajder JL, Scotti MM, Shin J, Taylor K, Ivankovic F, Nutter CA, et al. Loss of MBNL1 Induces RNA Misprocessing in the Thymus and Peripheral Blood. *Nat Commun* (2020) 11:2022. doi: 10.1038/s41467-020-15962-x

23. Xie RH, Chen X, Chen ZY, Huang M, Dong W, Gu P, et al. Polypyrimidine Tract Binding Protein 1 Promotes Lymphatic Metastasis and Proliferation of Bladder Cancer via Alternative Splicing of MEIS2 and PKM. *Cancer Lett* (2019) 449:31–44. doi: 10.1016/j.canlet.2019.01.041

24. Hu X, Harvey SE, Zheng R, Lyu J, Grzeskowiak CL, Powell E, et al. The RNA-Binding Protein AKAP8 Suppresses Tumor Metastasis by Antagonizing EMT-Associated Alternative Splicing. *Nat Commun* (2020) 11:486. doi: 10.1038/s41467-020-14304-1

25. Guo Z, Zhu HH, Xu WD, Wang X, Liu HT, Wu YL, et al. Alternative Splicing Related Genetic Variants Contribute to Bladder Cancer Risk. *Mol Carcinog* (2020) 59:923–9. doi: 10.1002/mc.23207

26. Zhang Y, Yan L, Zeng J, Zhou H, Liu H, Yu G, et al. Pan-Cancer Analysis of Clinical Relevance of Alternative Splicing Events in 31 Human Cancers. *Oncogene* (2019) 38:6678–95. doi: 10.1038/s41388-019-0910-7

27. Zhao XY, Si SS, Li XN, Sun WJ, Cui L. Identification and Validation of an Alternative Splicing-Based Prognostic Signature for Head and Neck Squamous Cell Carcinoma. *J Cancer* (2020) 11(15):4571–80. doi: 10.7150/jca.44746

28. Cao RY, Zhang JY, Jiang LB, Wang YT, Ren XY, Cheng B, et al. Comprehensive Analysis of Prognostic Alternative Splicing Signatures in Oral Squamous Cell Carcinoma. *Front Oncol* (2020) 10:1740:1740. doi: 10.3389/fonc.2020.01740

29. Wu SJ, Wang JC, Zhu XC, Chyr J, Zhou XB, Wu XM, et al. The Functional Impact of Alternative Splicing on the Survival Prognosis of Triple-Negative Breast Cancer. *Front Genet* (2021) 11:604262:604262. doi: 10.3389/fgene.2020.604262

30. Lou SH, Zhang J, Zhai Z, Yin X, Wang YM, Fang TY, et al. Development and Validation of an Individual Alternative Splicing Prognostic Signature in Gastric Cancer. *Aging* (2021) 17:13. doi: 10.18632/aging.202507

31. Lee SE, Alcedo KP, Kim JH, Snider NT. Alternative Splicing in Hepatocellular Carcinoma. *Cell Mol Gastroenterol Hepatol* (2020) 10(4):699–712. doi: 10.1016/j.jcmgh

32. Ladd AN, Charlet N, Cooper TA. The CELF Family of RNA Binding Proteins Is Implicated in Cell-Specific and Developmentally Regulated Alternative Splicing. *Mol Cell Biol* (2001) 21:1285–96. doi: 10.1128/mcb.21.4.1285-1296.2001

33. Dasgupta T, Ladd AN. The Importance of CELF Control: Molecular and Biological Roles of the CUG-BP, Elav-Like Family of RNA-Binding Proteins. *Wiley Interdiscip Rev RNA* (2012) 3:104–21. doi: 10.1002/wrna.107

34. Ajith S, Gazzara MR, Cole BS, Shankarling G, Martinez NM, Mallory MJ, et al. Position-Dependent Activity of CELF2 in the Regulation of Splicing and Implications for Signal-Responsive Regulation in T cells. *RNA Biol* (2016) 13:569–81. doi: 10.1080/15476286.2016.1176663

35. Chatrikhi R, Mallory MJ, Gazzara MR, Agosto LM, Zhu WS, Litterman AJ, et al. RNA Binding Protein CELF2 Regulates Signal-Induced Alternative Polyadenylation by Competing with Enhancers of the Polyadenylation Machinery. *Cell Rep* (2019) 28:2795–06.e3. doi: 10.1016/j.celrep.2019.08.022

36. New J, Subramaniam D, Ramalingam S, Enders J, Sayed AAA, Ponnurangam S, et al. Pleotropic Role of RNA Binding Protein CELF2 in Autophagy Induction. *Mol Carcinog* (2019) 58:1400–9. doi: 10.1002/mc.23023

37. Piqué L, Martinez de Paz A, Piñeyro D, Martínez-Cardús A, Castro de Moura M, Llinàs-Arias P, et al. Epigenetic Inactivation of the Splicing RNA-Binding Protein CELF2 in Human Breast Cancer. *Oncogene* (2019) 38:7106–12. doi: 10.1038/s41388-019-0936-x

38. Mallory MJ, McClory SP, Chatrikhi R, Gazzara MR, Ontiveros RJ, Lynch KW. Reciprocal Regulation of HnRNP C and CELF2 Through Translation and Transcription Tunes Splicing Activity in T cells. *Nucleic Acids Res* (2020) 48:5710–19. doi: 10.1093/nar/gkaa295

39. Fu X D, Ares MJr. Context-Dependent Control of Alternative Splicing by RNA-Binding Proteins. *Nat Rev Genet* (2014) 15:689–701. doi: 10.1038/nrg3778

40. Frankiw L, Baltimore D, Li G. Alternative mRNA Splicing in Cancer Immunotherapy. *Nat Rev Immunol* (2019) 19:675–87. doi: 10.1038/s41577-019-0195-7

41. Peng J, Shengqing G, Deng P, Fu JX, Sahu A, Hu XH, et al. Signatures of T Cell Dysfunction and Exclusion Predict Cancer Immunotherapy Response. *Nat Med* (2018) 24:1550–58. doi: 10.1038/s41591-018-0136-1

42. He RQ, Zhou XG, Yi QY, Deng CW, Gao JM, Chen G, et al. Prognostic Signature of Alternative Splicing Events in Bladder Urothelial Carcinoma Based on Spliceseq Data from 317 Cases. *Cell Physiol Biochem* (2018) 48:1355–68. doi: 10.1159/000492094

# 11

# Molecular Characterization and Clinical Relevance of Lysine Acetylation Regulators in Urological Cancers

*Jian Zhang[1†], Chunning Zhang[2†], Huali Jiang[3], Hualong Jiang[4*] and Yawei Yuan[1*]*

[1] Department of Radiation Oncology, Affiliated Cancer Hospital & Institute of Guangzhou Medical University, State Key Laboratory of Respiratory Diseases, Guangzhou Institute of Respiratory Disease, Guangzhou, China, [2] The First Tumor Department, Maoming People's Hospital, Maoming, China, [3] Department of Cardiovascularology, Tungwah Hospital of Sun Yat-sen University, Dongguan, China, [4] Department of Urology, Tungwah Hospital of Sun Yat-sen University, Dongguan, China

*Correspondence:*
*Yawei Yuan*
*yuanyawei@gzhmu.edu.cn*
*orcid.org/0000-0002-8761-1140*
*Hualong Jiang*
*hualongjiang@yahoo.com*

[†]These authors have contributed
equally to this work

**Background:** Lysine acetylation and deacetylation are posttranslational modifications that are able to link extracellular signals to intracellular responses. However, knowledge regarding the status of lysine regulators in urological cancers is still unknown.

**Methods:** We first systematically analyzed the genetic and expression alterations of 31 lysine acetylation regulators in urological cancers. The correlation between lysine acetylation regulators and activation of cancer pathways was explored. The clinical relevance of lysine acetylation regulators was further analyzed.

**Results:** We identified that there are widespread genetic alterations of lysine acetylation regulators, and that their expression levels are significantly associated with the activity of cancer hallmark-related pathways. Moreover, lysine acetylation regulators were found to be potentially useful for prognostic stratification. HDAC11 may act as a potential oncogene in cell cycle and oxidative phosphorylation of urological cancers.

**Conclusion:** Lysine acetylation regulators are involved in tumorigenesis and progression. Our results provide a valuable resource that will guide both mechanistic and therapeutic analyses of the role of lysine acetylation regulators in urological cancers.

Keywords: lysine acetyltransferase, lysine deacetylase, urological cancers, genetic alterations, cancer pathways

## INTRODUCTION

Acetylation is the most common type of post-translational modification (PTM) of proteins, and it plays crucial roles in the development and progression cancer (1–3). Lysine acetylation is a reversible epigenetic PTM that plays crucial roles in the eukaryotic cells, which is regulated by the antagonistic actions of two families of enzymes: lysine acetyltransferases (KATs) and lysine deacetylases (KDACs) (4–6). Protein lysine acetylation and deacetylation contribute to several processes that maintain the proper functioning of cells, including transcriptional regulation and metabolic functions. Therefore, acetylation and deacetylation by lysine acetylation regulators has emerged as a crucial PTM for a wide range of cellular processes and is involved in aging and the development of several diseases, including cancer (7, 8). In addition, acetylation of lysine residues mediated by these regulators has been shown to be involved in the development of several diseases (6, 9, 10). Thus, a comprehensive understanding of the genetic alterations and expression perturbations underlying cancer cell heterogeneity is necessary to elucidate protein acetylation-based therapeutic targets.

Urological cancers entail the management of prostate, bladder, kidney, and testis cancer. The Global Burden of Disease Study showed a 2.1-fold increase in kidney cancer, a 1.5-fold increase in bladder cancer, and a 3.2-fold increase in prostate cancer (11). Women comprise 23.2% of new cases and 27.4% of deaths for bladder cancer and 34.7% of new cases and 33.1% of deaths for kidney cancer (12). Aberrant acetylation and deacetylation of genes were involved in occurrence and development of tumor, especially urological cancers (13–15). However, the molecular alterations and clinical prognostic value of lysine acetylation regulators in urological cancers are still unclear.

In this study, we aimed to systematically characterize the molecular alterations and clinical relevance of lysine acetylation regulators in urological cancers. We identified that there exist widespread genetic alterations (including genetic mutations and copy number variations) in lysine acetylation regulators among urological tumors. We also assessed whether perturbations in the expression of lysine acetylation regulators was correlated with the activity of cancer pathways. Moreover, we further explored the clinical prognostic value of lysine acetylation regulators, and found that lysine acetylation regulators are potentially useful markers for prognostic stratification. Our analysis indeed the importance of lysine acetylation regulators in urological cancers development, and lays a foundation for the development of therapeutic strategies based on lysine acetylation.

## METHODS

### Collection of Lysine Acetylation Regulators

A flowchart of the study design is shown in **Figure 1**. 31 lysine acetylation regulators were collected from recently published review papers (16, 17), including 13 KATs and 18 KDACs. All these gene symbols were converted into Ensemble gene IDs and HGNC symbols by manually curated from GeneCards (https://www.genecards.org/).

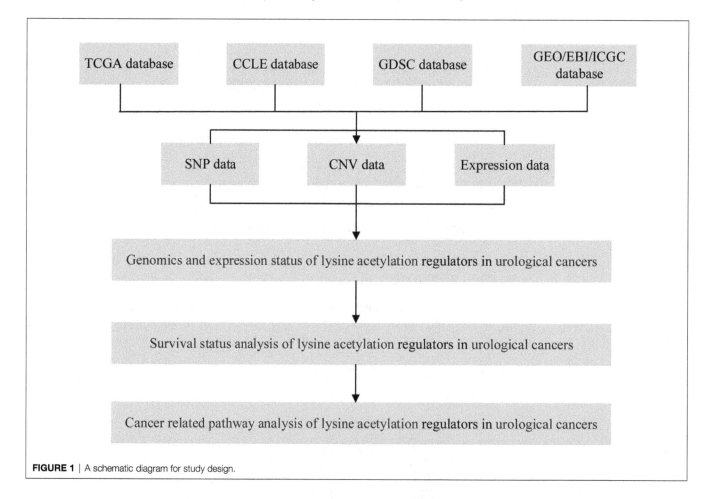

**FIGURE 1** | A schematic diagram for study design.

## Genome-Wide Omics Data Across Six Cancer Types

The omics datasets were downloaded from TCGA (http://cancergenome.nih.gov/). TCGA projects of six urological cancers, including kidney renal clear cell carcinoma (KIRC), kidney renal papillary cell carcinoma (KIRP), kidney chromophobe (KICH), bladder urothelial carcinoma (BLCA), prostate adenocarcinoma (PRAD) and testicular germ cell tumors (TGCT). All the somatic mutation data were obtained from TCGA database. The copy number variation data were downloaded from Broad GDAC Firehose (https://gdac.broadinstitute.org/). GISTIC was used to identify genomic regions that are significantly gained or lost across a set of tumors (18). RNA-seq data were obtained from the TCGA project *via* the R-package "TCGAbiolinks" (19), which is specifically developed for integrative analysis with GDC data. The clinical information for patients of urological cancer types were downloaded from TCGA project *via* the R-package "TCGAbiolinks".

## Genomic, Transcriptomic Data of Lysine Acetylation Regulators Across Cell Lines and Cancers

Genome-wide mutation data across cell lines were collected from the Broad Institute Cancer Cell Line Encyclopedia (CCLE) and the Genomics of Drug Sensitivity in Cancer database (GDSC) (20, 21). The cell lines were classified into different cancer types based on their annotations. In total, there were 14 cell lines across 2 cancer types from CCLE and 26 cell lines across 3 cancer types from GDSC. The mutation frequency of lysine acetylation regulators in each cancer type was defined as the proportion of cell lines with the regulator mutations. In addition, we also downloaded the copy number variation data for cell lines from CCLE and GDSC. There were 37 cell lines across 2 cancer types in CCLE and 47 cell lines in GDSC with CNV data. We calculated the CNV frequency in each cancer types as the proportion of cell lines with CNV amplification and deletion.

To validate the expression of lysine acetylation regulators across cancer types, we collected gene expression data across 778 samples representing 4 cancer types. These data were collected from Gene Expression Omnibus (GEO). To minimize inter-platform variation, only datasets generated from the Affymetrix Human Genome U133 Plus 2.0 Array were processed to develop the meta-dataset. Each dataset was preprocessed with RMA normalization, merged, and batch effect-corrected *via* Combat method (22).

## Identification of Differentially Expressed Genes

To identify differentially expressed genes in each cancer type, we used the Wilcox's rank sum test to identify differentially expressed genes. Genes with at least two-fold changes or less than half-fold changes and adjusted p-values <0.05 in expression were identified as differentially expressed genes using R package limma.

### Immunohistochemistry Analysis

To validate the protein expression of differentially expressed genes and activity of cell cycle and oxidative phosphorylation related pathway, as per the method described by our previous study (23), the protein of EP300, cyclin dependent kinases 2 (CDK2), cyclin A2 (CCNA2), NADH ubiquinone oxidoreductase complex assembly factor 8 of complex I (NDUFB8) and succinate dehydrogenase complex iron sulfur subunit B of complex II (SDHB) in TGCT, kidney_Tumor, BLCA and PRAD were clarified by immunohistochemistry analysis. All captured images were manually annotated by certified pathologists.

## Oncogenic Pathway Activity Across Cancer Types

To calculate the activity of cancer hallmark-related pathways, the FPKM-based gene expression was first transformed to Z-score by zFPKM package. To further estimate variation of gene set enrichment through the samples of an expression data set, the normalized gene expression were administered to Gene Set Variation Analysis (GSVA) (24). To identify the lysine acetylation regulators that were correlated with activation or inhibition of pathway, we calculated the Pearson Correlation Coefficient (PCC) between expression of lysine acetylation regulators and pathway activity. The regulator-pathway pairs with $|PCC|>0.5$ and adjusted p-value<0.01 were identified as significantly correlated lysine acetylation regulators.

## Clinical Relevance of Lysine Acetylation Regulators

To explore whether the expression of lysine acetylation regulators was associated with patient survival, we divided all the patients into two groups based on the median expression of HDAC9. The log-rank test was used to test the difference survival rates between two groups. This process was performed by the survival package in R program (https://cran.r-project.org/web/packages/survival/index.html). The p-values <0.05 were considered as significant.

## Validating the Clinical Association of Lysine Acetylation Regulators

We validated the clinical association of HDAC11 based on KIRC datasets from TCGA project. Patients were also divided into two groups based on the median expression of HDAC11, and the survival difference was tested by log-rank test.

## Validation of Lysine Acetylation Regulator-Pathway Correlation

To validate the lysine acetylation regulator-pathway correlation, we manually curated the TCGA database and collected KIRC gene expression data. The GSEA software tool (http://software.broadinstitute.org/gsea/index.jsp) was used to identify KEGG pathways (MSigDB, version 4.0) that show an overrepresentation of up- or downregulated genes between HDAC11 high expression and low expression. Briefly, an enrichment score was calculated for hallmark gene sets by ranking each gene and recording the maximum deviation from zero as the enrichment score.

## Statistical Analysis

Statistical analyses were performed using SPSS 17.0 (SPSS Inc., Chicago, IL, USA). All data shown are representative of at least three independent experiments, and values are expressed as the mean ± SD. Differences between two groups were analyzed using the two-tailed unpaired Student's *t*-test; *P*< 0.05 was considered significant.

## RESULTS

### Widespread Genetic Alterations of Lysine Acetylation Regulators Across Cancer Types

The numbers of lysine acetylation regulators have been identified from functions and mechanisms of non-histone protein

acetylation, and they can be broadly classified two groups: KATs and KDACs. We reviewed the literature and curated a catalog of 31 genes that function mainly as regulators of lysine acetylation, including 13 KATs and 18 KDACs (**Figure 2A**). We first determined the prevalence of lysine acetylation regulator alterations across 6 urological cancer types by integrating data on somatic mutations and copy number variations (CNVs). The overall average mutation frequency of lysine acetylation regulators was low, ranging from 0.0055-0.3443 (**Figure 2B** and **Table S1**). Cancer types with a higher global mutation burden (such as BLCA and KIRC) also exhibited a higher mutation frequency in lysine acetylation regulators. We identified that EP300 and CREBBP showed higher mutation

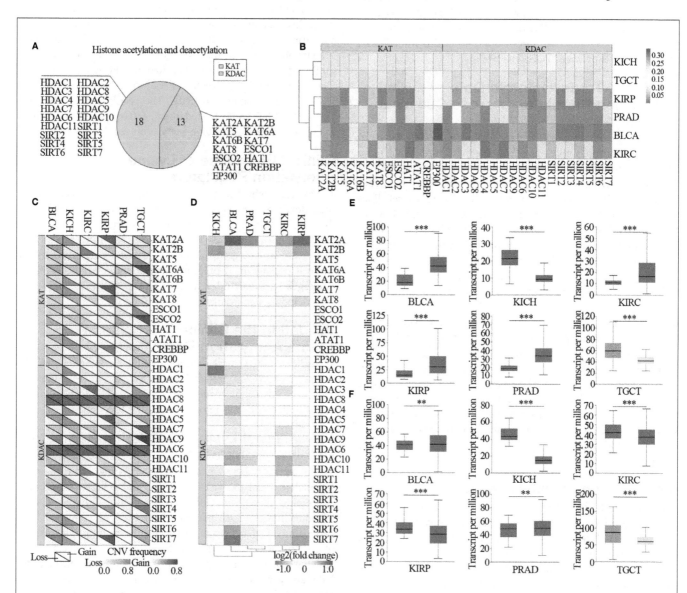

**FIGURE 2** | Urilogical tumors genetic and expression alterations of 31 lysine acetylation regulators. **(A)** The proportion of lysine acetylation regulators. **(B)** The mutation frequency of lysine acetylation regulators in 6 cancer types. **(C)** The CNV alteration frequency of lysine acetylation regulators in 6 cancer types. **(D)** The gene expression alterations of lysine acetylation regulators in TCGA database. **(E, F)** Box plots showing the expression distribution of KAT2A **(E)** and HAT1 **(F)** across tumor and normal samples in 6 cancer types. The blue color represents normal sample, the red color represents tumor sample, the blue color represents seminoma and the light green represents non-seminoma. **P < 0.01; ***P < 0.001.

frequencies (**Figure 2B**). Moreover, we found that lysine acetylation regulators in TGCT and KICH exhibited relatively few mutations compared to other cancers. Next the mutation data for 14 cell lines across 2 cancers from the Cancer Cell Line Encyclopedia (CCLE) and 26 cell lines across 3 cancers from the Genomics of Drug Sensitivity in Cancer (GDSC) database were collected. We identified that CREBBP had relatively high mutation frequencies across cancer types (**Figure S1** and **Tables S2, 3**).

The CNV alteration frequency for all lysine acetylation regulators, and found that CNV alterations are prevalent in urological cancers. CNV analysis showed that the CNV number of KAT2A, KAT2B, KAT7, KAT8, HDAC5, HDAC7, HDAC9, SIRT4 and SIRT7 were significantly increased in TCGT, KIRP, PRAD, KIRC and BLCA, while decreased in KICH. HDAC9 and SIRT7 showed widespread CNV amplification across cancer types (**Figure 2C**). While, ESCO2 had prevalent CNV deletions. Similarly, there were also prevalent CNV alterations in lysine acetylation regulators across cell lines (**Figure S2**). To further know whether these genetic alterations affect the expression of lysine acetylation regulators, we therefore analyzed the expression of lysine acetylation regulators across 6 cancer types. We found that CNV alterations are most likely one of the prominent mechanisms leading to perturbations in the expression of lysine acetylation regulators (**Figure 2D**).

The lysine acetylation regulators with CNV amplification showed significantly higher expression in cancer cells when compared to normal cells (e.g. KAT2A and ATAT1), while the regulators with CNV deletion showed significantly lower expression (e.g. SIRT6 and SIRT7). Meanwhile, we identified that KAT2A and HAT1 showed significantly differential expression, which was consistent with CNV variation in in 6 urological cancer types (**Figures 2E, F**). However, KAT2A was not significantly up-regulated in 800 samples based on GEO and EBI database (**Figure 3A** and **Table S4**), and EP300 was significantly up-regulated in kidney cancer, PRAD and TGCT (**Figure 3B**). To further validate the expression of EP300 in urological cancers, immunohistochemistry analysis showed that EP300 was significantly up-regulated in TGCT (100%, n = 12), kidney_tumor (100%, n = 11), BLCA (99%, n = 12) and PRAD (100%, n = 12) (**Figures 3C, D**). These results indicate that genetic and expression alteration landscape of lysine acetylation regulators across urological cancer types, suggesting that dysregulation of lysine acetylation regulator is involved in urological cancer contexts.

## Oncogenic Pathways Regulated by Lysine Acetylation Regulators

To further clarify the molecular mechanisms by which lysine acetylation regulators are involved in cancer, we examined the correlation between the expression of individual lysine acetylation regulators and the activity of 50 cancer hallmark-related pathways. We identified that the expression of lysine acetylation regulators is associated with the inhibition or activation of multiple oncogenic pathways (**Figure 4A** and

Table S3). The expression of KAT2A, KAT2B, SIRT3, SIRT5, SIRT6 and SIRT7 in KDACs, HDAC1, HDAC2, HDAC10 and HDAC11 in KATs were negatively correlated with a higher number of activated pathways, such as the MYC_targets, E2F_targets, Protein secretion and G2M checkpoint. In particular, we found that the EP300, ESCO2 and HDAC2 in KATs were correlated with the activation of several pathways (**Figure 4B**). Meanwhile, different KATs or KDACs were associated with distinct cancer pathway alterations, suggesting different functional effects of lysine acetylation regulators within the same functional class.

Moreover, to know the interaction of genetic alterations and expression correlation among lysine acetylation regulators, we found not only that genes within the same functional class showed significant co-occurrences of genetic alterations and highly correlated expression patterns, but that a high correlation also existed among KATs and KDACs (**Figure 4C**). For instance, the acetyltransferase KAT6B was significantly correlated with other acetyltransferases, such as, CREBBP and EP300. We also found that there were higher correlations among genes in the same protein complex, such as HDAC10 and SIRT7 (**Figure 2C**, R = 0.78 and P = 0). Meanwhile, we found that these KATs and KDACs interacted with each other frequently in protein-protein interaction networks (**Figure 4D**). There were an especially high number of interactions among the lysine acetylation regulators. Taken together, these results suggest that cross-talk among the KATs and KDACs of lysine acetylation, also mediates the abnormal expression of lysine acetylation regulators and plays critical roles in the development and progression of urological cancers.

## Clinical Relevance of Lysine Acetylation Regulators Across Cancer Types

To further explore the clinical relevance of lysine acetylation regulators, we first analyzed prognostic value of lysine acetylation regulators in urological cancers. We found that all of the lysine acetylation regulators were associated with the overall survival of patients in at least one cancer type (**Figure 5A**). Several lysine acetylation regulator genes showed oncogenic features, such as HDAC11 and SIRT4, and higher expression of these genes was associated with worse survival across cancer types.

In particular, high expression of HDAC11 was correlated with worse survival in 6 cancer types (**Figure 5B**), including BLCA (log-rank P = 0.002), KICH (log-rank P = 0.005), KIRC (log-rank P = 0), KIRP (log-rank P = 0), PRAD (log-rank P = 0.003) and TGCT (log-rank P = 0.006). Moreover, we collected another 4 datasets across three tissues from Gene Expression Omnibus (GEO) and International Cancer Genome Consortium (ICGC), and found that high expression of HDAC11 was associated with poor patient survival in GSE48075 and RECA-EU (ICGC) (**Figure 5C**). These observations indicate that HDAC11 might function as an oncogene across cancer types. In contrast, we found that several lysine acetylation regulators also showed features of tumor suppressors, such as ESCO2. Higher expression of ESCO2 was significantly associated with better survival in five cancer types.

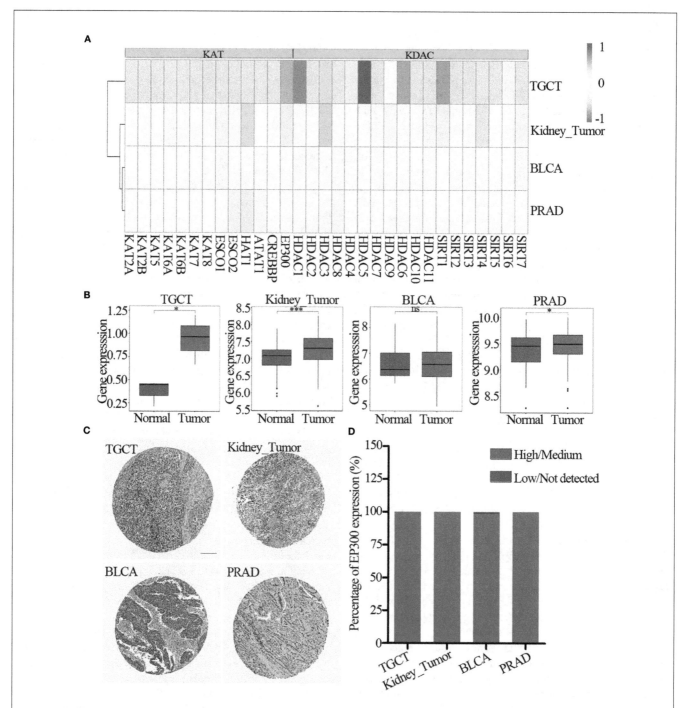

**FIGURE 3** | Expression of lysine acetylation regulators in GEO and EBI database. **(A)** Fold change of dysregulation genes. Red color represents upregulation genes and blue color represents downregulation genes. **(B)** The expression of EP300 in four cancer types. The blue color represents normal sample, the red color represents tumor sample. **(C)** Immunohistochemistry images of EP300 in TGCT, kidney_tumor, BLCA and PRAD. Scar bar = 200um. **(D)** Protein expression percentage of EP300 analyzed by immunohistochemistry. ns means not significant. *P < 0.05; ***P < 0.001.

Moreover, we found lysine acetylation regulators that were associated with patient survival in KIRC. We thus explored whether the expression of lysine acetylation regulators could contribute to the stratification of kidney cancer. Based on the global expression pattern of lysine acetylation regulators, we identified two subgroups of kidney cancer patient (**Figure 5D**).

The first subgroup consisted of 441 patients that showed higher expression of lysine acetylation regulators (Cluster 1), and the second of 86 patients with low expression (Cluster 2). Compared to the Cluster 2 subgroup, patients in the Cluster 1 subgroup had significantly better survival rates (**Figure 5E**, log-rank $P <$ 0.0001). To further validate the clinical implications of lysine

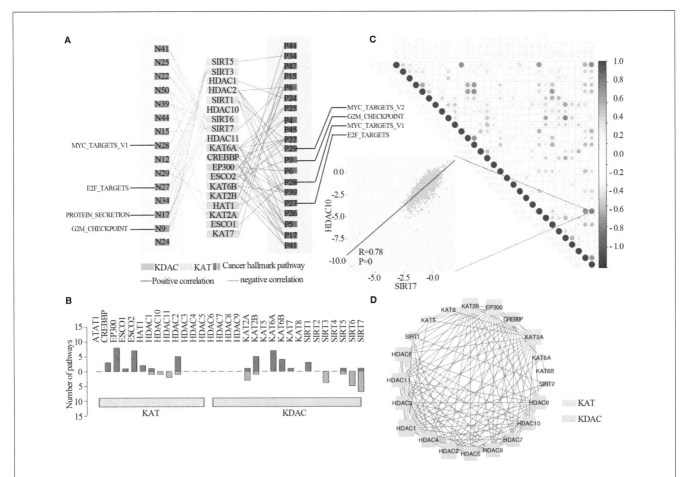

FIGURE 4 | Lysine acetylation regulators are associated with the activation and inhibition of cancer pathways. (A) Network diagram demonstrating the correlation between lysine acetylation regulators and cancer pathways. Red represents a positive correlation, and blue represents a negative correlation. The size of the nodes corresponds to the number of links. (B) The number of pathways is correlated with individual lysine acetylation regulators. The upper panel is for positively correlated pathways, and the bottom panel is for negatively correlated pathways. (C) Correlation among the expression of lysine acetylation regulators. The scatter plot shows the correlation between HDAC10 and SIRT7. (D) The protein-protein interactions among lysine acetylation regulators.

acetylation regulators, based on the mRNA expression of HDAC11 in KIRC, gene set enrichment analysis (GSEA) was performed to identify pathways potentially linked to HDAC11. Pathway analysis based on the KEGG database was performed, which identified 20 pathways with significant differences in gene expression (P < 0.05) (Figure 6A). GSEA analysis showed that hallmarks of cell cycle and oxidative phosphorylation were significantly enriched (Figures 6B, C). To further explore the activity of cell cycle and oxidative phosphorylation, the expression of CDK2 and CCNA2 in cell cycle pathway and the expression of NDUFB8 and SDHB in oxidative phosphorylation pathway were analyzed. The results showed that the high and medium expression percentage of CCNA2 in TCGT (36%, n = 11), kidney_tumor (17%, n = 12), BLCA (33%, n = 12) and PRAD (18%, n = 11) (Figures 6D, E), CDK2 in TCGT (0%, n = 11), kidney_tumor (0%, n = 12), BLCA (1%, n = 11) and PRAD (0%, n = 10) (Figures S3A, B) were up-regulated, while, the high and medium expression percentage of NDUFB8 in TCGT (58%, n = 12), kidney_tumor (73%, n = 11), BLCA (67%, n = 12) and PRAD (73%, n = 11) (Figures 6D, F), SDHB

in TCGT (100%, n = 10), kidney_tumor (83%, n = 12), BLCA (100%, n = 9) and PRAD (100%, n = 11) (Figures S3A, C) were up-regulated. The results indicated the cell cycle was significantly inactivated, however, oxidative phosphorylation was significantly activated in urological cancers. Together, these results suggest a diverse potential of lysine acetylation regulators in the prognostic stratification of specific types of urological cancer and in the development of targeted treatment strategies.

## DISCUSSION

This study demonstrates the prevalent genetic and expression alterations of lysine acetylation regulators across urological cancer types. These lysine acetylation regulators are significantly correlated with the activation and inactivation of cancer pathways, and are also associated with prognostically urological cancers. These results provide new mechanistic understanding of lysine acetylation regulators in urological cancers.

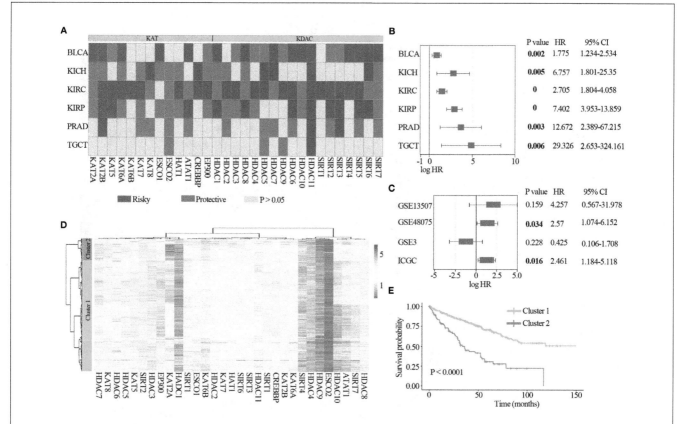

**FIGURE 5** | Clinical relevance of lysine acetylation regulators across 6 cancer types. **(A)** Summary of the correlation between expression of lysine acetylation regulators and patient survival. Red represents a higher expression of lysine acetylation regulator associated with worse survival, and blue represents an association with better survival. Only p values < 0.05 are shown. **(B)** The distribution of hazard ratios across 6 cancer types. **(C)** The distribution of hazard ratios across different GEO datasets. **(D)** Heat map showing the clustering for kidney renal clear cell carcinoma patients based on the expression of lysine acetylation regulators. **(E)** Kaplan-Meier survival plot of patients grouped by global expression pattern of lysine acetylation regulators.

KIRC, BLCA and PRAD are the most common urological cancers (25, 26). Despite improved primary prevention, detection, and treatment, the incidence of age-related cancers of the urinary tract is likely to rise as a result of global population ageing (27, 28). Therefore, it is vital to identify and address the most relevant perturbed genes/proteins for further early detection, investigation, and therapy of urological malignancies.

Dysfunctions in epigenetic and genomics regulation play critical roles in tumor development and progression. KATs and KDACs are functionally opposing epigenetic regulators, which control the activation status of tumor suppressor genes or oncogenes. Upregulation of HDAC activities could result in silencing of tumor suppressor genes and uncontrolled malignant characteristics in urological tumors (29–32). In this study, we comprehensively and systematically explored the genetic alterations and expression perturbations of KATs and KDACs. And we found that the mutation frequency of 31 lysine acetylation regulators, except for CREBBP and EP300, was completely low in KIRP, PRAD, BLCA and KIRC. CNV amplification of acetylation regulators were significantly increased in TCGT, KIRP, KIRC, BLCA and PRAD, while CNV deletion in KICH were found. However, the CNV of

HDAC8 and HDAC6 were unchanged in urological cancers. Expression analysis indicated that lysine acetylation regulators were downregulated in KICH, which may be associated with the CNV deletion, while upregulated in other 5 urological cancers, which may be associated with CNV amplification in cancers. However, the expression and prognostic roles of acetylation regulators in urological cancers were not completely consistent. Thus, abnormal expression of acetylation regulators was regulated not only CNV, but also interaction network between acetylation regulators. However, the concrete mechanism still need to be further explored.

Histone deacetylation describes the removal of acetyl groups regulated by KDACs. Widespread genetic alterations (including mutations and CNV) in lysine acetylation regulators were significantly associated with the activation of MYC_targets, E2F_targets, Protein secretion and G2M checkpoint. Histone deacetylase11 (HDAC11), one member of the KDACs family, is associated with condensed chromatin structures that in turn suppress transcription. HDAC11 were significantly up-regulated in 6 urological tumors, GSEA analysis found that dysregulation of HDAC11 was involved in cell cycle and oxidative phosphorylation pathways, which was consistent with hallmarks of acetylation regulators and other

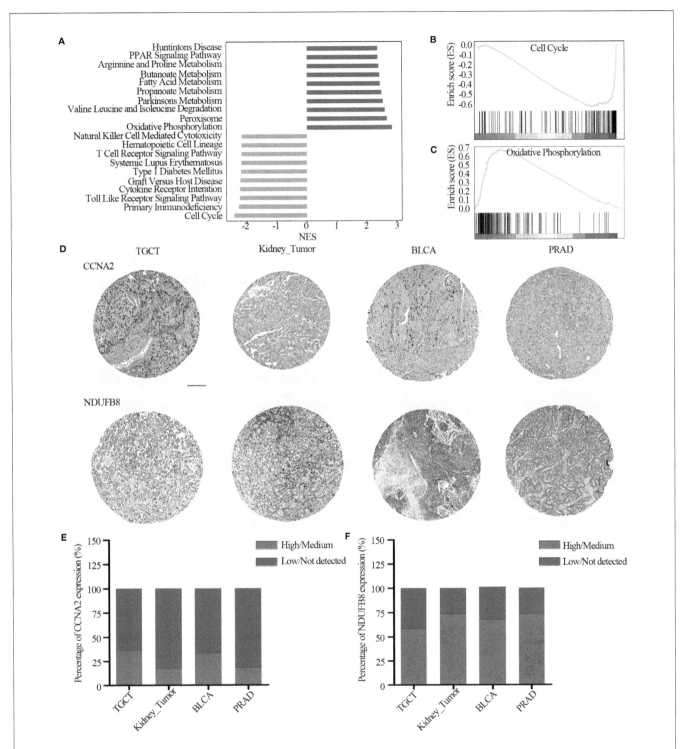

**FIGURE 6** | Pathways potentially regulated by HDAC11. **(A)** Distribution of normalized enrichment scores for pathways. The pathways colored in blue was the depleted pathways in HDAC11 downregulation, while the red one is enriched pathway. **(B, C)** GSEA-enrichment plot of the representative gene sets. **(B)** Cell cycle; **(C)** Oxidative phosphorylation. **(D)** Immunohistochemistry images of CCNA2 and NDUFB8 in TGCT, kidney_tumor, BLCA and PRAD. Scar bar = 200um. **(E, F)** Protein expression percentage of CCNA2 **(E)** and NDUFB8 **(F)** analyzed by immunohistochemistry.

studies (33–35). Our immunohistochemistry analysis also validated that cell cycle pathway (CDK2 and CCNA2) was significantly inactivated and oxidative phosphorylation pathway (NDUFB8 and SDHB) was significantly activated, which would may be associated with abnormal expression of acetylation regulators in urological cancers. However, the concrete mechanism of HDAC11 on urological tumors need be further explored.

## CONCLUSION

In summary, this systematic analysis of the landscape of molecular alterations and clinical relevance of lysine acetylation regulators clarifies a profound understanding the dysregulation of lysine acetylation regulators. It will also provide insights into the development of urological cancers.

## AUTHOR CONTRIBUTIONS

JZ, CZ, HualiJ, HualongJ, and YY conducted and designed experiments, performed data analysis, and drafted the manuscript. HualongJ and YY supervised the project, designed experiments, and edited the manuscript. All authors contributed to the article and approved the submitted version.

## REFERENCES

1. Audia JE, Campbell RM. Histone Modifications and Cancer. *Cold Spring Harb Perspect Biol* (2016) 8:a019521. doi: 10.1101/cshperspect.a019521
2. Narayan S, Bader GD, Reimand J. Frequent Mutations in Acetylation and Ubiquitination Sites Suggest Novel Driver Mechanisms of Cancer. *Genome Med* (2016) 8:55. doi: 10.1186/s13073-016-0311-2
3. Barneda-Zahonero B, Parra M. Histone Deacetylases and Cancer. *Mol Oncol* (2012) 6:579–89. doi: 10.1016/j.molonc.2012.07.003
4. Menzies KJ, Zhang H, Katsyuba E, Auwerx J. Protein Acetylation in Metabolism - Metabolites and Cofactors. *Nat Rev Endocrinol* (2016) 12:43–60. doi: 10.1038/nrendo.2015.181
5. Torres-Machorro AL, Pillus L. Bypassing the Requirement for an Essential MYST Acetyltransferase. *Genetics* (2014) 197:851–63. doi: 10.1534/genetics.114.165894
6. Iyer A, Fairlie DP, Brown L. Lysine Acetylation in Obesity, Diabetes and Metabolic Disease. *Immunol Cell Biol* (2012) 90:39–46. doi: 10.1038/icb.2011.99
7. Molehin D, Castro-Piedras I, Sharma M, Sennoune SR, Arena D, Manna PR, et al. Aromatase Acetylation Patterns and Altered Activity in Response to Sirtuin Inhibition. *Mol Cancer Res* (2018) 16:1530–42. doi: 10.1158/1541-7786.MCR-18-0047
8. Lee JV, Carrer A, Shah S, Snyder NW, Wei S, Venneti S, et al. Akt-Dependent Metabolic Reprogramming Regulates Tumor Cell Histone Acetylation. *Cell Metab* (2014) 20:306–19. doi: 10.1016/j.cmet.2014.06.004
9. Kaelin WGJr., McKnight SL. Influence of Metabolism on Epigenetics and Disease. *Cell* (2013) 153:56–69. doi: 10.1016/j.cell.2013.03.004
10. Min SW, Chen X, Tracy TE, Li Y, Zhou Y, Wang C, et al. Critical Role of Acetylation in Tau-Mediated Neurodegeneration and Cognitive Deficits. *Nat Med* (2015) 21:1154–62. doi: 10.1038/nm.3951
11. Dy GW, Gore JL, Forouzanfar MH, Naghavi M, Fitzmaurice C. Global Burden of Urologic Cancers, 1990-2013. *Eur Urol* (2017) 71:437–46. doi: 10.1016/j.eururo.2016.10.008
12. Siegel RL, Miller KD, Jemal A. Cancer Statistics, 2018. *CA Cancer J Clin* (2018) 68:7–30. doi: 10.3322/caac.21442
13. Zhang B, Ci X, Tao R, Ni JJ, Xuan X, King JL, et al. Klf5 Acetylation Regulates Luminal Differentiation of Basal Progenitors in Prostate Development and Regeneration. *Nat Commun* (2020) 11:997. doi: 10.1038/s41467-020-14737-8
14. Linehan WM, Rouault TA. Molecular Pathways: Fumarate Hydratase-Deficient Kidney Cancer–Targeting the Warburg Effect in Cancer. *Clin Cancer Res* (2013) 19:3345–52. doi: 10.1158/1078-0432.CCR-13-0304
15. Qu W, Kang YD, Zhou MS, Fu LL, Hua ZH, Wang LM. Experimental Study on Inhibitory Effects of Histone Deacetylase Inhibitor MS-275 and TSA on Bladder Cancer Cells. *Urol Oncol* (2010) 28:648–54. doi: 10.1016/j.urolonc.2008.11.018
16. Xia C, Tao Y, Li M, Che T, Qu J. Protein Acetylation and Deacetylation: An Important Regulatory Modification in Gene Transcription (Review). *Exp Ther Med* (2020) 20:2923–40. doi: 10.3892/etm.2020.9073

## SUPPLEMENTARY MATERIAL

**Supplementary Figure 1** | Mutation frequency distribution of lysine acetylation regulators across different urological cancer types. Left circos plot **(A)** showing the mutation frequency of lysine acetylation regulators in CCLE, and right circos **(B)** showing the mutation frequency in GDSC. Each circos represents one cancer type, which were shown in the bottom panel. *P < 0.05.

**Supplementary Figure 2** | CNV alterations of lysine acetylation regulators across cell lines in different urological cancer types. Left circos plot **(A)** showing the CNV frequency of lysine acetylation regulators in CCLE, and right circos **(B)** showing the CNV frequency in GDSC. Each circos represents one cancer type, which were shown in the bottom panel.

**Supplementary Figure 3** | **(A)** Immunohistochemistry images of CDK2 and SDHB in TGCT, kidney_tumor, BLCA and PRAD. Scar bar = 200um. **(B, C)** Protein expression percentage of CDK2 **(B)** and SDHB **(C)** analyzed by immunohistochemistry.

17. Di Martile M, Del Bufalo D, Trisciuoglio D. The Multifaceted Role of Lysine Acetylation in Cancer: Prognostic Biomarker and Therapeutic Target. *Oncotarget* (2016) 7:55789–810. doi: 10.18632/oncotarget.10048
18. Mermel CH, Schumacher SE, Hill B, Meyerson ML, Beroukhim R, Getz G. GISTIC2.0 Facilitates Sensitive and Confident Localization of the Targets of Focal Somatic Copy-Number Alteration in Human Cancers. *Genome Biol* (2011) 12:R41. doi: 10.1186/gb-2011-12-4-r41
19. Colaprico A, Silva TC, Olsen C, Garofano L, Cava C, Garolini D, et al. Tcgabiolinks: An R/Bioconductor Package for Integrative Analysis of TCGA Data. *Nucleic Acids Res* (2016) 44:e71. doi: 10.1093/nar/gkv1507
20. Ghandi M, Huang FW, Jane-Valbuena J, Kryukov GV, Lo CC, McDonald ER 3rd, et al. Next-Generation Characterization of the Cancer Cell Line Encyclopedia. *Nature* (2019) 569:503–8. doi: 10.1038/s41586-019-1186-3
21. Yang W, Soares J, Greninger P, Edelman EJ, Lightfoot H, Forbes S, et al. Genomics of Drug Sensitivity in Cancer (GDSC): A Resource for Therapeutic Biomarker Discovery in Cancer Cells. *Nucleic Acids Res* (2013) 41:D955–961. doi: 10.1093/nar/gks1111
22. Leek JT, Johnson WE, Parker HS, Jaffe AE, Storey JD. The Sva Package for Removing Batch Effects and Other Unwanted Variation in High-Throughput Experiments. *Bioinformatics* (2012) 28:882–3. doi: 10.1093/bioinformatics/bts034
23. Zhang J, Lin H, Jiang H, Jiang H, Xie T, Wang B, et al. A Key Genomic Signature Associated With Lymphovascular Invasion in Head and Neck Squamous Cell Carcinoma. *BMC Cancer* (2020) 20:226. doi: 10.1186/s12885-020-06728-1
24. Hanzelmann S, Castelo R, Guinney J. GSVA: Gene Set Variation Analysis for Microarray and RNA-seq Data. *BMC Bioinf* (2013) 14:7. doi: 10.1186/1471-2105-14-7
25. Capitanio U, Montorsi F. Renal Cancer. *Lancet* (2016) 387:894–906. doi: 10.1016/S0140-6736(15)00046-X
26. Clark PE, Agarwal N, Biagioli MC, Eisenberger MA, Greenberg RE, Herr HW, et al. Bladder Cancer. *J Natl Compr Canc Netw* (2013) 11:446–75. doi: 10.6004/jnccn.2013.0059
27. Chlosta PL, Golabek T, Nyirady P. New Insights Into Diagnosis and Treatment of Renal Cell Carcinoma, Bladder Cancer, and Prostate Cancer. *BioMed Res Int* (2017) 2017:6467072. doi: 10.1155/2017/6467072
28. Golabek T, Powroznik J, Chlosta P, Dobruch J, Borowka A. The Impact of Nutrition in Urogenital Cancers. *Arch Med Sci* (2015) 11:411–8. doi: 10.5114/aoms.2015.50973
29. Thoma C. Kidney Cancer: Combination of HDAC Inhibitor With IL-2 Promising. *Nat Rev Urol* (2017) 14:639. doi: 10.1038/nrurol.2017.171
30. Wang D, Li W, Zhao R, Chen L, Liu N, Tian Y, et al. Stabilized Peptide Hdac Inhibitors Derived From HDAC1 Substrate H3K56 for the Treatment of Cancer Stem-Like Cells In Vivo. *Cancer Res* (2019) 79:1769–83. doi: 10.1158/0008-5472.CAN-18-1421
31. Pinkerneil M, Hoffmann MJ, Schulz WA, Niegisch G. Hdacs and HDAC Inhibitors in Urothelial Carcinoma - Perspectives for an Antineoplastic

Treatment. *Curr Med Chem* (2017) 24:4151–65. doi: 10.2174/0929867324666170207142740

32. Shankar E, Pandey M, Verma S, Abbas A, Candamo M, Kanwal R, et al. Role of Class I Histone Deacetylases in the Regulation of Maspin Expression in Prostate Cancer. *Mol Carcinog* (2020) 59:955–66. doi: 10.1002/mc.23214

33. Thole TM, Lodrini M, Fabian J, Wuenschel J, Pfeil S, Hielscher T, et al. Neuroblastoma Cells Depend on HDAC11 for Mitotic Cell Cycle Progression

and Survival. *Cell Death Dis* (2017) 8:e2635. doi: 10.1038/cddis.2017.49

34. Bagui TK, Sharma SS, Ma L, Pledger WJ. Proliferative Status Regulates HDAC11 mRNA Abundance in Nontransformed Fibroblasts. *Cell Cycle* (2013) 12:3433–41. doi: 10.4161/cc.26433

35. Hurtado E, Nunez-Alvarez Y, Munoz M, Gutierrez-Caballero C, Casas J, Pendas AM, et al. HDAC11 is a Novel Regulator of Fatty Acid Oxidative Metabolism in Skeletal Muscle. *FEBS J* (2020) 288:902–19. doi: 10.1111/febs.15456

# 12

# Robust Prognostic Subtyping of Muscle-Invasive Bladder Cancer Revealed by Deep Learning-Based Multi-Omics Data Integration

Xiaolong Zhang [1,2,3†], Jiayin Wang [1*†], Jiabin Lu [4†], Lili Su [1], Changxi Wang [1], Yuhua Huang [2,4], Xuanping Zhang [1] and Xiaoyan Zhu [1]

[1] School of Electronic and Information Engineering, Xi'an Jiaotong University, Xi'an, China, [2] Sun Yat-sen University Cancer Center, State Key Laboratory of Oncology in South China, Collaborative Innovation Center for Cancer Medicine, Guangzhou, China, [3] School of Medicine, Shenzhen University, Shenzhen, China, [4] Department of Pathology, Sun Yat-sen University Cancer Center, Guangzhou, China

*Correspondence:
Jiayin Wang
wangjiayin@xjtu.edu.cn

†These authors share first authorship

Muscle-invasive bladder cancer (MIBC) is the most common urinary system carcinoma associated with poor outcomes. It is necessary to develop a robust classification system for prognostic prediction of MIBC. Recently, increasing omics data at different levels of MIBC were produced, but few integration methods were used to classify MIBC that reflects the patient's prognosis. In this study, we constructed an autoencoder based deep learning framework to integrate multi-omics data of MIBC and clustered samples into two different subgroups with significant overall survival difference ($P = 8.11 \times 10^{-5}$). As an independent prognostic factor relative to clinical information, these two subtypes have some significant genomic differences. Remarkably, the subtype of poor prognosis had significant higher frequency of chromosome 3p deletion. Immune decomposition analysis results showed that these two MIBC subtypes had different immune components including macrophages M1, resting NK cells, regulatory T cells, plasma cells, and naïve B cells. Hallmark gene set enrichment analysis was performed to investigate the functional character difference between these two MIBC subtypes, which revealed that activated IL-6/JAK/STAT3 signaling, interferon-alpha response, reactive oxygen species pathway, and unfolded protein response were significantly enriched in upregulated genes of high-risk subtype. We constructed MIBC subtyping models based on multi-omics data and single omics data, respectively, and internal and external validation datasets showed the robustness of the prediction model as well as its ability of prognosis ($P < 0.05$ in all datasets). Finally, through bioinformatics analysis and immunohistochemistry experiments, we found that KRT7 can be used as a biomarker reflecting MIBC risk.

Keywords: muscle-invasive bladder cancer, multi-omics, deep learning, subtyping, prognosis

# INTRODUCTION

Bladder urothelial carcinoma (BLCA) is one of the most common cancer types in human (1), while muscle-invasive bladder cancer (MIBC) accounts for the majority of patient mortality (2). Over the past tens of years, there is no practical option to improve the survival of MIBC patients. Unlike the high 5-year survival rate (95%) of bladder cancer that has not spread beyond the inner layer of the bladder wall, the 5-year survival rate of MIBC without distant metastasis dropped to 69%, and if cancer extends through the bladder to the surrounding tissue or has spread to nearby lymph nodes or organs, the 5-year survival rate is 35% (Approved by the Cancer.Net Editorial Board, 05/2019).

In recent years, many studies have characterized the molecular features at different omics levels and reported subclassification of bladder cancer into distinct subtypes based on unique molecular signatures (3–11). For example, The Cancer Genome Atlas (TCGA) consortium reported four clusters of MIBCs with gene expression profiling and two of which were also evident in microRNA (miRNA) sequencing and protein data (6). Robertson et al. (11) recruited many TCGA-MIBC samples and subtyped the MIBC patients referring to the mutation signature, the expression of mRNA, lncRNA, and miRNA, respectively, and revealed some of the subtypes related to a poor-survival phenotype.

Nevertheless, the previous studies investigated the molecular subtypes of bladder cancer only based on single omics level, and did not connect with the survival information during the process of defining subtypes. Thus, a subtyping method that could reflect

different survival profiles is valuable for the clinical application in guiding the treatment of MIBC patients.

Here, we employed a multi-omics-based utilized deep learning (DL) computational framework to stratify the MIBC patients into two subgroups concerning different risks of overall survival (OS) (**Figure 1**). We investigated feature differences between the two subgroups of MIBC, and derived prognostic models based on multi- or single-omics data to classify MIBC into different subgroups. Gene expression-based model were further validated by both in-group and out-group datasets. Besides, we figure out a cell surface marker—KRT7 (CK7), which is significantly differently expressed in high-risk and low-risk MIBC.

# MATERIALS AND METHODS

## Datasets and Study Design

The multi-omics data of TCGA-BLCA, including gene-level copy number variation (CNV) profile, mRNA and miRNA expression profile revealed by RNA-seq and miRNA-seq, and DNA methylation data profiled by Illumina Infinium HumanMethylation450 platform, were downloaded from the University of California Santa Cruz (UCSC) Xena database (https://xenabrowser.net/).

Only samples with tumor stage II/III/IV (MIBC) remained for downstream analysis. These TCGA-MIBC datasets were used in two ways: 1) All samples were used to perform subgroup stratification based on deep learning and clustering algorithm; 2)

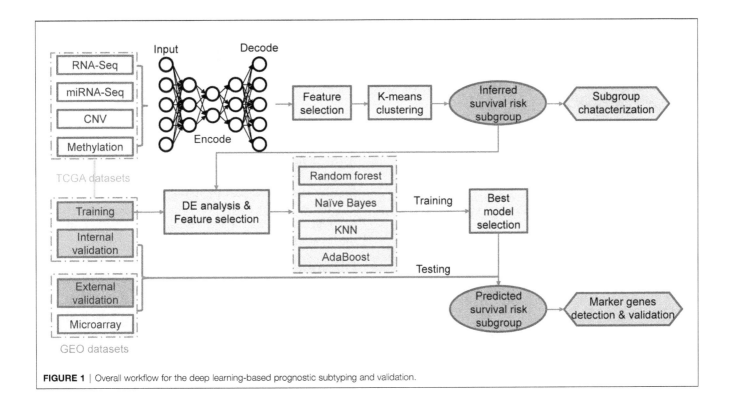

**FIGURE 1** | Overall workflow for the deep learning-based prognostic subtyping and validation.

samples were randomly split by 4:1, including a training dataset to train the classification model and an in-group testing dataset to validate the prediction accuracy. Three gene microarray matrices containing 43 MIBC patients (GSE19915), 62 MIBC patients (GSE48277-GPL14951), and 73 MIBC patients (GSE48277-GPL6947) were downloaded from Gene Expression Omnibus (GEO) database (https://www.ncbi.nlm.nih.gov/geo/), serving as out-group validation datasets. For these datasets, only samples with prognostic information were taken into consideration for downstream analysis.

## Multi-Omics Data Integration

The autoencoder framework was chosen as the implementation of deep learning for integrating the results derived from multi-omics data. The CNV, gene expression, miRNA expression, and methylation data extracted from TCGA-MIBC dataset served as an input for the autoencoders framework. The autoencoder was a dimensionality reduction method based on an unsupervised feed-forward, non-recurrent neural network, which is implemented in python with package Keras (https://github.com/fchollet/keras).

We build the autoencoder framework as previously reported (12), which could be briefly described as follows:

For a given input layer, the objective of an autoencoder reconstructed the input layer $x$ (sized as $d \times p$) into the same dimension output layer $y$ through an activation function $tanh$ (a hidden layer between $x$ and $y$). In this study, we used the four preprocessed data matrices of different level of omics data (features $\times$ samples) and stacked all features together into a merged big matrix. In total, 350,631 features were used for downstream analysis. All of the features except CNV features were scaled so that all values are within a similar distribution range. This step could be expressed as:

$$y_i = f_i(x) = tanh(W_i x + b_i)$$

where $b_i$ is an intercept vector of size p and $W_i.x = \Sigma_j W_{i,j}.x_j$, in which $x_j$ is the value of a single feature of $x$. When the autoencoder framework has $k$ layers,

$$y = F_{1 \to k}(x) = f_1 \circ \cdots f_{k-1} \circ f_k(x)$$

where $f_{k-1} \circ f_k(x) = f_{k-1}(f_k(x))$.

To train an autoencoder, the objective is to find the different weight vectors $W_i$ minimizing a specific objective function. We chose *binary crossentropy* as the objective function, which measures the error between the input $x$ and the output $y$:

$$binary\ crossentropy(x,y) = \sum_{k=1}^{d}(x_k log(y_k) + (1-x_k)log(1-y_k))$$

We added two regularization penalty $\alpha_w$ and $\alpha_a$ for both weight vector $W_i$ and node activities $F_{1 \to k}(x)$:

$$L(x,y) = binary\ crossentropy(x,y)$$
$$+ \sum_{i=1}^{d}(\alpha_w||W_i||_i + \alpha_a||F_{1 \to i}(x)||_2^2)$$

We set the three hidden layers in the autoencoder, which included 500, 100, and 500 nodes, respectively. The bottleneck layer of the autoencoder was adopted to generate novel characteristics from the four-level omics data. The penal values $\alpha_w$ and $\alpha_a$ were set as 0. 1 and $1 \times 10^{-7}$, respectively. Finally, the autoencoder was trained by the gradient descent algorithm with 10 epochs and a batch size of 64.

## Selection of the Transformed Features and Sample Clustering

One hundred novel features were derived from the omics data based on the deep learning algorithm. For each of these transformed features, we performed the univariate Cox proportional-hazards regression analysis to find out the OS-related features (log-rank test, $P < 0.05$). Subsequently, we used these selected features to cluster the MIBC samples into groups based on the K-means clustering algorithm. The hazard ratio and the p-value derived from log-rank test were used to evaluate the prognostic differences.

## Genomic Analysis of TCGA Data

Somatic mutation data of TCGA BLCA and copy number segment data were downloaded from UCSC Xena database (https://xenabrowser.net/datapages/), respectively, and MIBC samples were extracted for downstream analysis. The mutation data was converted into "maf" format and visualized by Maftools (13). The segmentation file contains the segmented data for all the samples separated into S1 and S2 subgroups, and the recurrent frequency of each segment in each subgroup was calculated using GISTIC2 (14). The frequency of each chromosome cytoband in S1 and S2 was calculated smoothly from the files named "scores.gistic", and then chi-square test was used to detect regions with significant differences in CNA frequency between S1 and S2 subtypes. Immune cell composition of MIBC was estimated from the expression data using the program CIBERSORT (15).

## Differential Expression Analysis and Functional Enrichment

Differentially expressed genes (DEGs) of TCGA data were detected by DESeq2 (16), and DEGs of microarray-based datasets were detected using the limma package (17) Hallmark gene set was downloaded from Molecular Signatures Database v7.0 (MSigDB, http://software.broadinstitute.org/gsea/msigdb/), and gene set enrichment analysis (GSEA) was performed using the R package "clusterProfiler" (18).

## Differential Methylation Analysis and Functional Enrichment

To test for differentially methylated CpG sites (DMS), we use the limma package. CpG site was defined as a DMS that |log2(fold-change)| of Beta value was more than 1 and adjusted p-value was less than 0.05. DMS located genes were extracted, and over-represent enrichment analysis was performed using the R package "clusterProfiler".

## Data Partitioning and Prognostic Subgroup Robustness Assessment

All TCGA MIBC samples were randomly separated into training/testing datasets following a 4:1 split. Then, we build a supervised classification model using random forest, Naïve Bayes, k-Nearest Neighbor, and Adaboost algorithms. For the training dataset, we normalized each omics layer and calculated the p-value (Wilcox test) of each feature between these two prognostic subgroups. Then, we selected top features (50 for CNV, 100 for mRNA, 50 for miRNA, and 50 for CpG methylation) that are most correlated with subgroup labels based on the p-values. Then, we conducted 10-fold cross-validation with 10-time repeat to evaluate the predictive ability of the selected features.

During each repetition, different algorithms were applied (mentioned above), and receiver operating characteristic (ROC) curves were executed. The area under the curve (AUC) in all the repeats would provide us the predictive value of the classification. Once the AUC value was less than 0.7, the whole dataset would be re-split and the analysis would be re-started till the satisfying results were obtained. Finally, we select the best classification model with the highest AUC.

We selected the same features of each omics data in the testing dataset and predicted the label of each sample based on the classification model. The univariate Cox proportional-hazards regression analysis was performed to test the survival risk difference between the predicted groups.

For the out-group validation dataset, which only has a gene expression profile, we just use the overlapped features with the 100 mRNAs mentioned above to fit the classification model. The same tests were performed on TCGA testing dataset.

## Immunohistochemical (IHC) Staining and Assessment

Twenty-two MIBC samples were selected from Sun Yat-sen University Cancer Center, Guangzhou, China, between January 2015 and December 2015. Only samples with overall survival less than 1.5 years or over 5 years were taken into consideration in this study. IHC staining was performed using BenchMark ULTRA automatic immunostaining device according to the manufacturer's instructions to analyze the KRT7 expression. In brief, the paraffin-embedded MIBC samples were sectioned and deparaffinized using EZ prep solution (BenchMark, Roche, Arizona, USA). The endogenous peroxidase activity was inhibited, and the sections were subjected to antigen retrieval in a cell-conditioning solution maintained at 95°C for 30 min. The sections with the primary antibody mouse anti-CK7 (MXB Biotechnologies Inc., Fuzhou, China, Kit-0021, 1:100 dilution) were incubated at 37°C for 1 h after adding Liquid crystal solution (BenchMark, Roche, Arizona, USA). A secondary antibody was then added at 37°C for 15 min, and signals were detected using the chromogen 3,3'-diaminobenzidine (DAB). The sections were counterstained with hematoxylin and then dehydrated and mounted on a coverslip. Staining proportion (0–100%) and staining strength (- to 4+) were measured for each sample, and an IHC score was calculated as follows:

$$S_{IHC} = S_{pro} + S_{str}$$

where $S_{pro}$ stands for the score of staining proportion (0%, $S_{pro}$ = 0; 1–20%, $S_{pro}$ = 1; 21–40%, $S_{pro}$ = 2; 41–60%, $S_{pro}$ = 3; 61–80%, $S_{pro}$ = 4; 81–100%, $S_{pro}$ = 5) and $S_{str}$ stands for the score of staining strength (-, $S_{str}$ = 0; +, $S_{str}$ = 1; ++, $S_{str}$ = 2; +++, $S_{str}$ = 3; + +++, $S_{str}$ = 4). The IHC score was used to measure the expression level of KRT7.

## RESULTS

### The Identification of OS-Related Subtypes Based on TCGA Multi-Omics Data

The multiple layers of genetic data were extracted from the TCGA database, and with the help of autoencoder-based deep learning algorithm, these data were stacked together (see *Materials and methods*). As a result, 100 new features were extracted from the bottleneck hidden layer, which represented the features of omics. We performed univariate Cox proportional-hazards regression analysis on these features and identified 98 features that were highly correlated with patients' OS ($P < 0.05$, log-rank test; **Supplementary Table S1**). Subsequently, the MIBC patients were assigned into different clusters using K-means clustering algorithm referring to these OS-related features. We chose 2 as the optimal number of clusters (**Figure 2A**). Then, we conducted a univariate Cox proportional-hazards regression on the grouping result and observed that these two subtypes show a significant difference in OS outcomes ($P = 8.11 \times 10^{-5}$, log-rank test, **Figure 2B**). Furthermore, we performed multi-variates cox regression analysis using general clinical characters as well as the predicted subtypes, and the result shows that this molecular classification can be used as an independent prognostic indicator compared to general clinical information (**Figure 2C**). We further analyzed the relationship between the molecular subtyping and clinical information, and found that all patients from S2 were of high grade (**Figure 2D**).

### Molecular Differences Between These Two Prognostic Subtypes

In order to analyze the molecular characteristics of the two molecular subtypes, we firstly compared the differences in mutation and CNA levels between the two groups. There is no significant difference between the two subtypes in terms of mutation burden (**Figure 3A**). Several genes were found significantly mutated in S1, including *NFE2L2*, *UGGT2*, *SCN3A*, *TGFBR3*, and *NPC1L1* (**Figure 3B**). Besides, regions located on chromosome 3p have a significantly higher frequency of deletion in S2 patients (**Figure 3C** and **Supplementary Table 2**; adjusted *P*-value < 0.05, chi-square test), which contains some important tumor suppressor genes (TSGs) including *FANCD2*, *VHL*, *RPARG*, *XPC*, *TGFBR2*, *MLH1*, *SETD2*, and *RHOA*. Interestingly, TGF-Beta receptors were significantly altered in S2 at both SNV and CNV levels. Considering that transforming growth factor (TGF)-b is a key executor of immune homeostasis

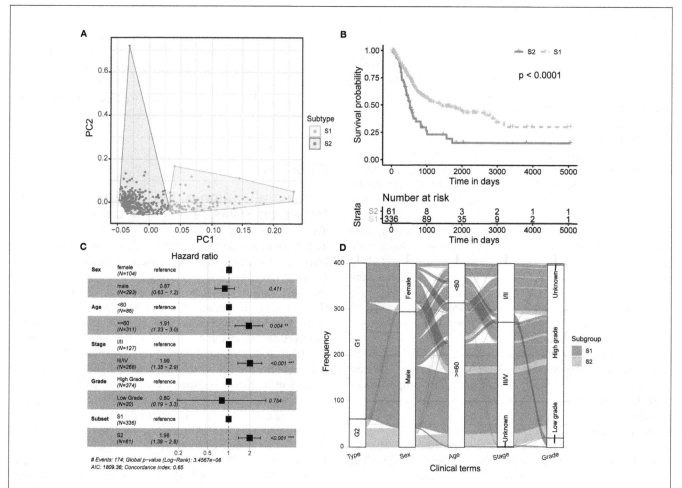

**FIGURE 2** | Two prognostic subtypes of MIBC were classified using multi-omics data-based deep learning framework. **(A)** Principal component analysis shows two distinguished MIBC subgroups clustered by K-means algorithm. **(B)** Kaplan-Meier curves show a significant difference of overall survival between MIBC subtypes. **(C)** Forest plot shows the multi-variates cox regression analysis result using general clinical characters as well as the predicted MIBC subtypes. **(D)** Distribution of the MIBC subtypes in various clinical phenotypes.

and tolerance, which can inhibit the expansion and function of many components of the immune system, we next performed immune decomposition for each sample and investigated the differences in immune components between the two molecular subtypes using CIBERSORT (15). As a result, tumors from S2 patients contained less M1 macrophages and resting NK cells, but more regulatory T cells, plasma cells, and naïve B cells (**Figure 3D**; $P < 0.05$, Wilcoxon signed-rank test).

Then, DEGs were derived by comparing the two prognostic subtypes, aiming to present the underlying mechanisms. A total of 6139 DEGs, including 2081 upregulated and 4058 downregulated genes, were detected with $\log_2$ fold change $> 1$ and FDR $< 0.05$ (**Figure 3E**). To investigate the functional difference between these two subtypes, we then performed Hallmark GSEA. In the top five most significantly enriched gene sets, we found that IL-6/JAK/STAT3 signaling, Interferon alpha response, reactive oxygen species, and unfolded protein response were activated in S2 subtype (high-risk group), while bile acid metabolism related genes were downregulated in this subtype (**Figure 3F** and **Supplementary Table 3**). Furthermore,

we also performed differential methylation analysis between these two subtypes of MIBC. As a result, 40 hypermethylated CpG sites and 34 hypomethylated CpG sites were found in S2 group compared with S1 (**Supplementary Figure 1A**). The hypermethylated CpG site located genes had significantly enriched functions such as cell mitosis, cell junction, protein binding, endocytosis, AMPK signaling pathway, and VEGF signaling pathway (**Supplementary Figure 1B**), while the hypomethylated CpG sites were in genes related to GTPase binding and Ras guanyl-nucleotide exchange factor activity (**Supplementary Figure S1C**).

## Internal and External Validation of the Subtyping of MIBC

To apply the identified classification into the prognosis of MIBC, we try to build a classification model of MIBC subtyping. We randomly selected 321 (80%) TCGA-MIBC cases as the training set and the other 81 (20%) MIBC cases as an internal validation set (**Table 1**). For the training set, we obtained the omics data at

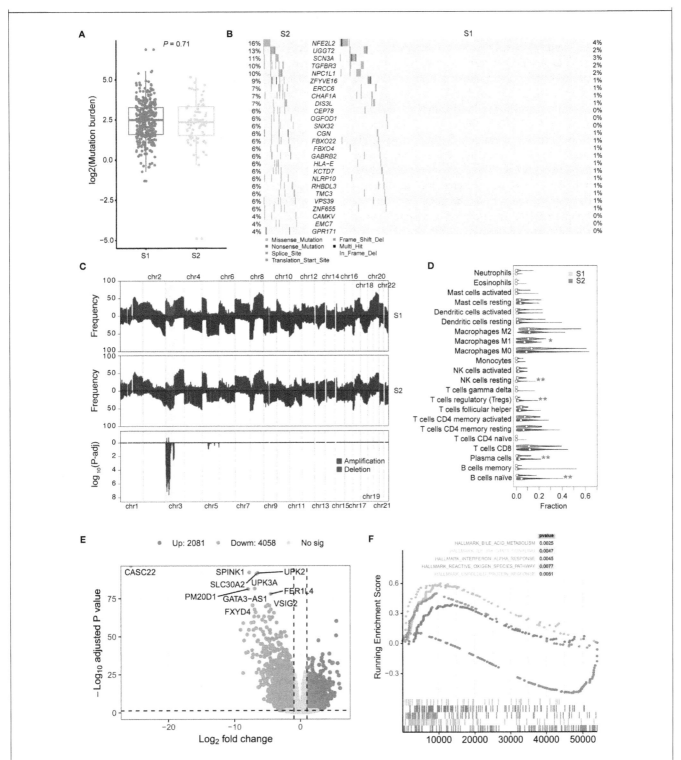

**FIGURE 3** | Molecular comparison between two prognostic MIBC subtypes. **(A)** Mutation burden of MIBCs for each tumor was compared in S1 and S2.
**(B)** Oncoplot shows differentially mutated genes between two MIBC subtypes. Chi-square test is performed, and genes with *P* < 0.05 are displayed. **(C)** Frequency
comparison between S1 and S2 of genome-wide copy number gain and loss. The CNV frequencies along genome of S1 and S2 are shown in top and middle
pattern, respectively. All amplifications in MIBC cohort are shown in red, and all deletions are shown in blue. Chi-square test is performed for each cytoband, and
the *P*-value distribution of each region was shown in the bottom module. Chromosome 3p, which contains all significant regions, is highlighted in orange.
**(D)** Comparison of the immune cell compositions in S1 and S2. The immune cell contents were decomposed using CIBERSORT. Wilcox test is performed for each
comparison, and significant entries are marked with asterisks (**P* < 0.01; *P* < 0.05). **(E)** Volcano plot shows the differentially expressed genes between high-
and low-risk subtypes. Ten most significantly expressed genes are marked. **(F)** Top five hallmark gene sets from gene set enrichment between high- and
low-risk subtypes.

four levels (CNV profile, gene expression profile by RNA-seq, miRNA expression profile by miRNA-seq, and DNA methylation profile) and calculated the p-value for each feature from each omics data profile between the two subtypes by Wilcox test, respectively. The top features (50 for CNV, 100 for mRNA, 50 for miRNA, and 50 for CpG methylation) were selected for model training, which were mostly different between the two subgroups of MIBC. We perform 10-fold cross-validation with 10-time repeat to evaluate the predictive ability of the selected features. In each repeat, different algorithms were used separately to build supervised classification model, and the best model with highest AUC was selected for the internal validation (see *Materials and methods*). The same features were extracted from the internal validation cohort, and samples were classified into two different groups according to the prediction model. Considering the previous subtype labels of samples from internal validation set, we construct the ROC curve to evaluate the robustness of the supervised classification model (**Figure 4A**). The AUC value (AUC = 0.784) indicated the reliable robustness of the model. Kaplan–Meier survival curve showed that the classification model using cluster labels was robust to predict the survival-specific clusters ($P = 0.031$, log-rank test; **Figure 4B**).

To expand the application of the prognostic subtyping, we also tested the stability of the identified classification using single-omics data from the internal validation dataset. We found the AUCs of gene expression data, miRNA expression profile, as well as methylation data were more than 0.8 (0.95, 0.90, and 0.87, respectively; **Figure 4C**), indicating the prediction robustness of these three single omics data. Then, we introduced three microarray-based gene expression datasets (GSE19915 and two subsets of GSE48277, **Table 1**) as external validation datasets to further validate our findings. Same expression features (the top 100 DEGs in training data) were extracted from each external

validation datasets, and the supervised prediction model is tested in the same way of internal validation, respectively. The predicted two subtypes of MIBC also show significant OS differences in all the three cohorts ($P = 0.026$, $P = 0.00094$, and $P = 0.00047$, respectively, log-rank test; **Figures 4D–F**). This result indicates that this subtyping method could be effectively applied to classify MIBC patients into different risk levels.

## KRT7 Is a Marker Gene to Classify High-Risk and Low-Risk MIBC

In order to further investigate potential marker genes that distinguish high-risk and low-risk MIBCs, we integrated the DEGs between high-risk group and low-risk group of MIBC from datasets of TCGA and two subsets of GSE48277 (the expression matrix data of GSE19915 was centralized so that it is not considered in this analysis). As shown in **Figure 5A**, only three upregulated genes (*NELL2*, *MDGA2*, and *CAMK4*) and two downregulated genes (*GGTLC1* and *KRT7*) are overlapped among these three datasets, respectively. We selected *KRT7* (also named as CK7) as a candidate marker to distinguish high-risk and low-risk MIBC. As expected, the expression level of *KRT7* was negatively correlated with risk-score of MIBC ($r = -0.47$, $P < 2.2 \times 10^{-16}$; **Figure 5B**). We further verified this candidate at the protein level. Firstly, we examined the KRT7 expression in bladder tumors on the webserver of The Human Protein Atlas (https://www.proteinatlas.org/) and found that KRT7 protein was highly expressed in the low-grade bladder cancer cells but medially or lowly expressed in high-grade bladder cancer cells (**Supplementary Figure 2**). We next selected 22 MIBC samples and separated them into two distinct groups with different risks: the high-risk group (12 samples) were samples that OS < 1.5 years and samples from the low-risk group (10 samples) were survived over 5 years. As expected, KRT7 was significantly highly expressed in the low-risk

**TABLE 1 |** Basic information of training and validation datasets for MIBC subtyping model.

|  | Training set | Validation sets | | | |
|---|---|---|---|---|---|
|  | TCGA | TCGA | GSE19915 | GSE48277-1 | GSE48277-2 |
| **Total** | 321 | 81 | 43 | 62 | 73 |
| **Sex** | | | | | |
| Female | 85 (26.5%) | 21 (25.9%) | 0 (0.0%) | 13 (21.0%) | 0 (0.0%) |
| Male | 236 (73.5%) | 60 (74.1%) | 0 (0.0%) | 49 (79.0%) | 0 (0.0%) |
| N/A | 0 (0.0%) | 0 (0.0%) | 43 (100.0%) | 0 (0.0%) | 73 (100.0%) |
| **Age** | | | | | |
| <60 | 72 (22.4%) | 14 (17.3%) | 0 (0%) | 16 (25.8%) | 13 (17.8%) |
| >=60 | 249 (77.6%) | 67 (82.7%) | 0 (0%) | 46 (74.2%) | 60 (82.2%) |
| N/A | 0 (0.0%) | 0 (0.0%) | 43 (100.0%) | 0 (0.0%) | 0 (0.0%) |
| **Stage** | | | | | |
| II | 106 (33.0%) | 23 (28.4%) | 19 (44.2%) | 46 (74.2%) | 42 (57.5%) |
| III | 111 (34.6%) | 27 (33.3%) | 21 (48.8%) | 15 (24.2%) | 23 (31.5%) |
| IV | 102 (31.8%) | 31 (38.3%) | 3 (7.0%) | 1 (1.6%) | 8 (11.0) |
| N/A | 2 (0.6%) | 0 (0.0%) | 0 (0.0%) | 0 (0.0%) | 0 (0.0%) |
| **Grade** | | | | | |
| High | 299 (93.1%) | 79 (97.5%) | 41 (95.3%) | 0 (0.0%) | 0 (0.0%) |
| Low | 19 (5.9%) | 2 (2.5%) | 2 (4.7%) | 0 (0.0%) | 0 (0.0%) |
| N/A | 3 (0.9%) | 0 (0.0%) | 0 (0.0%) | 62 (100.0%) | 73 (100.0%) |

*N/A, Not reported.*

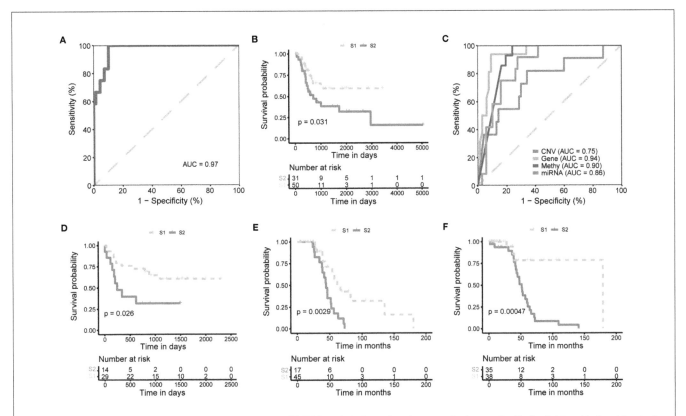

**FIGURE 4** | Internal and external validation of prognostic subtyping. **(A)** ROC analysis shows the robustness of subgroup classification in internal testing dataset using multi-omics data. **(B)** Kaplan-Meier curves show a significant difference of overall survival between subtypes predicted by multi-omics data in internal testing dataset. **(C)** ROC analysis shows the robustness of subgroup classification in internal testing dataset using each single omics data, respectively. **(D–F)**. Kaplan-Meier curves show a significant difference of overall survival between subtypes in external datasets, including GSE19915 **(D)** and two subsets of GSE48277 **(E, F)**, respectively.

MIBC (**Figures 5C, D** and **Supplementary Table 4**), which is further confirmed that KRT7 can be used as a marker to characterize MIBC risk.

## DISCUSSION

Different levels of omics data could present diverse tumor landscape from different angles. It is required to integrate multi-omics data to describe the relations between clinical outcomes and molecular characteristics, then get a comprehensively understanding of cancer. In the present study, we construct an autoencoder-based deep learning framework to integrate CNV, gene expression, miRNA expression, as well as CpG methylation results to classify MIBC into two prognostic subtypes. The subtype S2 shows a significantly higher risk on overall survival and some specific genetic characters compared with the other subtype. We construct a robustness MIBC subtyping model depending on different omics layers and assessed the prognostic value in both internal and external validation datasets. We also detected KRT7 as a biomarker to reflect the risk of MIBC.

We found that in the poor prognosis group, chromosome 3p had a significantly higher frequency of deletions. Many tumor suppressor genes are located on chromosome 3p, including *TP53, VHL, MLH1, TGFBR2, THRB, RARB,* and *FHIT.* Loss of one copy of chromosome 3p is one of the most frequent and early events in human cancer, found in 96% of lung tumors and 78% of lung preoplastic lesions (19). For cervical carcinoma (CC), researchers found that chromosome 3p deletions in precursor CIN lesions were smaller than the 3p losses found in the associated invasive CC (20). 3p arm loss has been associated with poorer prognosis for head and neck cancer as determined by reduced disease-free and overall survival of patients at early disease stage (21). These results suggest that the loss of chromosome 3p plays an important role in the occurrence and development of bladder cancer, and further analysis is needed. We detected 26 differentially mutated genes between S2 and S1. Some of these genes have been reported in previous tumor studies. For example, *NFE2L2* (the most significant gene that mutated in 16% of S2 but 4% in S1) has been reported in types of cancers. *NFE2L2* has long been considered a cytoprotective transcription factor, which is essential for the defense against oxidative stress, and activation of the *NFE2L2* pathway has been proposed as potential preventive strategy against carcinogenesis due to its function as a master regulator of the expression of antioxidant and detoxifying enzymes (22, 23). Reduced expression of *NFE2L2* are associated with poor outcome in breast cancer (24), ovarian cancer, and prostate cancer (25),

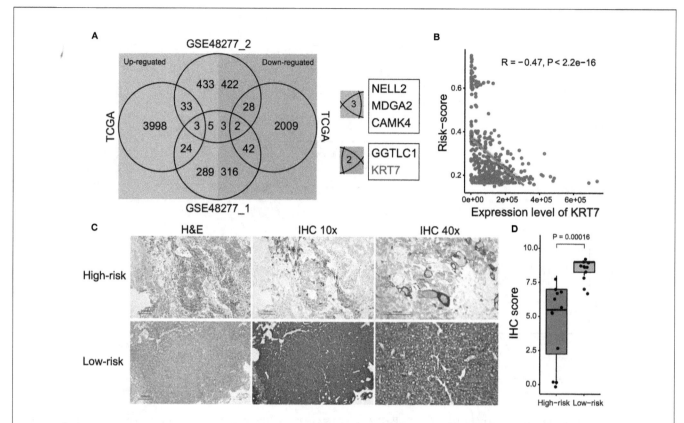

**FIGURE 5** | Detection and validation of risk-related markers of MIBCs. **(A)** Venn plot shows the overlaps of differentially expressed genes among TCGA and two subsets of GSE48277. **(B)** Correlation between tumor risk score and expression level of KRT7. TCGA data was used to perform this analysis. Both Pearson correlation coefficient (R) and P-value were calculated. **(C)** Representative images of KRT7 IHC staining in different risk types and corresponding H&E staining. **(D)** KRT7 protein expression was significantly decreased in high-risk MIBC specimens compared with low-risk MIBC tissues by IHC. For the details of calculating IHC score, please see *Materials and methods*.

but with favorable prognosis in cervical cancer (26), adrenocortical carcinoma, and kidney renal clear cell carcinoma (25), highlighting the dual role of *NFE2L2* in cancer. Remarkably, both mutation and CNA comparison show that TGF beta receptor was significantly altered in S2, indicating that the TGF-β signaling plays important roles in the prognostic impact in MIBC. One of the effects of this pathway is to enforce the immune homeostasis and tolerance, and disturbance of this pathway may influence the immune microenvironment of tumor. Interestingly, we found a variety of significant changes in immune cells between S1 and S2.

We investigate the gene expression and functional difference between the two prognostic subtypes. In the most significantly expressed genes shown in **Figure 3E**, lncRNA CASC22 has been reported that disrupting CASC22 was associated with a significantly increased risk of breast cancer (27). lncRNA FER1L4 also has been noticed as a favorable survival marker for endometrial carcinoma (28), colon cancer (29), and osteosarcoma (30). Interestingly, two UPK genes were significantly downregulated in high-risk MIBC subtype. UPK2 has been used as CTC markers of bladder cancer and got a satisfying result, which indicated a promising role for UPK2 mRNA detection using the circulatory blood of patients with

urothelial cancer as a new staging marker (31). This is not consistent with our results. Besides, the most enriched gene sets were also demonstrated prognostic in previous studies. For example, elevated levels of IL-6 stimulate hyperactivation of JAK/STAT3 signaling, which is often associated with poor patient outcomes in colorectal cancer (32), breast cancer (33), oral cancer (34), and myeloma (35). Elevated levels of reactive oxygen species are also a common hallmark of cancer progression and resistance to treatment (36), and unfolded protein response was also demonstrated to play an important role in the establishment and progression of several cancers (37). To our surprise, we found a significant activation of interferon alpha (IFN-α) response. IFN-α is usually used as an adjuvant with bacillus Calmette-Guérin (BCG) in the non-invasive bladder cancer treatment. However, there is still a lack of evidence to demonstrate its benefit in preventing recurrences in intermediate-risk and high-risk patients (38). Although we only analyzed MIBC in this study, this result reminds us to be cautious of adjuvant IFN-a therapy, especially for the high-risk bladder tumors.

To demonstrate the robustness of the subtyping classification, we built the prediction models at single- and multi-omics level and tested them in internal and external validation cohorts. Both results show an effective distinction of OS between predicted groups. In association with clinical characteristics, we noticed that the DL-based subtyping presented more prognostic efficiency than other clinical indexes. Comparing with other previous genetic feature-based prognostic models, the DL-based subtyping method is more flexible that we can use the model based on single or multiple levels of genomics data. Moreover, the ROC curve shows that our method is more powerful than previous studies in single genomic level, for instance, mRNA expression level [AUC = 0.954 *vs.* AUC = 0.761 (39, 40)] and miRNA expression level [AUC = 0.901 *vs.* AUC = 0.663 (40)].

KRT7 is a member of the keratin gene family and is specifically expressed in the simple epithelia lining the cavities of the internal organs and in the gland ducts and blood vessels. KRT7 was reported as a predictive factor of various types of cancer, such as colorectal cancer (41) and renal clear cell carcinoma (42), but bad prognostic factor in esophageal squamous cell carcinoma (43) and pancreatic adenocarcinoma (44). KRT7 was also reported to promote epithelial-mesenchymal transition (EMT) of ovarian cancer (45). To the best of our knowledge, few studies reveal the relationship between KRT7 and MIBC. In this study, we report that KRT7 can be used as a biomarker that reflects the prognostic risk of MIBC. This conclusion comes from the analysis of both RNA and protein levels, highlighting the value of KRT7 in the clinical application of MIBC. However, the underlying biological mechanism still needs further research.

## AUTHOR CONTRIBUTIONS

XLZ, LS, and CW performed bioinformatics analysis. JL and XLZ performed IHC experiments. YH provided pathology support. XLZ and JW designed the research study. XLZ performed paper drafting. XPZ and XYZ performed paper editing. All authors contributed to the article and approved the submitted version.

## SUPPLEMENTARY MATERIAL

**Supplementary Figure 1 |** Differential methylation analysis between S1 and S2. **(A)** Volcano plot shows differentially methylated CpG sites between S2 and S1. Sites with foldchange > 2 and adjusted *P*-value < 0.05 are considered to be significantly different. **(B)** Functional enrichment of hypermethylated CpG site related genes. Significantly enriched terms were defined as adjusted *P*-value < 0.05. Databases of GO, KEGG, Hallmark, and Reactome were included in this analysis, and top 10 most enriched terms of each database were shown in the figure. **(C)** Functional enrichment of hypomethylated CpG site related genes.

**Supplementary Figure 2 |** Immunohistochemical results show the expression level of KRT7 in low-grade **(A)** and high-grade **(B)** MIBC patients. The IHC figures were selected and downloaded from the webserver of The Human Protein Atlas (https://www.proteinatlas.org/) after a specific query.

## REFERENCES

1. Siegel RL, Miller KD, Jemal A. Cancer Statistics, 2018. *CA Cancer J Clin* (2018) 68:7–30. doi: 10.3322/caac.21442
2. Prasad SM, Decastro GJ, Steinberg GD, Medscape. Urothelial Carcinoma of the Bladder: Definition, Treatment and Future Efforts. *Nat Rev Urol* (2011) 8:631–42. doi: 10.1038/nrurol.2011.144
3. Volkmer JP, Sahoo D, Chin RK, Ho PL, Tang C, Kurtova AV, et al. Three Differentiation States Risk-Stratify Bladder Cancer Into Distinct Subtypes. *Proc Natl Acad Sci U S A.* (2012) 109:2078–83. doi: 10.1073/pnas.1120605109
4. Ho PL, Kurtova A, Chan KS. Normal and Neoplastic Urothelial Stem Cells: Getting to the Root of the Problem. *Nat Rev Urol* (2012) 9:583–94. doi: 10.1038/nrurol.2012.142
5. Sjodahl G, Lauss M, Lovgren K, Chebil G, Gudjonsson S, Veerla S, et al. A Molecular Taxonomy for Urothelial Carcinoma. *Clin Cancer Res* (2012) 18:3377–86. doi: 10.1158/1078-0432.CCR-12-0077-T
6. Cancer Genome Atlas Research N. Comprehensive Molecular Characterization of Urothelial Bladder Carcinoma. *Nature* (2014) 507:315–22. doi: 10.1038/nature12965
7. Choi W, Porten S, Kim S, Willis D, Plimack ER, Hoffman-Censits J, et al. Identification of Distinct Basal and Luminal Subtypes of Muscle-Invasive Bladder Cancer With Different Sensitivities to Frontline Chemotherapy. *Cancer Cell* (2014) 25:152–65. doi: 10.1016/j.ccr.2014.01.009
8. Damrauer JS, Hoadley KA, Chism DD, Fan C, Tiganelli CJ, Wobker SE, et al. Intrinsic Subtypes of High-Grade Bladder Cancer Reflect the Hallmarks of Breast Cancer Biology. *Proc Natl Acad Sci U S A* (2014) 111:3110–5. doi: 10.1073/pnas.1318376111
9. Rebouissou S, Bernard-Pierrot I, de Reynies A, Lepage ML, Krucker C, Chapeaublanc E, et al. EGFR as a Potential Therapeutic Target for a Subset of Muscle-Invasive Bladder Cancers Presenting a Basal-Like Phenotype. *Sci Transl Med* (2014) 6:244ra291. doi: 10.1126/scitranslmed.3008970
10. Biton A, Bernard-Pierrot I, Lou Y, Krucker C, Chapeaublanc E, Rubio-Perez C, et al. Independent Component Analysis Uncovers the Landscape of the Bladder Tumor Transcriptome and Reveals Insights Into Luminal and Basal Subtypes. *Cell Rep* (2014) 9:1235–45. doi: 10.1016/j.celrep.2014.10.035
11. Robertson AG, Kim J, Al-Ahmadie H, Bellmunt J, Guo G, Cherniack AD, et al. Comprehensive Molecular Characterization of Muscle-Invasive Bladder Cancer. *Cell* (2017) 171:540–556 e525. doi: 10.1016/j.cell.2017.09.007
12. Chaudhary K, Poirion OB, Lu L, Garmire LX. Deep Learning-Based Multi-Omics Integration Robustly Predicts Survival in Liver Cancer. *Clin Cancer Res* (2018) 24:1248–59. doi: 10.1158/1078-0432.CCR-17-0853
13. Mayakonda A, Lin DC, Assenov Y, Plass C, Koeffler HP. Maftools: Efficient and Comprehensive Analysis of Somatic Variants in Cancer. *Genome Res* (2018) 28:1747–56. doi: 10.1101/gr.239244.118
14. Mermel CH, Schumacher SE, Hill B, Meyerson ML, Beroukhim R, Getz G. GISTIC2.0 Facilitates Sensitive and Confident Localization of the Targets of Focal Somatic Copy-Number Alteration in Human Cancers. *Genome Biol* (2011) 12:R41. doi: 10.1186/gb-2011-12-4-r41
15. Newman AM, Liu CL, Green MR, Gentles AJ, Feng W, Xu Y, et al. Robust Enumeration of Cell Subsets From Tissue Expression Profiles. *Nat Methods* (2015) 12:453–7. doi: 10.1038/nmeth.3337
16. Love MI, Huber W, Anders S. Moderated Estimation of Fold Change and Dispersion for RNA-Seq Data With Deseq2. *Genome Biol* (2014) 15:550. doi: 10.1186/s13059-014-0550-8
17. Ritchie ME, Phipson B, Wu D, Hu Y, Law CW, Shi W, et al. limma Powers Differential Expression Analyses for RNA-Sequencing and Microarray Studies. *Nucleic Acids Res* (2015) 43:e47. doi: 10.1093/nar/gkv007
18. Yu G, Wang L-G, Han Y, He Q-Y. clusterprofiler: An R Package for Comparing Biological Themes Among Gene Clusters. *Omics: J Integr Biol* (2012) 16:284–7. doi: 10.1089/omi.2011.0118
19. Wistuba II, Behrens C, Virmani AK, Mele G, Milchgrub S, Girard L, et al. High Resolution Chromosome 3p Allelotyping of Human Lung Cancer and Preneoplastic/Preinvasive Bronchial Epithelium Reveals Multiple, Discontinuous Sites of 3p Allele Loss and Three Regions of Frequent Breakpoints. *Cancer Res* (2000) 60:1949–60.
20. Wistuba II, Montellano FD, Milchgrub S, Virmani AK, Behrens C, Chen H, et al. Deletions of Chromosome 3p are Frequent and Early Events in the Pathogenesis of Uterine Cervical Carcinoma. *Cancer Res* (1997) 57:3154–8.
21. Partridge M, Emilion G, Langdon JD. LOH at 3p Correlates With a Poor Survival in Oral Squamous Cell Carcinoma. *Br J Cancer* (1996) 73:366–71. doi: 10.1038/bjc.1996.62

22. Kwak MK, Kensler TW. Targeting NRF2 Signaling for Cancer Chemoprevention. *Toxicol Appl Pharmacol* (2010) 244:66–76. doi: 10.1016/j.taap.2009.08.028

23. Zhang Y, Gordon GB. A Strategy for Cancer Prevention: Stimulation of the Nrf2-ARE Signaling Pathway. *Mol Cancer Ther* (2004) 3:885–93.

24. Wolf B, Goebel G, Hackl H, Fiegl H. Reduced mRNA Expression Levels of NFE2L2 are Associated With Poor Outcome in Breast Cancer Patients. *BMC Cancer* (2016) 16:821. doi: 10.1186/s12885-016-2840-x

25. Ju Q, Li X, Zhang H, Yan S, Li Y, Zhao Y. NFE2L2 Is a Potential Prognostic Biomarker and Is Correlated With Immune Infiltration in Brain Lower Grade Glioma: A Pan-Cancer Analysis. *Oxid Med Cell Longev* (2020) 2020:3580719. doi: 10.1155/2020/3580719

26. Ma JQ, Tuersun H, Jiao SJ, Zheng JH, Xiao JB, Hasim A. Functional Role of NRF2 in Cervical Carcinogenesis. *PloS One* (2015) 10:e0133876. doi: 10.1371/journal.pone.0133876

27. Li N, Zhou P, Zheng J, Deng J, Wu H, Li W, et al. A Polymorphism Rs12325489c> T in the lincRNA-ENST00000515084 Exon was Found to Modulate Breast Cancer Risk *via* GWAS-Based Association Analyses. *PloS One* (2014) 9:e98251. doi: 10.1371/journal.pone.0098251

28. Kong Y, Ren Z. Overexpression of LncRNA FER1L4 in Endometrial Carcinoma is Associated With Favorable Survival Outcome. *Eur Rev Med Pharmacol Sci* (2018) 22:8113–8. doi: 10.26355/eurrev_201812_16502

29. Yue B, Sun B, Liu C, Zhao S, Zhang D, Yu F, et al. Long Non-Coding RNA Fer-1-Like Protein 4 Suppresses Oncogenesis and Exhibits Prognostic Value by Associating With miR-106a-5p in Colon Cancer. *Cancer Sci* (2015) 106:1323–32. doi: 10.1111/cas.12759

30. Fei D, Zhang X, Liu J, Tan L, Xing J, Zhao D, et al. Long Noncoding RNA FER1L4 Suppresses Tumorigenesis by Regulating the Expression of PTEN Targeting miR-18a-5p in Osteosarcoma. *Cell Physiol Biochem* (2018) 51:1364–75. doi: 10.1159/000495554

31. Lu J-J, Kakehi Y, Takahashi T, Wu X-X, Yuasa T, Yoshiki T, et al. Detection of Circulating Cancer Cells by Reverse Transcription-Polymerase Chain Reaction for Uroplakin II in Peripheral Blood of Patients With Urothelial Cancer. *Clin Cancer Res* (2000) 6:3166–71.

32. Kusaba T, Nakayama T, Yamazumi K, Yakata Y, Yoshizaki A, Inoue K, et al. Activation of STAT3 Is a Marker of Poor Prognosis in Human Colorectal Cancer. *Oncol Rep* (2006) 15:1445–51. doi: 10.3892/or.15.6.1445

33. Chen Y, Wang J, Wang X, Liu X, Li H, Lv Q, et al. STAT3, a Poor Survival Predictor, Is Associated With Lymph Node Metastasis From Breast Cancer. *J Breast Cancer* (2013) 16:40–9. doi: 10.4048/jbc.2013.16.1.40

34. Macha MA, Matta A, Kaur J, Chauhan S, Thakar A, Shukla NK, et al. Prognostic Significance of Nuclear Pstat3 in Oral Cancer. *Head Neck* (2011) 33:482–9. doi: 10.1002/hed.21468

35. Ludwig H, Nachbaur D, Fritz E, Krainer M, Huber H. Interleukin-6 Is a Prognostic Factor in Multiple Myeloma [Letter][See Comments]. *Blood* (1991) 77:2794–5. doi: 10.1182/blood.V77.12.2794.bloodjournal77122794

36. Kumari S, Badana AK, Malla R. Reactive Oxygen Species: A Key Constituent in Cancer Survival. *Biomarker Insights* (2018) 13:1177271918755391. doi: 10.1177/1177271918755391

37. Madden E, Logue SE, Healy SJ, Manie S, Samali A. The Role of the Unfolded Protein Response in Cancer Progression: From Oncogenesis to Chemoresistance. *Biol Cell* (2019) 111:1–17. doi: 10.1111/boc.201800050

38. Lamm D, Brausi M, O'Donnell MA, Witjes JA. Interferon Alfa in the Treatment Paradigm for Non–Muscle-Invasive Bladder Cancer *Urol Oncol* (2014) 32(1):35.e21–30. doi: 10.1016/j.urolonc.2013.02.010

39. Chen S, Zhang N, Shao J, Wang T, Wang X. A Novel Gene Signature Combination Improves the Prediction of Overall Survival in Urinary Bladder Cancer. *J Cancer* (2019) 10:5744–53. doi: 10.7150/jca.30307

40. Yin XH, Jin YH, Cao Y, Wong Y, Weng H, Sun C, et al. Development of a 21-miRNA Signature Associated With the Prognosis of Patients With Bladder Cancer. *Front Oncol* (2019) 9:729. doi: 10.3389/fonc.2019.00729

41. Harbaum L, Pollheimer MJ, Kornprat P, Lindtner RA, Schlemmer A, Rehak P, et al. Keratin 7 Expression in Colorectal Cancer–Freak of Nature or Significant Finding? *Histopathology* (2011) 59:225–34. doi: 10.1111/j.1365-2559.2011.03694.x

42. Mertz KD, Demichelis F, Sboner A, Hirsch MS, Dal Cin P, Struckmann K, et al. Association of Cytokeratin 7 and 19 Expression With Genomic Stability and Favorable Prognosis in Clear Cell Renal Cell Cancer. *Int J Cancer* (2008) 123:569–76. doi: 10.1002/ijc.23565

43. Oue N, Noguchi T, Anami K, Kitano S, Sakamoto N, Sentani K, et al. Cytokeratin 7 Is a Predictive Marker for Survival in Patients With Esophageal Squamous Cell Carcinoma. *Ann Surg Oncol* (2012) 19:1902–10. doi: 10.1245/s10434-011-2175-4

44. Li Y, Su Z, Wei B, Liang Z. KRT7 Overexpression is Associated With Poor Prognosis and Immune Cell Infiltration in Patients With Pancreatic Adenocarcinoma. *Int J Gen Med* (2021) 14:2677–94. doi: 10.2147/IJGM.S313584

45. An Q, Liu T, Wang MY, Yang YJ, Zhang ZD, Liu ZJ, et al. KRT7 Promotes Epithelialmesenchymal Transition in Ovarian Cancer *via* the TGFbeta/Smad2/3 Signaling Pathway. *Oncol Rep* (2021) 45:481–92. doi: 10.3892/or.2020.7886

# 13

# Identification of a Risk Stratification Model to Predict Overall Survival and Surgical Benefit in Clear Cell Renal Cell Carcinoma with Distant Metastasis

Jiasheng Chen [1,2†], Nailong Cao [2†], Shouchun Li [1*] and Ying Wang [2*]

[1] Department of Urology, The Affiliated Changzhou No.2 People's Hospital of Nanjing Medical University, Changzhou, China,
[2] Department of Urology, Shanghai Jiao Tong University Affiliated Sixth People's Hospital, Shanghai Eastern Institute of Urologic Reconstruction, Shanghai Jiao Tong University, Shanghai, China

*Correspondence:
Shouchun Li
lsc.8929@sohu.com
Ying Wang
sdzbbswangying@alumni.sjtu.edu.cn

† These authors have contributed equally to this work

**Background:** Clear cell renal cell carcinoma (ccRCC) is the main subtype of renal cell carcinoma and has different prognoses, especially in patients with metastasis. Here, we aimed to establish a novel model to predict overall survival (OS) and surgical benefit of ccRCC patients with distant metastasis.

**Methods:** Using data from the Surveillance, Epidemiology, and End Results (SEER) databases, we identified 2185 ccRCC patients with distant metastasis diagnosed from 2010 to 2015. Univariate and multivariate Cox analysis were used to identify significant prognostic clinicopathological variables. By integrating these variables, a prognostic nomogram was constructed and evaluated using C-indexes and calibration curves. The discriminative ability of the nomogram was measured by analyses of receiver operating characteristic (ROC) curve. A risk stratification model was built according to each patient's total scores. Kaplan-Meier curves were performed in the low-, intermediate- and high-risk groups to evaluate the survival benefit of surgery.

**Results:** Eight clinicopathological variables were included as independent prognostic factors in the nomogram: grade, marital status, T stage, N stage, bone metastasis, brain metastasis, liver metastasis, and lung metastasis. The nomogram had a better discriminative ability for predicting OS than Tumor-Node-Metastasis (TNM) stage. The C-index was 0.71 (95% CI 0.68–0.74) in the training cohort. The calibration plots demonstrated that the nomogram-based predictive outcomes had good consistency with the actual prognosis results. Total nephrectomy improved prognosis in both the low-risk and intermediate-risk groups, but partial nephrectomy could only benefit the low-risk group.

**Conclusions:** We constructed a predictive nomogram and risk stratification model to evaluate prognosis in ccRCC patients with distant metastasis, which was valuable for prognostic stratification and making therapeutic decisions.

Keywords: clear cell renal cell carcinoma, distant metastasis, nomogram, overall survival, surgical benefit

# INTRODUCTION

Renal cell carcinoma (RCC) is one of the most common malignant tumors in the genitourinary system. The latest cancer statistics report illustrated that more than 65,000 patients were diagnosed with RCC in the US, causing more than 15,000 deaths every year (1). Clear cell renal cell carcinoma (ccRCC) is the predominant histology of RCC, representing 75% of all cases (2). Among them, many patients with this disease are diagnosed with locally advanced disease or distant metastases despite improvements in the cancer control and survival rates. Clinically, approximately 16% of ccRCC patients have metastasis at diagnosis, and even one-third of localized ccRCC patients will develop metastatic lesions after tumor resection. The 5-year overall survival (OS) rate of metastatic ccRCC is only 12% (3). For RCC patients with distant metastasis, although the Memorial Sloan-Kettering Cancer Center (MSKCC) criteria and the International Metastatic RCC Database Consortium (IMDC) criteria can be used to evaluate the outcome of patient treatment, the impact of metastatic site and the overall tumor burden on survival is still missing (4, 5). Therefore, more practical tools and concise are required to improve the prognostic prediction of ccRCC patients with distant metastasis.

Cancer metastasis is a multistep process involving complex genetic alterations that drive the transformation of primary tumors into highly malignant and metastatic tumors (6, 7). To successfully metastasize, tumor cells must escape from the primary tumor, intravasate into circulatory and lymphatic systems, avoid immune attack, extravasate at distant capillary beds, and invade and proliferate in distant organs (8–10). For ccRCC, intensive studies demonstrated that different genes mediate tumor cell metastasis to different locations. The common metastasis sites of ccRCC include lung (in 50–60% of patients with metastases), bone (in 30–40%), liver (in 30–40%) and brain (in 5%) (11, 12).

The classic anatomical prognostic system is the tumor (T), node (N), and metastasis (M) classification, which is the most commonly used prognosis-predicting system for ccRCC patients (13). However, the TNM staging system lacks accuracy in predicting the prognostic of ccRCC patients, especially for ccRCC patients with distant metastasis (14). In ccRCC patients with distant metastasis, prognosis is further driven by the site of metastasis and the number of metastasis sites (15, 16). In addition, ccRCC patients with distant metastasis can be affected by clinical prognostic factors, including sex, age, marital status, race, and clinicopathological parameters such as grade, tumor size, and surgery treatment. Therefore, in consideration of all of these clinical factors, it is important to build a comprehensive prognostic model to accurately evaluate the prognosis of each patient. This predictive model can help doctors make therapeutic decisions.

Recently, nomogram has been accepted as a reliable tool to quantify risk by incorporating and evaluating important factors to assess prognostic outcome in multiple cancers (17–19). Several nomograms have been established to predict the risk of RCC recurrence and survival (20–22). However, there is no nomogram to estimate the prognostic outcome of ccRCC patients diagnosed with distant metastasis. In this study, we used data from the Surveillance, Epidemiology, and End Results (SEER) databases to establish and validate a nomogram that estimates the survival of ccRCC patients with distant metastasis.

# MATERIALS AND METHODS

## Data Source and Patient Selection

Patient data came from the Surveillance, Epidemiology, and End Results (SEER) database, which covers approximately 28% of the US population. In our study, patient selection based on the following inclusion and exclusion criteria. Inclusion criteria: (a) diagnosed between 2010 and 2015; (b) molecular subtype of clear cell carcinoma; and (c) diagnosed initially with at least one distant metastatic site. Exclusion criteria: (a) unknown metastatic status; (b) age at diagnosis under18 years; (c) incomplete demographic and clinical data, including race, marital status, T/N stage and grade; and (d) missing follow-up data.

## Nomogram Construction and Validation

We randomly divided the patients diagnosed from 2010 to 2013 into two cohorts, the training cohort and the validation I cohort, with a ratio of three to one, and we assigned the patients diagnosed from 2014 to 2015 as the validation II cohort. Categorical variables in the three cohorts were presented as frequencies and proportions. Univariate Cox regression analyses were used to calculate the influence of each variable on OS. Significant prognostic factors identified from the univariate analysis were further analyzed in a multivariate Cox proportional hazard model, and the corresponding 95% confidence interval (CI) for each potential risk factor was calculated. Based on the result of the multivariate model, a nomogram was built to predict 1-, 2- and 3-year OS. The discriminative ability of the nomogram was measured using the 1-, 2-, and 3-year survival area under curve (AUC) values from time-dependent receiver operating characteristic (ROC) curves. Predictive accuracy was assessed using the concordance index (C-index) and calibration plot. Additionally, a risk stratification model was established on the basis of each patient's total score in the nomogram, and all patients were divided into three prognostic groups.

## Statistical Analyses

Univariate and multivariate Cox regression analyses were performed to identify the prognostic factors. Kaplan-Meier curves was used to estimate the OS. The significance of differences in OS was assessed by log-rank test. Cox regression analysis, Kaplan-Meier curves, and the log-rank test were conducted by the *glmnet* and *survival* packages. The nomogram was established with the *rms* and *survival* packages. All statistical analyses were performed in R studio (version 3.6.2), and statistical significance was set at a *p*-value of <0.05.

# RESULTS

## Demographic and Clinical Characteristics of Patient Patients

Overall, 2,185 ccRCC patients with distant metastasis were included in this study. Among all patients, 1,027, 342, and 816 subjects were assigned to the training, validation I and validation II cohorts, respectively. The demographic and clinical characteristics of patients in each subgroup are demonstrated in **Table 1**. There was no significant difference in the distribution of the number of patients in different cohorts. Generally, most patients were male (1,523; 69.7%), aged 60–79 years (1,180; 54.0%), married (1,493; 68.3%), and white (1,891; 86.5%). Moreover, most patients underwent total nephrectomy (1,765; 80.8%).

In total, 30.2% (660), 10.0% (218), 11.0% (240), and 61.8% (1,350) of the patients had bone metastasis, brain metastasis, liver metastasis and lung metastasis, respectively. Additionally, 14.1% (307), 17.2% (375), 60.7% (1,327) and 8.1% (176) of the patients had stage T1, T2, T3, and T4 tumors, respectively. Furthermore, 76.5% (1,671) of the patients were negative for lymphatic metastasis, and 13.5% (295) and 10.0% (219) had N1 and N2 stage.

## Independent Prognostic Factors in the Training Set

Through univariate analysis and subsequent multivariate Cox analysis, marital status (divorced/separated: HR 1.219, 95% CI 0.971–1.531; widowed: HR 1.690, 95% CI 1.277–2.235; single: HR 1.094, 95% CI 0.889–1.347; married as a reference), grade (II: HR 1.126, 95% CI 0.931–1.363; III: HR 1.365, 95% CI 0.809–2.303; IV: HR 1.499, 95% CI 1.217–1.847; I as a reference), T stage (T2: HR 1.354, 95% CI 0.949–1.932; T3: HR 1.388, 95% CI 1.031–1.869; T4: HR 1.626, 95% CI 1.107–2.389; T1 as a reference), N stage (N1: HR 1.934, 95% CI 1.583–2.362; N2: HR 2.375, 95% CI 1.877–3.004; N0 as a reference), bone metastasis (metastasis: HR 1.621, 95% CI 1.378–1.907; no metastasis as a reference), brain metastasis (metastasis: HR 2.158, 95% CI 1.730–2.693; no metastasis as a reference), liver metastasis (metastasis: HR 1.538, 95% CI 1.217–1.943; no metastasis as a reference), and lung metastasis (metastasis: HR 1.709, 95% CI 1.454–2.008; no metastasis as a reference) were found to be statistically significant factors for OS, as shown in **Table 2**.

## Nomogram Construction and Validation

Considering the outcomes of the univariate and multivariate Cox regression analyses for OS, eight independent factors in the training cohort were included in the nomogram to predict the 1-, 2-, and 3-year OS rates (**Figure 1**). Among all included factors, N stage made the most significant contribution to the survival outcome, closely followed by brain metastasis. In addition, marital status, grade, T stage, and the presence of bone/liver/lung metastasis had a moderate impact on prognosis. The 1-, 2- and 3-year survival probabilities of

**TABLE 1** | Demographic and clinical characteristics of ccRCC patients with distant metastasis.

| | Training cohort (N = 1,027) | Validation I cohort (N = 342) | Validation II cohort (N = 816) | Overall (N = 2,185) |
|---|---|---|---|---|
| **Sex** | | | | |
| Male | 740 (72.1%) | 231 (67.5%) | 552 (67.6%) | 1,523 (69.7%) |
| Female | 287 (27.9%) | 111 (32.5%) | 264 (32.4%) | 662 (30.3%) |
| **Age (year)** | | | | |
| 18–39 | 11 (1.1%) | 2 (0.6%) | 11 (1.3%) | 24 (1.1%) |
| 40–59 | 448 (43.6%) | 143 (41.8%) | 280 (34.3%) | 871 (39.9%) |
| 60–79 | 521 (50.7%) | 180 (52.6%) | 479 (58.7%) | 1,180 (54.0%) |
| ≥80 | 47 (4.6%) | 17 (5.0%) | 46 (5.6%) | 110 (5.0%) |
| **Marital status** | | | | |
| Married | 704 (68.5%) | 229 (67.0%) | 560 (68.6%) | 1,493 (68.3%) |
| Divorced/Separated | 111 (10.8%) | 28 (8.2%) | 77 (9.4%) | 216 (9.9%) |
| Widowed | 65 (6.3%) | 38 (11.1%) | 62 (7.6%) | 165 (7.6%) |
| Single | 147 (14.3%) | 47 (13.7%) | 117 (14.3%) | 311 (14.2%) |
| **Race** | | | | |
| White | 889 (86.6%) | 304 (88.9%) | 698 (85.5%) | 1,891 (86.5%) |
| Black | 51 (5.0%) | 20 (5.8%) | 52 (6.4%) | 123 (5.6%) |
| Other | 87 (8.5%) | 18 (5.3%) | 66 (8.1%) | 171 (7.8%) |
| **Grade** | | | | |
| I | 24 (2.3%) | 14 (4.1%) | 20 (2.5%) | 58 (2.7%) |
| II | 262 (25.5%) | 92 (26.9%) | 181 (22.2%) | 535 (24.5%) |
| III | 458 (44.6%) | 139 (40.6%) | 340 (41.7%) | 937 (42.9%) |
| IV | 283 (27.6%) | 97 (28.4%) | 275 (33.7%) | 655 (30.0%) |
| **T stage** | | | | |
| T1 | 131 (12.8%) | 60 (17.5%) | 116 (14.2%) | 307 (14.1%) |
| T2 | 169 (16.5%) | 69 (20.2%) | 137 (16.8%) | 375 (17.2%) |
| T3 | 649 (63.2%) | 185 (54.1%) | 493 (60.4%) | 1,327 (60.7%) |
| T4 | 78 (7.6%) | 28 (8.2%) | 70 (8.6%) | 176 (8.1%) |
| **N stage** | | | | |
| N0 | 793 (77.2%) | 259 (75.7%) | 619 (75.9%) | 1,671 (76.5%) |
| N1 | 137 (13.3%) | 47 (13.7%) | 111 (13.6%) | 295 (13.5%) |
| N2 | 97 (9.4%) | 36 (10.5%) | 86 (10.5%) | 219 (10.0%) |
| **Bone metastasis** | | | | |
| No | 719 (70.0%) | 236 (69.0%) | 570 (69.9%) | 1,525 (69.8%) |
| Yes | 308 (30.0%) | 106 (31.0%) | 246 (30.1%) | 660 (30.2%) |
| **Brain metastasis** | | | | |
| No | 919 (89.5%) | 318 (93.0%) | 730 (89.5%) | 1,967 (90.0%) |
| Yes | 108 (10.5%) | 24 (7.0%) | 86 (10.5%) | 218 (10.0%) |
| **Liver metastasis** | | | | |
| No | 918 (89.4%) | 294 (86.0%) | 733 (89.8%) | 1,945 (89.0%) |
| Yes | 109 (10.6%) | 48 (14.0%) | 83 (10.2%) | 240 (11.0%) |
| **Lung metastasis** | | | | |
| No | 409 (39.8%) | 139 (40.6%) | 287 (35.2%) | 835 (38.2%) |
| Yes | 618 (60.2%) | 203 (59.4%) | 529 (64.8%) | 1,350 (61.8%) |
| **Size (mm)** | | | | |
| Size ≤ 40 | 63 (6.1%) | 23 (6.7%) | 50 (6.1%) | 136 (6.2%) |
| 40 < Size ≤ 70 | 220 (21.4%) | 84 (24.6%) | 191 (23.4%) | 495 (22.7%) |
| 70 < Size ≤ 100 | 358 (34.9%) | 108 (31.6%) | 283 (34.7%) | 749 (34.3%) |
| Size >100 | 386 (37.6%) | 127 (37.1%) | 292 (35.8%) | 805 (36.8%) |
| **Surgery** | | | | |
| No | 143 (13.9%) | 53 (15.5%) | 150 (18.4%) | 346 (15.8%) |
| Partial | 31 (3.0%) | 12 (3.5%) | 31 (3.8%) | 74 (3.4%) |
| Total | 853 (83.1%) | 277 (81.0%) | 635 (77.8%) | 1,765 (80.8%) |

**TABLE 2 |** Univariate and multivariate Cox analyses of overall survival in the training set.

| | Univariate analysis | | Multivariate analysis | |
|---|---|---|---|---|
| | HR (95%CI) | *P*-value | HR (95%CI) | *P*-value |
| **Sex** | | 0.113 | | |
| Female | Reference | | | |
| Male | 1.135 (0.971, 1.327) | | | |
| **Age (years)** | | 0.118 | | |
| 18–39 | Reference | | | |
| 40–59 | 1.214 (0.541, 2.722) | 0.638 | | |
| 60–79 | 1.254 (0.560, 2.809) | 0.582 | | |
| ≥80 | 1.753 (0.743, 4.137) | 0.200 | | |
| **Marital status** | | 0.036 | | 0.044 |
| Married | Reference | | Reference | |
| Divorced/Separated | 1.143 (0.913, 1.430) | 0.244 | 1.219 (0.971, 1.531) | 0.088 |
| Widowed | 1.443 (1.095, 1.902) | 0.009 | 1.690 (1.277, 2.235) | < 0.001 |
| Single | 1.145 (0.933, 1.405) | 0.194 | 1.094 (0.889, 1.347) | 0.394 |
| **Race** | | 0.166 | | |
| White | Reference | | | |
| Black | 1.042 (0.754, 1.439) | 0.804 | | |
| Other | 0.811 (0.622, 1.059) | 0.124 | | |
| **Grade** | | <0.001 | | < 0.001 |
| I | Reference | | Reference | |
| II | 1.268 (1.057, 1.522) | 0.011 | 1.126 (0.931, 1.363) | 0.222 |
| III | 1.221 (0.732, 2.037) | 0.445 | 1.365 (0.809, 2.303) | 0.244 |
| IV | 1.817 (1.493, 2.212) | <0.001 | 1.499 (1.217, 1.847) | < 0.001 |
| **T stage** | | <0.001 | | 0.016 |
| T1 | Reference | | Reference | |
| T2 | 1.448 (1.095, 1.916) | 0.009 | 1.354 (0.949, 1.932) | 0.094 |
| T3 | 1.561 (1.232, 1.978) | <0.001 | 1.388 (1.031, 1.869) | 0.031 |
| T4 | 2.349 (1.616, 3.253) | <0.001 | 1.626 (1.107, 2.389) | 0.013 |
| **N stage** | | <0.001 | | < 0.001 |
| N0 | Reference | | Reference | |
| N1 | 2.100 (1.724, 2.558) | <0.001 | 1.934 (1.583, 2.362) | < 0.001 |
| N2 | 2.454 (1.955, 3.081) | <0.001 | 2.375 (1.877, 3.004) | < 0.001 |
| **Bone metastasis** | | 0.013 | | < 0.001 |
| No | Reference | | Reference | |
| Yes | 1.213 (1.042, 1.412) | 0.013 | 1.621 (1.378, 1.907) | < 0.001 |
| **Brain metastasis** | | <0.001 | | < 0.001 |
| No | Reference | | Reference | |
| Yes | 2.063 (1.664, 2.559) | <0.001 | 2.158 (1.730, 2.693) | < 0.001 |
| **Liver metastasis** | | 0.010 | | < 0.001 |
| No | Reference | | Reference | |
| Yes | 1.343 (1.073, 1.680) | 0.010 | 1.538 (1.217, 1.943) | < 0.001 |
| **Lung metastasis** | | <0.001 | | < 0.001 |
| No | Reference | | Reference | |
| Yes | 1.554 (1.340, 1.803) | <0.001 | 1.709 (1.454, 2.008) | < 0.001 |
| **Tumor size (mm)** | | 0.023 | | 0.261 |
| Size ≤ 40 | Reference | | Reference | |
| 40 < Size ≤ 70 | 1.040 (0.743, 1.454) | 0.820 | 0.993 (0.706, 1.397) | 0.969 |
| 70 < Size ≤ 100 | 1.367 (0.995, 1.879) | 0.054 | 1.002 (0.700, 1.432) | 0.994 |
| Size > 100 | 1.274 (0.928, 1.750) | 0.135 | 0.855 (0.600, 1.218) | 0.385 |

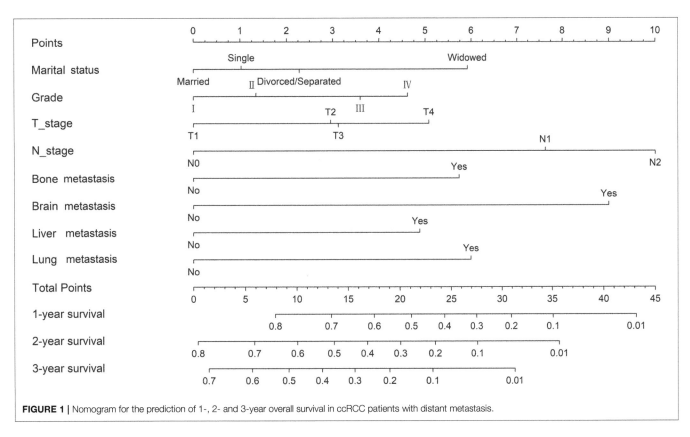

**FIGURE 1** | Nomogram for the prediction of 1-, 2- and 3-year overall survival in ccRCC patients with distant metastasis.

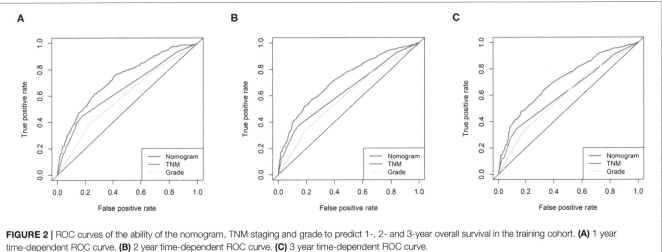

**FIGURE 2** | ROC curves of the ability of the nomogram, TNM staging and grade to predict 1-, 2- and 3-year overall survival in the training cohort. **(A)** 1 year time-dependent ROC curve. **(B)** 2 year time-dependent ROC curve. **(C)** 3 year time-dependent ROC curve.

each patient were obtained by adding the score of every prognostic factor.

The C-index in the training cohort (0.71, 95% CI 0.68–0.74) indicated reasonable predictive accuracy of the model. The discriminative ability of the nomogram was measured using the 1-, 2-, and 3-year survival AUC values from time-dependent ROC curve. In the training cohort, the nomogram was significantly superior to TNM staging or grade (1-year AUC: nomogram 0.73 vs. TNM 0.65 or grade 0.59; 2-year AUC: nomogram 0.72 vs. TNM 0.64 or grade 0.59; 3-year AUC: nomogram 0.71 vs. TNM 0.62 or grade 0.60; **Figure 2**). In addition, in a

validation cohort containing both the validation I + II cohorts, the nomogram AUC values for 1-, 2-, and 3-year survival were 0.67, 0.69, and 0.68, respectively. Moreover, the calibration plots in the training and validation cohorts demonstrated that the nomogram-based predictive results were mostly consistent with the actual prognosis results (**Figure 3**).

## Risk Stratification Model and Survival Benefit of Surgery

In addition, we built a risk stratification model based on each patient's total scores in the nomogram. According to

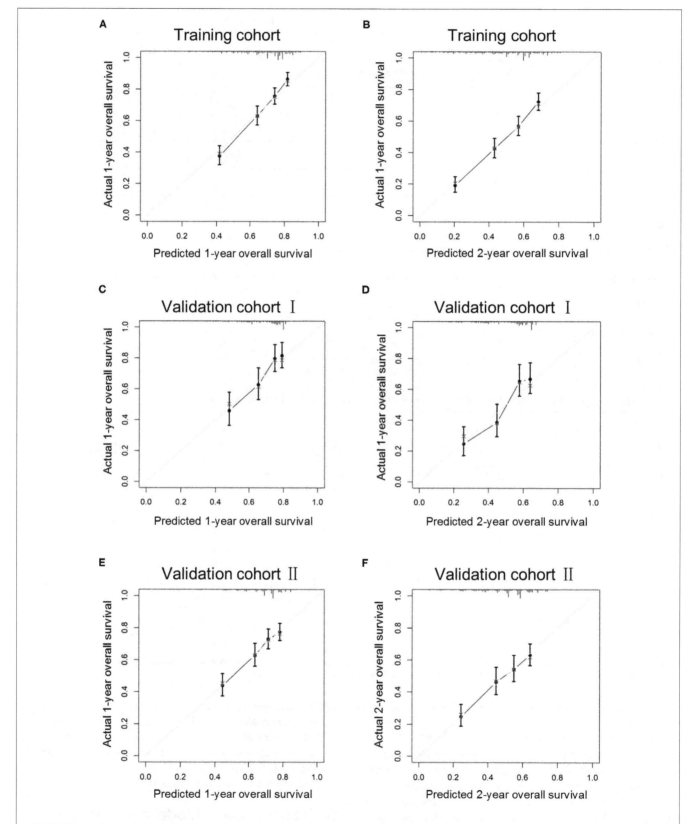

**FIGURE 3 |** Calibration curves of the ability of the nomogram to predict 1-year **(A)** and 2-year **(B)** overall survival in the training cohort, 1-year **(C)** and 2-year **(D)** overall survival in validation I cohort and 1-year **(E)** and 2-year **(F)** overall survival in validation II cohort.

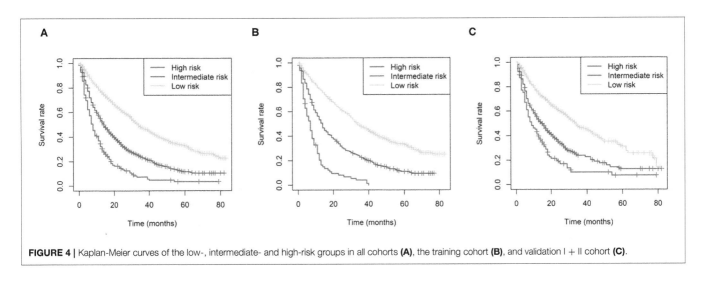

**FIGURE 4** | Kaplan-Meier curves of the low-, intermediate- and high-risk groups in all cohorts **(A)**, the training cohort **(B)**, and validation I + II cohort **(C)**.

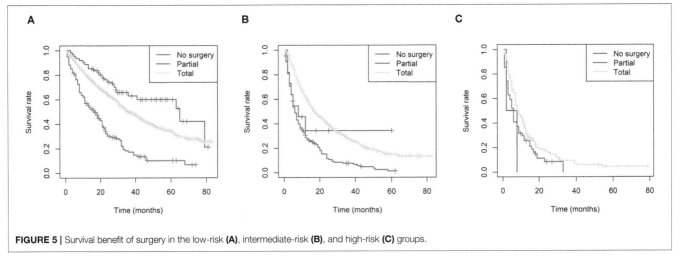

**FIGURE 5** | Survival benefit of surgery in the low-risk **(A)**, intermediate-risk **(B)**, and high-risk **(C)** groups.

the risk stratification model, all the patients were divided into three groups: low-risk group (1,289/2,185, 60.0%; total score < 15), intermediate-risk group (717/2,185, 32.8%; 15 ≤ total score < 25), and high-risk group (1,128/2,185, 51.6%, total score ≥ 25). Kaplan-Meier curves were performed in all cohorts and demonstrated that the risk stratification model can accurately distinguish survival in the three prognostic groups (**Figure 4**).

Furthermore, Kaplan-Meier curves were also performed in the stratified risk groups to assess the survival benefit of surgery (**Figure 5**). The results indicated that total nephrectomy could prolong overall survival in both the low- and intermediate-risk groups ($p < 0.0001$ and $p < 0.0001$, respectively); however, partial nephrectomy could only benefit the low-risk group ($p < 0.0001$). Interestingly, the low-risk group patients could benefit more in terms of prognosis from partial nephrectomy than total nephrectomy (p = 0.022). However, in the high-risk group, neither total nor partial nephrectomy could significantly improve the prognosis of patients.

## DISCUSSION

In this study, a nomogram was constructed and verified for predicting OS in 2,185 ccRCC patients with distant metastasis from the SEER database. We identified eight demographic and clinical characteristics as prognostic factors, including marital status, grade, T stage, N stage and bone, brain, liver and lung metastasis. In addition, the ROC curves and calibration curves demonstrated favorable discrimination and calibration. Moreover, we built a risk stratification model based on the total score of each patient in the nomogram, and analyzed the survival benefits of surgery choices in the classified risk groups. To our knowledge, this is the first large-cohort, comprehensive retrospective study to construct a nomogram for predicting the prognosis of ccRCC patients with distant metastasis. This predictive tool can be easily applied in clinical practice to predict the survival probability of each patient and help clinicians develop optimal therapy strategies for patients.

Regarding demographic features, marital status was an independent prognostic factor, which is consistent with previous studies (22, 23). Marriage may have a beneficial effect on RCC patients, as it can be associated with support from the spouse, such as helping in activities of daily life and medication reminders. The clinical characteristics grade, T stage, N stage and bone, brain, liver, and lung metastasis were significant for predicting overall survival. Among the sites of metastasis, brain metastasis was the worst factor affecting the prognosis, followed by lung, bone and liver metastasis. Consistently, previous studies have shown that the prognosis of patients with brain metastases is worse than that of patients without brain metastasis (24, 25). However, Abdel-Rahman (26) reported that metastatic RCC patients with liver metastasis seem to have worse outcomes than patients with other sites of metastasis. One explanation is that we mainly focused on clear cell histology rather than all subtypes of RCC. Therefore, the result must be further validated in many ongoing randomized studies.

According to the results of randomized controlled trials, cytoreductive nephrectomy has become the preferred treatment for metastatic RCC patients in the era of cytokine therapy, especially in patients with good performance status (27, 28). In 2005, the molecular-targeted agent sorafenib was approved for the treatment of advanced RCC, opening a new era of molecular-targeted therapy. Clinical data reported so far have clearly demonstrated that, compared with the era of cytokine therapy, the introduction of targeted therapy has significantly improved the prognosis of patients with metastatic RCC (29). However, in the era of targeted therapy, the role of cytoreductive nephrectomy in treating metastatic RCC has been brought into question. The result of CARMENA clinical trial showed that sunitinib alone was not inferior to nephrectomy followed by sunitinib in patients with intermediate- and high-risk metastatic RCC (30). Moreover, from a molecular genetic viewpoint, this intervention can only eliminate the easiest adversary (the main tumor) but cannot prevent cancer-related death. Therefore, the benefits and risks of cytoreductive nephrectomy must be carefully considered. Surgery may not be beneficial if treatment-induced morbidity would substantially affect the patient's quality of life. Thus, demographic and clinical characteristics need to be considered critically to make an optimal decision for each patient. Our study found that total nephrectomy could improve OS in both the low- and intermediate-risk groups, and partial nephrectomy could benefit only the low-risk group, which provides more accurate information for therapeutic decisions.

To our knowledge, this is the first study to generate a predictive nomogram for ccRCC patients with distant metastasis. Although Zheng et al. recently constructed a nomogram for patients with metastatic RCC by combining clinical and pathological characteristics derived from the SEER database (31). In our study, we only included patients with metastatic ccRCC and we stratified the age and tumor size of all patients. In addition, we constructed a training cohort and two validation cohorts to better verify the predictive ability of the nomogram. Moreover, we established a risk stratification model on the basis of each patient's total score from the nomogram and survival benefits of surgery was analyzed in the classified risk groups. As

we all know, in the past years both MSKCC and IMDC scores were used almost exclusively to define prognosis of patients with metastatic RCC. Even in the most recent immunotherapy era, their prognostic role was confirmed again and a potential predictive role has emerged (32, 33). Considering that the variables contributing to the IMDC or MSKCC risk model were not registered in the SEER database, there is no comparison in predictive accuracy was conducted between our nomogram and these two models. However, the predictive model proposed in our study is a nomogram, demonstrated to predict the OS more precisely. Regarding to the role of our model in immunotherapy era, it needs to be verified in further study.

The current study has several limitations that should be considered. First, the nomogram was built retrospectively using the SEER database, and it would be better if the nomogram could be verified in a prospective cohort or a clinical trial. Second, the database only contained information on distant metastasis. Some patients may have developed metachronous metastasis during follow-up, and such data are not available from the database. Third, we only focused on patients with ccRCC, and further studies are required to evaluate whether this nomogram is applicable to patients with other histological subtypes. In addition, there is a lack of information about the details of systemic treatment received. This is particularly important given the evidence-based role of targeted therapies in improving the outcomes of metastatic RCC. Finally, patients with missing data with respect to each of the variables were excluded from our cohort, which may lead to potential selection bias. Therefore, further prospective studies are necessary.

## CONCLUSIONS

We constructed a novel predictive nomogram and risk stratification model to predict the individual survival of ccRCC patients with distant metastasis. This prognostic model could assist clinicians to identify high-risk patients and make more individualized treatments for patients with different prognoses.

## AUTHOR CONTRIBUTIONS

YW and SL designed, conceived this study, and revised the paper. JC contributed to the literature search. JC and NC were involved in data extraction and wrote the manuscript. NC analyzed the data. All authors have approved the final edition of the manuscript.

## REFERENCES

1. Siegel RL, Miller KD, Jemal A. Cancer statistics, 2018. *CA Cancer J Clin.* (2018) 68:7–30. doi: 10.3322/caac.21442
2. Clark DJ, Dhanasekaran SM, Petralia F, Pan J, Song X, Hu Y, et al. Integrated proteogenomic characterization of clear cell renal cell carcinoma. *Cell.* (2019) 179:964–83. e31. doi: 10.1016/j.cell.2019.10.007
3. Capitanio U, Montorsi F. Renal cancer. *Lancet.* (2016) 387:894–906. doi: 10.1016/S0140-6736(15)00046-X

4. Motzer RJ, Mazumdar M, Bacik J, Berg W, Amsterdam A, Ferrara J. Survival and prognostic stratification of 670 patients with advanced renal cell carcinoma. *J Clin Oncol.* (1999) 17:2530–40. doi: 10.1200/JCO.1999.17.8.2530

5. Ko JJ, Xie W, Kroeger N, Lee JL, Rini BI, Knox JJ, et al. The international metastatic renal cell carcinoma database consortium model as a prognostic tool in patients with metastatic renal cell carcinoma previously treated with first-line targeted therapy: a population-based study. *Lancet Oncol.* (2015) 16:293–300. doi: 10.1016/S1470-2045(14)71222-7

6. Valastyan S, Weinberg RA. Tumor metastasis: molecular insights and evolving paradigms. *Cell.* (2011) 147:275–92. doi: 10.1016/j.cell.2011.09.024

7. Gomez-Cuadrado L, Tracey N, Ma R, Qian B, Brunton VG. Mouse models of metastasis: progress and prospects. *Dis Model Mech.* (2017) 10:1061–74. doi: 10.1242/dmm.030403

8. Steeg PS. Tumor metastasis: mechanistic insights and clinical challenges. *Nat Med.* (2006) 12:895–904doi: 10.1038/nm1469

9. Bacac M, Stamenkovic I. Metastatic cancer cell. *Annu Rev Pathol.* (2008) 3:221–47. doi: 10.1146/annurev.pathmechdis.3.121806.151523

10. Seyfried TN, Huysentruyt LC. On the origin of cancer metastasis. *Crit Rev Oncog.* (2013) 18:43–73. doi: 10.1615/critrevoncog.v18.i1-2.40

11. Gupta K, Miller JD, Li JZ, Russell MW, Charbonneau C. Epidemiologic and socioeconomic burden of metastatic renal cell carcinoma (mRCC): a literature review. *Cancer Treat Rev.* (2008) 34:193–205. doi: 10.1016/j.ctrv.2007.12.001

12. Lam JS, Leppert JT, Belldegrun AS, Figlin RA. Novel approaches in the therapy of metastatic renal cell carcinoma. *World J Urol.* (2005) 23:202–12. doi: 10.1007/s00345-004-0466-0

13. Sun M, Shariat SF, Cheng C, Ficarra V, Murai M, Oudard S, et al. Prognostic factors and predictive models in renal cell carcinoma: a contemporary review. Eur Urol. (2011) 60:644–61. doi: 10.1016/j.eururo.2011.06.041

14. Ficarra V, Galfano A, Mancini M, Martignoni G, Artibani W. TNM staging system for renal-cell carcinoma: current status and future perspectives. *Lancet Oncol.* (2007) 8:554–8. doi: 10.1016/S1470-2045(07)70173-0

15. Manola J, Royston P, Elson P, McCormack JB, Mazumdar M, Negrier S, et al. Prognostic model for survival in patients with metastatic renal cell carcinoma: results from the international kidney cancer working group. *Clin Cancer Res.* (2011) 17:5443–50. doi: 10.1158/1078-0432.CCR-11-0553

16. Klatte T, Fife K, Welsh SJ, Sachdeva M, Armitage JN, Aho T, et al. Prognostic effect of cytoreductive nephrectomy in synchronous metastatic renal cell carcinoma: a comparative study using inverse probability of treatment weighting. *World J Urol.* (2018) 36:417–25. doi: 10.1007/s00345-017-2154-x

17. Balachandran VP, Gonen M, Smith JJ, DeMatteo RP. Nomograms in oncology: more than meets the eye. *Lancet Oncol.* (2015) 16:e173–80. doi: 10.1016/S1470-2045(14)71116-7

18. Huang YQ, Liang CH, He L, Tian J, Liang CS, Chen X, et al. Development and validation of a radiomics nomogram for preoperative prediction of lymph node metastasis in colorectal cancer. *J Clin Oncol.* (2016) 34:2157–64. doi: 10.1200/JCO.2015.65.9128

19. Liang W, Zhang L, Jiang G, Wang Q, Liu L, Liu D, et al. Development and validation of a nomogram for predicting survival in patients with resected non-small-cell lung cancer. *J Clin Oncol.* (2015) 33:861–9. doi: 10.1200/JCO.2014.56.6661

20. Sorbellini M, Kattan MW, Snyder ME, Reuter V, Motzer R, Goetzl M, et al. A postoperative prognostic nomogram predicting recurrence for patients

with conventional clear cell renal cell carcinoma. *J Urol.* (2005) 173:48–51. doi: 10.1097/01.ju.0000148261.19532.2c

21. Karakiewicz PI, Briganti A, Chun FK, Trinh QD, Perrotte P, Ficarra V, et al. Multi-institutional validation of a new renal cancer-specific survival nomogram. *J Clin Oncol.* (2007) 25:1316–22. doi: 10.1200/JCO.2006.06.1218

22. Zhang G, Wu Y, Zhang J, Fang Z, Liu Z, Xu Z, et al. Nomograms for predicting long-term overall survival and disease-specific survival of patients with clear cell renal cell carcinoma. *Onco Targets Ther.* (2018) 11:5535–44. doi: 10.2147/OTT.S171881

23. Li Y, Zhu MX, Qi SH. Marital status and survival in patients with renal cell carcinoma. *Medicine (Baltimore).* (2018) 97:e0385. doi: 10.1097/MD.0000000000010385

24. Vickers MM, Al-Harbi H, Choueiri TK, Kollmannsberger C, North S, MacKenzie M, et al. Prognostic factors of survival for patients with metastatic renal cell carcinoma with brain metastases treated with targeted therapy: results from the international metastatic renal cell carcinoma database consortium. *Clin Genitourin Cancer.* (2013) 11:311–5. doi: 10.1016/j.clgc.2013.04.012

25. Vornicova O, Bar-Sela G. Do we have a "game changer" in treating patients with brain metastasis from renal cell carcinoma? *Ann Transl Med.* (2019) 7(Suppl 8):S360. doi: 10.21037/atm.2019.09.50

26. Abdel-Rahman O. Clinical correlates and prognostic value of different metastatic sites in metastatic renal cell carcinoma. *Future Oncol.* (2017) 13:1967–80. doi: 10.2217/fon-2017-0175

27. Flanigan RC, Salmon SE, Blumenstein BA, Bearman SI, Roy V, McGrath PC, et al. Nephrectomy followed by interferon alfa-2b compared with interferon alfa-2b alone for metastatic renal-cell cancer. *N Engl J Med.* (2001) 345:1655–9. doi: 10.1056/NEJM003013

28. Mickisch GH, Garin A, van Poppel H, de Prijck L, Sylvester R, European Organisation for R, et al. Radical nephrectomy plus interferon-alfa-based immunotherapy compared with interferon alfa alone in metastatic renal-cell carcinoma: a randomised trial. *Lancet.* (2001) 358:966–70. doi: 10.1016/s0140-6736(01)06103-7

29. Motzer RJ, Hutson TE, Tomczak P, Michaelson MD, Bukowski RM, Oudard S, et al. Overall survival and updated results for sunitinib compared with interferon alfa in patients with metastatic renal cell carcinoma. *J Clin Oncol.* (2009) 27:3584–90. doi: 10.1200/JCO.2008.20.1293

30. Mejean A, Ravaud A, Thezenas S, Colas S, Beauval JB, Bensalah K, et al. Sunitinib alone or after nephrectomy in metastatic renal-cell carcinoma. *N Engl J Med.* (2018) 379:417–27. doi: 10.1056/NEJMoa1803675

31. Zheng W, Zhu W, Yu S, Li K, Ding Y, Wu Q, et al. Development and validation of a nomogram to predict overall survival for patients with metastatic renal cell carcinoma. *BMC Cancer.* (2020) 20:1066. doi: 10.1186/s12885-020-07586-7

32. Motzer RJ, Tannir NM, McDermott DF, Aren Frontera O, Melichar B, Choueiri TK, et al. Nivolumab plus ipilimumab versus sunitinib in advanced renal-cell carcinoma. *N Engl J Med.* (2018) 378:1277–90. doi: 10.1056/NEJMoa1712126

33. Choueiri TK, Halabi S, Sanford BL, Hahn O, Michaelson MD, Walsh MK, et al. Cabozantinib versus sunitinib as initial targeted therapy for patients with metastatic renal cell carcinoma of poor or intermediate risk: the alliance a031203 CABOSUN trial. *J Clin Oncol.* (2017) 35:591–7. doi: 10.1200/JCO.2016.70.7398

# 14

# The Immune-Related Gene HCST as a Novel Biomarker for the Diagnosis and Prognosis of Clear Cell Renal Cell Carcinoma

Yongying Zhou [1†], Xiao Wang [2†], Weibing Zhang [1†], Huiyong Liu [3†], Daoquan Liu [1†], Ping Chen [1], Deqiang Xu [1], Jianmin Liu [1], Yan Li [1], Guang Zeng [1], Mingzhou Li [1], Zhonghua Wu [1], Yingao Zhang [1], Xinghuan Wang [1], Michael E. DiSanto [4] and Xinhua Zhang [1*]

[1] Department of Urology, Zhongnan Hospital of Wuhan University, Wuhan, China, [2] Department of Rehabilitation Medicine, Renmin Hospital of Wuhan University, Wuhan, China, [3] Department of Urology, Huanggang Central Hospital, Huanggang, China, [4] Department of Surgery and Biomedical Sciences, Cooper Medical School of Rowan University, Camden, NJ, United States

*Correspondence:
Xinhua Zhang
zhangxinhuad@163.com

[†] These authors have contributed equally to this work

Clear cell renal cell carcinoma (ccRCC) is the most common type of kidney tumor worldwide. Analysis of The Cancer Genome Atlas (TCGA) and Gene Expression Omnibus (GEO) databases showed that the immune-related gene (IRG) hematopoietic cell signal transducer (HCST) could provide guidance for the diagnosis, prognosis, and treatment of ccRCC. The RNA-seq data of ccRCC tissues were extracted from two databases: TCGA (https://www.cancer.gov/about-nci/organization/ccg/research/structural-genomics/tcga) and GEO (https://www.ncbi.nlm.nih.gov/geo/). Corresponding clinical information was downloaded from TCGA. Immune-related gene data were extracted from the IMMPORT website (https://www.immport.org/). Differential analysis with R software (https://www.r-project.org/) was used to obtain a prognosis model of ccRCC IRGs. The differences were combined with the clinical data to assess the usefulness of the HCST as a prognostic biomarker. Based on data obtained from the Oncomine (https://www.oncomine.org/), Human Protein Atlas (https://www.proteinatlas.org/), and PubMed (https://pubmed.ncbi.nlm.nih.gov/) databases, the expression levels of the HCST in ccRCC, clinical-pathological indicators of relevance, and influence on prognosis were analyzed. Regulation of the HCST gene in ccRCC was assessed by gene set enrichment analysis (GSEA). In TCGA/GEO databases, the high HCST expression in tumor tissues was significantly correlated to the TMN stage, tumor grade, invasion depth, and lymphatic metastasis ($p < 0.05$). The overall survival (OS) of patients with high HCST gene expression was significantly lower than that of patients with low HCST gene expression ($p < 0.001$). Multivariate Cox regression analysis suggested that the HCST expression level [hazard ratio (HR) = 1.630, 95% confidence interval (CI) = 1.042–2.552], tumor cell grade (HR = 1.829, 95% CI = 1.115–3.001), and distant metastasis (HR = 2.634, 95%, CI = 1.562–4.442) were independent risk factors affecting the OS of ccRCC patients (all, $p < 0.05$). The GSEA study showed that there was significant enrichment in cell adhesion, tumorigenesis, and immune and inflammatory responses in HCST high expression samples. Hematopoietic cell signal transducer expression was closely associated with the levels of infiltrating immune cells around ccRCC tissues, especially dendritic cells (DCs). In conclusion, the present study suggested that the HCST was interrelated to the clinicopathology and poor prognosis of ccRCC. High HCST expression was also closely correlated with the levels of tumor-infiltrating immune cells, especially DCs.

Keywords: prognosis, biomarker, clear cell renal cell carcinoma, HCST, immune-related gene

# INTRODUCTION

Renal carcinoma is one of the most common malignant tumors of the urinary system and accounts for 3% of all adult cancers. Clear cell renal cell carcinoma (ccRCC) is the most common pathological type of renal carcinoma, accounting for 70–85% of all cases (1). However, non-surgical treatments for ccRCC, such as chemotherapy and radiotherapy, are limited due to uncertain efficacy, heavy patient burden, frequent side effects, and poor prognosis. More effective treatments with fewer side effects have been actively sought (2). Indeed, target therapy and immunotherapy have recently become as first-line therapies for ccRCC (3, 4).

Since the last century, bacillus Calmette–Guerin vaccine, interferon-alpha, and interleukin-2 (IL-2) have been used for immunotherapy of cancer. The application of IL-2 in tumor therapy has confirmed the effectiveness of adaptive immunity for cancer control and revealed T-cell regulation as a new strategy for immunotherapy. In fact, chimeric antigen receptor-modified T cells and immune modulation using antibodies to block immune regulatory checkpoints were named as the "breakthrough of the year" by *Science* in 2013 (5). Currently, with an unprecedented sustained and stable antitumor response, immunotherapy cytotoxic T lymphocyte-associated antigen 4 (CTLA4) or programmed cell death protein 1 (PD-1)/PD-1 ligand 1 (PD-L1) has demonstrated remarkable efficacy against various types of cancer (6).

Previous studies have reported that ccRCC is prone to immune cell infiltration and, thus, is highly responsive to immunotherapies that inhibit the interactions between immune cells and tumor cells by targeting CTLA4, PD-1, and PD-L1 (2). The blood, immune cells, and stromal cells surrounding cancer tissue form an immune microenvironment containing receptor factors involved in immunosuppression tolerance (7). Other studies have found that some indicators in the ccRCC microenvironment, such as CD8+T-cell density and PD-1/PD-L1 expression in the tumor and invasive margin (8), can be used as indicators to evaluate the clinical effectiveness of PD-1 inhibitors (9, 10). Hence, the identification of molecules

as biomarkers that regulate the immune microenvironment is crucial to improving immunotherapy against ccRCC (11–13).

In the present study, analysis of public datasets identified 2,498 immune-related genes (IRGs) in ccRCC. Of these, hematopoietic cell signal transducer (HCST) was selected as the target gene. The HCST encodes a transmembrane signaling adaptor that forms part of the immune recognition receptor complex with the C-type lectin-like receptor NKG2D (14), which may have a role in cell survival and proliferation by activating dendritic cells (DCs), natural killer (NK) cells, and T cells (15). Thus, HCST may be a useful target for immunotherapy against ccRCC. Unfortunately, the HCST has not been studied in the field of kidney cancer.

Due to the limited understanding of the clinical significance and unique role of the HCST in ccRCC, the potential clinical value of the HCST was determined by assessment of relevant clinical data of factors and poor prognosis of ccRCC patients. Gene set enrichment analysis (GSEA) of the association between the HCST and immune cells indicated the potential role and prognostic value of the HCST in tumor immunology.

# MATERIALS AND METHODS
## Human Tissue Acquisition

Human ccRCC tissues were obtained from seven male and three female patients who underwent partial nephrectomy at Zhong Nan Hospital. All samples included tumor infiltrating tissues of renal parenchyma and adjacent para-cancerous tissues, which were identified by two separate pathologists. All human samples were obtained after the approval of the Hospital Committee for Investigation in Humans and after receiving written informed consent from all patients or their relatives. All human studies were conducted in accordance with the principles of the Declaration of Helsinki.

## Data Sources

A total of 2,498 IRGs were collected from the Tumor Immune Estimation Resource (TIMER) database (https://cistrome.shinyapps.io/timer/) in May 2020 (16). The mRNA expression profiles of 539 ccRCC samples and 72 para-cancer tissue samples, as well as relevant clinical data, were downloaded from The Cancer Genome Atlas (TCGA) database (https://www.cancer.gov/about-nci/organization/ccg/research/structural-genomics/tcga) (17), of which 537 patients had matching mRNA expression profiles and survival data. In addition, two ccRCC-associated

**Abbreviations:** ccRCC, Clear cell renal cell carcinoma; TCGA, The Cancer Genome Atlas; GEO, Gene Expression Omnibus; IRG, Immune-related gene; HCST, Hematopoietic cell signal transducer; GSEA, Gene set enrichment analysis; OS, Overall survival; CTLA4, Cytotoxic T lymphocyte-associated antigen 4; PD-1, Programmed cell death protein 1; PD-L1, Programmed death-2; DCs, Dendritic cells; NK cells, Natural Killer cells; TIMER, Tumor Immune Estimation Resource; TF, Transcription factors.

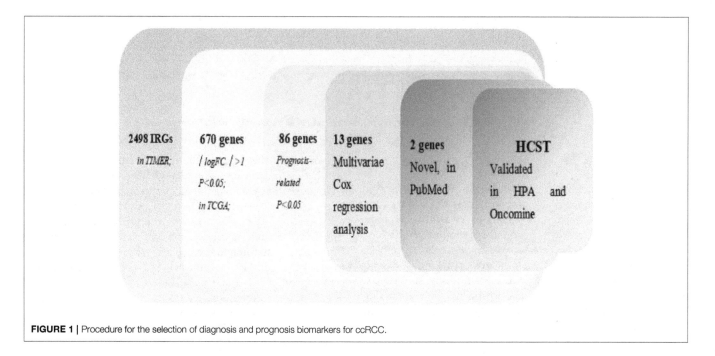

**FIGURE 1 |** Procedure for the selection of diagnosis and prognosis biomarkers for ccRCC.

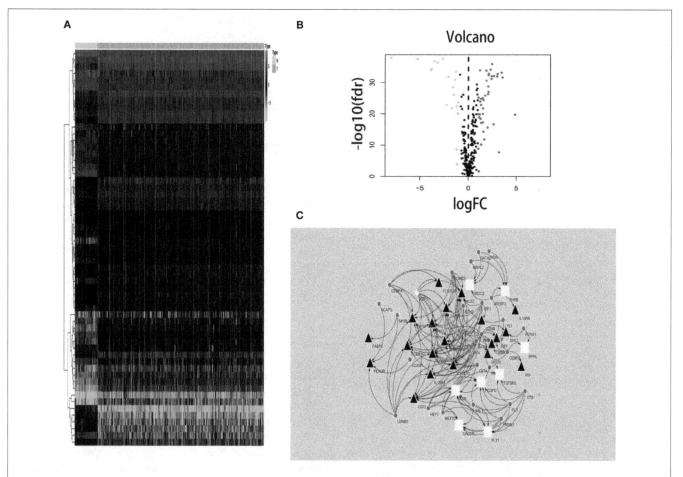

**FIGURE 2 |** TF-based regulatory network. Construction of a TF-based regulatory network. **(A)** A heatmap of TFs differentially expressed in the tissue samples. **(B)** A volcano plot of differentially expressed TFs. **(C)** A regulatory network constructed from potentially relevant TFs (red), low-risk IRGs (red), and high-risk IRGs (black). IRGs, immune-related genes; TFs, transcription factors.

datasets (GSE53757 and GSE66272) were downloaded from the Gene Expression Omnibus (GEO) database (https://www.ncbi.nlm.nih.gov/geo/) (18). In this study, the publication guidelines of TCGA and GEO were strictly followed.

## Differential Analysis of Immune-Related Genes

The "affy" and "limma" packages in R software (https://www.r-project.org/) were used to differentiate the specimens from the GSE53757 and GES66272 datasets, which included 72 and 27 pairs of ccRCC and normal kidney specimens, respectively. Differentially expressed Immune-Related Genes (DEIRGs) were screened using $t$-test in accordance with the following cut-off values: false discovery rate (FDR) < 0.05 and |log2 fold change| > 1.

## Selection of Prognostic Differentially Expressed Immune-Related Genes

Univariate ("futime" and "fustat") Cox regression analysis (19) identified 86 DEIRGs closely correlated with the overall survival (OS) of ccRCC patients ($p < 0.05$).

## Transcription Factor Regulatory Network

Cancer associated transcription factors (TFs) were downloaded from the Cistrome Project (http://cistrome.org/), which is a comprehensive resource for predicted transcription factor targets and enhancer profiles in cancers. The correlations between TFs and the expression patterns of PDEIRGs were analyzed in order to identify the mechanism(s) underlying the dysregulation of PDEIRG expression in ccRCC. A TF regulatory network was generated using the Cytoscape_3.7.1 software (https://cytoscape.org/).

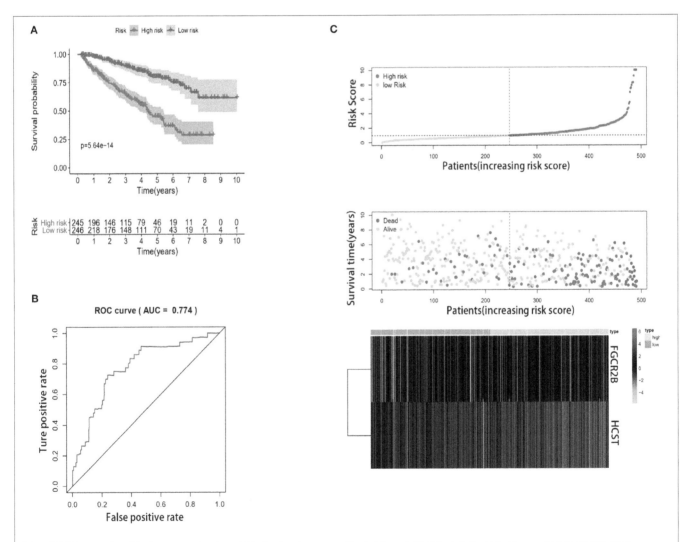

**FIGURE 3 |** Construction of the immune-system-based risk signature by means of the training set. **(A)** Patients in the high-risk group had shorter OS. **(B)** A receiver-operating characteristic curve illustrating the prognostic value of the risk signature. **(C)** Ranking of the risk signature and distribution of the risk groups, survival status of the patients in the low-risk and high-risk groups, and a heatmap of expression profiles of the included genes.

## Identification of Genes for Inclusion in a Prognostic Model

Based on the influence on the OS of ccRCC patients, the DEIRGs were screened using the Cox regression hazards model.

## Selection of the HCST Gene

Based on the data obtained from the Oncomine (https://www.oncomine.org/), Human Protein Atlas (https://www.proteinatlas.org/), and PubMed (https://pubmed.ncbi.nlm.nih.gov/) databases, the HCST gene was considered as a novel biomarker of ccRCC.

## RNA Extraction, Reverse Transcription, and Real-Time Quantitative PCR

The expression patterns of the HCST gene were assessed in matched ccRCC and para-cancerous tissues. Total RNA from tissues was isolated using the HiPurA™ Total RNA Miniprep Purification Kit (catalog no. R4111-03; Angen Biotech Co., Ltd., Guangzhou, China) in accordance with the manufacturer's instructions. The quantity of the isolated RNA was measured with a NanoDrop ND-1000 UV-Vis spectrophotometer (NanoDrop Technologies, LLC, Wilmington, DE, USA). Complementary DNA (cDNA) was synthesized from 1 μg of total RNA with the ABScript II RT Master Mix for qPCR (catalog no. RK20402; ABclonal Technology, Woburn, MA, USA). Each qPCR reaction consisted of 10 μl of 2× Universal SYBR Green Fast qPCR Mix (catalog no. RK21203; ABclonal Technology), 7 μl of ddH$_2$O, 1 μl of cDNA, 1 μl of the forward primer, and 1 μl of the reverse primer. Values were normalized to that of the glyceraldehyde 3-phosphate dehydrogenase gene. A gene-specific primer pair (forward: AGG CTC TTG TTC CGG ATG TG and reverse: TAG ACT TTG CCA TCT TGG GCG) was used for amplification of the HCST gene.

## Survival Analysis

Based on the median expression value, 537 ccRCC patients were allocated to the HCST high expression group or low expression group. The R software "survival" package, Kaplan–Meier method, and log-rank test were used to evaluate the effect of the HCST on the OS of ccRCC patients. In addition, the probability (p) values and 95% confidence intervals (CIs) were calculated, and a survival curve was plotted (20, 21).

## Correlation Analysis of the HCST Expression Patterns and Clinicopathological Features

Clinicopathological data [i.e., age, sex, grade, TNM stage, infiltration depth (T), distant metastasis (M), and lymph node metastasis (N)] of the ccRCC tissue specimens from the TCGA database were selected for further analysis. After exclusion of

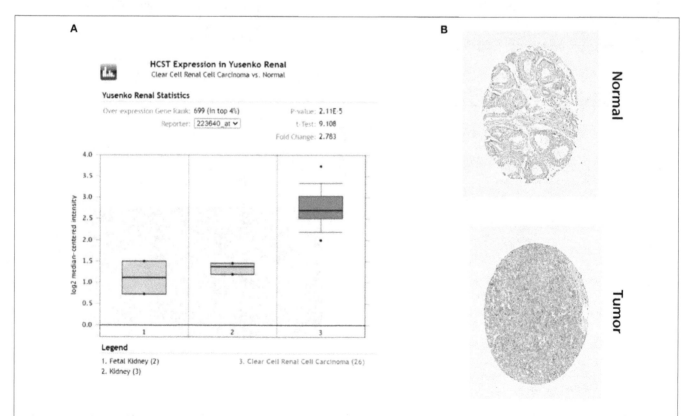

FIGURE 4 | HCST protein expression was significantly higher in ccRCC tissues than normal tissues. Representative IHC images of HCST (A) in normal (left) and ccRCC (right) tissues. Images were downloaded from the HPA database. Statistical analyses of the protein expression levels of the HCST according to the information of normal and ccRCC tissues (B) from Oncomine.

incomplete or defective clinical data, data from 226 patients were included for analysis. Independent sample *t*-test and paired *t*-test were used to identify correlations between HCST expression levels and clinical-pathological parameters.

## Statistical Analysis of Potential Prognostic Factors

Potential prognostic factors were identified using the R version 4.0.2 software ("survival" and "survminer" packages). Univariate Cox regression analysis was performed to identify several prognostic factors followed by multivariate Cox regression analysis to identify independent prognostic factors.

## Protein Interaction Network Analysis

The STRING database (https://string-db.org/) (22) was used to explore the known and predicted correlations between protein interactions and HCST expression patterns, and to screen proteins that interact with the HCST.

## GSEA

The GSEA software (23) was used to divide the high and low expression groups based on the median expression value of the HCST and to detect the highest ranking gene enrichment pathways in the two groups (Molecular Signatures Database c2. Cp. Kegg. V7.2. Symbols). The Gene Matrix Transposed function dataset was used as a reference gene set for all analyses. The number of genes was set to 1,000 for the calculation of the enrichment coefficient (enrichment score) and normalized enrichment score (NES). FDR < 0.05 was considered indicative of significant enrichment.

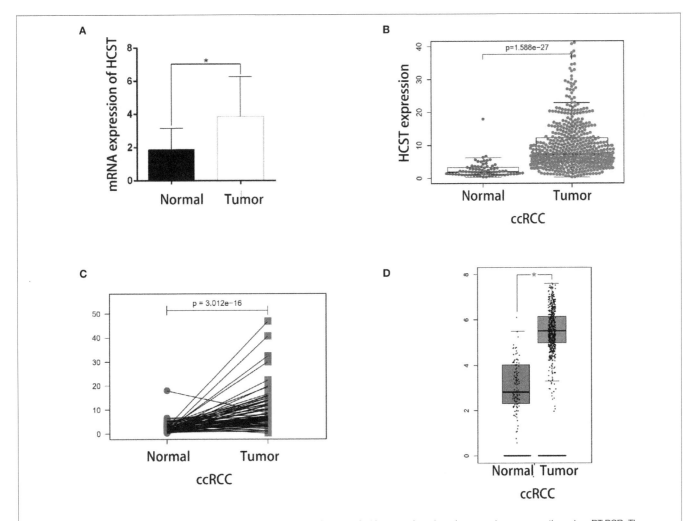

**FIGURE 5 |** Experimental validation. **(A)** Detection of HCST mRNA expression levels in 10 cases of renal carcinoma and para-cancer tissue by qRT-PCR. The glyceraldehyde 3-phosphate dehydrogenase gene was used as an internal control. HCST expression in cancer cells is clearly higher than normal kidney cells. **(B)** Statistical analyses of the mRNA expression levels of the HCST according to the information of normal and ccRCC tissues from R version 4.0.2 software matching TCGA data. **(C)** Statistical analyses of the mRNA expression levels of the HCST according to cancer and para-cancerous tissue from the same ccRCC patient from R version 4.0.2 software matching TCGA data. **(D)** Statistical analyses of the mRNA expression levels of the HCST according to the information of normal and ccRCC tissues from GEPIA 2 matching TCGA and GTEx data. *$p$ < 0.05.

## Correlation Analysis of HCST and Immune Cell Infiltration

The "cibersort" package (R version 4.0.2 software) was used to analyze the proportions of 22 immune cell types (LM22 gene signature) in CCRCC tissues. Then, the relationships between HCST expression levels and proportions of various immune cells were further quantified. Finally, the "ggplot2" and "limma" packages (R version 4.0.2 software) were used for analysis and plotting of the data. Meanwhile, the TIMER database was referenced for analysis of the tumor-infiltrating immune cells (i.e., CD8+ T cells, CD4+ T cells, B cells, macrophages, neutrophils, and DCs).

## Correlation Analysis of HCST and Immune-Related Genes PD-1

The expression of PD-1 is widely recognized as the most powerful predictive biomarker for anti-PD-1 therapy. The currently studied CD28 can be used as a biomarker for PD-1 expression (24). The correlations between the HCST and CD28, CD80, and CD86 were analyzed in the TIMER database to illustrate the role of the HCST as a biomarker of immunotherapy response. A correlation coefficient over 0.3 was considered statistically significant.

## Statistical Analysis

Statistical analyses were conducted using IBM SPSS Statistics for Windows, version 20.0 (IBM Corporation, Armonk, NY, USA) and R version 4.0.2. The gene expression data are presented as mean $\pm$ standard deviation. $t$-test was used to identify differences in HCST expression levels between the ccRCC and para-carcinoma tissues from the TCGA and GEO databases. Wilcoxon signed-rank test was used to analyze the interrelation between the HCST and clinical characteristic variables. Univariate and multivariate Cox analyses were used to calculate the hazard ratio and 95% CI. A $p$-value $< 0.05$ was considered statistically significant. FDR $< 0.05$ and $p < 0.01$ were considered indicative of significant enrichment.

## RESULTS

The process of screening target genes is shown in **Figure 1**.

## Expression Patterns of IRGs in ccRCC From Public Databases

The mRNA levels of 2,498 IRGs in 539 ccRCC samples and 72 normal renal tissue samples (TCGA) were analyzed. The same approach was applied to the GSE53757 and GES66272 datasets from the GEO database. Then, the data retrieved from two database were intersected. In total, 670 DEIRGs (554 upregulated and 116 downregulated) with an FDR $< 0.05$ and |log$_2$ fold change| $> 1$ were identified.

## Identification of PDEIRGs

Univariate Cox regression analysis identified 86 PDEIRGs significantly associated with the OS and disease-free survival (DFS) of ccRCC patients (all $p < 0.05$).

## TF Regulatory Network

In total, 318 TFs were downloaded from the Cistrome database (http://www.cistrome.com/). Sixty TFs were significantly different at the mRNA expression levels between the ccRCC ($n = 539$) and normal renal tissue ($n = 72$) samples ($r > 0.4$ and $p < 0.05$) (**Figures 2A,B**). Of those 60 TFs, 28 (46.7%) turned out to be closely related to abnormal expression of PDEIRGs by using a correlation coefficient $> 0.4$ and a $p$-value $< 0.05$ as the cut-off values. Based on these data, a TF regulatory network was generated using the Cytoscape 3.7.1 software (**Figure 2C**).

## Establishment and Validation of an IRG-Based Prognostic Model

In order to select the best gene model, multivariate Cox analysis was used to reduce the influence of genes on each other, and the genes with the best correlation with prognosis were selected and the risk score was calculated with the formula "Risk score (patient) $\sum_{i=1}^{N}$ (expression value of (gene)$^*$ coefficient (gene))". In this formula, "coefficient (gene)" is the estimated regression coefficient of gene from the Cox proportional hazards regression analysis. As is shown in **Supplementary Table 1**, a regression risk model identified 13 PDEIRGs. To verify the accuracy and significance of the model, an OS survival curve (**Figure 3A**), a receiver-operating characteristic curve (**Figure 3B**), and a risk curve of the IRG-based prognosis model (**Figure 3C**) were generated. A search of the PubMed database (performed on 2 May, 2020) revealed 11 genes associated with ccRCC in the model, which did not include the HCST and FCGR2.

**TABLE 1 |** Relationship between HCST expression level and clinicopathological variables in ccRCC patients.

| Classification | Total | HCST expression | t | P |
|---|---|---|---|---|
| **Age** | | | | |
| ≤60 | 142 | 10.530 ± 10.300 | 0.709 | 0.721 |
| >60 | 84 | 11.077 ± 11.169 | | |
| **Gender** | | | | |
| Male | 141 | 10.805 ± 12.080 | 0.897 | 0.292 |
| Female | 85 | 10.615 ± 7.637 | | |
| **TMN stage** | | | | |
| I–II | 122 | 9.068 ± 9.300 | 0.010 | 0.001 |
| III–IV | 104 | 12.630 ± 11.712 | | |
| **Grade** | | | | |
| G1–G2 | 98 | 9.013 ± 9.765 | 0.031 | 0.005 |
| G3–G4 | 128 | 12.075 ± 11.078 | | |
| **Invasion depth** | | | | |
| T1–T2 | 134 | 9.798 ± 9.897 | 0.110 | 0.018 |
| T3–T4 | 92 | 12.097 ± 11.489 | | |
| **Lymph node metastasis** | | | | |
| N0 | 213 | 10.126 ± 9.167 | <0.001 | 0.004 |
| N1 | 13 | 20.690 ± 22.631 | | |
| **Distant metastasis** | | | | |
| M0 | 186 | 10.479 ± 10.920 | 0.431 | 0.128 |
| M1 | 38 | 11.953 ± 9.005 | | |

$p < 0.05$, statistically significant.

According to the Beroukhim dataset derived from the Oncomine database, the fold change of these two genes was >2. But only HCST overexpression was ranked in the top 5% (**Figure 4A**). Analysis of 36 histological section images of ccRCC and normal kidney tissues from the HPA database showed that HCST protein expression was significantly increased in ccRCC

tissues (**Figure 4B**). Therefore, the HCST was chosen for further analysis.

## Experimental Validation

qRT-PCR analysis showed that HCST mRNA levels were significantly higher in ccRCC tissues than those in normal

**TABLE 2 |** Univariate analysis of the prognostic factors in ccRCC patients using a Cox regression model.

| Parameters OS | Univariate analysis | | Multivariate analysis | |
|---|---|---|---|---|
| | HR(95%CI) | p | HR(95%CI) | p |
| HCST expression High vs. Low | 1.853(1.210–2.839) | 0.004 | 1.630 (1.042–2.552) | 0.032 |
| Age ≥65 vs. <60 | 1.370(0.908–2.067) | 0.133 | 1.371 (0.893–2.105) | 0.149 |
| Female vs. male | 1.013(0.666–1.541) | 0.951 | 1.099 (0.709–1.704) | 0.673 |
| TMN stage III/IV vs. I/II | 3.676(2.366–5.711) | <0.001 | 1.295 (0.511–3.280) | 0.278 |
| Grade G1/2 vs. G3/4 | 2.629(1.655–4.176) | <0.001 | 1.829 (1.115–3.001) | 0.017 |
| Invasion depth T1/2 vs. T3/4 | 3.311(2.167–5.058) | <0.001 | 1.594 (0.699–3.634) | 0.268 |
| Lymph node metastasis | 2.932(1.516–2.839) | <0.001 | 1.273 (0.629–2.574) | 0.502 |
| Distant metastasis | 4.073(2.634–6.300) | 0.001 | 2.634 (1.562–4.442) | <0.001 |

*CI, confidence interval.*

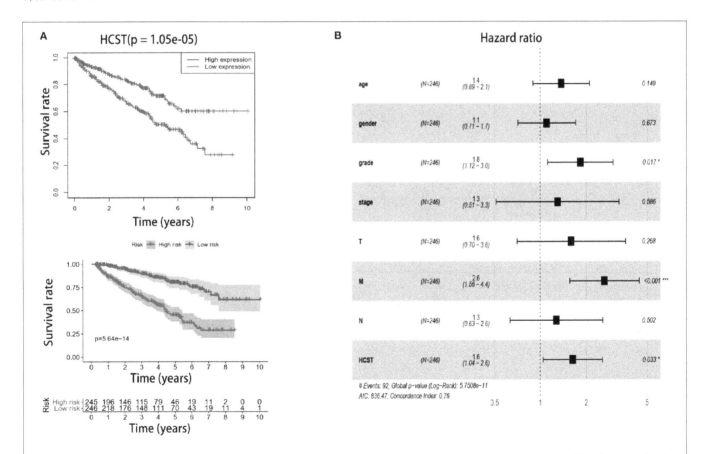

**FIGURE 6 |** High HCST expression is associated with poor survival of ccRCC patients. **(A,** Upper**)** OS of HCST (high) and HCST (low) ccRCC patients matching the TCGA database from R version 4.0.2 software. **(A,** Down**)** DFS of HCST (high) and HCST (low) patients from the GEPIA2 matching TCGA and GTEx data. **(B)** Multivariate Cox analysis showing the hazard ratios of different factors. The number of events for the number of tested factors was 92. The global *p*-value (log-rank) was 5.7508e−05, Akaike's information criterion was 836.47, and the concordance index was 0.76.

renal tissues (**Figure 5A**). Consistently, the HCST was observed upregulated with the R version 4.0.2 software analysis of TCGA data (**Figures 5B,C**), of which HCST mRNA levels of cancer and para-cancerous tissue are from the same ccRCC patients (**Figure 5C**). Matching TCGA and GTEx data, the Gene Expression Profiling Interactive Analysis (GEPIA2) (http://gepia.cancer-pku.cn/) found similarly elevated HCST expression (**Figure 5D**).

## Relationship Between HCST Gene Expression Levels and Clinicopathological Indices of Tumor Tissues

A median gene expression value of 6.436 was used to stratify the 537 TCGA-ccRCC patients into the low or high expression group. Analysis using TCGA clinical data and R version 4.0.2 showed

that HCST expression was correlated with grade ($p = 0.005$), TNM stage ($p = 0.001$), lymph node metastasis ($p = 0.004$), and invasion depth ($p = 0.018$), but not age ($p = 0.721$), sex ($p = 0.292$), or distant metastasis ($p = 0.218$) (**Table 1**).

## HCST Is an Independent Poor Prognostic Factor of ccRCC

The R software "survival" package, Kaplan–Meier method, and log-rank test were used to assess the effect of the HCST on the OS of ccRCC patients. The logarithmic rank $p$-value and 95% CI were calculated. Then, a survival curve was plotted. Univariate and multivariate Cox regression analyses were performed to investigate whether high expression of the HCST could be an independent adverse prognostic factor in patients with ccRCC. As shown in **Table 2**, Cox univariate survival analysis indicated

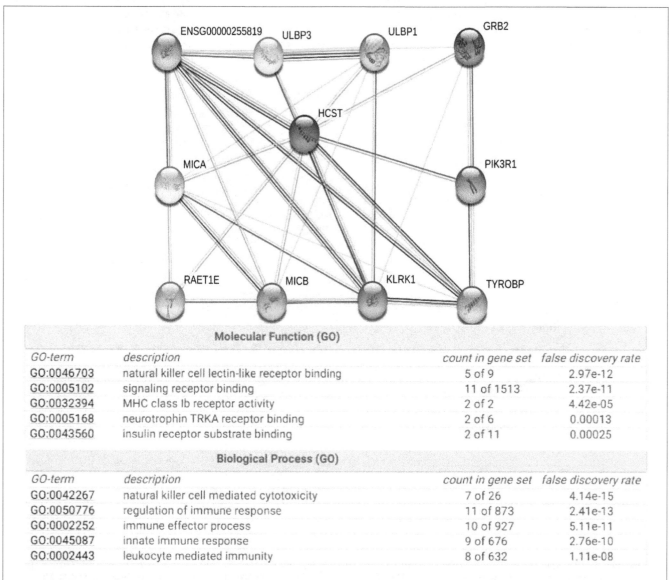

### Molecular Function (GO)

| GO-term | description | count in gene set | false discovery rate |
|---|---|---|---|
| GO:0046703 | natural killer cell lectin-like receptor binding | 5 of 9 | 2.97e-12 |
| GO:0005102 | signaling receptor binding | 11 of 1513 | 2.37e-11 |
| GO:0032394 | MHC class Ib receptor activity | 2 of 2 | 4.42e-05 |
| GO:0005168 | neurotrophin TRKA receptor binding | 2 of 6 | 0.00013 |
| GO:0043560 | insulin receptor substrate binding | 2 of 11 | 0.00025 |

### Biological Process (GO)

| GO-term | description | count in gene set | false discovery rate |
|---|---|---|---|
| GO:0042267 | natural killer cell mediated cytotoxicity | 7 of 26 | 4.14e-15 |
| GO:0050776 | regulation of immune response | 11 of 873 | 2.41e-13 |
| GO:0002252 | immune effector process | 10 of 927 | 5.11e-11 |
| GO:0045087 | innate immune response | 9 of 676 | 2.76e-10 |
| GO:0002443 | leukocyte mediated immunity | 8 of 632 | 1.11e-08 |

**FIGURE 7 |** Protein interaction network of HCST. An interaction network of the HCST protein with other proteins (i.e., TYROBP, KLRC4, MICA, MICB, ULBP3, ULBP1, RAET1E, GRB2, KLRK1, and PIK3R1). The interaction network was obtained from the STRING database.

that grade ($p < 0.001$), TNM stage ($p < 0.001$), lymph node metastasis ($p = 0.001$), invasion depth ($p < 0.001$), distant metastasis ($p < 0.001$), and HCST expression ($p = 0.005$) were important parameters affecting the duration of OS, while multivariate Cox survival analysis showed that grade, distant metastasis, and HCST expression were independent factors of a poor prognosis of ccRCC patients (all, $p < 0.05$) (**Figure 6**).

## Protein Interaction Network of HCST

The STRING database was used to explore the known and predicted protein–protein associations involving HCST. The top 10 predicted functional partners were TYROBP (score = 0.983), KLRC4 (score = 0.976), MICA (score = 0.966), MICB (score = 0.965), ULBP3 (score = 0.962), ULBP1 (score = 0.962), RAET1E (score = 0.951), GRB2 (score = 0.942), KLRK1 (score

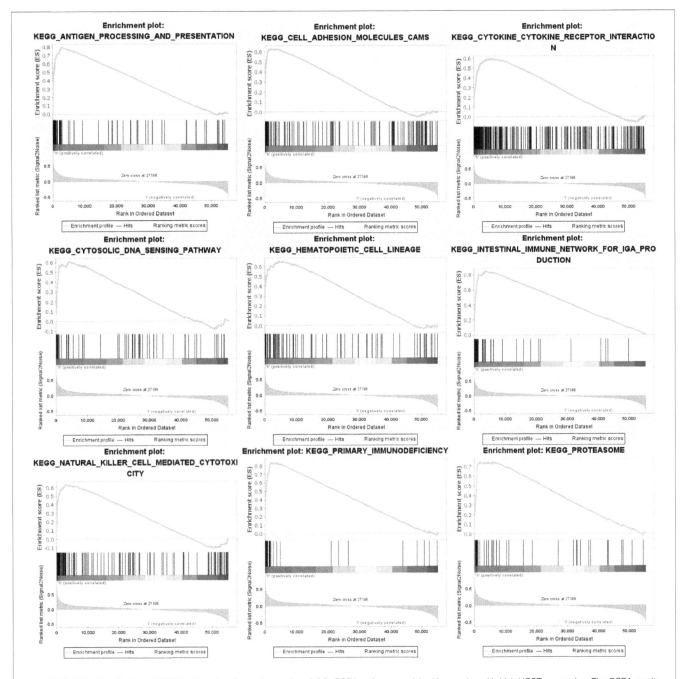

**FIGURE 8 |** GSEA identification of HCST-related signaling pathways in ccRCC. GSEA pathways enriched in samples with high HCST expression. The GSEA results showed that the terms "proteasome," "cytosolic DNA sensing pathway," "cell adhesion molecules cams," "cytokine receptor interaction," "primary immunodeficiency," "hematopoietic cell lineage," "natural killer cell-mediated cytotoxicity," "intestinal immune network for IGA production," and "antigen processing and presentation" were differentially enriched in GC samples with high BICC1. NES, normalized enrichment score.

= 0.923), and PIK3R1 (score = 0.870) (**Figure 7**). Function enrichment analysis of the HCST gene revealed that the most significant biological processes were "natural killer cell-mediated cytotoxicity," "regulation of immune response," "immune effector process," and "innate immune response." In regard to cellular components, the HCST gene was significantly enriched in "cell surface," "the plasma membrane," "membrane part," and "intrinsic component of plasma membrane."

## GSEA of HCST

GSEA identified 57 HCST-related signaling pathways that were upregulated in ccRCC, 17 of which were more obviously enriched (NOM $p < 0.05$, FDR < 0.1, and NES > 2.0) (**Figure 8**). As shown in **Table 3**, the terms "proteasome," "cytosolic DNA sensing pathway," "cell adhesion molecules cams," and "cytokine receptor interaction," whose function was involved in cell adhesion and tumorigenesis, were significantly enriched in the HCST high expression group. Meanwhile, the terms associated with immune and inflammatory responses included "hematopoietic cell lineage," "intestinal immune network for IGA production," "natural killer cell-mediated cytotoxicity," "antigen processing and presentation," and "primary immunodeficiency."

## Interrelation With Tumor-Infiltrating Immune Cells in ccRCC

Analysis with the CIBERSOFT software showed that HCST expression was correlated with tumor-filtrating immune cells, including naïve B cells, activated DCs, eosinophils, M2 macrophages, resting mast cells, monocytes, neutrophils, resting NK cells, plasma cells, activated CD4 memory T cells, resting CD4 memory T cells, CD8 T cells, follicular helper T cells, gamma delta T cells, and regulatory T cells (all, $p < 0.001$) (**Figure 9**). In addition, the TIMER database indicated that HCST expression was positively correlated to the levels of different infiltrating immune cells, including B cells ($r = 0.312$, $p = 8.04e{-}12$), CD8+ T cells ($r = 0.541$, $p = 1.11e{-}34$), and neutrophils ($r = 0.3.93$, $p = 2.33e{-}18$), and strongly correlated with DCs ($r = 0.576$, $p = 1.74e{-}41$) (**Figure 10A**).

## The Correlation Analysis of HCST and Immune-Related Genes PD-1

Our results showed that the HCST was positively correlated with the expression of CD80 in ccRCC (cor = 0.518, $p = 7.21e{-}38$, respectively); the HCST was positively correlated with the expression of CD86 in ccRCC (cor = 0.545, $p = 1.57e{-}42$, respectively); the HCST was positively correlated with the expression of CD28 in ccRCC (cor = 0.616, $p = 5.85e{-}57$, respectively) (**Figure 10B**).

## DISCUSSION

In recent years, due to the continuous and stable antitumor responses, immunotherapy has become the first-line therapy for ccRCC. Various studies of immunotherapy regimens have revealed that immune cell infiltration and IRGs play pivotal roles in carcinogenesis and tumor progression (25, 26). However, the relationship between IRGs and the mechanisms underlying tumorigenesis and progression is still not fully understood in ccRCC.

In the present study, IRG expression levels in ccRCC tissues were analyzed systematically. With a multistep selection and validation procedure, the HCST gene was chosen as the proposed IRG-based prognostic model. Firstly, R version 4.0.2 software was used to analyze the transcriptomic and clinical data retrieved from TCGA, which showed that patients had significantly shorter durations of OS and DFS with higher HCST mRNA levels. In addition, high HCST expression has been associated with grade ($p = 0.005$), TNM stage ($p = 0.001$), lymph node metastasis ($p = 0.004$), and invasion depth ($p = 0.018$) in ccRCC. Moreover, univariate and multivariate analyses demonstrated that the HCST was an independent poor prognostic biomarker of OS and DFS in ccRCC patients.

Subsequently, GSEA was performed with the STRING database to determine the molecular functions and potential mechanisms of the HCST. Protein–protein interaction analysis showed that the top 10 proteins associated with the HCST included TYROBP, KLRC4, MICA, MICB, ULBP3, ULBP1, RAET1E, GRB2, KLRK1, and PIK3R1, which are mainly involved in the immune response and tumorigenesis. Functional

---

**TABLE 3 |** GSEA pathways upregulated due to high expression of HCST.

| GS <br> follow link to MSigDB | ES | NES | p | FDR |
|---|---|---|---|---|
| KEGG_PROTEASOME | 0.75 | 2.09 | 0.004 | 0.004 |
| KEGG_CYTOSOLIC_DNA_SENSING_PATHWAY | 0.61 | 2.21 | <0.001 | 0.001 |
| KEGG_CELL_ADHESION_MOLECULES_CAMS | 0.63 | 2.30 | <0.001 | <0.001 |
| KEGG_CYTOKINE_CYTOKINE_RECEPTOR_INTERACTION | 0.59 | 2.47 | <0.001 | <0.001 |
| KEGG_PRIMARY_IMMUNODEFICIENCY | 0.84 | 2.20 | <0.001 | 0.001 |
| KEGG_NATURAL_KILLER_CELL_MEDIATED_CYTOTOXICITY | 0.63 | 2.38 | <0.001 | <0.001 |
| KEGG_INTESTINAL_IMMUNE_NETWORK_FOR_IGA_PRODUCTION | 0.85 | 2.51 | <0.001 | <0.001 |
| KEGG_ANTIGEN_PROCESSING_AND_PRESENTATION | 0.79 | 2.60 | <0.001 | <0.001 |
| KEGG_HEMATOPOIETIC_CELL_LINEAGE | 0.65 | 2.26 | <0.001 | 0.001 |

*NES, normalized enrichment score; NOM, nominal; FDR, false discovery rate. Gene sets with NOM p-value < 0.05 and FDR q-value < 0.1 are considered as significant.*

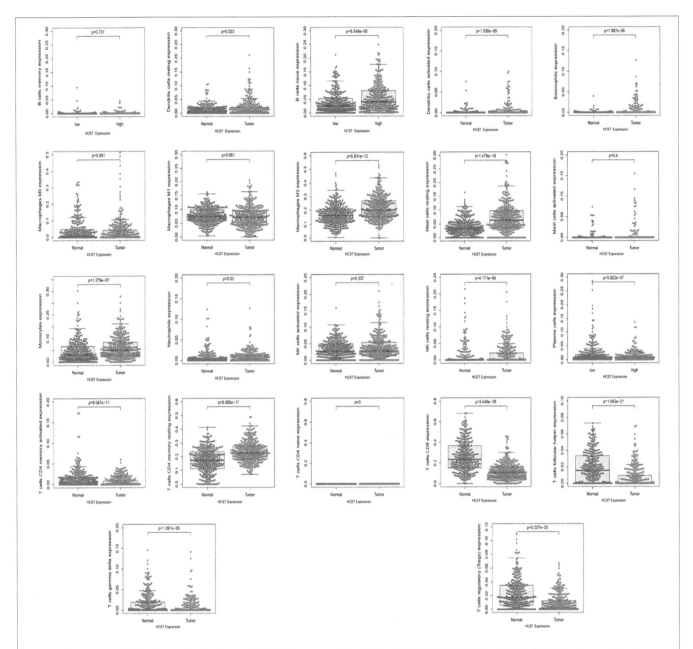

**FIGURE 9 |** HCST was significantly correlated with tumor-infiltrating immune cells in ccRCC. Analysis of the TCGA dataset via the LM22 signature matrix using CIBERSORT online. In total, 22 kinds of tumor-infiltrating immune cells are plotted according to the HCST expression level. There were significant differences in naïve B cells, activated DCs, eosinophils, M2 macrophages, resting mast cells, monocytes, neutrophils, resting NK cells, plasma cells, activated CD4 memory T cells, resting CD4 memory T cells, CD8 T cells, follicular helper T cells, gamma delta T cells, and regulatory T cells (all, $p < 0.001$).

enrichment analysis of these interaction partners at the gene level showed enrichment in the terms "immunoreaction" and "encoding a transmembrane signaling adaptor." For instance, PIK3R1 is a major regulatory isomer of PI3K, and dysregulation of the PI3K/PTEN pathway is a common cause of cancer (27). The HCST may be involved in tumorigenesis through synergistic action with these genes. The GSEA study further indicated that the pathways enriched in tissue samples with high HCST expression were mainly related to

cell adhesion, tumor formation, and the immune response. Of nine representative upregulated pathways, the enriched terms "proteasome," "cytosolic DNA sensing pathway," "cell adhesion molecules cams," and "cytokine receptor interaction" were associated with cell adhesion and tumorigenesis, while "hematopoietic cell lineage," "intestinal immune network for IGA production," "natural killer cell-mediated cytotoxicity," "antigen processing and presentation," and "primary immunodeficiency" were correlated to immune and inflammatory responses. Hence,

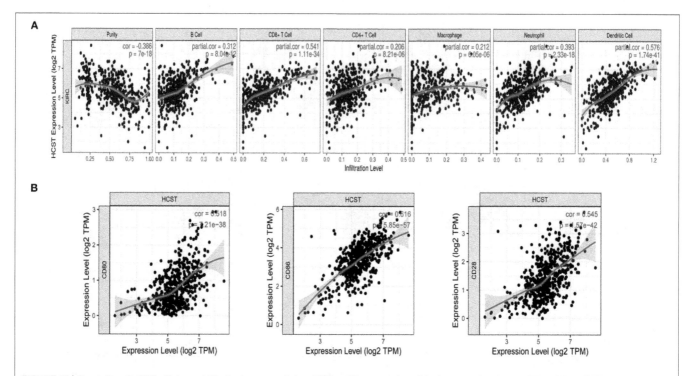

**FIGURE 10 |** Correlation of HCST with tumor-infiltrating immune cells in ccRCC and the expression of the immune-related genes PD-1. **(A)** In TIMER, HCST expression was correlated with B cells ($r = 0.312$, $p = 8.04e-12$), CD8+ T cells, **(A)** ($r = 0.541$, $p = 1.11e-34$) and neutrophils ($r = 0.3.93$, $p = 2.33e-18$), and strongly correlated with DCs ($r = 0.576$, $p = 1.74e-41$). **(B)** HCST with CD80, CD86, and CD28 in ccRCC.

these findings uncovered the molecular functions and underlying mechanisms of the HCST in ccRCC. High expression of the HCST influences the occurrence and development of ccRCC and contributes to the unfavorable prognosis of ccRCC patients.

Based on differential HCST expression, CIBERSORT analysis was used to evaluate the estimated proportions of tumor-infiltrating immune cells in ccRCC, which included naïve B cells, activated DCs, eosinophils, M2 macrophages, resting mast cells, monocytes, neutrophils, resting NK cells, plasma cells, activated CD4 memory T cells, resting CD4 memory T cells, CD8 T cells, follicular helper T cells, gamma delta T cells, and regulatory T cells. The expression level of the HCST influenced the proportions of these immune cells. Further analysis with the use of the TIMER database revealed that the HCST gene was prominently correlated with the tumor infiltration of B cells, CD8+ T cells, and neutrophils and strongly interrelated with DCs. Barry et al. found that intratumorally stimulatory DCs play important roles in the stimulation of cytotoxic T cells and driving the immune responses against cancer (28). Additionally, DCs were found to play a central role in the regulation of the balance between CD8 T-cell immunity vs. tolerance to tumor antigens (29–31). Of the antigen-presenting cells, DCs are the most effective in the activation of naïve T cells and induce an immune memory response in cancer (32). A number of effective tumor treatments related to DCs have been proposed, such as administration in conjunction with (neo)antigens, mobilization of endogenous DCs, and the use of stimulating adjuvants (33). However, improvements to treatment strategies are still required

to identify and understand biomarkers associated with DCs. Our study suggested that the HCST could influence the prognosis of ccRCC by affecting tumor-related immune cells, especially DCs.

Notably, T cell activation is dependent upon signals delivered through the antigen-specific T cell receptor and accessory receptors on the T cell. PD-1 is an inhibitory receptor with two B7-like ligands. A primary costimulatory signal is delivered through the CD28 receptor with combining its ligands, B7-1 (CD80) or B7-2 (CD86) (34). Therefore, CD28 can be used as a responsive biomarker to the expression of the IRGs PD-1. Therefore, the expression of the HCST can play roles in predicting the response to anti-PD-1 therapy in ccRCC.

Finally, we discovered, for the first time, the effect of the HCST on ccRCC. Consistently, Milioli et al. found that high HCST expression was associated with poor survival of patients with basal-like breast cancer, the cancer immune response, epithelial-mesenchymal transition, and the cell cycle (35). Qi et al. found that the HCST might be potential novel predictive markers for immunotherapy in non-small cell lung cancer (24). We performed a primary test using qRT-PCR to determine the expression of the HCST in renal cancer tissues and compared them with para-cancer tissues. Moreover, we conducted a survival analysis to verify the prognostic value of the HCST by extracting data from the TCGA database. However, a second cohort study will be more convincing if validated. Additionally, it is worth performing experimental studies on specific mechanisms. Therefore, further investigations are required.

In summary, the present study verified that overexpression of the HCST was interrelated to the clinicopathology and poor prognosis of ccRCC. High HCST expression was also closely correlated with the levels of tumor-infiltrating immune cells, especially DCs. However, further studies of the molecular function of the HCST are needed to identify new targets for immunotherapy of ccRCC, as well as new biomarkers for prognostic prediction.

## AUTHOR CONTRIBUTIONS

YZ, DL, XW, and HL designed the experiment. YZ wrote the first draft of the manuscript. YZ, XW, WZ, HL, and DL conducted most of the experiments and performed the analysis procedures. PC, DX, JL, GZ, ML, ZW, XW, and YGZ helped to analyze the results. MD and XZ critically revised drafts of the manuscript, provided important intellectual input, and approved the final version for publication. YZ and XZ contributed to the writing of the manuscript. All authors contributed to the article and approved the submitted version.

## ACKNOWLEDGMENTS

We thank the staff of Zhongnan Hospital of Wuhan University for their help in completing the study. We acknowledge the Oncomine, TIMER, and HPA databases for free use.

## REFERENCES

1. Siegel RL, Miller KD, Jemal A. Cancer statistics, 2020. *CA Cancer J Clin.* (2020) 70:7–30. doi: 10.3322/caac.21590
2. Barata PC, Rini BI. Treatment of renal cell carcinoma: current status and future directions. *CA Cancer J Clin.* (2017). 67:507–24. doi: 10.3322/caac.21411
3. Galon J, Bruni D. Approaches to treat immune hot, altered and cold tumors with combination immunotherapies. *Nat Rev Drug Discov.* (2019) 18:197–218. doi: 10.1038/s41573-018-0007-y
4. Miao D, Margolis CA, Gao W, Voss MH, Li W. Genomic correlates of response to immune checkpoint therapies in clear cell renal cell carcinoma. *Science.* (2018) 359:801–6. doi: 10.1126/science.aan5951
5. Ribas A, Wolchok JD. Cancer immunotherapy using checkpoint blockade. *Science.* (2018) 359:1350–5. doi: 10.1126/science.aar4060
6. Atkins MB, Tannir NM. Current and emerging therapies for first-line treatment of metastatic clear cell renal cell carcinoma. *Cancer Treat Rev.* (2018) 70:127–37. doi: 10.1016/j.ctrv.2018.07.009
7. Batlevi CL, Matsuki E, Brentjens RJ, Younes A. Novel immunotherapies in lymphoid malignancies. *Nat Rev Clin Oncol.* (2016) 13:25–40. doi: 10.1038/nrclinonc.2015.187
8. Tumeh PC, Harview CL, Yearley JH, Shintaku IP, Taylor EJ, Robert L, et al. PD-1 blockade induces responses by inhibiting adaptive immune resistance. *Nature.* (2014) 515:568–71. doi: 10.1038/nature13954
9. Locy H, de Mey S, de Mey W, De Ridder M, Thielemans K, Maenhout SK. Immunomodulation of the tumor microenvironment: turn foe into friend. *Front Immunol.* (2018) 9:2909. doi: 10.3389/fimmu.2018.02909
10. Hui L, Chen Y. Tumor microenvironment: sanctuary of the devil. *Cancer Lett.* (2015) 368:7–13. doi: 10.1016/j.canlet.2015.07.039
11. Senbabaoglu Y, Gejman RS, Winer AG, Liu M, Van Allen EM, de Velasco G, et al. Tumor immune microenvironment characterization in clear cell renal cell carcinoma identifies prognostic and immunotherapeutically relevant messenger RNA signatures. *Genome Biol.* (2016) 17:231.
12. Hakimi AA, Voss MH, Kuo F, Sanchez A, Liu M, Nixon BG, et al. Transcriptomic profiling of the tumor microenvironment reveals distinct subgroups of clear cell renal cell cancer: data from a randomized phase III trial. *Cancer Discov.* (2019) 9:510–25. doi: 10.1158/2159-8290.CD-18-0957
13. Giraldo NA, Becht E, Vano Y, Petitprez F, Lacroix L, Validire P, et al. Tumor-infiltrating and peripheral blood T-cell immunophenotypes predict early relapse in localized clear cell renal cell carcinoma. *Clin Cancer Res.* (2017) 23:4416–28. doi: 10.1158/1078-0432.CCR-16-2848
14. Schmiedel D, Mandelboim O. NKG2D ligands-critical targets for cancer immune escape and therapy. *Front Immunol.* (2018) 9:2040. doi: 10.3389/fimmu.2018.02040
15. Wang Q, Zhang J, Tu H, Liang D, Chang DW, Ye Y, et al. Soluble immune checkpoint-related proteins as predictors of tumor recurrence, survival, and T cell phenotypes in clear cell renal cell carcinoma patients. *J Immunother Cancer.* (2019) 7:334. doi: 10.1186/s40425-019-0810-y
16. Li T, Fan J, Wang B, Traugh N, Chen Q, Liu JS, et al. TIMER: a web server for comprehensive analysis of tumor-infiltrating immune cells. *Cancer Res.* (2017) 77:e108–10. doi: 10.1158/0008-5472.CAN-17-0307
17. Tomczak K, Czerwinska P, Wiznerowicz M. The Cancer Genome Atlas (TCGA): an immeasurable source of knowledge. *Contemp Oncol.* (2015), 19:A68–77. doi: 10.5114/wo.2014.47136
18. Oh SC, Sohn BH, Cheong JH, Kim SB, Lee JE, Park KC, et al. Clinical and genomic landscape of gastric cancer with a mesenchymal phenotype. *Nat Commun.* (2018) 9:1777.
19. Tian X, Xu W, Wang Y, Anwaier A, Wang H, Wan F, et al. Identification of tumor-infiltrating immune cells and prognostic validation of tumor-infiltrating mast cells in adrenocortical carcinoma: results from bioinformatics and real-world data. *Oncoimmunology.* (2020) 9:1784529. doi: 10.1080/2162402X.2020.1784529
20. Qu XM, Velker VM, Leung E, Kwon JS, Elshaikh MA, Kong I, et al. The role of adjuvant therapy in stage IA serous and clear cell uterine cancer: a multi-institutional pooled analysis. *Gynecol Oncol.* (2018) 149:283–90. doi: 10.1016/j.ygyno.2018.03.002
21. Ranstam J, Cook JA. Kaplan-Meier curve. *Br J Surg.* (2017) 104:442. doi: 10.1002/bjs.10238
22. Szklarczyk D, Franceschini A, Wyder S, Forslund K, Heller D, Huerta-Cepas J, et al. STRING v10: protein-protein interaction networks, integrated over the tree of life. *Nucleic Acids Res.* (2015) 43(Database issue):D447–52. doi: 10.1093/nar/gku1003
23. Powers RK, Goodspeed A, Pielke-Lombardo H, Tan AC, Costello JC. GSEA-InContext: identifying novel and common patterns in expression experiments. *Bioinformatics.* (2018) 34:i555–64. doi: 10.1093/bioinformatics/bty271
24. Qi X, Qi C, Wu T, Hu Y. CSF1R and HCST: novel candidate biomarkers predicting the response to immunotherapy in non-small cell lung cancer. *Technol Cancer Res Treat.* (2020) 19:1533033820970663. doi: 10.1177/1533033820970663
25. Desrichard A, Snyder A, Chan TA. Cancer neoantigens and applications for immunotherapy. *Clin Cancer Res.* (2016) 22:807–12. doi: 10.1158/1078-0432.CCR-14-3175
26. Ward EM, Flowers CR, Gansler T, Omer SB, Bednarczyk RA. The importance of immunization in cancer prevention, treatment, and survivorship. *CA Cancer J Clin.* (2017) 67:398–410. doi: 10.3322/caac.21407
27. Vallejo-Diaz J, Chagoyen M, Olazabal-Moran M, Gonzalez-Garcia A, Carrera AC. The opposing roles of PIK3R1/p85alpha and PIK3R2/p85beta in cancer. *Trends Cancer.* (2019) 5:233–44. doi: 10.1016/j.trecan.2019.02.009
28. Barry KC, Hsu J, Broz ML, Cueto FJ, Binnewies M, Combes AJ, et al. A natural killer-dendritic cell axis defines checkpoint therapy-responsive tumor microenvironments. *Nat Med.* (2018), 24:1178–91. doi: 10.1038/s41591-018-0085-8
29. Qi Y, Xia Y, Lin Z, Qu Y, Qi Y, Chen Y, et al. Tumor-infiltrating CD39(+)CD8(+) T cells determine poor prognosis and immune evasion in clear cell renal cell carcinoma patients. *Cancer Immunol. Immunother.* (2020) 69:1565–76. doi: 10.1007/s00262-020-02563-2

30. Curato C, Bernshtein B, Zupančič E, Dufner A, Jaitin D, Giladi A, et al. DC respond to cognate T cell interaction in the antigen-challenged lymph node. *Front Immunol.* (2019) 10:863. doi: 10.3389/fimmu.2019. 00863

31. Fu C, Jiang A. Dendritic cells and CD8 T cell immunity in tumor microenvironment. *Front Immunol.* (2018) 9:3059. doi: 10.3389/fimmu.2018.03059

32. Theisen DJ, Davidson JT IV, Briseno CG, Gargaro M, Lauron EJ, Wang Q, et al. WDFY4 is required for cross-presentation in response to viral and tumor antigens. *Science.* (2018) 362:694–9. doi: 10.1126/science. aat5030

33. Wculek SK, Cueto FJ, Mujal AM, Melero I, Krummel MF, Sancho D. Dendritic cells in cancer immunology and immunotherapy. *Nat Rev Immunol.* (2020) 20:7–24. doi: 10.1038/s41577-019-0210-z

34. Zhao Y, Lee CK, Lin CH, Gassen RB, Xu X, Huang Z, et al. PD-L1:CD80 cis-heterodimer triggers the co-stimulatory receptor CD28 while repressing the inhibitory PD-1 and CTLA-4 pathways. *Immunity.* (2019) 51:1059.e9–73.e9. doi: 10.1016/j.immuni.2019.11.003

35. Milioli HH, Tishchenko I, Riveros C, Berretta R, Moscato P. Basal-like breast cancer: molecular profiles, clinical features and survival outcomes. *BMC Med Genomics.* (2017). 10:19. doi: 10.1186/s12920-017-0250-9

# 15

# Neoadjuvant Cabozantinib in an Unresectable Locally Advanced Renal Cell Carcinoma Patient Leads to Downsizing of Tumor Enabling Surgical Resection

Mehmet A. Bilen [1,2*†], James F. Jiang [3†], Caroline S. Jansen [3], Jacqueline T. Brown [1,2], Lara R. Harik [4], Aarti Sekhar [5], Haydn Kissick [3], Shishir K. Maithel [6], Omer Kucuk [1,2], Bradley Carthon [1,2] and Viraj A. Master [2,3*]

[1] Department of Hematology and Medical Oncology, Emory University, Atlanta, GA, United States, [2] Winship Cancer Institute of Emory University, Atlanta, GA, United States, [3] Department of Urology, Emory University, Atlanta, GA, United States, [4] Department of Pathology, Emory University, Atlanta, GA, United States, [5] Department of Radiology, Emory University, Atlanta, GA, United States, [6] Department of Surgery, Emory University, Atlanta, GA, United States

*Correspondence:
Mehmet A. Bilen
mbilen@emory.edu
Viraj A. Master
vmaster@emory.edu

[†]These authors have contributed equally to this work

**Introduction:** Cabozantinib (XL-184) is a small molecule inhibitor of the tyrosine kinases c-Met, AXL, and VEGFR2 that has been shown to reduce tumor growth, metastasis, and angiogenesis. After the promising results from the METEOR and CABOSUN trials, cabozantinib was approved for use in the first- and second-line setting in patients with advanced RCC. Previously, targeted therapies have been used in the neoadjuvant setting for tumor size reduction and facilitating nephrectomies. The increased response rates with cabozantinib in metastatic renal cell carcinoma (mRCC), along with the other neoadjuvant TKI data, strongly support an expanded role for cabozantinib in the neoadjuvant setting.

**Case Description:** We report on a 59-year-old gentleman presenting with an unresectable 21.7 cm left renal cell carcinoma (RCC) with extension to soft tissue and muscles of the thoracic cage, psoas muscle, posterior abdominal wall, tail of pancreas, splenic flexure of colon, and inferior margin of spleen. Presurgical, neoadjuvant systemic therapy with cabozantinib was initiated for 11 months in total. Initially after 2 months of cabozantinib, magnetic resonance imaging (MRI) revealed a significant reduction (44.2%) in tumor diameter from 21.7 to 12.1 cm with decreased extension into adjacent structures. After 11 months total of cabozantinib, the corresponding MRI showed grossly stable size of the tumor and significant resolution of invasion of adjacent structures. After washout of cabozantinib, radical resection, including nephrectomy, was successfully performed without any major complications, either intra-operative or perioperative. Negative margins were achieved.

**Conclusions:** This is a report of neoadjuvant cabozantinib downsizing a tumor and enabling surgical resection in this patient with locally advanced RCC. Our findings demonstrate that neoadjuvant cabozantinib to facilitate subsequent surgical resection may be a feasible option for patients presenting with unresectable RCC.

**Keywords: cabozantinib, renal cell carcinoma, neoadjuvant therapy, radical nephrectomy, case report**

## INTRODUCTION

Cabozantinib is a potent multikinase agent that inhibits, in addition to VEGF receptors, MET, and AXL, both of which are associated with resistance to VEGF-directed therapy. The METEOR phase 3 clinical trial results proved that treatment with cabozantinib increased overall survival, delayed disease progression, and improved the objective response compared with everolimus in advanced renal cell carcinoma (RCC) patients (1). These promising results led to initial approval of cabozantinib treatment for advanced renal cell carcinoma. In the CABOSUN phase 2 clinical trial, cabozantinib treatment demonstrated a significant clinical benefit in progression free survival and objective response rate over standard-of-care sunitinib as first-line therapy in patients with intermediate- or poor-risk metastatic RCC (2). Thus, recently, cabozantinib has been approved for use in the first- and second-line setting in patients with advanced RCC (3). Therefore, cabozantinib was selected to be administered for this patient with locally advanced RCC.

Targeted therapies, primarily inhibitors of the VEGF receptor tyrosine kinase and rapamycin pathways, have changed the management of advanced RCC. Over the past 10 years, studies have established efficacy and have led to approval of sorafenib, sunitinib, temsirolimus, everolimus, pazopanib, axitinib, and also cabozantinib. These agents have significantly improved progression-free survival, with certain therapies achieving a median overall survival of >2 years in advanced RCC patients (4, 5). Most recently, trials on novel multikinase inhibitors, such as cabozantinib, and PD-1 inhibitors, such as nivolumab, have demonstrated significantly prolonged progression free survival and increases in overall survival, compared to standard therapy in metastatic RCC patients (2, 3). Using these agents in the neoadjuvant setting has emerged as a treatment option for locally advanced RCC patients. Neoadjuvant therapy can potentially downsize advanced tumors, enabling surgical interventions when they may not otherwise have been feasible or safe due to unresectable locoregional disease. We describe here, a patient presenting with initially unresectable locally advanced RCC treated with neoadjuvant cabozantinib, downsizing the tumor and enabling surgical resection.

## CASE DESCRIPTION

A 59-year-old man with an Eastern Cooperative Oncology Group (ECOG) status of 0 presented with a left renal mass in

March 2018. Computed tomography (CT) scans of the chest, abdomen, and pelvis revealed a locally invasive 21-cm left renal mass inseparable from the soft tissue of the thorax, psoas muscle, posterior abdominal wall, tail of pancreas, splenic flexure of colon, and inferior margin of spleen with no evidence of nodal involvement or metastatic disease. In April 2018, magnetic resonance imaging (MRI) supported these findings showing a 21.7 cm renal mass invading the renal hilum and adjacent structures described above (**Figure 1A**). In April 2018, patient underwent a CT-guided renal biopsy that confirmed renal cell carcinoma (RCC). The tumor was deemed unresectable at our multidisciplinary genitourinary tumor board, and systemic treatment was recommended. In April 2018, patient was seen in genitourinary medical oncology clinic, and cabozantinib 60 mg daily was started. In June 2018, after 2 months of treatment, MRI revealed a significant decrease in tumor size from 21.7 to 12.1 cm with marked decrease of extension into the psoas muscle, posterior abdominal wall, tail of the pancreas, splenic flexure of the colon, and inferior margin of the spleen (**Figures 1** and **2**). After 11 months of therapy, the corresponding MRI showed grossly stable size of the tumor but resolved invasion of adjacent structures (**Figures 1C, 2**, and **3**).

During cabozantinib therapy, the patient developed hypertension, secondary to cabozantinib, which was well controlled with lisinopril and amlodipine. Otherwise, there were no adverse events during drug therapy, besides mild hand-foot disease, and patient did not require any dose reduction. The patient was therefore scheduled for surgery after a 3-weeks washout from systemic therapy in March 2019.

In April 2019, patient underwent *en bloc* left radical nephrectomy, left adrenalectomy, retroperitoneal lymph node dissection, omentoplasty, distal pancreatectomy, splenectomy, and resections of quadratus lumborum, left psoas muscle, left crus muscle, and diaphragm with negative margins. Final pathology confirmed a 13.7 cm T4N0M0 grade 3 clear cell renal cell carcinoma invading the renal vein, renal sinus fat, perinephric fat, and psoas/diaphragm muscle and surgical margins were negative (**Figure 4**). The patient was discharged in a stable clinical status 9 days after surgery. When we wrote this report, the patient was still alive and well, and no evidence of recurrence on imaging.

Correlative studies were performed on resected tumor samples. **Figure 5** shows this patient's flow cytometry and pre-operative lab results compared to a cohort of renal cell carcinoma patients. The patient's intraoperative sample was processed to obtain a single cell suspension, which was analyzed using flow cytometry. This allowed for enumeration of tumor infiltrating T lymphocytes (**Figure 5A**). The patient's tumor had extremely few infiltrating CD8 T cells (0.061% CD8 T cells) (**Figure 5B**), which has been reported to suggest a poor prognosis (6). The patient's

---

**Abbreviations:** VEGF, vascular endothelial growth factor; RCC, renal cell carcinoma; CT, computed tomography; MRI, magnetic resonance imaging; TLS, tertiary lymphoid structure.

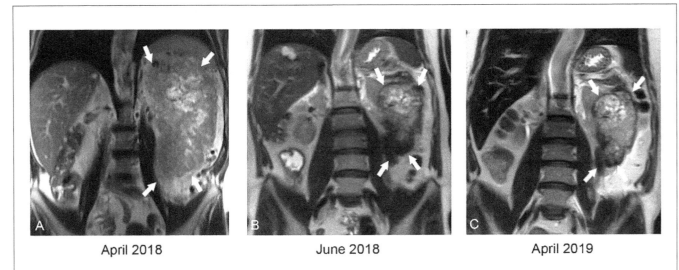

**FIGURE 1** | Coronal T2 weighted MRI at baseline **(A)** demonstrates a large 21.7 cm mass (white arrows) replacing the entire left kidney with central areas of necrosis. After just 2 months of cabozantinib therapy **(B)**, the mass had decreased to 12.1 cm (white arrows). After 12 months of cabozantinib **(C)**, the mass was stable in size.

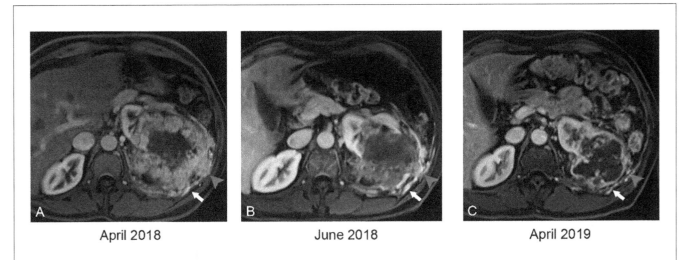

**FIGURE 2** | Axial T1 weighted MR with contrast at baseline **(A)** demonstrates tumor invasion into the intercostal space (red arrowhead) and neovascularity (white arrow). By 2 months of therapy **(B)**, the invasion has retracted (red arrowhead). By 12 months **(C)**, the invasion has resolved and vascularity has decreased significantly.

neutrophil to lymphocyte ratio were within the first quartile of the cohort's results (**Figure 5C**). His pre-operative C-reactive protein level and albumin level were within the second quartile (**Figures 5D, E**).

Correlative studies were also performed on the formaldehyde fixed paraffin embedded pathology specimens from the tumor resection. Immunofluorescence imaging showed sparse CD8 T cell infiltration in two distinct specimens from the resected tumor lesion (**Figures 6A, B**), consistent with flow cytometry results (**Figures 5A, B**). The presence of CD31+ endothelium throughout the tumor specimen was also evident on immunofluorescence imaging (**Figures 6A, B**). Interestingly, tertiary lymphoid structures (TLS) were identified in both

specimens examined (**Figures 6C, D**), despite the paucity of CD8 T cells identified on flow cytometry and immunofluorescence imaging, which is consistent with a report that there does not appear to be a correlation between CD8 T cell infiltration and the presence of TLS in RCC tumors (6).

Next generation sequencing testing was performed on intra-operative resected tumor samples. No microsatellite instability was detected. No genes with pathogenic or likely pathogenic alternations were detected in the sample. Of note, there were no mutations detected in MET, VHL, PBRM1, BAP1, SETD2, or RET. Immunohistochemistry results were positive for MLH1 (2+, 80%), MSH2 (2+, 90%), MSH6 (1+, 60%), and PMS2 (1+, 80%) and were negative for PD-L1 (SP142).

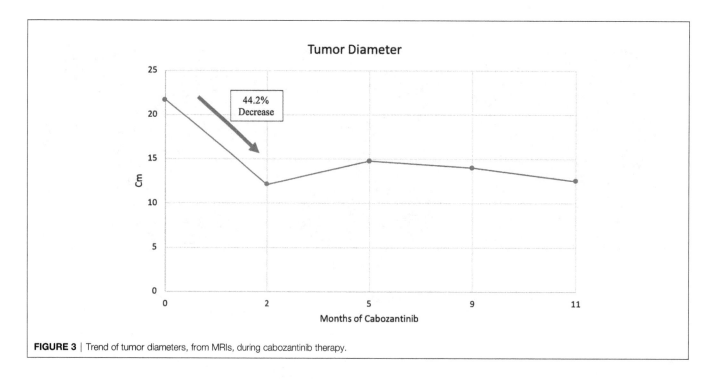

**FIGURE 3** | Trend of tumor diameters, from MRIs, during cabozantinib therapy.

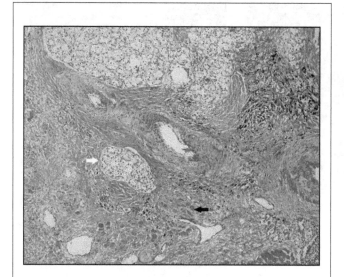

**FIGURE 4** | Clear cell renal cell carcinoma (white arrow) infiltrating into skeletal muscle (black arrow), representing psoas muscle and diaphragm. The background is fibrotic with extensive hemosiderin laden macrophages, possibly representing therapy related changes (H&E-10x).

## DISCUSSION

We reported a patient presenting with initially unresectable locally advanced RCC treated with neoadjuvant cabozantinib, downsizing the tumor, and enabling surgical resection. This case study demonstrates important points about cabozantinib for patients with advanced RCC.

In patients presenting with initially unresectable advanced RCC, neoadjuvant cabozantinib may be of benefit for downsizing tumors to enable surgical resections that otherwise wouldn't be possible. We also showed that this approach is feasible and safe prior to surgery. Reduction of tumor size was rapid, as the tumor diameter decreased by 44.2% after only 2 months of cabozantinib, a partial response on the Response Evaluation Criteria for Solid Tumors (RECIST). In the following 9 months, of 11 months total, of cabozantinib therapy, tumor size, appearance, and involvement of surrounding tissues remained stable. It has been suggested that one mechanism of cabozantinib's efficacy is modulation of the immune microenvironment in the tumor (7–9), so it is interesting that this patient had a strong response to cabozantinib, despite a sparsely immune infiltrated tumor.

Although neoadjuvant therapy shows reduction of tumor size, it is yet not clear whether a prolonged survival can be achieved for patients. Several studies of neoadjuvant therapy for RCC have demonstrated consistent primary tumor size reduction to enable surgical resection (10–13). Rini *et al.* were the first to report response (28% median reduction in primary tumor size) of advanced primary renal tumors to treatment with neoadjuvant sunitinib. Of 28 patients with advanced RCC deemed unsuitable for initial nephrectomy, 13 (45%) were able to undergo nephrectomy following sunitinib (12). Emerging data from recent prospective phase II trials have also reported consistent tumor size reduction facilitating nephrectomies (13–16). In a literature review of neoadjuvant therapy to facilitate nephrectomy for locally advanced disease, Bindayi *et al.* found that 12 of 14 of the studies investigated neoadjuvant sunitinib or sorafenib (17). In a prospective phase 2 clinical trial, Karam *et al.* reported that axitinib, when given prior to surgery, resulted in significant shrinking of kidney cancers, facilitating surgical resections (13). Most recently, Roy et al. reported two patients with unresectable RCCs that were treated with cabozantinib, and

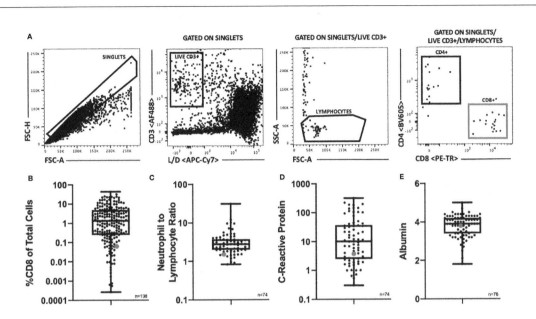

FIGURE 5 | (A) Flow cytometry gating scheme. Samples were gated to exclude doublets and cell aggregates and to include only single cells for further analysis. This single cell population was then gated to include only live, CD3+ cells, then to include only lymphocyte sized cells. These gates insured as pure of a T lymphocyte population as possible for further analysis. T lymphocytes were then divided into CD4+ and CD8+ populations. (B) Distribution of %CD8 of total cells by flow cytometry among a cohort of renal cell carcinoma patients, n = 198. (C) Distribution of pre-operative neutrophil to lymphocyte ratio among a cohort of renal cell carcinoma patients (n=74). (D) Distribution of pre-operative C-reactive protein level (mg/L) among a cohort of renal cell carcinoma patients (n=74). (E) Distribution of pre-operative albumin level (g/dl) among a cohort of renal cell carcinoma patients (n=76). (B–E) Patient of interest highlighted in red. Box plots show middle 50% with the median at the center and the whiskers extending to minimum and maximum values.

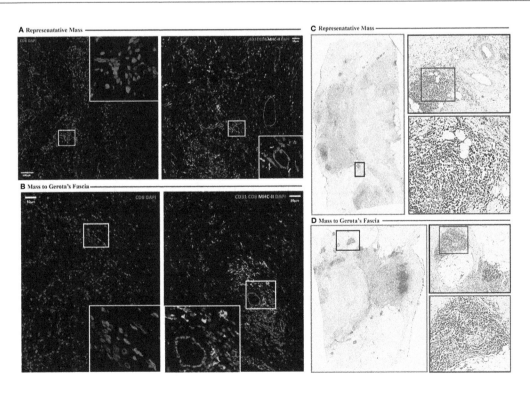

FIGURE 6 | (A, B) Immunofluorescence imaging illustrating sparse CD8 T cell infiltration (A, B, left) and presence of CD31+ endothelium (A, B, right) in resected tumor specimens (A representative. Mass, B mass to Gerota's fascia). (C, D) Hematoxylin and eosin staining shows presence of tertiary lymphoid structures (highlighted in insets) (C representative mass, D mass to Gerota's fascia).

achieved >50% tumor shrinkage which allowed surgical resection (18).

In summary, we present a patient with locally advanced RCC, treated with neoadjuvant cabozantinib downsizing a tumor and enabling surgical resection in this patient. Our findings demonstrate that neoadjuvant cabozantinib to facilitate subsequent surgical resection may be a feasible option for patients presenting with unresectable RCC. There is still a need for more effective neoadjuvant agents that might improve outcome of kidney cancer patients. Currently, we are conducting a neoadjuvant cabozantinib clinical trial at our institution (NCT04022343), with multiple correlative studies to facilitate identification of the patients most likely to respond.

# AUTHOR CONTRIBUTIONS

MB and VM conceived and designed the study. JJ, MB, CJ, and VM wrote the manuscript. MB, VM, JB, LH, AS, SM, OK, and BC provided the study materials or patients. LH, HK, CJ, and VM performed the experiments. MB managed the cabozantinib therapy. VM and SM performed the surgery. All authors contributed to the article and approved the submitted version.

# ACKNOWLEDGMENTS

The authors would like to thank the patients and their families, and all members of the study team.

# REFERENCES

1. Choueiri TK, Escudier B, Powles T, Tiinar N, Mainwaring P, Rini B, et al. Cabozantinib versus everolimus in advanced renal cell carcinoma (METEOR): final results from a randomised, open-label, phase 3 trial. *Lancet Oncol* (2016) 17(7):917–27. doi: 10.1016/S1470-2045(16)30107-3

2. Choueiri TK, Halabi S, Sanford BL, Hahn O, Michaelson M, Walsh M, et al. Cabozantinib Versus Sunitinib As Initial Targeted Therapy for Patients With Metastatic Renal Cell Carcinoma of Poor or Intermediate Risk: The Alliance A031203 CABOSUN Trial. *J Clin Oncol* (2017) 35(6):591–7. doi: 10.1200/JCO.2016.70.7398

3. Desai A, Small EJ. Treatment of advanced renal cell carcinoma patients with cabozantinib, an oral multityrosine kinase inhibitor of MET, AXL and VEGF receptors. *Future Oncol* (2019) 12:3741–9. doi: 10.2217/fon-2019-0021

4. Escudier B, Eisen T, Stadler WM, Szczylik C, Oudard S, Siebels M, et al. Sorafenib in advanced clear-cell renal-cell carcinoma. *N Engl J Med* (2007) 356(2):125–34. doi: 10.1056/NEJMoa060655

5. Motzer RJ, Hutson TE, Tomczak P, Michaelson M, Bukowski R, Oudard S, et al. Overall survival and updated results for sunitinib compared with interferon alfa in patients with metastatic renal cell carcinoma. *J Clin Oncol* (2009) 27(22):3584–90. doi: 10.1200/JCO.2008.20.1293

6. Jansen CS, Prokhnevska N, Master VA, Sanda M, Carlisle J, Bilen M, et al. An intra-tumoral niche maintains and differentiates stem-like CD8 T cells. *Nature* (2019) 576(7787):465–70. doi: 10.1038/s41586-019-1836-5

7. Patnaik A, Swanson KD, Csizmadia E, Solanki A, Landon-Brace N, Gehring M, et al. Cabozantinib Eradicates Advanced Murine Prostate Cancer by Activating Antitumor Innate Immunity. *Cancer Discovery* (2017) 7(7):750–65. doi: 10.1158/2159-8290.CD-16-0778

8. Lu X, Horner JW, Paul E, Shang X, Troncoso P, Deng P, et al. Effective combinatorial immunotherapy for castration-resistant prostate cancer. *Nature* (2017) 543(7647):728–32. doi: 10.1038/nature21676

9. Kwilas AR, Ardiani A, Donahue RN, Aftab DT, Hodge JW. Dual effects of a targeted small-molecule inhibitor (cabozantinib) on immune-mediated killing of tumor cells and immune tumor microenvironment permissiveness when combined with a cancer vaccine. *J Transl Med* (2014) 12:294. doi: 10.1186/s12967-014-0294-y

10. Amin C, Wallen E, Pruthi RS, Calvo BF, Godley PA, Rathmell WK. Preoperative tyrosine kinase inhibition as an adjunct to debulking nephrectomy. *Urology* (2008) 72(4):864–8. doi: 10.1016/j.urology.2008.01.088

11. Kondo T, Hashimoto Y, Kobayashi H, Iizuka J, Nishikawa T, Nakano T, et al. Presurgical targeted therapy with tyrosine kinase inhibitors for advanced renal cell carcinoma: clinical results and histopathological therapeutic effects. *Jpn J Clin Oncol* (2010) 40(12):1173–9. doi: 10.1093/jjco/hyq150

12. Rini BI, Garcia J, Elson P, Wood L, Shah S, Stephenson A, et al. The effect of sunitinib on primary renal cell carcinoma and facilitation of subsequent surgery. *J Urol* (2012) 187(5):1548–54. doi: 10.1016/j.juro.2011.12.075

13. Karam JA, Devine CE, Urbauer DL, Lozano M, Maity T, Ahrar K, et al. Phase 2 trial of neoadjuvant axitinib in patients with locally advanced nonmetastatic clear cell renal cell carcinoma. *Eur Urol* (2014) 66(5):874–80. doi: 10.1016/j.eururo.2014.01.035

14. Cowey CL, Amin C, Pruthi RS, Wallen E, Nielson M, Grigson G, et al. Neoadjuvant clinical trial with sorafenib for patients with stage II or higher renal cell carcinoma. *J Clin Oncol* (2010) 28(9):1502–7. doi: 10.1200/JCO.2009.24.7759

15. Hatiboglu G, Hohenfellner M, Arslan A, Hadaschik B, Teber D, Radtke J, et al. Effective downsizing but enhanced intratumoral heterogeneity following neoadjuvant sorafenib in patients with non-metastatic renal cell carcinoma. *Langenbecks Arch Surg* (2017) 402(4):637–44. doi: 10.1007/s00423-016-1543-8

16. Hellenthal NJ, Underwood W, Penetrante R, Litwin A, Zhang S, Wilding G, et al. Prospective clinical trial of preoperative sunitinib in patients with renal cell carcinoma. *J Urol* (2010) 184(3):859–64. doi: 10.1016/j.juro.2010.05.041

17. Bindayi A, Hamilton ZA, McDonald ML, Yim K, Millard F, McKay R, et al. Neoadjuvant therapy for localized and locally advanced renal cell carcinoma. *Urol Oncol* (2018) 36(1):31–7. doi: 10.1016/j.urolonc.2017.07.015

18. Roy AM, Briggler A, Tippit D, Dawson K, Verma R. Neoadjuvant Cabozantinib in Renal-Cell Carcinoma: A Brief Review. *Clin Genitourin Cancer* (2020) 18(6):e688–91. doi: 10.1016/j.clgc.2020.04.003

# 16

# High SAA1 Expression Predicts Advanced Tumors in Renal Cancer

Sen Li[1,2,3], Yongbiao Cheng[1,2], Gong Cheng[1,2], Tianbo Xu[1,2], Yuzhong Ye[1,2], Qi Miu[1,2], Qi Cao[1,2], Xiong Yang[1,2], Hailong Ruan[1,2]* and Xiaoping Zhang[1,2]*

[1] Department of Urology, Union Hospital, Tongji Medical College, Huazhong University of Science and Technology, Wuhan, China, [2] Institute of Urology, Union Hospital, Tongji Medical College, Huazhong University of Science and Technology, Wuhan, China, [3] Key Lab for Biological Targeted Therapy of Education Ministry and Hubei Province, Union Hospital, Tongji Medical College, Huazhong University of Science and Technology, Wuhan, China

*Correspondence:
Hailong Ruan
hlruan2018@hust.edu.cn
Xiaoping Zhang
xzhang@hust.edu.cn

Renal cell carcinoma (RCC) is the most frequent malignant tumor of the kidney. 30% of patients with RCC are diagnosed at an advanced stage. Clear cell renal cell carcinoma (ccRCC) is the most common pathological subtype of RCC. Currently, advanced ccRCC lacks reliable diagnostic and prognostic markers. We explored the potential of SAA1 as a diagnostic and prognostic marker for advanced ccRCC. In this study, we mined and analyzed the public cancer databases (TCGA, UALCAN and GEPIA) to conclude that SAA1 was up-regulated at mRNA and protein levels in advanced ccRCC. We further found that hypomethylation of SAA1 promoter region was responsible for its high expression in ccRCC. Receiver operating characteristic curve (ROC) indicated that high SAA1 levels could distinguish advanced ccRCC patients from normal subjects ($p <$ 0.0001). Kaplan-Meier curve analysis showed that high SAA1 levels predicted poor overall survival time ($p < 0.0001$) and poor disease-free survival time ($p = 0.0003$). Finally, the functional roles of SAA1 were examined using a si-SAA1 knockdown method in RCC cell lines. Our results suggest that SAA1 may possess the potential to serve as a diagnostic and prognostic biomarker for advanced ccRCC patients. Moreover, targeting SAA1 may represent as a novel therapeutic target for advanced ccRCC patients.

Keywords: SAA1, diagnosis, prognosis, biomarker, renal cancer

## INTRODUCTION

In the United States, renal cancer represents respectively the 6th and 8th most common malignancy in men and in women, accounting for about 3% of cancer deaths (1). Cancer statistics show that approximately 73,820 new cases of renal cancer and expected 14,770 deaths happened in the United States in 2019 (1). Clear cell renal cell carcinoma (ccRCC) is clinically divided into localized ccRCC (L-ccRCC), locally advanced ccRCC (LA-ccRCC), and metastatic ccRCC (M-ccRCC). L-ccRCC and LA-ccRCC can achieve clinical curative effect through nephron-sparing surgery or nephrectomy. M-ccRCC requires comprehensive medical treatment, including cytoreductive nephrectomy, molecular targeted therapy and immunotherapy (2–6). Although surgical treatment, targeted therapy and immunotherapy have acquired great progress in recent years, there are still many patients with advanced ccRCC or M-ccRCC die from this disease due to treatment tolerance (7, 8). Therefore, the progress and metastatic mechanisms of locally advanced ccRCC and M-ccRCC are the primary tasks of current research.

SAA1 protein belongs to a member of the serum amyloid A family of apolipoproteins. SAA1 is a major acute-phase protein whose expression is upregulated when the body is stressed by inflammation and tissue damage (9). In addition, SAA1 expression also can be induced following surgery or in advanced malignancies (10). SAA1 also plays a critical role in high-density lipoprotein metabolism and cholesterol homeostasis (11, 12). Extensive literatures have reported that SAA1 could contribute to cancer development and accelerate tumor progression and distant metastasis (10). For example, SAA1 enhances plasminogen activation to promote colon cancer progression (13). SAA1 may interact with the extracellular matrix to change its affinity to cells, leading to cell metastasis (14). In addition, a large number of studies have confirmed the positive correlation between SAA1 concentrations and tumor stage (15, 16). In a sample of 233 different tumor patients, higher SAA1 levels appeared in more advanced tumor patients (17). Moreover, the up-regulation of SAA1 could be used as a biomarker for a variety of malignant tumors (18–20). Most importantly, serum SAA1 was identified as a biomarker of distant metastases but not as an early tumor marker in RCC patients (21). However, the diagnostic and prognostic potential of SAA1 at the tumor tissue level and its biological function in ccRCC have not been reported.

In this study, we were committed to exploring the diagnostic and prognostic value of SAA1 in ccRCC, especially in advanced ccRCC, and strived to explore the therapeutic potential of targeting SAA1.

## MATERIALS AND METHODS

### Data Download
We downloaded the GSE11151 (22), GSE6344 (23) and GSE781 (24) datasets from the GEO database (https://www.ncbi.nlm.nih.gov/geo/), which is a public and shared cancer database. We took the top ten up-regulated genes in these three datasets to analyze the intersection genes.

### Data Processing
The differentially expressed genes (DEGs) of GSE11151, GSE6344 and GSE781 datasets were identified using GEO2R (https://www.ncbi.nlm.nih.gov/geo/geo2r/), an available online analysis software for the GEO database, which was dependent on R language programming. According to the criteria of logFC ≥2 or logFC ≤-2 and adjusted p value < 0.05, DEGs from the three datasets were identified. We used the Wayne diagram to screen the intersection of three datasets with the top 10 up-regulated DEGs.

### TCGA Database
The mRNA expression data of SAA1 in ccRCC tissues and para-cancer tissues and clinicopathological features including gender, age, T stage, tumor grade, M stage, N stage, histopathological stage, overall survival (OS) were downloaded from TCGA-KIRC datasets (https://xenabrowser.net/heatmap/). Kaplan-Meier curves and ROC curves were analyzed using mRNA levels from TCGA-KIRC dataset.

### UALCAN Online Analysis
SAA1 mRNA, protein expression and promoter methylation levels were evaluated using the UALCAN online analysis software (http://ualcan.path.uab.edu/index.html) (25).

### GEPIA
SAA1 mRNA, overall survival and disease-free survival were also evaluated using GEPIA online analysis software (http://gepia.cancer-pku.cn/) (26).

### ROC Curves Analysis of SAA1
The potential diagnostic value of SAA1 was evaluated using the receiver operating characteristic (ROC) curves by Graphpad Prism software.

### Cell Culture and Transfection
Human RCC cell lines 786-O, ACHN, A-498, Caki-1 and normal renal tubular epithelial cells HK-2 were obtained from ATCC. OS-RC-2 cell line was a gift from the Department of Urology of Wuhan Tongji Hospital. All cell lines were cultured in DMEM medium containing 1% penicillin-streptomycin and 10% FBS. Small interfering RNA (si-RNA) against SAA1 and corresponding negative control (si-NC) were purchased from Ribobio Biological Co., Ltd. (Guangzhou, China). si-SAA1 sequences and si-NC sequences were transfected into cells using Lipofectamine 2000 reagent.

### Immunohistochemistry (IHC), Transwell Migration and Invasion, and Western Blotting (WB) Assays
ccRCC tissues and adjacent normal tissues were fixed in 10% formalin, dehydrated, and embedded in paraffin sequentially. The paraffin sections were incubated with anti-SAA1 antibody overnight at 4°C. Transwell migration and invasion were performed using 24-well transwell chambers. The specific details of these experiments were previously described (27).

### ccRCC Tissue Samples
We collected ccRCC tissues and adjacent normal tissues of 30 case patients who were subjected to partial nephrectomies or nephrectomies at Wuhan Union Hospital between 2018 and 2019. All patients had signed an informed consent form. This study was approved by the Ethics Committee of Huazhong University of Science and Technology.

### Statistical Analysis
SPSS statistical software and Graphpad Prism 7.0 were used for statistical analysis. The SAA1 mRNA levels were analyzed among different clinicopathological features of ccRCC using the Mann-Whitney test. Pearson's chi-square test was used to analyze the correlation between SAA1 expression levels and clinicopathological features of ccRCC. The ROC curve was used to distinguish ccRCC patients and obtain the area under the curve (AUC). The Kaplan-Meier curve was used to analyze the relationship between the expression level of SAA1 and the overall survival and progression-free survival of ccRCC patients. Each group of data is presented as mean ± SD. The p value<0.05 was considered statistically significant.

# RESULTS

## Screening and Prognostic Analysis of Up-Regulated Target Genes in ccRCC Patients

By analyzing three public cancer datasets, we found two intersection genes, SAA1 and CCL20, in these three datasets (**Figure 1A**). Next, we analyzed the correlation between the expression levels of these two genes and the overall and disease-free survival of patients with ccRCC. We found that

only SAA1 expression was associated with prognosis in patients with ccRCC and high SAA1 expression indicated a worse prognosis (**Figures 1B, C**).

## SAA1 Is Highly Expressed and Predicts High Tumor Stage in Advanced and Metastatic ccRCC Patients

To verify the reliability of the above three studies, we analyzed the expression of SAA1 and its association with clinical pathological parameters in the TCGA database. As shown in

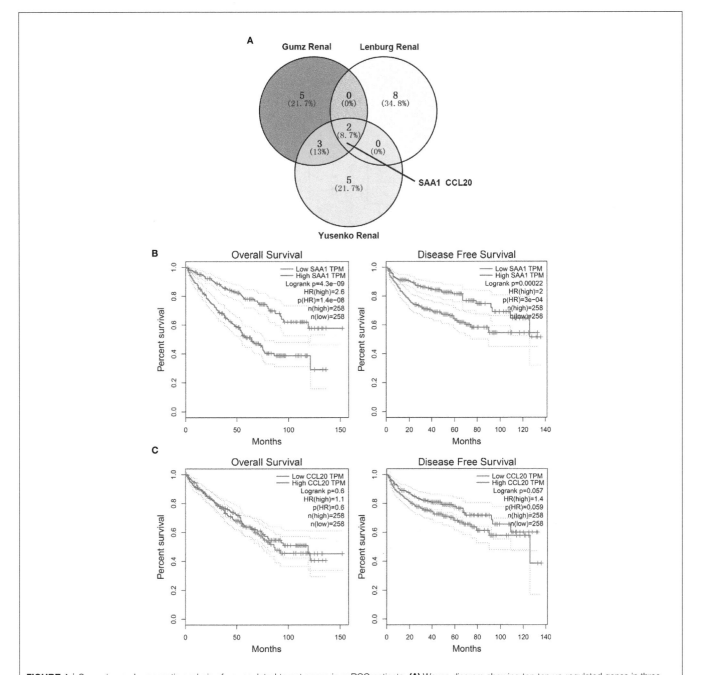

**FIGURE 1** | Screening and prognostic analysis of up-regulated target genes in ccRCC patients. **(A)** Wayne diagram showing top ten up-regulated genes in three public databases. **(B)** Kaplan Meier curve analysis for the effect of SAA1 expression on the prognosis of ccRCC patients. **(C)** Kaplan Meier curve analysis for the effect of CCL20 expression on the prognosis of ccRCC patients.

**Figure 2A**, SAA1 expression in tumor tissues is upregulated at mRNA levels. Next, we analyzed the mRNA expression levels of SAA1 against T stage, N stage, M stage, Grade classification, histopathological stage and its correlation with these clinicopathological parameters in patients with ccRCC (**Figures 2B–F** and **Table 1**). Our analysis found that the mRNA expression of SAA1 was positively correlated with these clinicopathological parameters and that the mRNA expression of SAA1 increased significantly in higher tumor stages but did not increase or show a downward trend in early tumor stages (**Figures 2B–F**). These results suggested that elevated mRNA expression of SAA1 was predictive of advanced tumor stages. To

make our study more precise, we also analyzed the expression of SAA1 in the UALCAN and GEPIA online tumor database websites. As shown in **Figures 3A–F**, high SAA1 expression mainly occurred in patients with advanced and metastatic ccRCC, which were consistent with the analysis results of the TCGA database. Similarly, we also analyzed the expression of SAA1 at the protein level, and the results showed that SAA1 protein expression increased significantly in patients with advanced ccRCC (**Figures 4A–C**). The above results indicate that SAA1 is highly expressed at mRNA and protein levels and predicts high stage risk in patients with advanced and metastatic ccRCC.

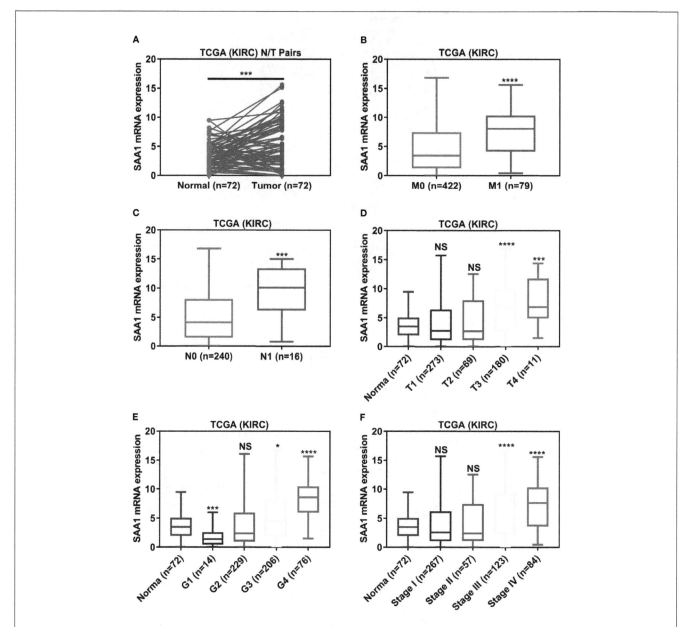

**FIGURE 2** | Analysis of SAA1 mRNA expression using TCGA database. **(A)** The mRNA expression levels of SAA1 were up-regulated in ccRCC samples, which were downloaded from TCGA-KIRC database containing 72 paired ccRCC samples. The expression levels of SAA1 mRNA were compared in various tumor stages: **(B)** M stage, **(C)** N stage, **(D)** T stage, **(E)** tumor grade, **(F)** TNM stage. (****P <0.0001, ***P <0.001, *P <0.05, NS means no significance, compared with the respective control).

**TABLE 1** | Association of SAA1 mRNA expression with clinicopathological parameters in ccRCC patients.

| Parameters | | Number | SAA1 mRNA expression | | |
|---|---|---|---|---|---|
| | | | Low (n=124) | High (n=124) | P value |
| Age | < 60 | 104 | 51 | 53 | |
| | >= 60 | 144 | 73 | 71 | 0.797 |
| Gender | female | 97 | 58 | 39 | |
| | male | 151 | 66 | 85 | 0.013 |
| T stage | T1 + T2 | 146 | 88 | 58 | |
| | T3 + T4 | 102 | 36 | 66 | 0.000 |
| N stage | N0 | 233 | 121 | 112 | |
| | N1 | 15 | 3 | 12 | 0.017 |
| M stage | M0 | 207 | 113 | 94 | |
| | M1 | 41 | 11 | 30 | 0.001 |
| G stage | G1 + G2 | 111 | 72 | 39 | |
| | G3 + G4 | 137 | 52 | 85 | 0.000 |
| TNM stage | I + II | 134 | 86 | 48 | |
| | III + IV | 114 | 38 | 76 | 0.000 |

## SAA1 Gene Promoter Region Is Hypomethylated in Patients With Advanced and Metastatic ccRCC

DNA methylation modification is an important component of epigenetics, which can silence the expression of methylated genes. To understand the cause of SAA1 overexpression in advanced and metastatic ccRCC, we analyzed the methylation status of SAA1 gene through the UALCAN online database. As shown in **Figure 5A**, the SAA1 gene was hypomethylated in ccRCC tissues, while it was hypermethylated in normal kidney tissues. Moreover, with the increase of tumor stage and grade, the degree of SAA1 gene methylation decreased accordingly, which means that the degree of SAA1 gene methylation was inversely

related to the tumor's stage (**Figures 5B–D**). These results indicate that the upregulation of SAA1 expression is due to the low methylation levels of the SAA1 promoter region in ccRCC and its methylation levels are inversely correlated with tumor stage and grade.

## SAA1 Possesses Diagnostic Value for Advanced and Metastatic ccRCC

Biomarkers for tumor progression are still lacking in ccRCC patients. We found that SAA1 expression was significantly up-regulated at the mRNA and protein levels in patients with advanced and metastatic ccRCC. We wondered whether SAA1 could accurately diagnose patients with advanced and metastatic

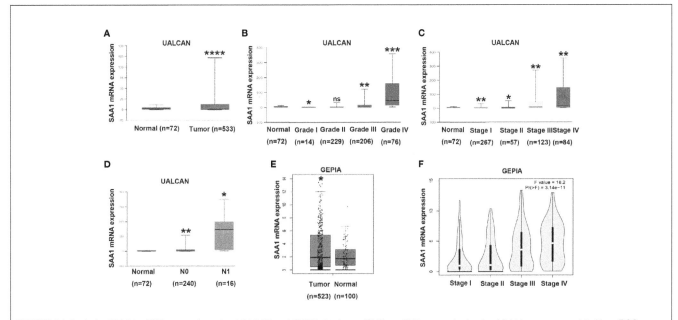

**FIGURE 3** | Analysis of SAA1 mRNA expression using UALCAN and GEPIA database. **(A)** The mRNA expression levels of SAA1 were up-regulated in ccRCC samples from UALCAN database. **(B)** The expression levels of SAA1 mRNA were compared in tumor grade from UALCAN database. **(C)** The expression levels of SAA1 mRNA were compared in TNM stage from UALCAN database. **(D)** The expression levels of SAA1 mRNA were compared in N stage from UALCAN database. **(E)** The mRNA expression levels of SAA1 were up-regulated in ccRCC samples from GEPIA database. **(F)** The expression levels of SAA1 mRNA were compared in TNM stage from GEPIA database. (****P<0.0001, ***P<0.001, **P<0.01, *P<0.05, NS means no significance, compared with the respective control).

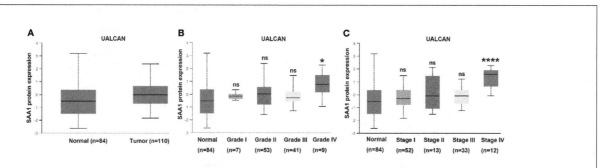

**FIGURE 4** | Analysis of SAA1 protein expression using UALCAN database. **(A)** The protein expression analysis of SAA1 in ccRCC samples from UALCAN database. **(B)** The protein expression levels of SAA1 were compared in tumor grade from UALCAN database. **(C)** The protein expression levels of SAA1 were compared in TNM stage from UALCAN database. (****$P<0.0001$, *$P<0.05$, NS means no significance, compared with the respective control).

ccRCC. To determine the diagnostic value of SAA1, we performed ROC curve analysis between tumor tissues with different stage or grade and normal tissues. As shown in **Figures 6A–D**, high SAA1 levels could effectively distinguish advanced and metastatic ccRCC tissues from normal tissues (Normal/T4 (**Figure 6A**, AUC = 0.8157, p = 0.0008); Normal/N1 (**Figure 6B**, AUC = 0.8481, p < 0.0001); Normal/M1 (**Figure 6B**, AUC = 0.7917, p < 0.0001); Normal/G4 (**Figure 6C**, AUC = 0.8862, p < 0.0001); Normal/Stage IV (**Figure 6D**, AUC = 0.7737, p < 0.0001), but could not distinguish early ccRCC tissues from normal tissues. These results suggested that

SAA1 could serve as a new diagnostic marker for patients with advanced and metastatic ccRCC. We wondered whether SAA1 predicts a similar prognosis in ccRCC patients with different stages and clinical parameters.

## SAA1 Possesses Prognostic Value for ccRCC Patients Regardless of Early and Advanced Tumors

Our previous results have confirmed that high expression of SAA1 predicts poor overall and disease-free survival in patients with ccRCC (**Figure 1B**). Moreover, our COX regression analysis

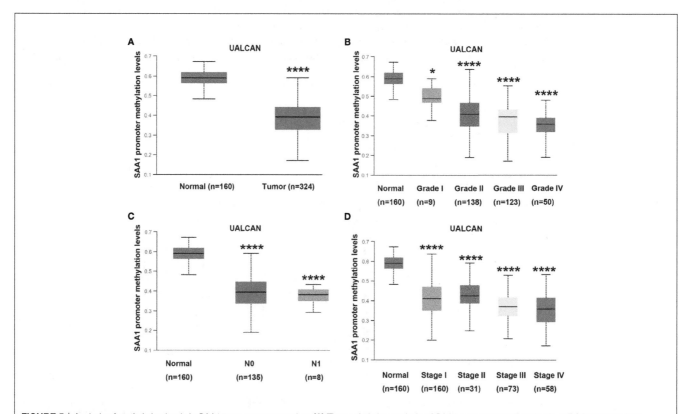

**FIGURE 5** | Analysis of methylation levels in SAA1 gene promoter region. **(A)** The methylation analysis of SAA1 gene promoter region in ccRCC samples from UALCAN database. **(B)** The methylation levels of SAA1 gene promoter region were compared in tumor grade from UALCAN database. **(C)** The methylation levels of SAA1 gene promoter region were compared in N stage from UALCAN database. **(D)** The methylation levels of SAA1 gene promoter region were compared in TNM stage from UALCAN database. (****$P<0.0001$, *$P<0.05$, compared with the respective control).

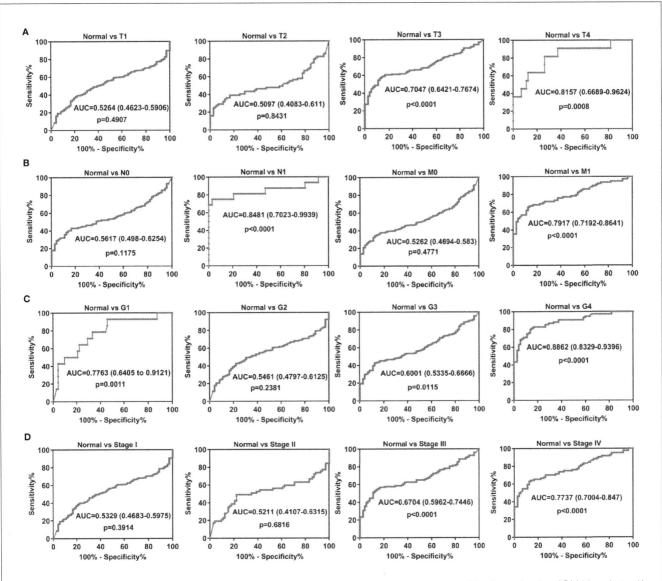

**FIGURE 6** | Analysis of the diagnostic value of SAA1 for advanced and metastatic ccRCC. **(A)** ROC curve analysis of the diagnostic value of SAA1 in patients with ccRCC at T stage. **(B)** ROC curve analysis of the diagnostic value of SAA1 in patients with ccRCC at N and M stages. **(C)** ROC curve analysis of the diagnostic value of SAA1 in patients with ccRCC at tumor grade. **(D)** ROC curve analysis of the diagnostic value of SAA1 in patients with ccRCC at TNM stage.

found that SAA1 could be used as an independent prognostic factor for ccRCC (**Table 2**). We wondered whether SAA1 predicted a similar prognosis in ccRCC patients with different stages and clinical parameters. Therefore, we performed Kaplan Meier curve analysis towards the expression of SAA1 in ccRCC patients with different stages and clinical parameters (**Figures 7A–L**). Our results indicated that high SAA1 expression could serve as a potential prognostic factor for ccRCC patients with T1 + T2 stage (**Figure 7A**, p = 0.0002), T3 + T4 stage (**Figure 7B**, p = 0.0030), N0 stage (**Figure 7C**, p < 0.0001), M0 stage (**Figure 7D**, p < 0.0001), G1 + G2 stage (**Figure 7E**, p = 0.0088), G3 + G4 stage (**Figure 7F**, p = 0.0014), Stage I+II (**Figure 7G**, p = 0.0004), Stage III+IV (**Figure 7H**, p = 0.0081), Female (**Figure 7I**, p < 0.0001), Male (**Figure 7J**, p = 0.0009), Age ≥ 60 years (**Figure 7K**, p < 0.0001), Age < 60 years (**Figure 7L**, p = 0.0044).

## The Protein Levels of SAA1 Were Examined in RCC Cell Lines and Tissues

To further confirm the results of the UALCAN, GEPIA and TCGA databases, SAA1 was subjected to western blotting in RCC cell lines and tissues. As shown in **Figures 8A, B**, the protein levels of SAA1 in RCC cell lines were significantly up-regulated compared with normal renal epithelial cell HK-2, and the protein levels of SAA1 in ccRCC tissues was also obviously overexpressed compared with adjacent normal tissues. The protein levels of SAA1 were also examined by immunohistochemistry (IHC) in paired ccRCC tissues, and the IHC results were consistent with the results of western blotting (**Figure 8C**). These results indicate that SAA1 is up-regulated in ccRCC cell lines and tissues, consistent with the results of UALCAN, GEPIA and TCGA database.

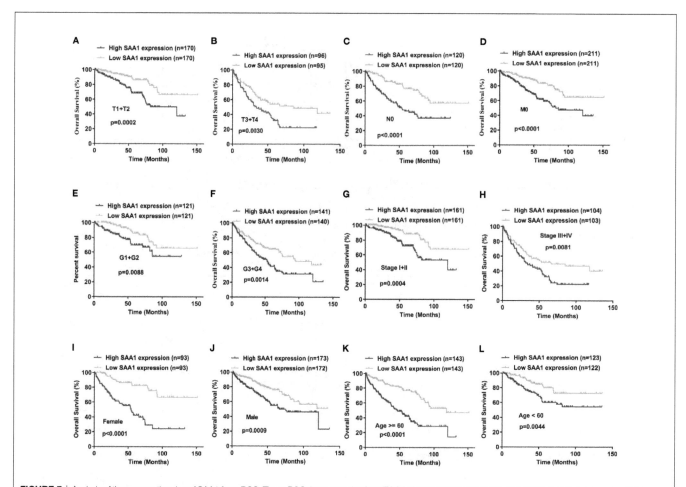

**FIGURE 7** | Analysis of the prognostic value of SAA1 for ccRCC. The ccRCC tissue samples from TCGA database were divided into low SAA1 expression group and high SAA1 expression group according to the median expression value of SAA1 mRNA level. The correlation between SAA1 expression and overall survival time of ccRCC patients was analyzed by Kaplan-Meier. (A-L) Overall survival analysis towards the expression of SAA1 mRNA was performed in subgroups of ccRCC patients: **(A)** T1+T2 stage, **(B)** T3+T4 stage, **(C)** N0 stage, **(D)** M0 stage, **(E)** G1+G2 stage, **(F)** G3+G4 stage, **(G)** Stage I+II, **(H)** Stage III+IV, **(I)** Female, **(J)** Male, **(K)** Age≥60 years, **(L)** Age<60 years.

**TABLE 2** | COX regression analysis between prognostic risk factors and overall survival of ccRCC patients.

| Risk factors | Univariate analysis | | | Multivariate analysis | | |
|---|---|---|---|---|---|---|
| | HR | 95% CI | P value | HR | 95% CI | P value |
| Age | 1.803 | 1.318-2.468 | 0.000 | 1.579 | 1.147-2.175 | 0.005 |
| Gender | 0.948 | 0.697-1.290 | 0.736 | | | |
| T stage | 3.120 | 2.306-4.220 | 0.000 | 0.827 | 0.453-1.511 | 0.537 |
| N stage | 3.823 | 2.070-7.061 | 0.000 | 2.029 | 1.073-3.835 | 0.029 |
| M stage | 4.346 | 3.192-5.918 | 0.000 | 2.144 | 1.474-3.117 | 0.000 |
| G stage | 2.639 | 1.885-3.697 | 0.000 | 1.542 | 1.067-2.228 | 0.021 |
| TNM stage | 3.794 | 2.767-5.202 | 0.000 | 2.263 | 1.140-4.493 | 0.020 |
| SAA1 expression | 2.433 | 1.770-3.346 | 0.000 | 1.538 | 1.094-2.162 | 0.013 |

*HR, Hazard ratio; CI, Confidence interval.*

## SAA1 Knockdown Inhibits Migration and Invasion of RCC cells *In Vitro*

To investigate whether SAA1 affects the migration and invasion of RCC cells, we performed the transwell assays. As shown in **Figures 9A, B**, knockdown of SAA1 significantly impaired the migration and invasion capability of 786-O and ACHN cells. These results reversely suggest that SAA1 promotes migration and invasion of RCC cells.

## DISCUSSION

The most common malignant tumor of the kidney is renal cell carcinoma (RCC), and ccRCC is the most common pathological subtype of RCC. The surrounding abundant vascularization causes ccRCC to grow easily and metastasize through the blood (28). It is reported that about 15% of RCC patients have distant metastases at the time of diagnosis (29). Moreover,

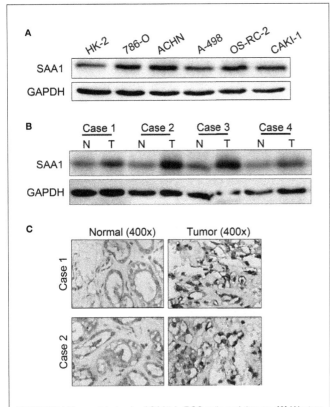

**FIGURE 8** | The protein levels of SAA1 in RCC cells and tissues. **(A)** Western blotting analysis of SAA1 expression levels in RCC cell lines (786-O, ACHN, A-498, OS-RC-2, Caki-1) and renal normal epithelial cells (HK-2). **(B)** Western blotting analysis of SAA1 protein levels in 4 pairs of ccRCC tissues (N, normal tissue; T, tumor tissue). **(C)** IHC analysis of SAA1 protein levels in normal renal tissues and ccRCC tissues.

treatment options for patients with advanced and metastatic ccRCC are limited and their survival prognosis is poor. Therefore, biomarkers screening for ccRCC progression is the key to improve the diagnosis and treatment of advanced and metastatic ccRCC. However, there is still a lack of clinical biomarkers for ccRCC progression and therapeutic targets for biomarkers.

SAA1 is currently recognized as an acute phase protein. When the body suffers from inflammation, trauma, surgery or advanced malignant tumors, the expression of SAA1 is significantly up-regulated (30). SAA1 has been reported to play a critical role in high-density lipoprotein metabolism and cholesterol homeostasis (11, 12). In addition, the role of SAA1 in tumor progression and its potential as a biomarker have also been extensively studied. For example, a large number of studies have reported that SAA1 promotes tumor progression and accelerates distant metastasis (31, 32). High SAA1 expression could be used as a potential biomarker for a variety of malignant tumors (18–20). Previous studies reported that SAA1 possessed the potential to become a prognostic marker of RCC (33, 34). Moreover, another study reported that serum SAA1 has been identified as a biomarker of distant metastases but not as an early tumor marker in RCC patients (21). These studies, unfortunately, did not detect the

expression of SAA1 at the level of tumor cells and tissues. In addition, studies on SAA1 as a diagnostic and prognostic marker for advanced and metastatic ccRCC lack the support of extensive public research data.

In this study, we used three publicly published ccRCC GSE datasets to mine the top ten up-regulated genes and used the Wayne diagram to take the intersection in the three datasets. As a result, we screened out two candidate genes, SAA1 and CCL20. Next, we performed a prognostic analysis of these two genes using data from the TCGA database and found that only SAA1 possessed a predictive significance for ccRCC patients. So we used SAA1 as our target gene. To verify the accuracy of our screened genes, we analyzed SAA1 expression using publicly available TCGA, UALCAN and GEPIA databases. The results indicate that SAA1 is upregulated not only at the mRNA level but also at the protein level in ccRCC patients and exhibits higher expression levels in advanced and metastatic ccRCC. Next, we analyzed the reasons for the upregulation of SAA1 in ccRCC and found that the methylation levels of the promoter region of SAA1 gene were reduced, especially in advanced and metastatic ccRCC. ROC curve analysis found that SAA1 could only distinguish patients with advanced and metastatic ccRCC from the normal population, while Kaplan Meier curve analysis indicated that high SAA1 expression always predicted a worse prognosis regardless of tumor stage. Functionally, SAA1 knockdown significantly inhibits the migration and invasion of RCC cells *in vitro*.

Collectively, we found that SAA1 expression was up-regulated in kidney cancer tissues and its high expression was predictive of advanced tumor stage. In addition, SAA1 could serve as a biomarker for the diagnosis and prognosis of advanced and metastatic renal cell carcinoma at the tumor tissue level. Targeted SAA1 therapy might provide new treatment directions and good prognosis for patients with advanced and metastatic ccRCC.

Unsatisfactorily, there are some flaws in our research. Such as, the specific mechanism and molecular pathways of SAA1-mediated ccRCC metastasis remain unclear. The functions of SAA1 *in vivo* are still unclear. Moreover, our prediction data on tumor diagnosis and prognosis are mainly derived from cancer databases, and there is a lack of clinical and prognostic data for metastatic renal cell carcinoma patients, such as the International Metastatic Renal-Cell Carcinoma Database Consortium (IMDC) risk score. In addition, the SAA1 expression level in tissue specimens of metastatic renal cell carcinoma and its relationship with the prognosis of patients are still unclear. In subsequent experiments, we will continue to carry out relevant studies on these shortcomings. However, our study confirms that SAA1 expression is significantly up-regulated in advanced and metastatic ccRCC and can effectively distinguish patients with advanced and metastatic ccRCC from the normal population.

In summary, for the first time, we have demonstrated that SAA1 expression is significantly upregulated at the mRNA and protein levels in advanced and metastatic ccRCC. Moreover,

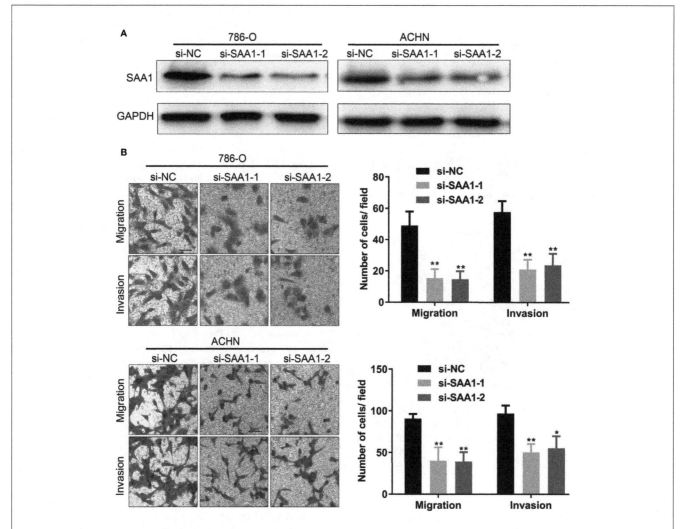

**FIGURE 9** | SAA1 knockdown significantly inhibits migration and invasion of RCC cells *in vitro*. **(A, B)** Transwell assays analysis of the effect of SAA1 knockdown on cell migration and invasion of 786-O and ACHN. (**P<0.01, *P<0.05, compared with si-NC group).

SAA1 has great potential as a diagnostic and prognostic marker for advanced and metastatic ccRCC. In addition, targeted SAA1 therapy provides a new treatment and strategy for patients with advanced and metastatic ccRCC.

## AUTHOR CONTRIBUTIONS

All authors contributed to the article and approved the submitted version.

## REFERENCES

1. Siegel RL, Miller KD, Jemal A. Cancer Statistics, 2019. *CA Cancer J Clin* (2019) 69:7–34. doi: 10.3322/caac.21551
2. Motzer RJ, Bacik J, Schwartz LH, Reuter V, Russo P, Marion S, et al. Prognostic Factors for Survival in Previously Treated Patients With Metastatic Renal Cell Carcinoma. *J Clin Oncol* (2004) 22:454–63. doi: 10.1200/JCO.2004.06.132
3. Flanigan RC, Mickisch G, Sylvester R, Tangen C, Van Poppel H, Crawford ED. Cytoreductive Nephrectomy in Patients With Metastatic Renal Cancer: A Combined Analysis. *J Urol* (2004) 171:1071–6. doi: 10.1097/01.ju.000011 0610.61545.ae
4. Motzer RJ, Hutson TE, Tomczak P, Michaelson MD, Bukowski RM, Rixe O, et al. Sunitinib Versus Interferon Alfa in Metastatic Renal-Cell Carcinoma. *N Engl J Med* (2007) 356:115–24. doi: 10.1056/NEJMoa065044
5. Escudier B, Eisen T, Stadler WM, Szczylik C, Oudard S, Siebels M, et al. Sorafenib in Advanced Clear-Cell Renal-Cell Carcinoma. *N Engl J Med* (2007) 356:125–34. doi: 10.1056/NEJMoa060655
6. Garje R, An J, Greco A, Vaddepally RK, Zakharia Y. The Future of Immunotherapy-Based Combination Therapy in Metastatic Renal Cell Carcinoma. *Cancers (Basel)* (2020) 12. doi: 10.3390/cancers12010143
7. Park K, Lee JL, Park I, Park S, Ahn Y, Ahn J-H, et al. Comparative Efficacy of Vascular Endothelial Growth Factor (VEGF) Tyrosine Kinase Inhibitor (TKI) and Mammalian Target of Rapamycin (mTOR) Inhibitor as Second-Line Therapy in Patients With Metastatic Renal Cell Carcinoma After the Failure of First-Line VEGF TKI. *Med Oncol* (2012) 29:3291–7. doi: 10.1007/s12032-012-0227-7
8. Ascierto ML, McMiller TL, Berger AE, Danilova L, Anders RA, Netto GJ, et al. The Intratumoral Balance Between Metabolic and Immunologic Gene Expression is Associated With Anti-PD-1 Response in Patients With Renal Cell Carcinoma. *Cancer Immunol Res* (2016) 4:726–33. doi: 10.1158/2326-6066.CIR-16-0072

9. Gabay C, Kushner I. Acute-Phase Proteins and Other Systemic Responses to Inflammation. *N Engl J Med* (1999) 340:448–54. doi: 10.1056/NEJM19990211 3400607

10. Malle E, Sodin-Semrl S, Kovacevic A. Serum Amyloid A: An Acute-Phase Protein Involved in Tumour Pathogenesis. *Cell Mol Life Sci* (2009) 66:9–26. doi: 10.1007/s00018-008-8321-x

11. Prufer N, Kleuser B, van der Giet M. The Role of Serum Amyloid A and Sphingosine-1-Phosphate on High-Density Lipoprotein Functionality. *Biol Chem* (2015) 396:573–83. doi: 10.1515/hsz-2014-0192

12. Deetman PE, Bakker SJ, Dullaart RP. High Sensitive C-reactive Protein and Serum Amyloid A are Inversely Related to Serum Bilirubin: Effect-Modification by Metabolic Syndrome. *Cardiovasc Diabetol* (2013) 12:166. doi: 10.1186/1475-2840-12-166

13. Michaeli A, Finci-Yeheskel Z, Dishon S, Linke RP, Levin M, Urieli-Shoval S. Serum Amyloid A Enhances Plasminogen Activation: Implication for a Role in Colon Cancer. *Biochem Biophys Res Commun* (2008) 368:368–73. doi: 10.1016/j.bbrc.2008.01.079

14. Urieli-Shoval S, Shubinsky G, Linke RP, Fridkin M, Tabi I, Matzner Y. Adhesion of Human Platelets to Serum Amyloid a. *Blood* (2002) 99:1224–9. doi: 10.1182/blood.V99.4.1224

15. Biran H, Friedman N, Neumann L, Pras M, Shainkin-Kestenbaum R. Serum Amyloid A (SAA) Variations in Patients With Cancer: Correlation With Disease Activity, Stage, Primary Site, and Prognosis. *J Clin Pathol* (1986) 39:794–7. doi: 10.1136/jcp.39.7.794

16. Liu DH, Wang XM, Zhang LJ, Dai S-W, Liu L-Y, Liu J-F, et al. Serum Amyloid A Protein: A Potential Biomarker Correlated With Clinical Stage of Lung Cancer. *BioMed Environ Sci* (2007) 20:33–40.

17. Raynes JG, Cooper EH. Comparison of Serum Amyloid A Protein and C-reactive Protein Concentrations in Cancer and non-Malignant Disease. *J Clin Pathol* (1983) 36:798–803. doi: 10.1136/jcp.36.7.798

18. Chan DC, Chen CJ, Chu HC, Chang W-K, Yu J-C, Chen Y-J, et al. Evaluation of Serum Amyloid A as a Biomarker for Gastric Cancer. *Ann Surg Oncol* (2007) 14:84–93. doi: 10.1245/s10434-006-9091-z

19. Moshkovskii SA, Serebryakova MV, Kuteykin-Teplyakov KB, Tikhonova OV, Goufman EI, Zgoda VG, et al. Ovarian Cancer Marker of 11.7 kDa Detected by Proteomics is a Serum Amyloid A1. *Proteomics* (2005) 5:3790–7. doi: 10.1002/pmic.200401205

20. Yokoi K, Shih LC, Kobayashi R, Koomen J, Hawke D, Li D, et al. Serum Amyloid A as a Tumor Marker in Sera of Nude Mice With Orthotopic Human Pancreatic Cancer and in Plasma of Patients With Pancreatic Cancer. *Int J Oncol* (2005) 27:1361–9. doi: 10.3892/ijo.27.5.1361

21. Ramankulov A, Lein M, Johannsen M, Schrader M, Miller K, Loening SA, et al. Serum Amyloid A as Indicator of Distant Metastases But Not as Early Tumor Marker in Patients With Renal Cell Carcinoma. *Cancer Lett* (2008) 269:85–92. doi: 10.1016/j.canlet.2008.04.022

22. Yusenko MV, Kuiper RP, Boethe T, Ljungberg B, van Kessel AG, Kovacs G. High-Resolution DNA Copy Number and Gene Expression Analyses Distinguish Chromophobe Renal Cell Carcinomas and Renal Oncocytomas. *BMC Cancer* (2009) 9:152. doi: 10.1186/1471-2407-9-152

23. Gumz ML, Zou H, Kreinest PA, Childs AC, Belmonte LS, LeGrand SN, et al. Secreted Frizzled-Related Protein 1 Loss Contributes to Tumor Phenotype of Clear Cell Renal Cell Carcinoma. *Clin Cancer Res* (2007) 13:4740–9. doi: 10.1158/1078-0432.CCR-07-0143

24. Lenburg ME, Liou LS, Gerry NP, Frampton GM, Cohen HT, Christman MF. Previously Unidentified Changes in Renal Cell Carcinoma Gene Expression Identified by Parametric Analysis of Microarray Data. *BMC Cancer* (2003) 3:31. doi: 10.1186/1471-2407-3-31

25. Chandrashekar DS, Bashel B, Balasubramanya SAH, Creighton CJ, Ponce-Rodriguez I, Chakravarthi BVSK, et al. UALCAN: A Portal for Facilitating Tumor Subgroup Gene Expression and Survival Analyses. *Neoplasia* (2017) 19:649–58. doi: 10.1016/j.neo.2017.05.002

26. Tang Z, Li C, Kang B, Gao G, Li C, Zhang Z. GEPIA: A Web Server for Cancer and Normal Gene Expression Profiling and Interactive Analyses. *Nucleic Acids Res* (2017) 45:W98–102. doi: 10.1093/nar/gkx247

27. Ruan H, Yang H, Wei H, Xiao W, Lou N, Qiu B, et al. Overexpression of SOX4 Promotes Cell Migration and Invasion of Renal Cell Carcinoma by Inducing Epithelial-Mesenchymal Transition. *Int J Oncol* (2017) 51:336–46. doi: 10.3892/ijo.2017.4010

28. Cutz JC, Guan J, Bayani J, Yoshimoto M, Xue H, Sutcliffe M, et al. Establishment in Severe Combined Immunodeficiency Mice of Subrenal Capsule Xenografts and Transplantable Tumor Lines From a Variety of Primary Human Lung Cancers: Potential Models for Studying Tumor Progression-Related Changes. *Clin Cancer Res* (2006) 12:4043–54. doi: 10.1158/1078-0432.CCR-06-0252

29. Siegel RL, Miller KD, Jemal A. Cancer Statistics, 2018. *CA Cancer J Clin* (2018) 68:7–30. doi: 10.3322/caac.21442

30. Cheng N, Liang Y, Du X, Ye RD. Serum Amyloid A Promotes LPS Clearance and Suppresses LPS-induced Inflammation and Tissue Injury. *EMBO Rep* (2018) 19. doi: 10.15252/embr.201745517

31. Lin CY, Yang ST, Shen SC, Hsieh Y-C, Hsu F-T, Chen C-Y, et al. Serum Amyloid A1 in Combination With Integrin alphaVbeta3 Increases Glioblastoma Cells Mobility and Progression. *Mol Oncol* (2018) 12:756–71. doi: 10.1002/1878-0261.12196

32. Hansen MT, Forst B, Cremers N, Quagliata L, Ambartsumian N, Grum-Schwensen B, et al. A Link Between Inflammation and Metastasis: Serum Amyloid A1 and A3 Induce Metastasis, and are Targets of Metastasis-Inducing S100A4. *Oncogene* (2015) 34:424–35. doi: 10.1038/onc.2013.568

33. Vermaat JS, van der Tweel I, Mehra N, Sleijfer S, Haanen JB, Roodhart JM, et al. Two-Protein Signature of Novel Serological Markers apolipoprotein-A2 and Serum Amyloid Alpha Predicts Prognosis in Patients With Metastatic Renal Cell Cancer and Improves the Currently Used Prognostic Survival Models. *Ann Oncol* (2010) 21:1472–81. doi: 10.1093/annonc/mdp559

34. Junker K, von Eggeling F, Muller J, Steiner T, Schubert J. Identification of Biomarkers and Therapeutic Targets for Renal Cell Cancer Using ProteinChip Technology. *Urologe A* (2006) 45:305–8. doi: 10.1007/s00120-006-1001-2

# 17

# Low Expression Levels of SLC22A12 Indicates a Poor Prognosis and Progresses Clear Cell Renal Cell Carcinoma

Jiaju Xu[1†], Yuenan Liu[1†], Jingchong Liu[1], Yi Shou[1], Zhiyong Xiong[1], Hairong Xiong[2], Tianbo Xu[1], Qi Wang[1], Di Liu[1], Huageng Liang[1], Hongmei Yang[2], Xiong Yang[1*] and Xiaoping Zhang[1,3*]

[1] Department of Urology, Union Hospital, Tongji Medical College, Huazhong University of Science and Technology, Wuhan, China, [2] Department of Pathogenic Biology, School of Basic Medicine, Huazhong University of Science and Technology, Wuhan, China, [3] Shenzhen Huazhong University of Science and Technology Research Institute, Shenzhen, China

*Correspondence:
Xiong Yang
yangxiong1368@hust.edu.cn
Xiaoping Zhang
xzhang@hust.edu.cn

[†]These authors have contributed equally to this work

Clear cell renal cell carcinoma (ccRCC) accounts for approximately 4/5 of all kidney cancers. Accumulation of minor changes in the cellular homeostasis may be one cause of ccRCC. Therefore, we downloaded the RNA sequencing and survival data of the kidney renal cell carcinoma (KIRC) cohort from the Cancer Genome Atlas (TCGA) database. After the univariate and multivariate Cox regression analyses, 19 kidney-specific differentially expressed genes (DEGs) were found. Solute Carrier Family 22 Member 12 (SLC22A12) resulted in an independent prognostic predictor for both overall survival (OS) and disease-free survival (DFS). SLC22A12 expression was lower in tumoral tissue compared to normal tissue. Moreover, patients in the SLC22A12 low expression group had a higher pathological stage and worse survival than the high expression group. Additionally, qRT-PCR assay, immunoblotting test (IBT), and immunohistochemical (IHC) analyses of cancer tissues/cells and the corresponding normal controls verified that SLC22A12 is downregulated in ccRCC. Receiver operator characteristic (ROC) curves showed that the low expression level of SLC22A12 could be a good diagnostic marker for ccRCC (AUC=0.7258; p <0.0001). Gene set enrichment analysis (GSEA) showed that SLC22A12 expression levels are related to metabolism, cell cycle, and tumor-related signaling pathways. GO and KEGG analyses revealed that SLC22A12 transports multiple organic compounds, ions, and hormones and participates in the extracellular structure organization. Furthermore, SLC22A12 over-expression in vitro inhibited the proliferation, migration, and invasion of renal cancer cells by regulating PI3K/Akt pathways. Such effects were reversed when knocking out SLC22A12. In summary, as a transporter for many vital metabolites, SLC22A12 may affect tumor cell survival through its impacts on the mentioned metabolites. In conclusion, this study uncovered that SLC22A12 is a promising prognostic and diagnostic biomarker for ccRCC.

Keywords: cellular homeostasis, renal cell carcinoma, biomarker, gene set enrichment analysis, metastasis, solute carrier family, bioinformatic analysis, signal pathway

# INTRODUCTION

Kidney cancer, also called renal cancer, represents a significant threat to human health, as it develops fatal metastasis in the lung or brain. Kidney cancer mainly includes renal cell cancer (RCC), transitional cell cancer (TCC), and Wilms tumor. RCC accounts for roughly 4/5 of kidney cancers, while most of the other renal cancer are TCC (1–3). According to the American Cancer Society, 73,750 new kidney and renal pelvis cancer cases were estimated in the United States in 2020. Among the diagnosed, 520 were males and 28,230 females, with an estimated 14,830 deaths, including 9,860 males and 4,970 females (4). The five-year survival rate is 93% for patients with localized kidney cancer, 70% with surrounding lymph nodes spread, and 12% with distant metastasis (5). Surgery is the typical treatment for kidney cancer due to the slight response to radiation and chemotherapy. Target therapy is growing, but its capacity to limit the progression is restricted. Therefore, it is crucial to investigate the biological functions and molecular mechanisms involved in kidney cancer in order to find new therapeutic targets.

Maintaining homeostasis is essential for a healthy body, and the same happens in the constituent cells. Complex intracellular reactions occur to maintain the level of various biological macromolecules, including multiple enzymes, transporters, kinases, and cytokines. The environment where epithelial cells live is more complicated than normal cells. Since there is an active exchange of substances, a considerable accumulation of metabolic waste, and a distinctive osmotic pressure difference, it is more challenging to maintain cellular homeostasis. During the adaptation to this harsh environment, epithelial cells have developed a cloning strategy to replace the exfoliated cells. This strategy contributes to dyshomeostasis, tumorigenesis, and differential protein expression profile. Unfortunately, the connection between cellular homeostasis and tumorigenesis has not been thoroughly studied. Since we consider this a critical pathophysiological aspect, we aim to study oncogenes or tumor suppressor genes specifically expressed in the kidney. Finding differentially expressed genes in kidney cancer will contribute to a deeper understanding of this cancer and could also help to identify new prognostic biomarkers. Moreover, potential new drugs against these targets may be safer since they will not harm other organs and tissues.

**Abbreviations:** RCC, renal cell cancer; TCC, transitional cell cancer; SLC22A12, Solute Carrier Family 22 Member 12; URAT1, Urate Transporter 1; RST, Renal-Specific Transporter; PPI, protein-protein interaction; DEG, differently expressed gene; TCGA, the Cancer Genome Atlas; ICGC, International Cancer Genome Consortium; RNA-seq, RNA sequencing; KIRC, kidney renal clear cell carcinoma; AJCC, American Joint Committee on Cancer; GO, Gene Ontology; qRT-PCR, reverse transcription-quantitative PCR; FBS, fetal bovine serum; IBT, immunoblotting test; RIPA, radio immunoprecipitation assay; PVDF, polyvinylidene difluoride; ECL, Electrochemiluminescence; BLAST, Basic Local Alignment Search Tool; CCK-8, Cell Counting Kit-8; GSEA, gene set enrichment analysis; KEGG, Kyoto Encyclopedia of Genes and Genomes; PID, Pathway Interaction Database; FDR, false discovery rate; ROC, Receiver operator characteristic; AUC, areas under the curve; OS, overall survival; DFS, disease-free survival; KIRP, kidney renal papillary cell carcinoma; KICH, kidney chromophobesarcoma; SARC, sarcoma; NES, normalized enrichment score; ccRCC, clear-cell renal cell carcinoma; pRCC, papillary RCC; chRCC, chromophobe RCC.

We found that Solute Carrier Family 22 Member 12 (SLC22A12), a tissue-specific gene, played an important role in the occurrence and development of kidney cancer. SLC22A12, also known as Urate Transporter 1(URAT1) or Renal-Specific Transporter (RST), is a membrane protein located in epithelial cells of the kidney proximal tubule. Initially, it was considered a urate transporter (6–10); however, later studies proved that it is involved in pharmacodynamics (11–14). It can transport glucose and other sugars, bile salts and organic acids, metal ions and amine compounds (10, 13, 15–18). To the best of our knowledge, the relationship between SLC22A12 and ccRCC has not been disclosed yet.

We screened the TCGA data set to discover differentially expressed genes (DEGs) in kidney cancer. As a result, we found 19 kidney-specific genes that regulate cell homeostasis. Using Cox regression analyses, we discovered that SLC22A12 has a significant impact on patient survival. Our results demonstrate that SLC22A12 low expression predicted a poor prognosis in ccRCC. Additionally, an *in vitro* experiment confirmed its role as a tumor suppressor. Gene set enrichment analysis, and protein-protein interaction (PPI) network strengthened the hypothesis that SLC22A12 contributes to the homeostasis regulation in ccRCC.

# MATERIALS AND METHODS

## Dataset

The data were gathered from the Cancer Genome Atlas (TCGA) project (https://portal.gdc.cancer.gov/), cBioPortal for Cancer Genomics (http://www.cbioportal.org/), UCSC Xena browser (https://xenabrowser.net/), and International Cancer Genome Consortium (ICGC, https://dcc.icgc.org/), including gene expression datasets (RNA sequencing, RNA-seq) on kidney renal clear cell carcinoma (KIRC) patients, as well as corresponding demographic (age, gender), clinicopathological [American Joint Committee on Cancer (AJCC) T stage, N stage, M stage, G stage and clinical stage] and survival (overall survival, disease-free survival) information (19, 20). Patients without survival information were eliminated from further evaluation.

## Screening of the Critical Gene Involved in Cellular Homeostasis in ccRCC

The gene set of cellular homeostasis was downloaded from the Gene Ontology (GO) Resource (http://geneontology.org/). Kidney-specific gene set was gathered from the Human Protein Atlas (https://www.proteinatlas.org/). Differential expressed gene set was acquired by "limma" package (21–23) with a cut-off value of p<0.05 by R 4.0.2. Then a Venn diagram was depicted to obtain the intersection of three gene sets for further study. Pan-cancer profile of SLC22A12 was gathered from Gene Expression Profiling Interactive Analysis (GEPIA, http://gepia.cancer-pku.cn/) (24).

## ccRCC Tissue Samples

A total of 120 pairs of ccRCC and their adjacent normal renal tissues were sampled from patients aged 22-79 years old between

May 2015 and May 2018 at the Department of Urology, Union Hospital, Tongji Medical College, Huazhong University of Science and Technology (Wuhan, China). The adjacent normal renal tissues were collected more than 2 cm away from the edge of the tumor site. The proteins extracted from 16 pairs of these resected samples were analyzed *via* immunoblotting test. The RNAs extracted from 20 pairs of samples were analyzed *via* reverse transcription-quantitative PCR (qRT-PCR). Two pairs of tissues were analyzed *via* immunohistochemistry (IHC). Three pairs of tissues were analyzed by whole transcriptome sequencing in 2017. The basic clinical characteristics (age, gender, tumor size, tumor location and tumor stage) of the patients are presented in **Table S2** (25). No patients had received any adjuvant anticancer therapy prior to or following surgery. The present study was approved by the Human Research Ethics Committee of Huazhong University of Science and Technology. Written informed consent was provided by the patients or the patients' family. The study methodologies conformed to the standards set by the Declaration of Helsinki.

## Cell Culture

The human renal proximal tubular epithelial cell line HK-2, and five types of human renal cell carcinoma cell lines purchased from the American Type Culture Collection (ATCC, USA), including 786-O, ACHN, A-498, OSRC-2 and Caki-1, were employed in the present study. The cells were cultured in high glucose Dulbecco's Modified Eagle's Medium (DMEM; Gibco, USA) containing 10% fetal bovine serum (FBS; Gibco, USA) and 1% penicillin-streptomycin solution (Servicebio, China) and incubated in a humidified atmosphere with 5% $CO_2$ at 37°C.

## Immunoblotting Test (IBT)

Cells and tissues were lysed in Radio Immunoprecipitation Assay (RIPA) Lysis Buffer (Beyotime, China) containing protease inhibitors. Then the protein concentration of each sample was measured using a BCA Protein Assay Kit (Beyotime, China). For IBT, 15 μg proteins were separated *via* SDS-PAGE (12% gel) at 90-120 mV for 90 min and transferred to a polyvinylidene difluoride (PVDF) membrane (Invitrogen, USA) at 300 mA for 60 min. Afterwards, the PVDF membranes were blocked with 2.5% bovine serum albumin (BSA) for 2 h at room temperature and then incubated with specific primary antibodies overnight at 4°C. The primary antibody used in this paper: anti-SLC22A12 (14937-1-AP), 1:1,000, Proteintech, China; anti-GAPDH (AC002), 1:5,000, Abclonal, China; anti-PI3K(PAB43806), 1:2,000, Bioswamp, China; anti-p-PI3K(PAB43641-P), 1:2,000, Bioswamp, China; anti-AKT1(A17909), 1:3,000, Proteintech, China; anti-p-AKT1(ab81283), 1:3,000, Abcam, US. Following incubation with the primary antibodies, the membranes were incubated with specie-matched secondary antibodies (AS014/AS003, 1:3,000; Abclonal, China) for 2 h at room temperature following washing with PBST for 30 min. Finally, the protein bands were visualized with Electrochemiluminescence (ECL) Western Blotting Substrate (Ultra sensitivity; Biosharp, China) using ChemiDoc-XRS+ (Bio-Rad, China).

## RNA Extraction and qRT-PCR

Total RNA was isolated from tissues or cells using Ultrapure RNA Kit (CoWin Biosciences, China) directed by the manufacturer's protocols. The concentration and purity of the RNA solution were detected using Tecan's Infinite M200 Pro (Thermo Fisher Scientific, USA). Extracted RNA was then reverse transcribed into cDNA using PrimeScript™ RT Master Mix (Takara, Japan) according to the manufacturer's protocols. The reaction conditions were as follows: 37°C for 15 min; 85°C for 5 sec. Subsequently, the cDNA was diluted at a proper concentration and subjected to qPCR using AceQ® qPCR SYBR Green Master Mix (Vazyme, China) on CFX Connect Real-Time PCR Detection System (Biorad, China) according to the manufacturer's protocols. The qPCR conditions were as follows: pre-denaturation at 95°C for 5 min; 40 cycles of denaturation at 95°C for 10 sec; annealing and extension at 60°C for 30 sec. The housekeeping gene, GAPDH, was used to normalize the relative expression of SLC22A12 as an endogenous control by the comparative Ct (threshold cycle) method ($2^{-\Delta\Delta Ct}$). All qRT-PCR reactions were performed in duplicate. The primers used to amplify SLC22A12 and GAPDH were chemically synthesized by TSINGKE, China. The primer sequences were as follows: SLC22A12: 5′- TCT CCA CGT TGT GCT GGT TC -3′ (forward) and 5′- GGA TGT CCA CGA CAC CAA TGA -3′(reverse); GAPDH: 5′- CGT GGA AGG ACT CAT GAC CA -3′ (forward) and 5′- GCC ATC ACG CCA CAG TTT C -3′ (reverse).

## Immunohistochemistry (IHC) Assay

The IHC assay was performed as previously described. Briefly, ccRCC tissues and adjacent normal tissues were sequentially fixed in formalin at room temperature for 12 h, dehydrated and embedded in paraffin. Tissue sections were then incubated with a rabbit antibody against SLC22A12 overnight at 4°C. They were then rinsed three times with PBS and incubated with secondary antibodies that were conjugated to horseradish peroxidase at room temperature for 2 h. Finally, tissues were observed in three randomly selected fields under a light microscope (Olympus CX41-32C02; Olympus, Japan) at 40, 100, and 200× magnification.

## Transient Transfection for Overexpression and Knockdown of SLC22A12

Plasmids overexpressing SLC22A12 and a negative control (Vector) were constructed by Vigene Biosciences (Shandong, China). Small interfering RNA (siRNA) oligonucleotide sequences specifically targeting SLC22A12 (si-SLC22A12) and a negative control (si-NC) siRNA were synthesized by Guangzhou RiboBio and verified no off-target effects by Basic Local Alignment Search Tool (BLAST, https://blast.ncbi.nlm.nih.gov/Blast.cgi). For transient transfection, ACHN and 786-O cell lines were incubated in 6-well plates until they reached 70% confluence. 10μg per well of plasmids (vector or SLC22A12) or 0.1 nmol per well of siRNAs (si-SLC22A12 or si-NC) were transfected with Invitrogen Lipofectamine® 2000 (Thermo Fisher Scientific, USA) according to the manufacturer's protocol. Cells were collected for subsequent experiments 48 h post-transfection. The si-SLC22A12 sequence was as follows: 5'-TCA CCT GCA TCA CCA TCT A -3'.

## Colony Formation Assay

ACHN and 786-O cells had been transfected with plasmids or siRNAs for 48 h before subsequent experimentation. Cells were inoculated on 6-well plates at a cell density of $1\times10^3$ cells per well with 2 mL of medium. After culture for 10 days, cells were fixed with methanol for 10 min and stained with crystal violet for 20 min. After PBS wash and air drying, colonies (>50 cells) were manually counted. All experiments were independently repeated in duplicate.

## 5-Ethynyl-2′-deoxyuridine (EdU) Assay

EdU assay was implemented in ACHN and 786-O cells according to manufacturer's protocol by use of the BeyoClick™ EdU-647 Cell Proliferation Kit (Beyotime, China). After transfection, cells ($1 \times 10^5$ per well) were seeded into 6-well plates. 24 h later, 10μM EdU medium was added into cells for 2 h. Next, 4% paraformaldehyde (PFA) was added for 15-min fixing. After three-time rinse by washing buffer (3% BSA), cells were washed by permeabilization buffer (0.3% Triton X-100) for 15 min. After one-time rinse by washing buffer, Click additive reaction system was added to label the proliferated cells and Hoechst 33342 was added for cell counting. Finally, cells were visualized using fluorescence microscope (Olympus, Japan). Each independent experiment was carried out in duplicate.

## Cell Counting Kit-8 (CCK8) Assay

ACHN and 786-O cells had been transfected with plasmids or siRNAs for 48 h before subsequent experimentation. Cells were inoculated on 96-well plates at a cell density of $1\times10^3$ cells per well with 100 μl of medium. A cell proliferation assay was performed using Cell Counting Kit-8 (CCK8; MedChemExpress, USA) at a concentration of 10μl in 100μl serum-free medium every 24 h for four days according to the manufacturer's protocols. After incubation for 2 h at 37°C, the optical density of each well was measured at 450 nm with a spectrophotometer to measure the quantity of living cells. Finally, the absorbance of cells over four days were plotted in a graph for a reflection of cell proliferation rate.

## Cell Migration and Invasion Assays

ACHN and 786-O cells had been transfected with plasmids or siRNAs for 48 h before subsequent experimentation. Prior to the assays, cells were incubated in serum-free DMEM for 6-8 h. Boyden Transwell chambers and 24-well plates (Corning, USA) with 8-μm membrane filters were used in the migration and invasion assays. Serum-starved cells ($1\times10^5$) were seeded into the upper chambers in serum-free medium, and the lower chambers were filled with DMEM containing 10% FBS. After incubation for 24 h at 37°C, the lower chamber was washed twice with PBS and fixed with 100% methanol for 10 min at room temperature and stained with 0.1% crystal violet dye for 20 min at room temperature. Following washing the chamber again three times with PBS, non-migrated and non-invaded cells were carefully removed from the upper chamber with a cotton bud. Migrated cells in lower chambers

were observed in five randomly selected fields under a light microscope (Olympus CX41-32C02; Olympus, Japan) at 400× magnification. Based on the migration assay, a cell invasion assay was performed in Matrigel-coated Transwell insert chambers (BD Biosciences, USA), which had already been incubated at 37°C for 6-8 h, with double cell numbers. The remaining procedure was the same as described for the cell migration assays.

## Bioinformatics Analyses

The median of SLC22A12 expression was set as the cutoff point for dividing patients into high and low expression groups. To determine which SLC22A12 signaling pathways were involved in the pathogenesis of ccRCC, a gene set enrichment analysis (GSEA; http://www.broadinstitute.org/gsea) was used with the curated gene sets (c2.all.v7.1.symbols.gmt) that integrate Kyoto Encyclopedia of Genes and Genomes (KEGG), Biocarta Pathways dataset, Reactome Pathway Database and Pathway Interaction Database (PID). For the enriched gene sets, after performing 1,000 permutations, the false discovery rate (FDR) value <0.25 and the p<0.05 were considered statistically significant enriched pathways (26). The KEGG and Gene Ontology (GO) analyses of DEGs between high and low SLC22A12 expression groups were conducted by R 4.0.2.

## Statistical Analyses

As seen in the previous article (27), statistical analyses were performed using GraphPad Prism version 7.0. The numerical data of each group are presented as the mean ± standard deviation. The significant differences in SLC22A12 expression between each ccRCC subgroup were analyzed using a Student's t-test. A paired Student's t-test was used to analyze SLC22A12 expression in tumor tissues and matched normal kidney tissues. The associations between SLC22A12 expression and clinicopathological characteristics in patients with ccRCC were evaluated using Pearson's $\chi^2$ test. Receiver operator characteristic (ROC) curves and areas under the curve (AUC) were used to calculate the diagnostic values of SLC22A12 expression in patients with ccRCC. The association between SLC22A12 expression and OS was investigated using Kaplan-Meier curves with log-rank tests. p<0.05 was considered a statistically significant difference.

## RESULTS

### SLC22A12 Is an Essential Kidney-Specific Tumor Suppressor Gene That Maintains Cell Homeostasis

One of the aims of this work was to identify the critical genes for cellular homeostasis in ccRCC. For that purpose, we screened three independent gene sets: DEGs set in TCGA datasets, kidney-specific gene sets, and cellular homeostasis gene sets. As a result, we found that only 19 genes belonged to the three gene sets (**Figure 1A**). Next, univariate Cox regression analyses were performed to explore the relationship between the gene expression levels and patient survivals. As shown in **Figures 1B, C**, among all 19 genes, only SLC22A12, PTH1R, MT1G, and SLC34A1 expression significantly

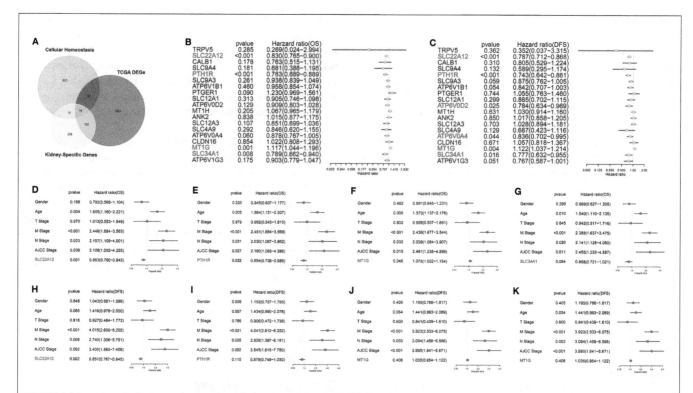

**FIGURE 1** | Screening of critical genes involved in cellular homeostasis in ccRCC. **(A)** Venn diagram selects 19 kidney-specific DEGs involved in cellular homeostasis. **(B, C)** Univariate Cox regression analyses of 19 selected genes select SLC22A12, PTH1R, MT1G and SLC34A1 as four prognostic biomarkers. Left: OS; right: DFS. **(D–K)** Multivariate Cox regression analyses of four candidate prognostic biomarkers along with clinicopathological characteristics select SLC22A12 as the critical gene. Middle row: OS; bottom row: DFS.

impacted overall survival (OS) and disease-free survival (DFS). Multivariate Cox analyses (**Figures 1D–K**) and clinicopathological data confirmed that SLC22A12 is an independent risk factor in both OS and DFS and has a better prognostic value. No other cancer transcriptome profile included SLC22A12, except for two sarcoma samples (SARC) (**Figures 2A, B**) (24). Apart from that, SLC22A12 was only expressed in the kidney (KIRC: Kidney renal clear cell carcinoma; KIRP: Kidney renal papillary cell carcinoma; KICH: Kidney Chromophobe). From the results above, SLC22A12 was selected as the principal gene for further investigation.

## SLC22A12 Downregulation Is Associated With Various Types of Clinicopathological Characteristics in ccRCC

Data of SLC22A12 mRNA expression levels in ccRCC tissues and para-cancer tissues were downloaded from the TCGA database to understand the role of SLC22A12 expression in tumorigenesis. The results suggest that SLC22A12 expression in tumor tissues was significantly lower than in para-cancer tissues (**Figures 2C, D**). Similar results were found in the ICGC database (**Figures S1A, B**). In addition, we studied the connection between SLC22A12 expression and the clinicopathological characteristics. We found that a decrease in the gene expression was associated with increasing primary tumor (T stage), regional lymph node (N stage), distant metastasis (M stage), histologic grade (G stage), and AJCC prognostic stage (**Figures 2F–M**). Also, SLC22A12 expression was lower in females (**Figure 2E**).

## SLC22A12 Downregulation Indicates a Poor Clinical Prognosis

Kaplan-Meier survival analysis with log-rank test was applied to determine the association between patients' survival and SLC22A12 expression. From the TCGA database, 522 patients with ccRCC were divided into two groups using the SLC22A12 mRNA expression median as the cutoff criteria. The results revealed that the lower SLC22A12 expression group had the poorest OS and DFS (**Figures 3A, B**). The survival data from the ICGC-RECA cohort showed a similar pattern of results (**Figure S1C**). Kaplan-Meier survival analyses regarding SLC22A12 expression in ccRCC patients with different clinicopathological characteristics were in line with the previous results (**Figures 3C–Q**). The present findings indicate that SLC22A12 could have a prognostic value in ccRCC since its decreased expression resulted in poor patient outcomes.

## SLC22A12 Expression Levels Could Be Valuable for ccRCC Clinical Diagnosis

To explore the diagnostic value of SLC22A12 in ccRCC, ROC curves were plotted to assess the clinicopathological characteristics of the patients. In general, ccRCC could be properly differentiated from normal tissues using SLC22A12 expression levels with an AUC of 0.7258 (p < 0.0001; **Figure 4A**) in the TCGA-KIRC cohort and 0.8926( p< 0.0001; **Figure S1D**) in the ICGC-RECA cohort. Furthermore, the diagnostic value of SLC22A12 expression levels was analyzed between clinicopathological subgroups: male vs. female (AUC=0.6706; p < 0.0001; **Figure 4B**); $T_1 + T_2$ vs. $T_3 +$

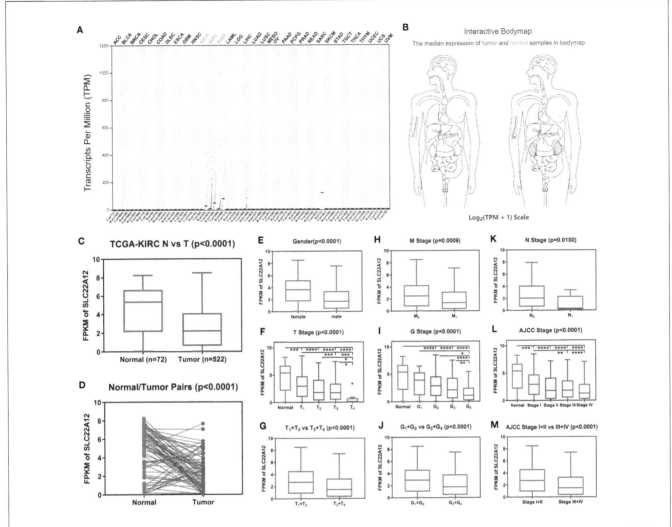

**FIGURE 2** | Transcriptome profile of SLC22A12 of kidney cancer in TCGA database. **(A)** Transcriptome profile of SLC22A12 in multiple types of cancers and their corresponding normal tissues in TCGA database. **(B)** Distribution of SLC22A12 RNA expression levels across organs. The mRNA expression levels of SLC22A12 were lower in **(C)** 522 ccRCC tissues than in 72 para-cancer tissues, **(D)** 72 ccRCC tissues than in 72 corresponding adjacent normal tissues. SLC22A12 expression was lower in **(E)** male, **(F, G)** higher T stage, **(H)** higher M stage, **(I, J)** higher G stage, **(K)** higher N stage, and **(L, M)** higher AJCC clinical stage. *$p < 0.05$, **$p < 0.01$, ***$p < 0.001$, ****$p < 0.0001$.

$T_4$ stage (AUC=0.6129; $p < 0.0001$; **Figure 4C**); $N_0$ vs. $N_1$ stage (AUC=0.6959; p=0.0110; **Figure 4D**); $M_0$ vs. $M_1$ stage (AUC=0.6189; p=0.0009; **Figure 4E**); AJCC stage I + II vs. stage III + IV (AUC=0.6145; $p < 0.0001$; **Figure 4F**); $G_1+G_2$ vs. $G_3+G_4$ (AUC=0.0.6007; $p < 0.0001$; **Figure 4G**). Conclusively, SLC22A12 may be a potential diagnostic biomarker for clear cell renal cell carcinoma.

## SLC22A12 Is Down-Regulated in ccRCC Cells and Tissues

qRT-PCR and IBT were performed to verify the expression levels of SLC22A12 in RCC cells. SLC22A12 mRNA and protein expression levels in RCC cell lines (786-O, ACHN, A-498, OSRC-2, and Caki-1) were decreased compared to the normal cell line HK-2 (**Figures 5D, E**). In contrast, SLC22A12 expression levels were notably elevated in ccRCC tissues compared to their corresponding adjacent normal tissues (**Figures 5A–C**). Our own RNA-Seq cohort also suggested a SLC22A12 downregulation in tumoral tissues(**Figure 5F**). Furthermore, IHC results from cancer/para-cancer pairs (**Figures 5G** and **S2**) suggest that SLC22A12 was primarily located in the plasma membranes of both cancer and normal renal tubular epithelial cells; however, it was down-regulated in cancer cells. Generally, these results collectively indicate that SLC22A12 is under-expressed in kidney cancer cells.

## SLC22A12 Restricts the Proliferation, Invasion, and Migration of RCC Cells *In Vitro*

RCC cell lines were transfected with SLC22A12 plasmid or si-SLC22A12 to investigate the function of SLC22A12 on the pathobiology of renal cancer. The mRNA and protein

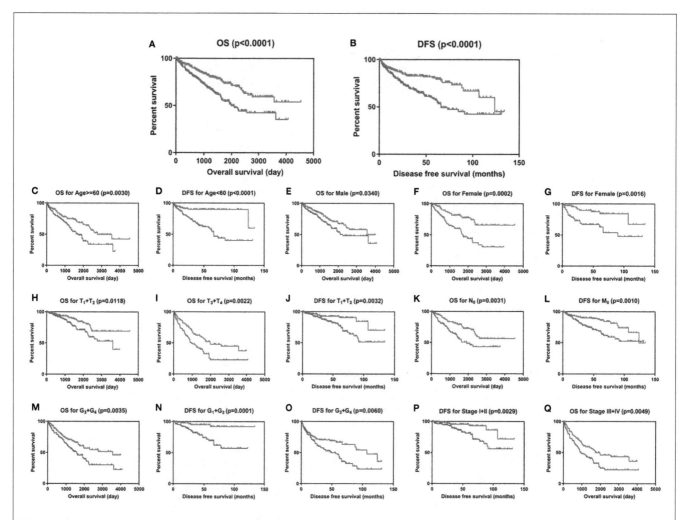

**FIGURE 3** | Low SLC22A12 mRNA expression is associated with both poor OS and DFS in patients with ccRCC. Patients with lower SLC22A12 mRNA expression levels harbor worse **(A)** OS and **(B)** DFS. The similar results were obtained from **(C–Q)** subgroup of patients with ccRCC.

expression levels increased or decreased significantly in ACHN and 786-O cells compared with the corresponding negative control (**Figures 6A–C**). Cell viability was analyzed by colony formation (**Figures 6D**), EdU (**Figures 6E, F**) and CCK-8 assays (**Figure 6G**) in both cell lines, where we observed that SLC22A12 silencing promoted cell proliferation. Moreover, transwell assays verified that the SLC22A12 expression level negatively correlates with the cells' ability to migrate and invade (**Figures 6H**). Collectively, these results provide us with solid evidence suggesting that SLC22A12 suppresses RCC cell proliferation, migration, and invasion, which play an essential role in tumor metastasis.

## SLC22A12 Is Involved in Multiple Biological Pathways That Regulate Cellular Homeostasis and ccRCC Pathogenesis

Multiple functional enrichment analyses were performed using the TCGA-KIRC cohort to study the SLC22A12 role in ccRCC pathogenesis. As demonstrated in **Figures 7A–C**, activated gene sets are associated with multiple metabolic pathways (**Figure 7A**),

cell cycle (**Figure 7B**), and tumor-related signaling pathways (**Figure 7C**). The enrichment of metabolic pathways, including glycerolipid [normalized enrichment score(NES)=-2.15, p<0.001, FDR=0.053], fatty acid (NES=-2.23, p<0.001, FDR=0.047), glucose (NES=-2.02, p=0.008, FDR=0.070), amino acids and derivatives (NES=-2.20, p=0.002, FDR=0.046), and steroids (NES=-1.90, p<0.001, FDR=0.104) indicated that the role of SLC22A12 on the transport of metabolites may also partially regulate metabolic processes. The enrichment of tumor-related pathways, including Akt pathway (NES=-2.04, p=0.004, FDR=0.068), Wnt pathway (NES=-1.95, p=0.008, FDR=0.087), p53 pathway (NES=1.95, p=0.012, FDR=0.243), mTOR signaling pathway (NES=-1.74, p=0.021, FDR=0.141), MAPK (NES=-1.89, p=0.014, FDR=0.107) pathway, Hedgehog signaling pathway (NES=-1.79, p=0.042, FDR=0.129) and ERKs pathway(NES=-2.03, p=0.008, FDR=0.068), suggested that abnormally expressed SLC22A12 may activate various cancer pathways that promote ccRCC occurrence or development. The activation of PI3K and Akt pathways in SLC22A12 down-regulated cells was validated by IBT (**Figure S5**). The GO and KEGG analyses indicate that SLC22A12 is involved in the transport of multiple organic

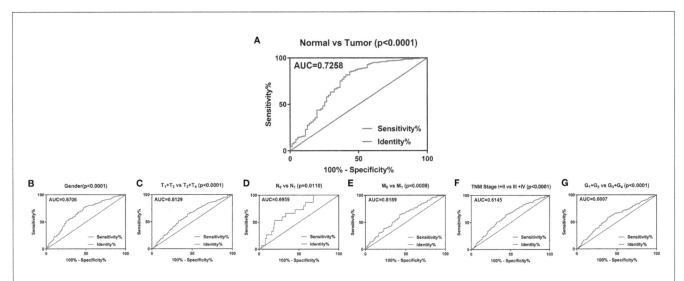

FIGURE 4 | SLC22A12 expression may be a diagnostic predictor in patients with ccRCC. (A) SLC22A12 effectively discriminated between ccRCC and normal tissues. Receiver operating characteristic curve subanalysis were performed for the following subgroups of patients with ccRCC: (B) gender, (C) T stage, (D) N stage, (E) M stage, (F) AJCC clinical stage, (G) G stage. AUC, area under curve; OS, overall survival; DFS, disease-free survival.

compounds, ions, and hormones, as well as extracellular structure organization (**Figures 7D, E**).

## SLC22A12 Interacts With Various Proteins That Regulate Cellular Homeostasis

To further investigate how SLC22A12 affects cellular homeostasis, we performed a PPI network analysis on the String database (https://string-db.org/) and selected the 20 proteins with the highest confidence. As shown in **Figure S3** and **Table S1**, most of the proteins are related to homeostasis maintenance. For example, SLC2A5 and SLC2A9 are involved in glucose and fructose transportation; SLC38A3 transports amino acids, while SLC5A8 and SLC16A9 transport various monocarboxylates. Also, many ion pumps essential for the exchange of substances are associated with SLC22A12. Moreover, heatmap of those genes that associated to SLC22A12 showed that most of them were expressed differentially in tumoral tissue compared to normal tissue, suggesting a completely different profile of cellular homeostasis in ccRCC (**Figure S4**). Altogether, SLC22A12 may interact with these proteins that regulate tumor cell homeostasis, thereby affecting cell proliferation, invasion, and migration.

## DISCUSSION

RCC is among the 3% of the cancers with the highest morbidity in western countries (28). During the last two decades, RCC mortality worldwide has increased 2% per year. As a result, in 2018 within the European Union, 99,200 new cases and 39,100 kidney cancer-specific deaths were estimated (28). Regionally localized RCC has a 65–90% five-year survival rate, decreasing considerably as the tumor spread. Clear-cell RCC (ccRCC), the principal cause of renal cell carcinoma, is named after its microscopic characteristics. ccRCC cells contain a clear cytoplasm surrounded by a distinct cell membrane and round and uniform nucleus. Generally, ccRCC

has a worse prognosis than papillary RCC (pRCC) and chromophobe RCC (chRCC) (29, 30), which is a big hazard for human beings. At the moment, surgery is considered the most effective treatment, although it cannot treat metastatic cancer (31–33). Targeted therapy that activates the immune system or inhibits growth factors is also employed in ccRCC patients, but drug resistance development restricts its use (34). Nevertheless, researchers have been working on new tumor-related targets involved in multiple biological processes (25, 35–42)since there is still a need for new therapeutic targets.

An ideal therapeutic target has high specificity. The idea is to attack tumor cells without affecting normal cells and target diseased organs without affecting healthy organs. Considering this, we used proteomics to study kidney-specific genes that are differentially expressed in the kidney. This means the target selected in this study is distinctive of ccRCC and has great potential as a specific drug target.

Maintenance of internal homeostasis is an essential aspect of a normal cell. Tumoral cells alter their homeostasis to adapt to their intense function, including proliferation, invasion, migration, etc. Additionally, homeostasis alterations may also support tumor development. A cellular homeostasis gene set was applied in this study that comprises various enzymes, transporters, kinases, and cytokines.

Herein, in order to find the overlapping functions of SLC22A12, we analyzed three gene sets: kidney-specific genes, cellular homeostasis genes, and survival-related DEGs. From the 19 overlapping genes, 13 were transporters, including TRPV5, SLC22A12, SLC9A4, SLC9A3, ATP6V1B1, SLC12A1, ATP6V0D2, SLC12A3, SLC4A9, ATP6V0A4, CLDN16, SLC34A1, and ATP6V1G3. It is well-known that kidney epithelial cells frequently exchange substances through diverse transporters located in the plasma membrane to preserve cellular homeostasis. The results show that kidney cell tumorigenesis is associated with cellular transporters changes.

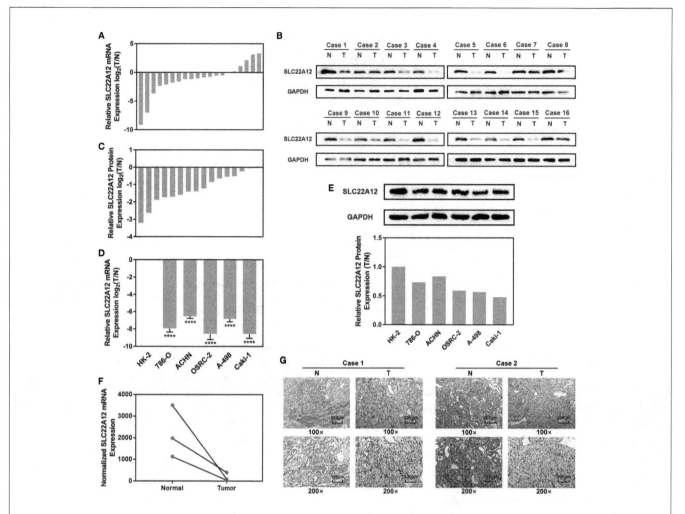

**FIGURE 5** | SLC22A12 was down-regulated in RCC cells and tissues compared to their corresponding control. Relative mRNA expression of SLC22A12 was lower in RCC **(A)** tissues and **(D)** cells than their normal control measured by qRT-PCR assays. Relative protein expression of SLC22A12 was lower in RCC **(B, C)** tissues and **(E)** cells than their normal control measured by immunoblotting tests. **(F)** Transcriptomic levels of SLC22A12 in normal and tumoral tissues gathered from Wuhan Union Hospital's cohort. **(G)** Representative images of immunohistochemical analyses suggested a lower SLC22A12 expression in tumoral tissue. ****$p < 0.0001$.

Using univariate and multivariate Cox regression analyses, SLC22A12 came out as an effective prognostic biomarker, independent of other clinicopathological features. RCC prognosis depends on clinicopathological characteristics that include clinical symptoms, pathology, and histology; hence, transcriptomic data should also be evaluated. Our further experiments preliminarily verified the inhibitory effect of SLC22A12 expression on ccRCC.

Previous studies on SLC22A12 focused on its function as uric acid transporter. Mutations in the SLC22A12 gene are associated with diseases with abnormal serum uric acid levels, including hypouricemia (43, 44), hyperuricemia (45–47), gout (43, 45, 48), and nephrolithiasis (49). Nevertheless, SLC22A12 is not the only uric acid transporter, and it does not transport solely uric acid. Although urate processing is affected when SLC22A12 is knocked out in mice (15, 50), it was soon discovered that this effect was limited since SLC2A9 and ABCG2 played a central role in uric acid transport (50–52). Metabolomic and transcriptomic studies on SLC22A12 knockout mice revealed that URAT1 has a

broader role in metabolism than previously recognized. According to Eraly et al., SLC22A12 directly interacted with urate, acetoacetate, lactate, 2-oxoglutarate, and pyruvate and affected the levels of many other essential substances, including calcium, norepinephrine, dopamine, D-fructose, glycerol, and cytidine (15). GO and KEGG analyses further proved that DEGs related to the expression of SLC22A12 were involved in the transportation of organic acid/anion, (mono)carboxylic acid, and sodium ion and hormone metabolic processes, which can affect cellular homeostasis. A similar pattern of results was obtained in the PPI network, where a strong confidence correlation was found between SLC22A12 and a large number of other transport proteins. SLC22A12 affects the organization of collagen-containing extracellular matrix. This may alter tumor growth and promote ccRCC cell proliferation, invasion, and migration, as well as activation of angiogenesis, which collectively determine the phenotype of the tumor. In summary, SLC22A12 may affect tumor progression and metastasis by affecting its cellular homeostasis.

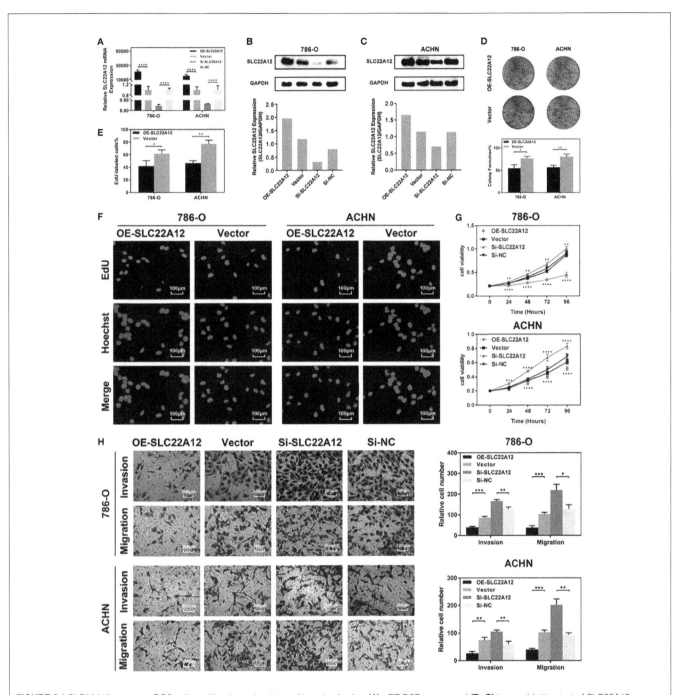

**FIGURE 6** | SLC22A12 promotes RCC cells proliferation, migration and invasion *in vitro*. **(A)** qRT-PCR assays and **(B, C)** immunoblotting test of SLC22A12 overexpression and knockdown in 786-O and ACHN cells. **(D)** Colony formation assays and **(E, F)** representative images (400X) of EdU assays of SLC22A12 overexpression in 786-O and ACHN cells. **(G)** CCK-8 assays examined the proliferation ability of 786-O and ACHN cells after SLC22A12 overexpression or knockdown with their corresponding negative controls. **(H)** Representative images (200X) of invasion and migration assays of 786-O and ACHN cells after SLC22A12 overexpression or knockdown with their corresponding negative controls. Data are presented as the mean ± standard deviation from three independent experiments. *p < 0.05; **p < 0.01; ***p < 0.001; ****p < 0.0001.

To the best of our knowledge, the present study is the first to disclose that SLC22A12 may be a potential diagnostic and prognostic biomarker that inhibits tumor progression in ccRCC. Furthermore, this study showed that SLC22A12 up-regulation attenuates RCC cell proliferation, migration, and invasion, further proving that SLC22A12 could be used as a therapeutic target for ccRCC. However, the present study presents some limitations. First, we only verified the anti-tumor effect of SLC22A12 through *in silico* and *in vitro* experiments, without relevant *in vivo* data. Second, we have not thoroughly studied the mechanism by which

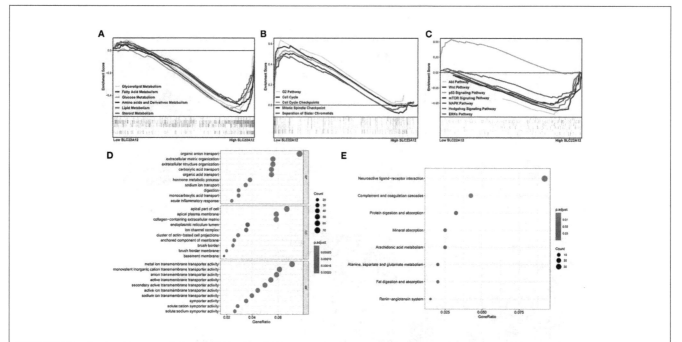

**FIGURE 7** | Functional enrichment analysis of SLC22A12 in ccRCC. Gene set enrichment analysis show that the activated genes are related to **(A)** multiple metabolic pathways, **(B)** cell cycle, **(C)** classic cancer-related signaling pathways. The functional differences between high-SLC22A12 and low- groups by **(D)** Gene Ontology analysis and **(E)** Kyoto Encyclopedia of Genes and Genomes.

SLC22A12 exerts its tumor suppressor effect. Our future research will be focused on overcoming such limitations.

In conclusion, this is the first study that demonstrates that high expression levels of SLC22A12 are associated with poor survival and low clinicopathological stage in patients with ccRCC. Furthermore, high expression levels of SLC22A12 may decrease the proliferation, migration, and invasion ability of RCC cells *in vitro*. The above results suggest that SLC22A12 is an important renal cancer biomarker and a potential highly-specific therapeutic target. SLC22A12 downregulation may impact cellular homeostasis, altering the survival of the tumor cells.

## AUTHOR CONTRIBUTIONS

XZ and XY designed the study. JX and YL carried out data acquisition and analysis. JX, YL, and JL performed the majority of the experiments. JX wrote the manuscript. JX, YS, TX and QW conducted immunohistochemistry analyses. DL, HL and XZ collected the clinical samples and managed the clinical data. JL and YS contributed to bioinformatics analysis. JX, ZX and HX supplemented the experiment based on the comments made by the reviewers. XZ and XY were involved in project management. HY and XZ supervised the study. All authors contributed to the article and approved the submitted version.

## REFERENCES

1. EAU Guidelines Office. European Association of Urology Guidelines on Renal Cell Carcinoma. Ljungberg B, Albiges L, Bedke J, Bex A, Capitanio U, Giles R, et al. *Arnhem* (2021). ISBN 978-94-92671-13-4
2. Srigley JR, Delahunt B, Eble JN, Egevad L, Epstein JI, Grignon D, et al. The International Society of Urological Pathology (ISUP) Vancouver Classification of Renal Neoplasia. *Am J Surg Pathol* (2013) 37(10):1469–89. doi: 10.1097/PAS.0b013e318299f2d1
3. Moch H, Cubilla AL, Humphrey PA, Reuter VE, Ulbright TM. The 2016 WHO Classification of Tumours of the Urinary System and Male Genital Organs-Part a: Renal, Penile, and Testicular Tumours. *Eur Urol* (2016) 70(1):93–105. doi: 10.1016/j.eururo.2016.02.029
4. Siegel RL, Miller KD, Jemal A. Cancer Statistics, 2020. *CA Cancer J Clin* (2020) 70(1):7–30. doi: 10.3322/caac.21590
5. *Cancer Stat Facts: Kidney and Renal Pelvis Cancer*. Available at: https://seer.cancer.gov/statfacts/html/kidrp.html.
6. Nakanishi T, Ohya K, Shimada S, Anzai N, Tamai I. Functional Cooperation of URAT1 (SLC22A12) and URATv1 (SLC2A9) in Renal Reabsorption of Urate. *Nephrol Dial Transplant* (2013) 28(3):603–11. doi: 10.1093/ndt/gfs574

7. Nigam SK. The SLC22 Transporter Family: A Paradigm for the Impact of Drug Transporters on Metabolic Pathways, Signaling, and Disease. *Annu Rev Pharmacol Toxicol* (2018) 58:663–87. doi: 10.1146/annurev-pharmtox-010617-052713
8. Lu Y, Nakanishi T, Tamai I. Functional Cooperation of SMCTs and URAT1 for Renal Reabsorption Transport of Urate. *Drug Metab Pharmacokinet* (2013) 28(2):153–8. doi: 10.2133/dmpk.DMPK-12-RG-070
9. Bobulescu IA, Moe OW. Renal Transport of Uric Acid: Evolving Concepts and Uncertainties. *Adv Chronic Kidney Dis* (2012) 19(6):358–71. doi: 10.1053/j.ackd.2012.07.009
10. Enomoto A, Endou H. Roles of Organic Anion Transporters (Oats) and a Urate Transporter (URAT1) in the Pathophysiology of Human Disease. *Clin Exp Nephrol* (2005) 9(3):195–205. doi: 10.1007/s10157-005-0368-5
11. Martovetsky G, Tee JB, Nigam SK. Hepatocyte Nuclear Factors 4alpha and 1alpha Regulate Kidney Developmental Expression of Drug-Metabolizing Enzymes and Drug Transporters. *Mol Pharmacol* (2013) 84(6):808–23. doi: 10.1124/mol.113.088229
12. Martovetsky G, Bush KT, Nigam SK. Kidney versus Liver Specification of SLC and ABC Drug Transporters, Tight Junction Molecules, and Biomarkers. *Drug Metab Dispos* (2016) 44(7):1050–60. doi: 10.1124/dmd.115.068254

13. Engelhart DC, Granados JC, Shi D, Saier MH, Baker ME, Abagyan R, et al. Systems Biology Analysis Reveals Eight SLC22 Transporter Subgroups, Including OATs, OCTs, and OCTNs. *Int J Mol Sci* (2020) 21(5):1791. doi: 10.3390/ijms21051791

14. Wempe MF, Lightner JW, Miller B, Iwen TJ, Rice PJ, Wakui S, et al. Potent human uric acid transporter I inhibitors: in vitro and in vivo metabolism and pharmacokinetic studies. *Drug Des Dev Ther* (2012) 6:323–39. doi: 10.2147/DDDT.S35805

15. Eraly SA, Liu HC, Jamshidi N, Nigam SK. Transcriptome-Based Reconstructions From the Murine Knockout Suggest Involvement of the Urate Transporter, URAT1 (slc22a12), in Novel Metabolic Pathways. *Biochem Biophys Rep* (2015) 3:51–61. doi: 10.1016/j.bbrep.2015.07.012

16. Ohtsu N, Anzai N, Fukutomi T, Kimura T, Sakurai H, Endou H. Human Renal Urate Transpoter URAT1 Mediates the Transport of Salicylate. *Nihon Jinzo Gakkai shi* (2010) 52(4):499–504.

17. Miura D, Anzai N, Jutabha P, Chanluang S, He X, Fukutomi T, et al. Human urate transporter 1 (hURAT1) mediates the transport of orotate. *J Physiol Sci* (2011) 61(3):253–7. doi: 10.1007/s12576-011-0136-0

18. Yang CH, Glover KP, Han X. Characterization of Cellular Uptake of Perfluorooctanoate Via Organic Anion-Transporting Polypeptide 1A2, Organic Anion Transporter 4, and Urate Transporter 1 for Their Potential Roles in Mediating Human Renal Reabsorption of Perfluorocarboxylates. *Toxicol Sci* (2010) 117(2):294–302. doi: 10.1093/toxsci/kfq219

19. Amin MB. American Joint Committee on Cancer. *American Cancer Society. AJCC cancer staging manual. Eight edition.* MB Amin, SB Edge, DM Gress, LR Meyer, editors. Chicago IL: American Joint Committee on Cancer, Springer (2017). p. xvii, 1024.

20. Edge SB. American Joint Committee on Cancer. *AJCC cancer staging manual. 7th ed.* New York: Springer (2010). p. xiv, 648.

21. Phipson B, Lee S, Majewski IJ, Alexander WS, Smyth GK. Robust Hyperparameter Estimation Protects Against Hypervariable Genes and Improves Power to Detect Differential Expression. *Ann Appl Stat* (2016) 10 (2):946–63. doi: 10.1214/16-AOAS920

22. Ritchie ME, Phipson B, Wu D, Hu YF, Law CW, Shi W, et al. limma powers differential expression analyses for RNA-sequencing and microarray studies. *Nucleic Acids Res* (2015) 43(7):e47. doi: 10.1093/nar/gkv007

23. Law CW, Chen YS, Shi W, Smyth GK. Voom: Precision Weights Unlock Linear Model Analysis Tools for RNA-seq Read Counts. *Genome Biol* (2014) 15(2):R29. doi: 10.1186/gb-2014-15-2-r29

24. Tang ZF, Li CW, Kang BX, Gao G, Li C, Zhang ZM. GEPIA: A Web Server for Cancer and Normal Gene Expression Profiling and Interactive Analyses. *Nucleic Acids Res* (2017) 45(W1):W98–W102. doi: 10.1093/nar/gkx247

25. Liu Y, Cheng G, Song Z, Xu T, Ruan H, Cao Q, et al. RAC2 acts as a prognostic biomarker and promotes the progression of clear cell renal cell carcinoma. *Int J Oncol* (2019) 55(3):645–56. doi: 10.3892/ijo.2019.4849

26. Subramanian A, Tamayo P, Mootha VK, Mukherjee S, Ebert BL, Gillette MA, et al. Gene set enrichment analysis: a knowledge-based approach for interpreting genome-wide expression profiles. *Proc Natl Acad Sci U S A* (2005) 102(43):15545–50. doi: 10.1073/pnas.0506580102

27. Xu J, Liu Y, Liu J, Xu T, Cheng G, Shou Y, et al. The Identification of Critical m(6)A RNA Methylation Regulators as Malignant Prognosis Factors in Prostate Adenocarcinoma. *Front Genet* (2020) 11:602485. doi: 10.3389/fgene.2020.602485

28. Ferlay J, Steliarova-Foucher E, Lortet-Tieulent J, Rosso S, Coebergh JW, Comber H, et al. Cancer incidence and mortality patterns in Europe: estimates for 40 countries in 2012. *Eur J Cancer* (2013) 49(6):1374–403. doi: 10.1016/j.ejca.2012.12.027

29. Capitanio U, Cloutier V, Zini L, Isbarn H, Jeldres C, Shariat SF, et al. A critical assessment of the prognostic value of clear cell, papillary and chromophobe histological subtypes in renal cell carcinoma: a population-based study. *Bju Int* (2009) 103(11):1496–500. doi: 10.1111/j.1464-410X.2008.08259.x

30. Keegan KA, Schupp CW, Chamie K, Hellenthal NJ, Evans CP, Koppie TM. Histopathology of Surgically Treated Renal Cell Carcinoma: Survival Differences by Subtype and Stage. *J Urol* (2012) 188(2):391–7. doi: 10.1016/j.juro.2012.04.006

31. Sun M, Bianchi M, Trinh QD, Hansen J, Abdollah F, Hanna N, et al. Comparison of partial vs radical nephrectomy with regard to other-cause mortality in T1 renal cell carcinoma among patients aged >/=75 years with multiple comorbidities. *Bju Int* (2013) 111(1):67–73. doi: 10.1111/j.1464-410X.2012.11254.x

32. Zini L, Perrotte P, Jeldres C, Capitanio U, Duclos A, Jolivet-Tremblay M, et al. A Population-Based Comparison of Survival After Nephrectomy vs Nonsurgical Management for Small Renal Masses. *Bju Int* (2009) 103 (7):899–904. doi: 10.1111/j.1464-410X.2008.08247.x

33. Xing M, Kokabi N, Zhang D, Ludwig JM, Kim HS. Comparative Effectiveness of Thermal Ablation, Surgical Resection, and Active Surveillance for T1a Renal Cell Carcinoma: A Surveillance, Epidemiology, and End Results (SEER)-Medicare-Linked Population Study. *Radiology* (2018) 288(1):81–90. doi: 10.1148/radiol.2018171407

34. Motzer RJ, Hutson TE, Tomczak P, Michaelson MD, Bukowski RM, Oudard S, et al. Overall survival and updated results for sunitinib compared with interferon alfa in patients with metastatic renal cell carcinoma. *J Clin Oncol* (2009) 27(22):3584–90. doi: 10.1200/JCO.2008.20.1293

35. Liu Y, Cheng G, Huang Z, Bao L, Liu J, Wang C, et al. Long noncoding RNA SNHG12 promotes tumour progression and sunitinib resistance by upregulating CDCA3 in renal cell carcinoma. *Cell Death Dis* (2020) 11 (7):515. doi: 10.1038/s41419-020-2713-8

36. Xiong Z, Xiao W, Bao L, Xiong W, Xiao H, Qu Y, et al. Tumor Cell "Slimming" Regulates Tumor Progression through PLCL1/UCP1-Mediated Lipid Browning. *Adv Sci (Weinh)* (2019) 6(10):1801862. doi: 10.1002/advs.201801862

37. Xiao W, Xiong Z, Xiong W, Yuan C, Xiao H, Ruan H, et al. Melatonin/PGC1A/UCP1 promotes tumor slimming and represses tumor progression by initiating autophagy and lipid browning. *J Pineal Res* (2019) 67(4):e12607. doi: 10.1111/jpi.12607

38. Meng T, Huang R, Zeng Z, Huang Z, Yin H, Jiao C, et al. Identification of Prognostic and Metastatic Alternative Splicing Signatures in Kidney Renal Clear Cell Carcinoma. *Front Bioeng Biotechnol* (2019) 7:270. doi: 10.3389/fbioe.2019.00270

39. Barth DA, Drula R, Ott L, Fabris L, Slaby O, Calin GA, et al. Circulating Non-coding RNAs in Renal Cell Carcinoma-Pathogenesis and Potential Implications as Clinical Biomarkers. *Front Cell Dev Biol* (2020) 8:828. doi: 10.3389/fcell.2020.00828

40. Ha M, Moon H, Choi D, Kang W, Kim JH, Lee KJ, et al. Prognostic Role of TMED3 in Clear Cell Renal Cell Carcinoma: A Retrospective Multi-Cohort Analysis. *Front Genet* (2019) 10:355. doi: 10.3389/fgene.2019.00355

41. Buder-Bakhaya K, Hassel JC. Biomarkers for Clinical Benefit of Immune Checkpoint Inhibitor Treatment-a Review From the Melanoma Perspective and Beyond. *Front Immunol* (2018) 9:1474. doi: 10.3389/fimmu.2018.01474

42. Zhao X, Ma Y, Cui J, Zhao H, Liu L, Wang Y, et al. FLCN Regulates HIF2alpha Nuclear Import and Proliferation of Clear Cell Renal Cell Carcinoma. *Front Mol Biosci* (2020) 7:121. doi: 10.3389/fmolb.2020.00121

43. So A, Thorens B. Uric Acid Transport and Disease. *J Clin Invest* (2010) 120 (6):1791–9. doi: 10.1172/JCI42344

44. Ichida K, Hosoyamada M, Kamatani N, Kamitsuji S, Hisatome I, Shibasaki T, et al. Age and origin of the G774A mutation in SLC22A12 causing renal hypouricemia in Japanese. *Clin Genet* (2008) 74(3):243–51. doi: 10.1111/j.1399-0004.2008.01021.x

45. Reginato AM, Mount DB, Yang I, Choi HK. The Genetics of Hyperuricaemia and Gout. *Nat Rev Rheumatol* (2012) 8(10):610–21. doi: 10.1038/nrrheum.2012.144

46. Ichida K, Hosoyamada M, Hisatome I, Enomoto A, Hikita M, Endou H, et al. Clinical and molecular analysis of patients with renal hypouricemia in Japan-influence of URAT1 gene on urinary urate excretion. *J Am Soc Nephrol* (2004) 15(1):164–73. doi: 10.1097/01.ASN.0000105320.04395.D0

47. Iwai N, Mino Y, Hosoyamada M, Tago N, Kokubo Y, Endou H. A High Prevalence of Renal Hypouricemia Caused by Inactive SLC22A12 in Japanese. *Kidney Int* (2004) 66(3):935–44. doi: 10.1111/j.1523-1755.2004.00839.x

48. Pavelcova K, Bohata J, Pavlikova M, Bubenikova E, Pavelka K, Stiburkova B. Evaluation of the Influence of Genetic Variants of SLC2A9 (GLUT9) and SLC22A12 (URAT1) on the Development of Hyperuricemia and Gout. *J Clin Med* (2020) 9(8):2510. doi: 10.3390/jcm9082510

49. Fu W, Li Q, Yao J, Zheng J, Lang L, Li W, et al. Protein expression of urate transporters in renal tissue of patients with uric acid nephrolithiasis. *Cell Biochem Biophysics* (2014) 70(1):449–54. doi: 10.1007/s12013-014-9939-y

50. Eraly SA, Vallon V, Rieg T, Gangoiti JA, Wikoff WR, Siuzdak G, et al. Multiple organic anion transporters contribute to net renal excretion of uric acid. *Physiol Genomics* (2008) 33(2):180 92. doi: 10.1152/physiolgenomics.00207.2007

# 18

# RNA Modification of N6-Methyladenosine Predicts Immune Phenotypes and Therapeutic Opportunities in Kidney Renal Clear Cell Carcinoma

Huihuang Li[1†], Jiao Hu[1†], Anze Yu[1,2], Belaydi Othmane[1], Tao Guo[1], Jinhui Liu[1], Chunliang Cheng[1], Jinbo Chen[1*] and Xiongbing Zu[1*]

[1] Department of Urology, Xiangya Hospital, Central South University, Changsha, China, [2] Immunobiology & Transplant Science Center, Houston Methodist Research Institute, Texas Medical Center, Houston, TX, United States

*Correspondence:
Xiongbing Zu
zuxbxyyy@126.com
Jinbo Chen
chenjinbo1989@yahoo.com

[†] These authors have contributed equally to this work

RNA modification of N6-methyladenosine (m6A) plays critical roles in various biological processes, such as cancer development, inflammation, and the anticancer immune response. However, the role played by a comprehensive m6A modification pattern in regulating anticancer immunity in kidney renal clear cell carcinoma (KIRC) has not been fully elucidated. In this study, we identified two independent m6A modification patterns with distinct biological functions, immunological characteristics, and prognoses in KIRC. Next, we developed an m6A score algorithm to quantify an individual's m6A modification pattern, which was independently validated in external cohorts. The m6A cluster 1 and low m6A score groups were characterized by a hot tumor microenvironment with an increased infiltration level of cytotoxic immune cells, higher tumor mutation burden, higher immune checkpoint expression, and decreased stroma-associated signature enrichment. In general, the m6A cluster 1 and low m6A score groups reflected an inflammatory phenotype, which may be more sensitive to anticancer immunotherapy. The m6A cluster 2 and high m6A score groups indicated a non-inflammatory phenotype, which may not be sensitive to immunotherapy but rather to targeted therapy. In this study, we first identified m6A clusters and m6A scores to elucidate immune phenotypes and to predict the prognosis and immunotherapy response in KIRC, which can guide urologists for making more precise clinical decisions.

Keywords: kidney renal clear cell carcinoma, N6-methyladenosine, immune phenotype, immune checkpoint blockade, tumor microenvironment

## INTRODUCTION

Kidney renal clear cell carcinoma (KIRC) is a common urinary cancer with increasing incidence (1). Despite advances in targeted therapy, the prognosis of patients with advanced KIRC remains extremely poor (1). The emergence of anticancer immune checkpoint blockade (ICB) therapy has revolutionized the treatment of advanced KIRC and significantly improved survival status (2–4). However, response rates to ICB in advanced KIRC are low, even though KIRC is an immunogenic cancer characterized by a high tumor mutation burden (TMB) (5). These low response rates indicated that there were some primary or secondary resistance mechanisms to ICB. Hence, to decrease adverse events and economic burden and identify the best candidates to receive ICB treatment, it is necessary to explore these resistance mechanisms and identify reliable predictors for response to ICB response.

RNA modification of N6-methyladenosine (m6A) is the most prominent and abundant RNA modification pattern in eukaryotic cells (6). M6A modification is a dynamically reversible process regulated by methyltransferases (writers), demethylases (erasers), and binding proteins (readers) (6, 7). Moreover, it plays a critical role in various biological processes, such as cancer occurrence, progression and inflammation (8, 9). Recently, m6A modification has been found to play an essential role in anticancer immune regulation (10). Wang et al. elucidated that depletion of METTL3/14 promoted secretion of IFN-γ, CXCL9, and CXCL10, subsequently inducing infiltration of CD8+ T cells, which overcomes resistance to ICB (11). In contrast, another study reported that METTL3 activates dendritic cells by increasing m6A levels of CD40, CD80, and TLR4, priming cytotoxic T lymphocyte activation (12). Interestingly, the same m6A writer gene (METTL3) exerted the opposite role in regulating anticancer immunity. FTO, an m6A eraser gene, promoted tumor immune evasion by increasing expression of immune checkpoint genes, such as LILRB4 and PD-1 (13, 14). Genetic depletion or pharmacological inhibition of FTO reactivates immune surveillance and overcomes resistance to ICB. Furthermore, Han et al. revealed the potential of YTHDF1 as a promising therapeutic target in anticancer immunotherapy (15). They demonstrated that genetic depletion of YTHDF1 significantly enhanced tumor antigen cross-presentation and CD8+ T cell priming. Therefore, m6A modification represents a potential emerging immunotherapy target and predictor of response to ICB response.

However, all of the studies above are confined to only one or two m6A modification genes because of technical limitations. As we all known, antitumor effect and tumor microenvironment (TME) can be regulated by numerous factors (16). Therefore, comprehensive analysis of multiple m6A regulators will improve our understanding of antitumor effect and TME. In this study, we comprehensively analyzed m6A modification patterns based on 24 m6A genes in KIRC. To the best of our knowledge, the number of m6A genes included in this manuscript is the largest reported to date. Additionally, we correlated m6A modification patterns with the immune phenotype and response to ICB for the first time.

## MATERIALS AND METHODS

**Figure 1** illustrates the mechanism diagram of our study and **Supplementary Figure 1** shows the workflow of our study.

### Data Retrieval and Preprocessing
#### Cancer Genome Altas (TCGA) Data
RNA sequencing data (FPKM value), mutation profiles, and clinical data for TCGA-KIRC were downloaded from the Genomic Data Commons (GDC, https://portal.gdc.cancer.gov/) using the R package TCGAbiolinks (17). The FPKM value was transformed into transcripts per kilobase million (TPM) value. After removing duplicated patients, we included 530 KIRC patients with full clinical information and 72 normal tissues for further analysis. The copy number variation (CNV) data, processed with the GISTIC algorithm, were downloaded from the UCSC Xena data portal (http://xena.ucsc.edu/). Somatic mutation data were analyzed using VarScan2 and used to calculate the tumor mutation burden (TMB). Microsatellite instability (MSI) data were collected from the supplementary files of Bonneville's study (18).

### Other Data Sources
A KIRC cohort (GSE22541) with detailed survival data and an RNA expression matrix was downloaded from GEO (https://www.ncbi.nlm.nih.gov/geo/). After removing 44 samples collected from pulmonary metastasis of KIRC, we included 24 samples collected from primary KIRC for further analysis. An immunotherapy cohort (PMID29301960) containing 33 KIRC patients was collected from the supplementary files of Miao's study (19). Based on the Creative Commons 3.0 License, an immunotherapy cohort (IMvigor210) containing 348 bladder cancer patients was obtained from http://research-pub.gene. com/IMvigor210CoreBiologies/ (20). Another immunotherapy cohort of melanoma (GSE78220) was downloaded from GEO. After removing one duplicated patient and one patient without follow-up time, we included 26 patients of GSE78220 for further analysis.

Detailed information on these cohorts is summarized in **Supplementary Table 1**.

## Unsupervised Clustering for 24 m6A Regulator Genes
We systematically identified 24 m6A regulator genes in our study from previous studies (16, 21). These m6A genes included eight writers (METTL3, METTL14, RBM15, RBM15B, WTAP, KIAA1429, CBLL1, and ZC3H13), two erasers (ALKBH5 and FTO), and 14 readers (YTHDC1, YTHDC2, YTHDF1, YTHDF2, YTHDF3, IGF2BP1, IGF2BP2, IGF2BP3, HNRNPA2B1, HNRNPC, FMR1, LRPPRC, ELAVL1, and EIF3A). Unsupervised clustering analysis was then conducted to comprehensively identify differential m6A modification patterns using the ConsensuClusterPlus package (22). Finally, the TCGA-KIRC cohort was classified into several clusters with different biological functions using a consensus clustering algorithm.

## Functional Analysis Between Different m6A Clusters
First, we downloaded 50 hallmark pathways from the MSigDB database (23). These 50 pathways systematically reflect the majority of the biological functions of humans. The GSVA algorithm was applied to calculate the enrichment scores of these pathways using the "GSVA" R package (24). Then, we analyzed difference in these pathways between different m6A clusters using the LIMMA algorithm (25). An adjusted $P < 0.05$ was considered statistically significant. Second, the limma R package's empirical Bayesian approach was applied to determine differentially expressed genes (DEGs) between different m6A

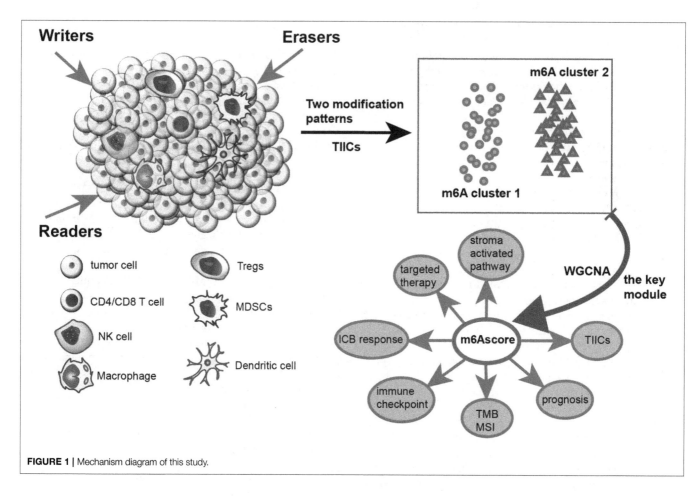

**FIGURE 1 |** Mechanism diagram of this study.

clusters. The significance criteria for determining DEGs were set as an adjusted $P < 0.05$ and $|logFC|>1$. Finally, we performed Gene Ontology (GO) and Kyoto Encyclopedia of Genes and Genomes (KEGG) analyses using the ClusterProfiler R package based on these DEGs.

## Depicting Immunological Characteristics of the TME in KIRC

The anticancer immune response, also called the cancer immunity cycle, is composed of seven key steps in the TME: the release and presentation of cancer cell antigens (Steps 1 and 2), the priming and activation of the immune system (Step 3), trafficking and infiltration of immune cells into tumors (Steps 4 and 5), and recognition and killing of cancer cells by T cells (Steps 6 and 7) (26). The activities of these seven steps were downloaded from http://biocc.hrbmu.edu.cn/TIP/ (27). Then, the single-sample gene-set enrichment analysis (ssGSEA) algorithm was used to quantify the relative abundance of tumor-infiltrating immune cells (TIICs) in the TME based on specific immune cell gene sets obtained from the study of Charoentong (**Supplementary Table 2**) (28). In addition, to avoid calculation errors caused by different algorithms and mark gene sets, we validated the infiltration level of TIICs using Cibersort-ABS, xCell and TIMER algorithm (29–31).

Mariathasan et al. revealed a set of gene signatures related to immune processes and stromal pathways, such as the CD8 T-effector signature, epithelial-mesenchymal transition (EMT) markers, and the panfibroblast TGF-b response signature (Pan-FTBRS) (20). We also collected 19 gene signatures related to the clinical response to the anti-PD-L1 agent atezolizumab (**Supplementary Table 3**). The ssGSEA algorithm was used to calculate the enrichment score of individuals.

## Generation of Co-expression Module Networks

The R package "WGCNA" was used to develop the gene co-expression network and to identify the m6A cluster-related module (32). First, TPM data from the TCGA-KIRC dataset were tested to determine whether they were good genes or samples. Then, the filtered genes were used to calculate the connection strength and to develop a scale-free network. The gradient method was used to test the scale independence and modules' average connectivity degree. The degree of independence was set as 0.85, and then we chose a suitable power value when the connectivity degree was relatively higher (33). Next, scale-free gene co-expression networks were generated using the selected power value. A heatmap was drawn to describe the interactions between different modules and clinical characteristics, and we chose the module that had the strongest relationship with the m6A cluster.

## Generation of m6A Score

An m6A score was developed to quantify the m6A modification pattern in an individual patient with KIRC. First, we conducted univariate Cox analysis on genes of the module that had the strongest relationship with the m6A cluster and subsequently identified those genes with prognostic value. Similar to previous studies, we then performed principal component analysis (PCA) on these prognostic genes to calculate principal component 1, which was used for m6A score calculation (16, 34).

$$m6A\ score = \sum PC1_i$$

where i is the selected gene.

## External Validation and Drug Sensitivity Analysis

To confirm the robustness of this m6A score, we validated the prognostic value and the association between the m6A score and immunological characteristics of the TME in an independent KIRC cohort (GSE22541).

The functions significantly differed among m6A clusters. We further compared the drug sensitivities between different m6A clusters. First, we collected 184 common anticancer drugs and their target genes from the DrugBank database (www.drugbank.ca). In addition, we validated the predictive value of the m6A score for the response to ICB in three external immunotherapy cohorts.

## Statistical Analysis

Correlations between m6A regulators, m6A score and cancer immunity cycle and m6A score and pathways related to the ICB response were explored by Spearman coefficients and distance correlation analyses. Continuous variables fitting a normal distribution between binary groups were compared using a $t$-test and presented as mean $\pm$ standard deviation (SD). Otherwise, the Mann-Whitney U test was applied. Chi-square or Fisher exact tests were used to compare differences between categorical variables. The "survcutpoint" function for the maximum rank statistic was applied to determine the optimal cutoff value of the m6A score. The survival curves for prognostic analyses of categorical variables were generated using the Kaplan-Meier method, while the log-rank test was applied to estimate the statistical significance. The hazard ratio (HR) for m6A regulators was calculated using univariate Cox regression model. The independent prognostic factor of m6A score was conducted using multivariate Cox regression model and the forestplot R package was used to visualize the results. The receiver operating characteristic (ROC) curve and area under the curve (AUC) were conducted to assess the specificity and sensitivity of m6A score using time ROC R package. The mutations of m6A regulators and mutation profiles between high and low m6A score groups were visualized using maftools R package. The level of significance was set at $P < 0.05$, and all statistical tests were two-sided. Finally, all statistical data analyses were implemented using R software, version 3.6.3 (http://www.r-project.org).

## RESULTS

## Multi-Omics Analysis of m6A Genes in KIRC

We first analyzed the expression patterns of 24 m6A genes in KIRC and normal tissues. Interestingly, the majority of m6A writers and readers, such as METTL14, EIF3A, YTHDC1, YTHDF1, and YTHDF2, were significantly downregulated in KIRC compared to normal tissues. In contrast, expression of two m6A eraser genes (FTO and ALKBH5) was significantly higher in KIRC (**Figure 2A**). This expression imbalance between m6A writer and eraser genes may lead to abnormal m6A modification patterns and consequently promote the development of KIRC. Similarly, most of the m6A genes were prognostic factors. METTL14, RBM15, KIAA1429, CBLL1, YTHDC2, ZC3H13, FMR1, RBM15B, YTHDC1, FTO, LRPPRC, YTHDF2, YTHDF3, and EIF3A were favorable prognostic factors. On the other hand, METTL3, IGF2BP1, IGF2BP2, IGF2BP3, and HNRNPA2B1 were adverse prognostic factors (**Figure 2B**). Based on the expression of these 24 m6A genes, we could completely distinguish KIRC samples from normal samples (**Figure 2C**). These results suggested that m6A genes are potential diagnostic and prognostic predictors in KIRC.

Next, we assessed the CNV and mutation profiles of 24 m6A genes. Analysis of CNV data revealed prevalent CNV alterations in 24 m6A genes, and most were focused on amplification of YTHDC2, while RBM15 and RBM15B had the highest frequency of CNV deletion (**Figure 2D**). However, mutations of m6A genes were not frequent. Among 417 KIRC samples, only 66 (15.83%) exhibited mutations in m6A genes. ZC3H13 exhibited the highest mutation frequency at 4%, followed by YTHDC2 (2%) (**Figure 2E**). Finally, the close connections between the majority of m6A genes laid the foundation for the subsequent m6A clustering analysis (**Figure 2F**, **Supplementary Table 4**).

## Depicting m6A Clusters and Correlating Them With Biological Functions

**Figure 3A** shows the comprehensive landscapes of 24 m6A genes concerning their prognostic value, correlations, and groups. Most of them were prognostic factors and were significantly correlated with each other, which prompted us to perform a comprehensive unsupervised clustering analysis based on these 24 m6A gene expression profiles. The results were robust when the TCGA-KIRC cohort was divided into two independent clusters. One hundred six patients were classified into m6A cluster 1, whereas the remaining 423 patients were classified into m6A cluster 2. m6A cluster 1 exhibited a significantly poorer prognosis ($P = 0.00057$) (**Figure 3B**). The DEGs between m6A clusters are displayed in a heatmap and volcano plot (**Figures 3C,D**, **Supplementary Table 5**). The results of GO analysis suggested that these DEGs were enriched in several biological processes, including organic anion transport, metal ion transmembrane transporter activity,

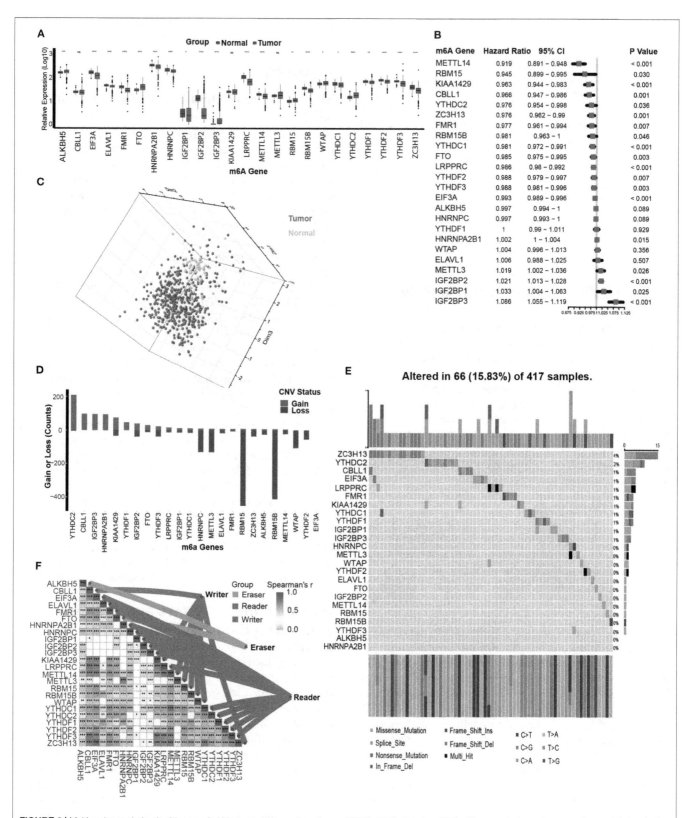

**FIGURE 2 |** Multi-omics analysis of m6A genes in kidney renal clear cell carcinoma (KIRC). **(A)** Expression of 24 m6A genes between tumor and normal tissues in the TCGA-KIRC dataset. Tumor, red; Normal, blue. **(B)** The prognostic analyses for 24 m6A genes in the TCGA-KIRC dataset using the univariate Cox regression model. **(C)** Principal component analysis (PCA) of the expression profiles of 24 m6A genes between tumor and normal tissues in the TCGA-KIRC dataset. Tumor, red;

*(Continued)*

FIGURE 2 | Normal, green. **(D)** The copy number variation (CNV) frequency of 24 m6A genes in the TCGA-KIRC dataset. The height of the column represents the count, and the color represents gains or losses. Gains, red; Losses, blue. **(E)** The mutation frequency of 24 m6A genes in 417 patients with kidney clear cell carcinoma from the TCGA-KIRC cohort. Column presents individual patients. The upper bar plot represents TMB. The number on the right represents the mutation frequency in each regulator. The right bar plot represents the proportion of each variant type. The stacked bar plot below represents the fraction of conversions in each sample. **(F)** Expression correlations between 24 m6A regulators in the TCGA-KIRC dataset using Spearman analyses. Eraser, green; Reader, brown; Writer, purple (ns, Not Significant; *$P < 0.05$; **$P < 0.01$; ***$P < 0.001$; ****$P < 0.0001$).

collagen-containing extracellular matrix, and cellular divalent inorganic cation homeostasis (**Supplementary Figures 2A–C, Supplementary Table 6**). The results of KEGG analysis indicated that these DEGs were enriched in pathways such as neuroactive ligand-receptor interaction, bile secretion, vascular smooth muscle contraction, mineral absorption, complement and coagulation cascades, serotonergic synapse, protein digestion and absorption, and leukocyte transendothelial migration (**Supplementary Figure 2D, Supplementary Table 7**). Finally, the enrichment scores of many hallmark signatures significantly differed between the two clusters. As shown in **Figure 3E**, TGF-beta signaling, Wnt-beta catenin signaling, protein secretion, PI3K-Akt-Mtor signaling, androgen response, heme metabolism, mitotic spindle, and Notch signaling were enriched in m6A cluster 2. In contrast, spermatogenesis, estrogen response late, and KRAS signaling DN were enriched in m6A cluster 1 (**Figure 3E, Supplementary Table 8**).

## m6A Clusters Correlate With Immune Phenotypes and Immunotherapy-Related Signatures

We next comprehensively correlated the m6A clusters with immune phenotypes. First, we focused on the activities of anticancer immunity cycles. The activity of priming and activation of the immune system of m6A cluster 1 was significantly higher than that of m6A cluster 2, while the activities of releasing and presenting cancer cell antigens were lower (**Figure 4A**). In addition, the activities of T cell recruiting, B cell recruiting, and dendritic cell recruiting were consistently higher in m6A cluster 1 (**Figure 4A**). Finally, activities of recognition of cancer cells by T cells were higher in m6A cluster 1. To confirm these findings, we directly compared the infiltration level of tumor-infiltrating immune cells between m6A clusters. As expected, the abundance of several antitumor immune cells, such as activated CD8 T cells, activated CD4 T cells, CD56bright natural killer cells and type 17 T helper cell, was significantly higher in m6A cluster 1 than in m6A cluster 2 (**Figure 4B**). However, the abundance of the most recognized protumor immune cells, including regulatory T cells, immature dendritic cells, and plasmacytoid dendritic cells, was significantly downregulated in m6A cluster 1 (**Figure 4B**). Based on these results, we proposed that m6A cluster 1 may be an inflammatory immune phenotype, while m6A cluster 2 may be a non-inflammatory phenotype. Previous research demonstrated that stroma-associated pathways, such as EMT and Pan-FTBRS signatures, inhibited the anticancer immunity in TME (20). Here, EMT1, EMT3, and Pan-F-TBRS enrichment

scores were significantly downregulated in m6A cluster 1 (**Figure 4C**).

Inflammatory tumor phenotypes are more sensitive to ICB (35, 36). Consistently, pathways that were positively related to the ICB response, such as RNA degradation, the cell cycle, and DNA replication, were enriched in m6A cluster 1 (inflammatory phenotype). In contrast, the pathway cytokine-cytokine receptor interaction negatively related to the ICB response was enriched in m6A cluster 2 (non-inflammatory phenotype) (**Figure 4D**). Therefore, we confirmed that m6A cluster 1 might represent an inflamed phenotype from the aspect of immunotherapy response.

## Developing m6A Scores and Correlating Them With Immune Phenotypes

All tumor data from the TCGA-KIRC dataset were used to develop the gene co-expression network and to identify m6A cluster-related modules. All KIRC samples with full clinical characteristics were included in the co-expression analysis (**Figure 5A**). The "WGCNA" package was used to allocate genes with similar expression patterns into different modules. In this study, we chose the soft threshold as 7 (scale-free $R^2 = 0.85$) to develop a scale-free network. As shown in **Figure 5B**, a total of 29 modules were recognized. The modules with the most significant association with clinical characteristics had the greatest biological meanings. The turquoise module was found to have the highest association with the m6A cluster ($r = 0.64$, $p = 4e-64$; **Figure 5C**). We chose the turquoise module to be analyzed in the subsequent steps, and the turquoise module was also related to tumor grade and stage. The genes in the turquoise modules were significantly co-expressed (cor = 0.81, $P < 1e-200$; **Figure 5D**). Among these genes, 2,214 were significantly related to prognosis (**Supplementary Table 9**). Then, the m6A score was calculated for individuals using the PCA algorithm.

m6A score was lower in m6A cluster 1 (**Figure 6A**). Similar to the performance of m6A cluster 1, patients in the low m6A score group exhibited poorer prognosis than patients in the high m6A score group (**Figure 6B**). Also, m6A score still remained an independent prognosis factor in multivariate Cox regression analysis ($p = 0.01$, **Supplementary Figure 3A**). The Q-Q plot of the model showed that the residuals are approximately normally distributed (**Supplementary Figure 3B**) and the AUC at 5 years showed that the predictive accuracy of m6a score was comparative to tumor stage (**Supplementary Figure 3C**). There were consistent correlations between the m6A score and the immune phenotype. The CD8 T effector signatures were enriched in the low m6A score group (**Figure 6C**). The abundance of antitumor immune cells, including activated CD8 T cells, activated CD4 T cells, activated dendritic cells, CD56bright natural killer cells, central memory CD4 T cells,

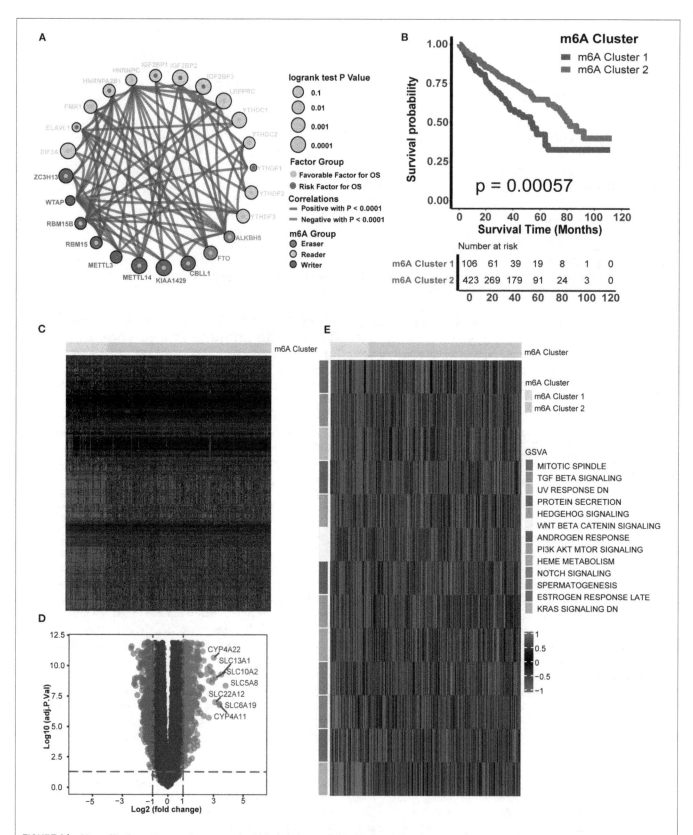

**FIGURE 3 |** m6A modification patterns and corresponding biological characteristics. **(A)**. Correlations between 24 m6A genes in KIRC. The size of the circle represents the prognosis of each gene, and values were calculated by the log-rank test, which ranged from 0.1 to 0.0001. Green dots represent favorable factors for

*(Continued)*

FIGURE 3 | overall survival, while purple dots in the circle represent risk factors for overall survival. The color of the lines shows the correlation between regulators. Negative correlation, blue; Positive correlation, red. **(B)** Survival analysis for m6A clusters from the TCGA-KIRC dataset. m6A cluster 1 is shown in blue and m6A cluster 2 is shown in red. **(C)** A heatmap was drawn based on the differentially expressed genes between m6A clusters 1 and 2. Differentially expressed genes with higher expression are shown in red, and genes with lower expression are shown in blue. **(D)** A volcano plot was drawn based on the differentially expressed genes between m6A clusters 1 and 2. Differentially expressed genes with log2(fold change) higher than 1 were shown in red while the genes lower than −1 were shown in blue, and the genes without different expression were shown in gray. **(E)** GSVA analysis showed the activation (red) or inhibition (blue) of biological pathways between m6A modification patterns.

natural killer T cells, type 1 T helper cells, and type 17 T helper cells was significantly upregulated in the low m6A score group (**Figure 6D**). However, the abundance of protumor immune cells, including immature dendritic cells and plasmacytoid dendritic cells, was downregulated in the low m6A score group (**Figure 6D**). We validated the infiltration level of TIICs using Cibersort-ABS, xCell, and TIMER algorithm (**Supplementary Figures 4–6**). Generally, most of the algorithms showed that m6A score was negatively correlated with anti-tumor immune cells, including CD8 T cells, CD4 T cells, and natural killer T cell. Except TIMER algorithm showed that CD8 T cells was positively correlated with m6A score. This could be the calculation errors caused by different algorithms and mark gene sets. In addition, the EMT1 and EMT3 pathways were enriched in the high m6A score group (**Figure 6E**). Meanwhile, the m6A score was negatively related to the activities of several critical anticancer immunity cycles, such as priming and activation, T cell recruiting, CD8 T cell recruiting, CD4 T cell recruiting, dendritic cell recruiting, Th17 cell recruiting, and infiltration of immune cells into tumors (**Figure 6F, Supplementary Table 10**). These findings suggested that the low m6A score group may have an inflammatory phenotype.

As expected, m6A scores were negatively correlated with pathways that were positively related to the ICB response, such as RNA degradation, cell cycle, and DNA replication. In contrast, the m6A score was positively related to the cytokine-cytokine receptor interaction pathway, which was negatively related to the ICB response (**Figure 6F, Supplementary Table 11**). Finally, several common immune checkpoints, such as CTLA-4, PD-1, LAG-3, LAALS3, and TIGIT, were highly expressed in the low m6A score group (**Figure 6G**).

In summary, the m6A score predicts the immune phenotype and clinical response to ICB.

## Mutation Profiles of m6A Score Groups

Genomic mutations are a prominent factor in initiating malignancy. Here, we analyzed distribution differences in the top 20 somatic mutations between m6A score groups using the maftools R package. The most common mutations in KIRC were VHL and PBRM1. There was no difference in the VHL mutation between the m6A score groups (**Figure 7A**). The mutation frequencies of TTN (32 vs. 23%), SETD2 (19 vs. 9%), BAP1 (16 vs. 7%), and MUC16 (15 vs. 7%) were markedly higher in the low m6A score group suggesting that these mutations may be m6A score-specific mutations in KIRC. In general, a more extensive tumor mutation burden was presented in the low m6A score group than in the high m6A score group (97.4 vs. 90.67%) (**Figure 7A**). Consequently, the TMB quantification

analysis revealed that the low m6A score group was markedly correlated with a higher TMB (**Figure 7B**). However, there was no difference in MSI status between the two m6A score groups (**Figure 7C**).

## External Validation of the m6A Score in GSE22541

Similar to the performance of the m6A score in the TCGA-KIRC cohort, we found that the low m6A score group had a poorer prognosis in the GSE22541 cohort as well (**Figure 8A**). Meanwhile, the m6A score was negatively correlated with the activities of many anticancer immunity cycles, such as the recognition of cancer cells by T cells (**Figure 8B, Supplementary Table 12**). Furthermore, the infiltration levels of activated CD8 T cells, activated CD4 T cells, activated dendritic cells, central memory CD8 T cells, natural killer T cells, type 1 T helper cells, and type 17 T helper cells were significantly higher in the low m6A score group (**Figure 8C**). Finally, the m6A score was negatively related to most pathways that predicted higher ICB response rates (**Figure 8B, Supplementary Table 13**). These results confirmed that the m6A score might be a robust predictor of immune phenotype, prognosis, and ICB response.

## Role of the m6A Score in Predicting the Response to Targeted Therapy and Immunotherapy

We further explored the role of the m6A score in guiding clinical decision making in KIRC. First, we found that the sensitivities of many anticancer drugs were significantly different between m6A score groups (**Supplementary Table 14**). Targeted therapy was the first-line treatment option for advanced KIRC. Here, we collected the targeted therapy drugs used in KIRC and their targeted genes from the DrugBank database: sorafenib with its targeted genes including BRAF, FLT1, FLT3, FLT4, KDR, KIT, and RAF1; sunitinib with its targeted genes including CSF1R, FLT1, FLT3, FLT4, KDR, and RET; pazopanib with its targeted gene SH2B3; and bevacizumab with its targeted gene VEGFA. Interestingly, all targeted therapy drug sensitivities were significantly lower in the low m6A score group (**Figure 9A**). These results indicate that the m6A score may identify suitable candidates to receive targeted therapy.

Although findings from TCGA-KIRC and GSE22541 cohorts suggested that the m6A score predicts ICB response, it would be more convincing to validate these results in cohorts that received ICB. First, in a KIRC cohort that received anti-PD-1 therapy (nivolumab), we demonstrated that the clinical benefit rate was higher in the low m6A score group than in the high m6A score group ($p = 0.26$; **Figure 9B**). Regrettably, because of

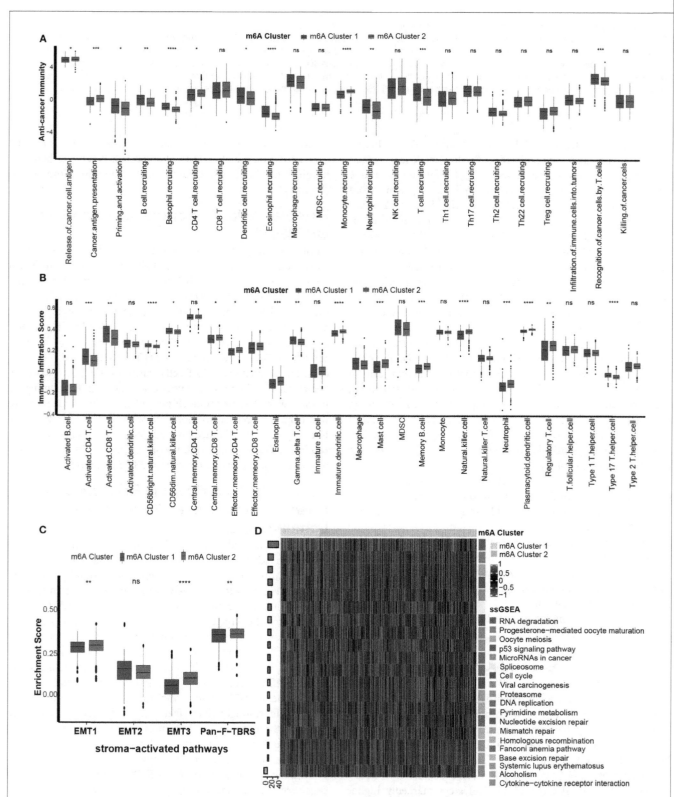

**FIGURE 4** | Differences in immunological characteristics between m6A clusters. **(A)** Activities of cancer immunity cycles between the two distinct m6A modification patterns. m6A cluster 1, blue; m6A cluster 2, red. **(B)** TME immune cell infiltration scores between the two distinct m6A modification patterns. m6A cluster 1, blue; m6A cluster 2, red. **(C)** Differences in stroma-activated pathways between the two distinct m6A modification patterns. m6A cluster 1, blue; m6A cluster 2, red. **(D)** Differences in immunotherapy-predicted pathways between the two m6A clusters. Left bar plots represent log10 p-values, red bars represent activated pathways, and blue bars represent inhibited pathways. The colors of the right bar plots represent different pathways, as shown in the legend (ns, Not Significant; *$P < 0.05$; **$P < 0.01$; ***$P < 0.001$; ****$P < 0.0001$).

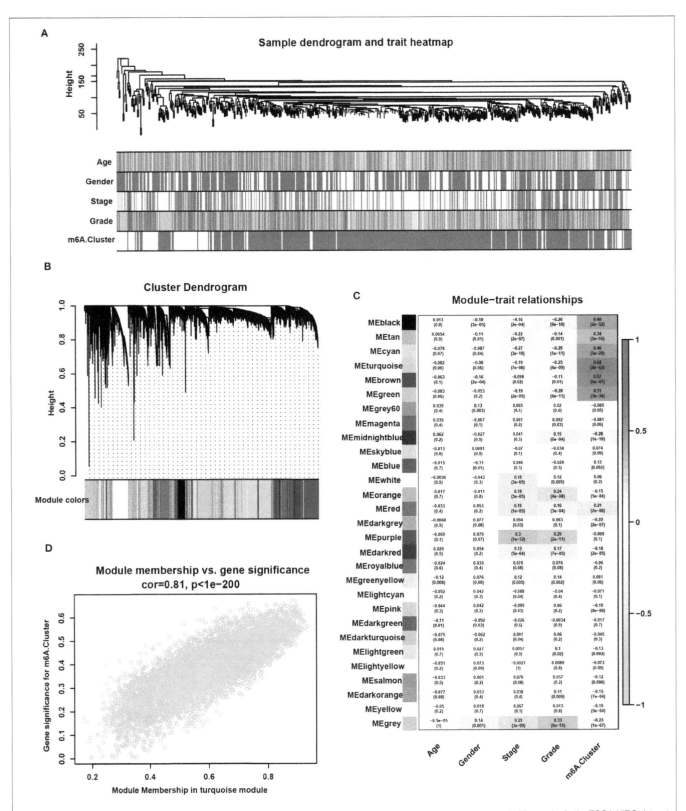

**FIGURE 5 |** Detection and validation of m6A modification pattern-related modules by WGCNA. **(A)** Clustering dendrogram of 530 samples in the TCGA-KIRC dataset and heatmaps of clinical traits. The color intensity was related to older age, male sex, higher tumor stage, higher tumor grade, and m6A cluster 2. **(B)** Clustering dendrogram of differentially expressed genes. The dissimilarity was based on the topological overlap, and different modules were assigned to different colors. **(C)** Heatmap of the correlation between different gene modules and clinical characteristics. Red represents a positive correlation, and blue represents a negative correlation. **(D)** Scatter plot of membership in the turquoise module.

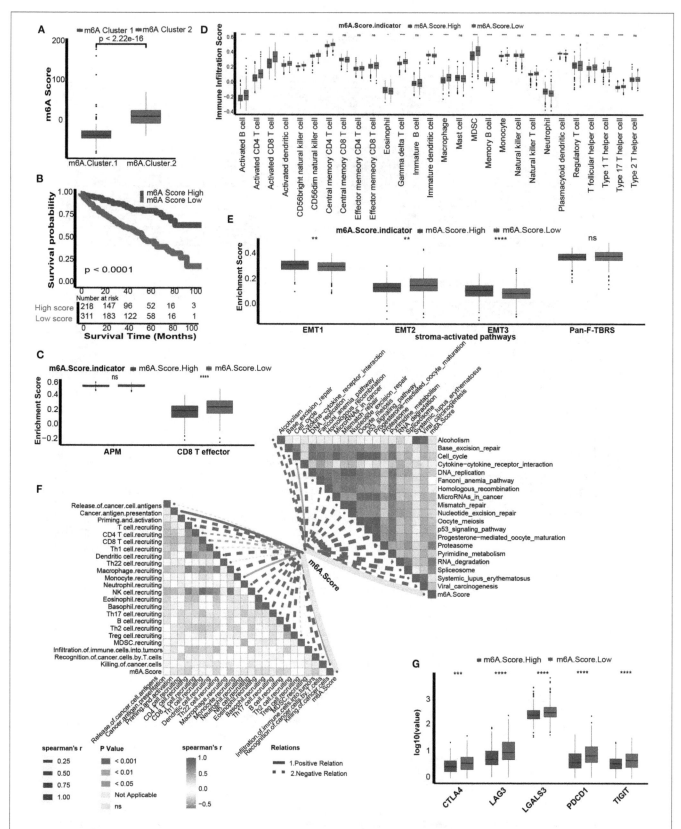

**FIGURE 6 |** Differences in prognosis and immunological characteristics between the m6A score groups. **(A)** The m6A score in the two distinct m6A modification patterns. Kruskal-Wallis tests to calculate significant differences. **(B)** Survival analyses for the low (311 cases) and the high (218 cases) m6A score patient groups in

*(Continued)*

FIGURE 6 | the TCGA-KIRC cohort using Kaplan-Meier curves. m6A Score High, blue; m6A Score Low, red. (C) Activation of antigen processing machinery (APM) and CD8T effector pathways between the m6A Score group. M6A Score High, blue; m6A Score Low, red. (D) TME immune cell infiltration scores between the m6A score groups. M6A Score High, blue; m6A Score Low, red. (E) Activation of stroma-activated pathways in the m6A score group. M6A Score High, blue; M6A Score Low, red. (F) Spearman correlation analysis of m6A scores with activities of cancer immunity cycles (left) and immune-related pathways analyzed by ssGSEA (right). The thickness of the lines represents the relation strength. The different colors of the lines represent different p-values. The red bar plots represent a positive correlation, and the blue bar plots represent a negative correlation. (G) The histogram of immune checkpoint gene expression between the m6A score groups. M6A Score High, blue; m6A Score Low, red (ns, Not Significant; *P < 0.05; **P < 0.01; ***P < 0.001; ****P < 0.0001).

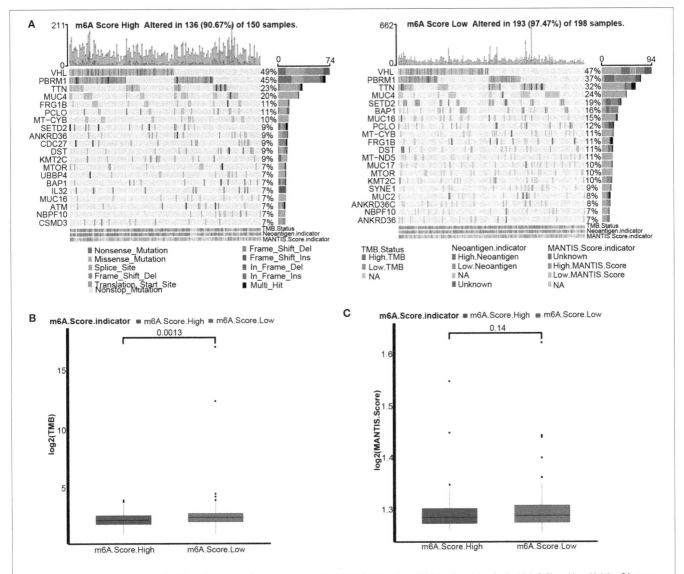

FIGURE 7 | Tumor mutation burden (TMB) analyses of m6A score groups in the TCGA-KIRC cohort. (A) Mutation status in the high (left) and low (right) m6A score groups of the TCGA-KIRC dataset. Each column is related to individual patients. Upper bar plots represent TMB, right bar plots represent variant type proportions, and lower bar plots represent conversions or each sample. (B) The histogram of log2(TMB) between the m6A score groups. M6A Score High, blue; m6A Score Low, red. (C) The histogram of log2(MANTIS Score) between the m6A score groups. M6A Score High, blue; m6A Score Low, red.

the small sample size, we didn't find significantly differences. The prognosis of the low m6A score group was better than in the high m6A score group ($p = 0.039$; **Figure 9C**). It is worth noting that this survival outcome was contrary to the results showing that the prognosis of the low m6A score group was worse in the TCGA-KIRC and GSE22541 cohorts. These differences in outcome were

due to the response rate of immunotherapy being more likely to determine the prognosis of an immunotherapy cohort when compared to other prognostic risk factors, such as the m6A score. Additionally, we successfully validated the role of the m6A score in predicting the response to ICB in two other cancer cohorts, including the IMvigor210 cohort (bladder cancer) and GSE78220

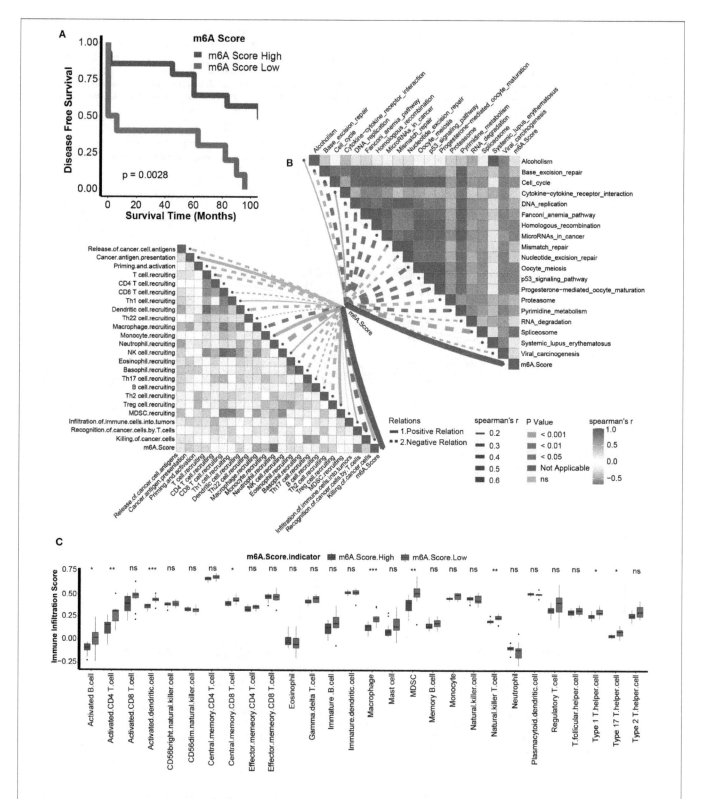

**FIGURE 8** | Validation of m6A score in the GSE22541 dataset. **(A)** Survival analyses for the low and high m6A score patient groups in the GSE22541 dataset using Kaplan-Meier curves. M6A Score High, blue; m6A Score Low, red. **(B)** Spearman correlation analysis of m6A scores with activities of cancer immunity cycles (left) and immune-related pathways analyzed by ssGSEA (right) in the GSE22541 dataset. The thickness of the lines represents the relation strength. The different colors of the lines represent different *p*-values. The red bar plots represent a positive correlation, and the blue bar plots represent a negative correlation. **(C)** TME immune cell infiltration scores between the m6A score groups in the GSE22541 dataset. M6A Score High, blue; m6A Score Low, red (ns, Not Significant; *P < 0.05; **P < 0.01; ***P < 0.001).

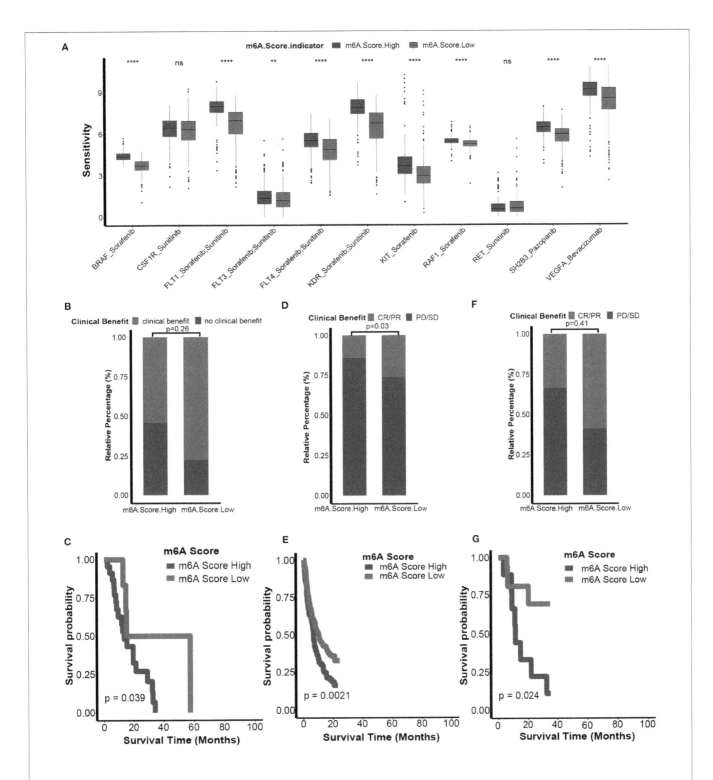

**FIGURE 9 |** Role of m6A score in predicting sensitivities of targeted therapy and immunotherapy. **(A)** The differences in sensitivities of targeted therapy between m6A score groups by analyzing data from the DrugBank dataset. m6A Score High, blue; m6A Score Low, red. **(B)** Proportion of patients with clinical benefit to immunotherapy between the different m6A score groups in an RCC immunotherapy dataset (PMID29301960). **(C)** Survival analyses for the low and high m6A score patient groups in the RCCICI dataset using Kaplan-Meier curves. **(D)** Proportion of patients with clinical benefit to immunotherapy between the different m6A score groups in IMvigor210 dataset. **(E)** Survival analyses for the low and high m6A score patient groups in the IMvigor210 dataset using Kaplan-Meier curves. **(F)** Proportion of patients with clinical benefit to immunotherapy between the different m6A score groups in the GSE78220 dataset. **(G)** Survival analyses for the low and high m6A score patient groups in the GSE78220 dataset using Kaplan-Meier curves (CR, complete response; PR, partial response; SD, stable disease; PD, progressive disease; ns, Not Significant; $^{**}P < 0.01$; $^{****}P < 0.0001$).

cohort (melanoma) (**Figures 9D–G**). These findings revealed that this m6A score may represent a generalized predictor for response to ICB in other cancer types as well.

## DISCUSSION

m6A modification plays a critical role in regulating the immune status of the TME in various cancers (10). However, the role of m6A in modifying immune characteristics in KIRC needs to be further explored. In this manuscript, we identified two independent m6A modification patterns with distinct biological functions, immunological characteristics, and prognoses. Then, we developed an m6A score algorithm to quantify an individual's m6A modification pattern, which was independently validated in external cohorts.

There are some studies reporting the function of m6A modification in the progression, prognosis and the TME in KIRC, indicating the potential key role of m6A regulators in KIRC. Strick et al. reported that ALKBH5 and FTO were significantly downregulated in KIRC compared to normal tissues, and their low expression predicted poorer prognosis (37). However, Zhang et al. found that ALKBH5 was highly expressed in KIRC compared to normal tissues, and high expression of ALKBH5 promoted progression of KIRC (38). Notably, a simple analysis of a single m6A gene in KIRC may lead to obvious contradictory results. These differences in results might be because m6A modification is an extremely complex process that is regulated by writers, erasers, and readers. Therefore, systematic analysis of all m6A genes may more comprehensively reflect the m6A modification pattern in the TME. To date, there are some studies performing systematic analysis of multiple m6A genes using bioinformatics algorithms and reported that the m6A modification pattern predicted progression and prognosis of KIRC. Chen et al. systematically analyzed the global m6A modification pattern in KIRC and correlated it with cancer-related gene expressions (39). Zhou et al. found a close relationship between genetic alterations of m6A regulators with clinical characteristics in KIRC (40). Zhang et al. (41), Wang et al. (42), and Chen et al. (43) systematically analyzed the m6A regulators in KIRC and developed a METTL3 and METTL14 based risk score for the prognosis of KIRC. Zhao et al. developed a risk score based on three m6A regulators, including METTL3, METTL14, and HNRNPA2B1 (44). However, all of them have not correlated m6A regulators with TME. Fang et al. systematically analyzed 16 m6A regulators and correlated them with TME. Also, they developed a four-m6A-regulators based risk score only for the prognosis (45). But they have not analyzed the relationship between m6A regulators and ICB response. In addition, their risk score can't predict the immune phenotypes of KIRC and quantify the m6A modification pattern of an individual patient.

Abnormal m6A modification patterns promote the development of cancers (8). In our study, we found that the expression profiles between m6A writers and m6A erasers were imbalanced. Theoretically, these imbalanced expression profiles may cause abnormal m6A modification patterns and consequently lead to KIRC development. In addition,

the majority of m6A genes were related to prognosis. More importantly, these m6A genes were related to each other and formed a close interaction network. These findings prompted us to perform a comprehensive clustering analysis instead of analyzing the role of a single m6A gene.

Zhang et al. identified three different m6A clusters in gastric cancer based on 21 m6A genes. After analyzing the landscapes of immunological characteristics, prognosis, and other functions, they connected the three m6A clusters to different immune phenotypes, including inflammatory, excluded, and deserted phenotypes (16). Indeed, the excluded and deserted phenotypes can be unified into a non-inflammatory phenotype. In our study, we similarly identified two m6A clusters that reflected different immune phenotypes.

The TME is a complex system composed of cancer cells, various TIICs, and an extracellular matrix. These TIICs play a distinct role in regulating anticancer immunity. In general, CD8 T cells and natural killer cells were the most important cytotoxic cells that killed tumor cells. Other antitumor TIICs included CD4 T cells, type 1 T helper cells, and type 17 T helper cells (46). Regulatory T cells are recognized as the most important protumor TIICs (46). In addition, there are various immunomodulators, including chemokines, MHC, immune stimulators, immune inhibitors, and receptors (28). The comprehensive effects of these different TIICs and immunomodulators determine the direction of the anticancer immune response. The activities of the anticancer immune response determine the fate of cancer cells. In this study, T cell recruitment activity was higher in m6A cluster 1. Consequently, activated CD8 T cells, activated CD4 T cells, natural killer cells, and type 17 T helper cells were enriched in m6A cluster 1. In contrast, regulatory T cells were enriched in m6A cluster 2. Stromal pathways, such as EMT and Pan-FTBRS signatures, may inhibit anticancer immunity (20). Consistently, the enrichment score of these immune-inhibiting pathways was lower in m6A cluster 1. This evidence indicates that the m6A cluster 1 belongs to an inflammatory phenotype, while m6A cluster 2 reflected a non-inflammatory phenotype. Additionally, pathways that were positively related to the ICB response were enriched in the m6A cluster 1. Therefore, m6A cluster 1 was theoretically more sensitive to ICB.

We developed the m6A score using WGCNA and PCA algorithms. The WGCNA algorithm identified gene sets that are highly related to the specific biological behavior and clinical phenotype of a cohort (32). Genes in these sets are highly correlated with each other. Based on this, the PCA algorithm further calculated the score of genes with the highest correlation with the m6A cluster, while decreasing the contributions from other factors (16, 34). As a result, the m6A score accurately reflected the m6A clusters. In our study, the low m6A score group indicated m6A cluster 1, while the high m6A score group indicated m6A cluster 2. We then evaluated the value of the m6A score in predicting immune phenotypes, prognosis, and ICB response. In general, the m6A score was negatively related to anticancer immunity in the TME. Therefore, the low m6A score group indicated an inflamed phenotype. As a result, the

RNA Modification of N6-Methyladenosine Predicts Immune Phenotypes and Therapeutic Opportunities in Kidney...

209

m6A score was negatively related to pathways that were positively related to ICB response.

Theoretically, patients with an inflammatory phenotype may have a better prognosis. However, we found that patient prognosis in the low m6A score group was worse, even though the low m6A score group had an inflammatory phenotype. This could be because several critical inhibitor immune checkpoints, including CTLA-4, PD-1, LAG-3, LAALS3, and TIGIT, were significantly highly expressed in the low m6A score group. Higher expression of these immune checkpoints may limit cytotoxic immune cell activities in the TME, such as CD8 T cells, causing these cytotoxic cells to be in an exhausted functional state (47, 48). Finally, the robustness of the m6A score was invalidated in external cohorts.

Both targeted therapy and ICB have been recommended as first-line treatments for advanced KIRC (2–4). However, it is difficult to determine an individual's optimal treatment option, which prompted us to explore more accurate predictive biomarkers. Here, the m6A score may be a potential biomarker to guide clinical decision-making and help us achieve individualized and precision treatment. First, we identified a highly consistent result that all targeted therapy drugs' sensitivities were significantly lower in the low m6A score group, indicating that patients with high m6A scores might be suitable candidates to receive targeted therapy. In contrast, patients with low m6A scores may be the optimal candidates to receive ICB. More importantly, we demonstrated that this m6A score may be a generalized predictor for the response to ICB in other cancer types.

Several inevitable shortcomings exist in this study. First, all conclusions came from public databases, including validations. This weakens the use of these conclusions for the future. Therefore, it is necessary to validate these findings with experiments *in vivo* and *in vitro* and more data from our center in the future. Second, in order to enlarge our sample size and verify our results, we pooled data from TCGA and GEO together. However, despite the inevitable analysis error caused by different sequencing platforms, we found that the results found in TCGA can be successfully verified in multiple independent external datasets, which enhanced the reliability of our results. Third, it is difficult to unify the same cutoff value of the m6A score in different cohorts due to the differences in sequencing platform and batch effects. Alternatively, we used the survcutpoint function to calculate the optimal cutoff values.

In conclusion, this work revealed that m6A modification patterns played significant role in regulating the TME of KIRC, including immunological characters, mutation profiles and other functional pathways. Based on the comprehensive m6A patterns, we first identified m6A clusters and m6A scores to elucidate immune phenotypes and to predict the prognosis and immunotherapy response in KIRC. Finally, the m6A clusters and m6A scores can guide urologists for making more precise clinical decision.

## AUTHOR CONTRIBUTIONS

HL and JH performed analyses and drafted the manuscript. AY, BO, and TG searched and downloaded the original datasets from TCGA and GEO. HL, JH, and JL contributed to statistical analyses. JL and CC collected and assembled clinical data. HL, TG, and JC edited the pictures. XZ and JC conceived and supervised the study. All authors contributed to writing the manuscript and reviewed and approved the final manuscript.

## ACKNOWLEDGMENTS

We sincerely thank all participants in the study.

## SUPPLEMENTARY MATERIAL

**Supplementary Figure 1 |** The workflow of the study design.

**Supplementary Figure 2 |** GO and KEGG analysis of differentially expressed genes between m6A cluster 1 and 2. **(A)** Biological process. **(B)** Cellular component. **(C)** Molecular function. **(D)** KEGG analysis.

**Supplementary Figure 3 |** Prognosis value of m6A score in multivariate regression model. **(A)** Forest plot of age, gender, tumor grade, tumor stage, and m6A score in multivariate regression model; **(B)** Q-Q plot of the multivariate regression model; **(C)** The five-year predictive value of m6A score, tumor stage, tumor grade, and age in TCGA-KIRC.

**Supplementary Figure 4 |** Correlations between m6A score and tumor-infiltrating immune cells calculated with Cibersort-ABS algorithm.

**Supplementary Figure 5 |** Correlations between m6A score and tumor-infiltrating immune cells calculated with xCell algorithm.

**Supplementary Figure 6 |** Correlations between m6A score and tumor-infiltrating immune cells calculated with TIMER algorithm.

**Supplementary Table 1 |** Information for datasets selected in this study.

**Supplementary Table 2 |** The gene sets for TME cell infiltration enrichment analysis.

**Supplementary Table 3 |** The signatures related to response of immunotherapy.

**Supplementary Table 4 |** Spearman correlation values for 24 regulators in renal cell carcinoma.

**Supplementary Table 5 |** Differentially expressed genes between m6A cluster 1 and 2.

**Supplementary Table 6 |** Functional annotation of differentially expressed genes between m6a cluster 1 and 2 (GO).

**Supplementary Table 7 |** Functional annotation of differentially expressed genes between m6a cluster 1 and 2 (KEGG).

**Supplementary Table 8 |** Differences in HALLMARK pathway GSVA enrichment between m6A Cluster 1 and 2.

**Supplementary Table 9 |** Prognosis-related genes from WGCNA between m6A cluster 1 and 2.

**Supplementary Table 10 |** Correlations between m6A score and anticancer immunity.

**Supplementary Table 11 |** Correlations between m6A score and immunotherapy associated signatures.

**Supplementary Table 12 |** Correlations between m6A score and anticancer immunity in GSE22541.

**Supplementary Table 13** | Correlations between m6A Score and immunotherapy associated signatures in GSE22541.

**Supplementary Table 14** | Differences in the expression of target genes of antitumor drugs between high and low m6A score groups.

# REFERENCES

1. Ljungberg B, Albiges L, Abu-Ghanem Y, Bensalah K, Dabestani S, Fernández-Pello S, et al. European association of urology guidelines on renal cell carcinoma: the 2019 update. *Euro Urol.* (2019) 75:799–810. doi: 10.1016/j.eururo.2019.02.011

2. McGregor BA, McKay RR, Braun DA, Werner L, Gray K, Flaifel A, et al. Results of a multicenter Phase II study of atezolizumab and bevacizumab for patients with metastatic renal cell carcinoma with variant histology and/or sarcomatoid features. *J Clin Oncol.* (2020) 38:63–70. doi: 10.1200/JCO.19.01882

3. Diab A, Tannir NM, Bentebibel SE, Hwu P, Papadimitrakopoulou V, Haymaker C, et al. Bempegaldesleukin (NKTR-214) plus nivolumab in patients with advanced solid tumors: Phase I Dose-Escalation study of safety, efficacy, and immune activation (PIVOT-02). *Cancer Discov.* (2020) 10:1158–73. doi: 10.1158/2159-8290.CD-19-1510

4. Ravi P, Mantia C, Su C, Sorenson K, Elhag D, Rathi N, et al. evaluation of the safety and efficacy of immunotherapy rechallenge in patients with renal cell carcinoma. *JAMA Oncol.* (2020) 6:1606–10. doi: 10.1001/jamaoncol.2020.2169

5. Kandoth C, McLellan MD, Vandin F, Ye K, Niu B, Lu C, et al. Mutational landscape and significance across 12 major cancer types. *Nature.* (2013) 502:333–9. doi: 10.1038/nature12634

6. Zaccara S, Ries RJ, Jaffrey SR. Reading, writing and erasing mRNA methylation. *Nat Rev Mol Cell Biol.* (2019) 20:608–24. doi: 10.1038/s41580-019-0168-5

7. Yang Y, Hsu PJ, Chen YS, Yang YG. Dynamic transcriptomic m(6)A decoration: writers, erasers, readers and functions in RNA metabolism. *Cell Res.* (2018) 28:616–24. doi: 10.1038/s41422-018-0040-8

8. Deng X, Su R, Weng H, Huang H, Li Z, Chen J. RNA N(6)-methyladenosine modification in cancers: current status and perspectives. *Cell Res.* (2018) 28:507–17. doi: 10.1038/s41422-018-0034-6

9. Hou J, Zhang H, Liu J, Zhao Z, Wang J, Lu Z, et al. YTHDF2 reduction fuels inflammation and vascular abnormalization in hepatocellular carcinoma. *Mol Cancer.* (2019) 18:163. doi: 10.1186/s12943-019-1082-3

10. Shulman Z, Stern-Ginossar N. The RNA modification N(6)-methyladenosine as a novel regulator of the immune system. *Nat Immunol.* (2020) 21:501–12. doi: 10.1038/s41590-020-0650-4

11. Wang L, Hui H, Agrawal K, Kang Y, Li N, Tang R, et al. m A RNA methyltransferases METTL3/14 regulate immune responses to anti-PD-1 therapy. *EMBO J.* (2020) 39:e104514. doi: 10.15252/embj.202010 4514

12. Wang H, Hu X, Huang M, Liu J, Gu Y, Ma L, et al. Mettl3-mediated mRNA mA methylation promotes dendritic cell activation. *Nat Commun.* (2019) 10:1898. doi: 10.1038/s41467-019-09903-6

13. Su R, Dong L, Li Y, Gao M, Han L, Wunderlich M, et al. Targeting FTO suppresses cancer stem cell maintenance and immune evasion. *Cancer Cell.* (2020) 38:79–96.e11. doi: 10.1016/j.ccell.2020.04.017

14. Yang S, Wei J, Cui Y-H, Park G, Shah P, Deng Y, et al. mA mRNA demethylase FTO regulates melanoma tumorigenicity and response to anti-PD-1 blockade. *Nat Commun.* (2019) 10:2782. doi: 10.1038/s41467-019-10669-0

15. Han D, Liu J, Chen C, Dong L, Liu Y, Chang R, et al. Anti-tumour immunity controlled through mRNA m(6)A methylation and YTHDF1 in dendritic cells. *Nature.* (2019) 566:270–4. doi: 10.1038/s41586-019-0916-x

16. Zhang B, Wu Q, Li B, Wang D, Wang L, Zhou YL. m(6)A regulator-mediated methylation modification patterns and tumor microenvironment infiltration characterization in gastric cancer. *Mol Cancer.* (2020) 19:53. doi: 10.1186/s12943-020-01170-0

17. Colaprico A, Silva TC, Olsen C, Garofano L, Cava C, Garolini D, et al. TCGAbiolinks: an R/Bioconductor package for integrative analysis of TCGA data. *Nucleic Acids Res.* (2016) 44:e71. doi: 10.1093/nar/gkv1507

18. Bonneville R, Krook MA, Kautto EA, Miya J, Wing MR, Chen HZ, et al. Landscape of microsatellite instability across 39 cancer types. *JCO Precision Oncol.* (2017) 1:PO.17.00073. doi: 10.1200/PO.17.00073

19. Miao D, Margolis CA, Gao W, Voss MH, Li W, Martini DJ, et al. Genomic correlates of response to immune checkpoint therapies in clear cell renal cell carcinoma. *Science.* (2018) 359:801–6. doi: 10.1126/science.aan5951

20. Mariathasan S, Turley SJ, Nickles D, Castiglioni A, Yuen K, Wang Y, et al. TGFβ attenuates tumour response to PD-L1 blockade by contributing to exclusion of T cells. *Nature.* (2018) 554:544–8. https://dx.doi.org/10.1038 %2Fnature25501

21. Chen YT, Shen JY, Chen DP, Wu CF, Guo R, Zhang PP, et al. Identification of cross-talk between m(6)A and 5mC regulators associated with onco-immunogenic features and prognosis across 33 cancer types. *J Hematol Oncol.* (2020) 13:22. doi: 10.1186/s13045-020-00854-w

22. Wilkerson MD, Hayes DN. ConsensusClusterPlus: a class discovery tool with confidence assessments and item tracking. *Bioinformatics.* (2010) 26:1572–3. doi: 10.1093/bioinformatics/btq170

23. Liberzon A, Birger C, Thorvaldsdóttir H, Ghandi M, Mesirov JP, Tamayo P. The Molecular Signatures Database (MSigDB) hallmark gene set collection. *Cell Syst.* (2015) 1:417–25. doi: 10.1016/j.cels.2015.12.004

24. Hänzelmann S, Castelo R, Guinney J. GSVA: gene set variation analysis for microarray and RNA-seq data. *BMC Bioinform.* (2013) 14:7. doi: 10.1186/1471-2105-14-7

25. Ritchie ME, Phipson B, Wu D, Hu Y, Law CW, Shi W, et al. limma powers differential expression analyses for RNA-sequencing and microarray studies. *Nucleic Acids Res.* (2015) 43:e47. doi: 10.1093/nar/gkv007

26. Chen DS, Mellman I. Oncology meets immunology: the cancer-immunity cycle. *Immunity.* (2013) 39:1–10. doi: 10.1016/j.immuni.2013.07.012

27. Xu L, Deng C, Pang B, Zhang X, Liu W, Liao G, et al. TIP: a web server for resolving tumor immunophenotype profiling. *Cancer Res.* (2018) 78:6575–80. doi: 10.1158/0008-5472.CAN-18-0689

28. Charoentong P, Finotello F, Angelova M, Mayer C, Efremova M, Rieder D, et al. Pan-cancer immunogenomic analyses reveal genotype-immunophenotype relationships and predictors of response to checkpoint blockade. *Cell Rep.* (2017) 18:248–62. doi: 10.1016/j.celrep.2016.12.019

29. Newman AM, Liu CL, Green MR, Gentles AJ, Feng W, Xu Y, et al. Robust enumeration of cell subsets from tissue expression profiles. *Nat Methods.* (2015) 12:453–7. doi: 10.1038/nmeth.3337

30. Aran D, Hu Z, Butte AJ. xCell: digitally portraying the tissue cellular heterogeneity landscape. *Genome Biol.* (2017) 18:220. doi: 10.1186/s13059-017-1349-1

31. Li T, Fu J, Zeng Z, Cohen D, Li J, Chen Q, et al. TIMER2.0 for analysis of tumor-infiltrating immune cells. *Nucleic Acids Res.* (2020) 48:W509–w14. doi: 10.1093/nar/gkaa407

32. Langfelder P, Horvath S. WGCNA: an R package for weighted correlation network analysis. *BMC Bioinform.* (2008) 9:559. doi: 10.1186/1471-2105-9-559

33. Chen L, Yuan L, Wang Y, Wang G, Zhu Y, Cao R, et al. Co-expression network analysis identified FCER1G in association with progression and prognosis in human clear cell renal cell carcinoma. *Int J Biol Sci.* (2017) 13:1361–72. doi: 10.7150/ijbs.21657

34. Zeng D, Li M, Zhou R, Zhang J, Sun H, Shi M, et al. Tumor microenvironment characterization in gastric cancer identifies prognostic and immunotherapeutically relevant gene signatures. *Cancer Immunol Res.* (2019) 7:737–50. doi: 10.1158/2326-6066.CIR-18-0436

35. Ji RR, Chasalow SD, Wang L, Hamid O, Schmidt H, Cogswell J, et al. An immune-active tumor microenvironment favors clinical response to ipilimumab. *Cancer Immunol Immunother.* (2012) 61:1019–31. doi: 10.1007/s00262-011-1172-6

36. Gajewski TF, Corrales L, Williams J, Horton B, Sivan A, Spranger S. Cancer immunotherapy targets based on understanding the t cell-inflamed versus non-T Cell-inflamed tumor microenvironment. *Adv Exp Med Biol.* (2017) 1036:19–31. doi: 10.1007/978-3-319-67577-0_2

37. Strick A, von Hagen F, Gundert L, Klümper N, Tolkach Y, Schmidt D, et al. The N(6) -methyladenosine (m(6) A) erasers alkylation repair homologue 5 (ALKBH5) and fat mass and obesity-associated protein (FTO) are prognostic biomarkers in patients with clear cell renal cell carcinoma. *BJU Int.* (2020) 125:617–24. doi: 10.1111/bju.15019

38. Zhang X, Wang F, Wang Z, Yang X, Yu H, Si S, et al. ALKBH5 promotes the proliferation of renal cell carcinoma by regulating AURKB expression in an m(6)A-dependent manner. *Ann Trans Med.* (2020) 8:646. doi: 10.21037/atm-20-3079

39. Chen Y, Zhou C, Sun Y, He X, Xue D. m(6)A RNA modification modulates gene expression and cancer-related pathways in clear cell renal cell carcinoma. *Epigenomics.* (2020) 12:87–99. doi: 10.2217/epi-2019-0182

40. Zhou J, Wang J, Hong B, Ma K, Xie H, Li L, et al. Gene signatures and prognostic values of m6A regulators in clear cell renal cell carcinoma - a retrospective study using TCGA database. *Aging.* (2019) 11:1633–47. doi: 10.18632/aging.101856

41. Zhang QJ, Luan JC, Song LB, Cong R, Ji CJ, Zhou X, et al. m6A RNA methylation regulators correlate with malignant progression and have potential predictive values in clear cell renal cell carcinoma. *Exp Cell Res.* (2020) 392:112015. doi: 10.1016/j.yexcr.2020.112015

42. Wang J, Zhang C, He W, Gou X. Effect of m(6)A RNA Methylation regulators on malignant progression and prognosis in renal clear cell carcinoma. *Front Oncol.* (2020) 10:3. doi: 10.3389/fonc.2020.00003

43. Chen J, Yu K, Zhong G, Shen W. Identification of a m(6)A RNA methylation regulators-based signature for predicting the prognosis of clear cell renal carcinoma. *Cancer Cell Int.* (2020) 20:157. doi: 10.1186/s12935-020-01238-3

44. Zhao Y, Tao Z, Chen X. Identification of a three-m6A related gene risk score model as a potential prognostic biomarker in clear cell renal cell carcinoma. *PeerJ.* (2020) 8:e8827. doi: 10.7717/peerj.8827

45. Fang J, Hu M, Sun Y, Zhou S, Li H. Expression profile analysis of m6A RNA methylation regulators indicates they are immune signature associated and can predict survival in kidney renal cell carcinoma. *DNA Cell Biol.* (2020) 39:2194–211. doi: 10.1089/dna.2020.5767

46. Li X, Wen D, Li X, Yao C, Chong W, Chen H. Identification of an immune signature predicting prognosis risk and lymphocyte infiltration in colon cancer. *Front Immunol.* (2020) 11:1678. doi: 10.3389/fimmu.2020.01678

47. Dong H, Strome SE, Salomao DR, Tamura H, Hirano F, Flies DB, et al. Tumor-associated B7-H1 promotes T-cell apoptosis: a potential mechanism of immune evasion. *Nat Med.* (2002) 8:793–800. doi: 10.1038/nm730

48. Sanmamed MF, Chen L. A paradigm shift in cancer immunotherapy: from enhancement to normalization. *Cell.* (2018) 175:313–26. doi: 10.1016/j.cell.2018.09.035

# 19

# Urinary Markers in Bladder Cancer

*Giorgio Santoni[1]\*, Maria B. Morelli[1,2], Consuelo Amantini[2] and Nicola Battelli[3]*

[1] Immunopathology Laboratory, School of Pharmacy, University of Camerino, Camerino, Italy, [2] Immunopathology Laboratory, School of Biosciences, Biotechnology and Veterinary Medicine, University of Camerino, Camerino, Italy, [3] Oncology Unit, Macerata Hospital, Macerata, Italy

*\*Correspondence:*
*Giorgio Santoni*
*giorgio.santoni@unicam.it*

Bladder cancer (BC) is ones of the most common cancer worldwide. It is classified in muscle invasive (MIBC) and muscle non-invasive (NMIBC) BC. NMIBCs frequently recur and progress to MIBCs with a reduced survival rate and frequent distant metastasis. BC detection require unpleasant and expensive cystoscopy and biopsy, which are often accompanied by several adverse effects. Thus, there is an urgent need to develop novel diagnostic methods for initial detection and surveillance in both MIBCs and NMIBCs. Multiple urine-based tests approved by FDA for BC detection and surveillance are commercially available. However, at present, sensitivity, specificity and diagnostic accuracy of these urine-based assays are still suboptimal and, in the attend to improve them, novel molecular markers as well as multiple-assays must to be translated in clinic. Now there are growing evidence toward the use of minimally invasive "liquid biopsy" to identify biomarkers in urologic malignancy. DNA- and RNA-based markers in body fluids such as blood and urine are promising potential markers in diagnostic, prognostic, predictive and monitoring urological malignancies. Thus, circulating cell-free DNA, DNA methylation and mutations, circulating tumor cells, miRNA, lncRNA and mRNAs, cell-free proteins and peptides, and exosomes have been assessed in urine specimens. However, proteomic and genomic data must to be validated in well-designed multicenter clinical studies, before to be employed in clinic oncology.

Keywords: urinary biomarkers, bladder cancer, liquid biopsy, microRNA, exosomes

## INTRODUCTION

Bladder cancer (BC) represents the 9th and 4th most common cancer worldwide and in men in the USA, respectively (1, 2). Its main histological type is urothelial carcinoma (UC). About 70–80% of BC is diagnosed as non-muscle invasive BC (NMIBC) and 20–30% as muscle invasive (MIBC). Because 10–30% of patients with NMIBC progress to invasive disease (3–8), early diagnosis and early detection of recurrence are very important. BC diagnosis requires cystoscopy and biopsy, which are unpleasant and costly procedures (9). It is necessary to develop new diagnostic methods less invasive and expensive for BC diagnosis and surveillance. The Food and Drug Administration (FDA) has approved the use of multiple urine-based tests that are commercially available. However, none of these tests has been routinely used and incorporated in the American Urological Association or in the European Association of Urology clinical guidelines for BC treatment (10). In this mini-review we discuss the clinical implementation by the use of novel molecular approaches and liquid biopsy in BC.

At present, the gold standard methods for BC diagnosis are urine cytology and cystoscopy. Cytopathology of urine specimens is the widely used non-invasive test for detection and surveillance of BC (11–13). Cytology is very specific (about 86%), but it is low sensitive (48%) limiting its use in low-grade BC (14–16). Diagnostic accuracy of urinary cytology is subjective, depending on cytopathologist expertise (17). Thus, new molecular-based urinary tests for reducing or substituting, the endoscopy frequency in BC recurrence patients, are required (18, 19).

Advanced technology utilizes patients' urine as samples instead of primary BC tissues to identify novel predictive biomarkers. At present, the major problem is to translate the extensive proteomic and genomic data in clinical practice and to validate the expression of these biomarkers in well-designed multicenter clinical studies (20).

## PROTEOMIC AND PEPTIDOMIC ANALYSIS

Proteomic analyses have opened a new horizon for cancer biomarker discovery (21). At present, seven tests are available: FDA approved six on seven of these tests, and the last one is in agree with the Clinical Laboratory Improvement Act standards. NMP22, NMP22 BladderChek, and UroVysion have FDA approval for BC diagnosis and surveillance; immunocytology (uCyt+), BTA-TRAK, and BTA-STAT have been approved only for surveillance (22–26).

In order to improve sensitivity, specificity and diagnostic accuracy in BC diagnosis, novel protein markers, waiting to be approved, are used experimentally. BCLA-1 and BCLA-4 are nuclear matrix proteins specifically targeting BC tissues, with no interference with infection, smoking, catheterization or cystitis (27). In patients with hematuria, aurora A kinase (AURKA) discriminates between low-grade BC vs. normal patients (28). The Aura Tek FDP Test™ in urine can detect BC recurrence (29). The activated leukocyte cell adhesion molecule (ALCAM), a cell adhesion molecule (30), positively correlates with tumor stage and overall survival (OS), after adjusting for patients, clinical features and Bacillus Calmette-Guerin treatment (31). Nicotinamide N-methyltransferase is high in BC patients and correlate with histological grade (32). Apurinic/apyrimidinic endonuclease 1/redox factor-1 (APE/Ref-1) levels are higher in BC, respect to non-BC, and correlate with tumor grade and stage; moreover it is high also in patients with recurrence history of BC (33). The cytokeratin-20 (CK20) urine RT-PCR assay shows 78–87% sensitivity and 56–80% specificity for urothelial BC detection, with improved diagnostic accuracy in tumor progression (34) but it has poor performance for low-grade tumors. Higher levels of CK8 and CK18 was detected in the urine by UBC Rapid test in high- vs low-grade BC (35).

As multiple markers for BC detection, increased urinary levels of apolipoprotein A1, A2, B, C2, C3, *E* (APOA1, APOA2, APOB, APOC2, APOC3, APOE) were found in BC relative to healthy controls (36, 37). A signature of 4 urinary fragments of uromodulin, collagen α-1 (I), collagen α-1 (III), and membrane-associated progesterone receptor component 1 seems

to discriminate MIBCs from NMIBCs (38). Other panel employs IL-8, MMP-9/10, ANG, APOE, SDC-1, α1AT, PAI-1, VEGFA, and CA9 to diagnose BC starting from urine samples (39). The advantage of these multi-urinary protein biomarkers was evident in high- and low-grade and high- and low-stage disease (39). The combination of urinary markers such as midkine (MDK) and synuclein G or MDK, ZAG2 and CEACAM1 (40), angiogenin and clusterin (41) evaluated by immunoassay and urine cytology increases the sensitivity and specificity in NMIBC diagnosis (40). Increased CK20 and Insulin Like Growth Factor II (IGFII) levels were detected in the urine sediments of NMIBC patients compared to controls (42). Increased levels of urinary HAI-1 and Epcam evaluated by ELISA, are prognostic biomarkers in high-risk NMIBC patients (43). Urinary survivin evaluated by chemiluminescence enzyme immunoassay correlates with tumor stage, lymph node and distant metastases and represents a potential marker for preliminary BC diagnosis (44). Snail overexpression represents an independent prognostic factor for tumor recurrence in NMIBC (45). Finally, specific glycoproteins were identified by glycan-affinity glycoproteomics nanoplatforms in the urine of low- and high-grade NMIBC; among these, increased urinary CD44 levels were evidenced in high-grade MIBC (46).

Urinary metabolomics signature could also be useful in early BC. By ultra-performance liquid chromatography time and mass spectrometry, imidazole-acetic acid was evidenced in BC (47). Moreover, acid trehalose, nicotinuric acid, AspAspGlyTrp peptide were upregulated; inosinic acid, ureidosuccinic acid and GlyCysAlaLys peptide were downregulated in BC, but not in normal cohort (48). A metabolite panel with indolylacryloylglycine, N2-galacturonyl-L-lysine and aspartyl-glutamate permits to discriminate high- vs. low-grade BC (49). In addition, the alteration of phenylalanine, arginine, proline and tryptophan metabolisms was evidenced by UPLC-MS in NMBIC (50).

## CIRCULATING TUMOR AND CELL-FREE DNA

Tumors release DNA fragments into circulation, called circulating tumor DNA (ctDNA) containing tumor-specific mutations, variations of copy number and alterations in DNA methylation status. This ctDNA reflects the heterogeneity of tumor subclones. In BC patients, ctDNA is detectable in over 70% of urine samples (51) and it allows to discriminate between BC patients and control subjects (52). CtDNA measures about 180 and 200 base pairs. It is easily accessible, but it is rapidly cleared from circulation following systemic therapy (53). PCR-based approaches, and more recently, digital-PCR and genome sequencing, represent the methods of choice for cell-free DNA (cfDNA) analysis.

### DNA Methylation

The methylation status of tumor-related genes represents a very important epigenetic alteration affecting cancer initiation and progression. Hyper- and hypo-methylated regions are identified in BC and in premalignant lesions. Alterations in DNA methylation status are chemically stable, develop early during tumorigenesis and can be assessed in circulating cfDNA fragments and in cells shed into the urine (54). A significant prevalence of methylated genes, for example APC and cyclin D2, was found in the urine from malignant vs. benign cases (55). Hyper-methylation in GSTP1 and RARβ2 and APC genes has been identified in the urine from BC patients (56). The evaluation of Twist Family BHLH Transcription Factor 1 (TWIST1) and NID2 genes methylation status in urine permits to differentiate primary BC patients from controls with 90% sensitivity and 93% specificity (57). In addition, the evaluation of the methylation status of NID2 and TWIST1 or CFTR, SALL3 and TWIST1 genes in urinary cells in combination with cytology, has been found to increase sensitivity and high negative predictive value in BC patients (58, 59). The analysis of 1,370 loci specific DNA methylation patterns seem to permit to distinguish NMIBC from MIBC (60). Sun and coworkers demonstrated higher recurrence predictivity than urine cytology and cystoscopy (80 vs. 35 vs. 15%) by using SOX-1, IRAK3, and Li-MET genes methylation status from urine sediments of BC patients (54). POU4F2 and PCDH17 methylation levels in urine distinguish BC from normal controls with 90% sensitivity and 94% specificity (61). Promoter hyper-methylation of HS3ST2, SEPTIN9 and SLIT2 genes combined with FGFR3 mutation showed 97.6% sensitivity and 84.8% specificity for diagnosis, surveillance and risk stratification in low- or high-risk NMIBC patients (62). Finally, the methylation status of p14ARF, p16INK4A, RASSF1A, DAPK, and APC tumor suppressor genes has been found to correlate with BC grade and stage (63).

Altogether, although promising results were obtained, accuracy of urinary methylated DNA is variable and results still await validation studies and complementary markers for clinical implementation (64, 65). In this regard, the recent introduction of the methylation-sensitive High Resolution Melting and Methylated CpG Island Recovery methods could further increases the sensitivity for the detection of methylome in BC urine (Table 1) (72, 73).

## cfDNA, Mutation and Microsatellite Alterations

Since tumor-derived DNA can be released into circulation and mutations in cfDNA can be detected in various biological fluids, their use as non-invasive cancer biomarkers has been proposed. Urinary TERT promoter mutations, that occur early in urothelial neoplasia, FGFR3 mutation and telomere length correlate with high-risk BC recurrence (66, 67). TERT, evaluated by telomeric repeat amplification protocol, in combination with FGF3 and OTX1 shows high sensitivity in NMIBCs as well as in pT1 tumors and in high-grade BC (68). In addition, increased FGFR3 and PIK3CA mutated DNA levels in urine has been found to be indicative of progression and metastasis in NMIBC (69). Microsatellite analysis in circulating DNA of BC patients targets highly polymorphic, short tandem repeats. Loss of heterozygosity (LOH) analysis is more sensitive than urine cytology (97 vs. 79%), particularly for low-grade BC diagnosis. It also significantly

improves the detection of low-grade and low-stage BC, with 95% sensitivity for G1-G2 grades and 100% for pTis and pTa tumors (Table 1) (74).

## Histone Tail Modifications

The levels of histone methylation are lower in advanced tumors respect to controls and correlated to poor survival. Thus, increased levels of HAK20me3 were evidenced in a MIBC subset (70); furthermore high H3K27me3 levels correlate with worse survival after cystectomy in pT1-3 and pN- BC patients (71). H2AFX1 gene methylation was detected in paraffin-embedded BC and its expression correlated with increased recurrence rates (Table 1) (75).

## URINARY TUMOR RNA

Several RNA classes, messenger RNAs (mRNAs), microRNAs (miRs) and long non-coding RNAs (lncRNAs), have been recognized as potential non-invasive cancer biomarkers (76). Altered levels of circulating RNAs in cancer, which returned to normal following surgery have been reported (77), suggesting release of RNA molecules from tumors.

## miRNAs (miRNAs)

miRNAs are short (21–23 nucleotides length) non-coding RNAs regulating gene expression by pairing to the 3′untranslated region (UTR) of their target mRNA. Several miRNAs have been found to play an important role in tumorigenesis, progression and metastasis of cancer cells (78, 79). Urine seems to be a good source for miRNA detection for its content of cell-free nucleic acid in supernatant or sediments (80). However, the diagnostic significance in the detection of miRs in urine as respect to blood of BC patients is controversial (81). MiR-126 urinary levels were found to be enhanced in BC compared to healthy controls (82). Urine miR-146a-5p is significantly increased in high-grade BC (77). Low miR-200c expression correlates with tumor progression in NMIBCs (83). Chen et al. detected 74 miRNAs, of which 33 upregulated and 41 downregulated in BC compared to healthy patients (84). The most interesting are let-7miR, mir-1268, miR-196a, miR-1, miR-100, miR-101, and miR-143 (84). MiR-200 was identified as epithelial–mesenchymal transition regulator in BC cells by targeting Zinc Finger E-Box Binding Homeobox 1 (ZEB1), ZEB2 and Epidermal growth factor receptor (EGFR) (85). Some miRNAs have been associated with hemolysis including miR-451a, miR-16, miR-486-5p, and miR-92a (86). Eissa et al. by screening BC patients with negative cystoscopy, identified miR-96 and miR-210 in BC (87). Sapre et al., by using a panel of 12 miRNA, reduced the cystoscopy rates by 30% by increasing sensitivity and specificity (88). MiR-125b, miR-30b, miR-204, miR-99a, and miR-532-3p were downregulated in BC patient's urine supernatant, with miR-125 levels (95.7% specificity, 59.3% sensitivity) (89). MiR-9, miR-182 and miR-200b correlated with MIBC aggressiveness, recurrence-free and OS (90). MiR-145 distinguishes NMIBCs from non-BCs (91). MiR-144-5p inhibited BC proliferation, affecting CCNE1, CCNE2, CDC25A, PKMYT1 target genes (92). Cell-free urinary miR-99a and miRNA-125b were found to be downregulated

**TABLE 1 |** Urinary tumor-derived DNAs as biomarkers in BCs.

| Urinary tumor-derived DNA | Gene | Application | References |
|---|---|---|---|
| CfDNA | TERT and FGFR3 | Recurrence | (66, 67) |
| | TERT, FGFR3/OTX1 | BC diagnosis | (68) |
| | FGFR3 and PIK3CA | Progression/metastasis | (69) |
| Histone modifications | HAK20me3 | Poor survival | (70) |
| | H3K27me3 | Poor survival | (71) |
| DNA methylation status | GSTP1 and RARb2 and APC | BC diagnosis | (56) |
| | TWIST1 and NID2 | BC diagnosis | (57) |
| | SOX-1, IRAK3, and Li-MET | Recurrence | (54) |
| | POU4F2 and PCDH17 | BC diagnosis | (61) |
| | HS3ST2, SEPTIN9, SLIT2/FGFR3 | surveillance, low vs. high risk | (62) |
| | NID2 and TWIST1 | BC diagnosis | (58) |
| | CFTR, SALL3/TWIST1 | BC diagnosis | (59) |
| | p14ARF, p16INK4A, RASSF1A | BC grade and stage | (63) |
| | DAPK and APC | | |

*BC, Bladder cancer; CfDNA, circulating-free DNA.*

in the urine supernatants of BC patients (sensitivity 86.7%; specificity 81.1%) (93). Urinary levels of miR-618 and miR-1255b-5p in MIBC patients were increased in comparison to controls (94). Multiple miRNA assay shows higher diagnostic performance than single RNA assay (95). By whole genome analysis increased miR-31-5p, miR-191-5p and miR-93-5p levels were identified in the urine of BC patients as compared to controls (96).

Recently, a miRNA profile, identified in urine by next-generation sequencing (NGS) analysis, has been capable to stratify different BC subtypes (97). In NMIBC G1/G2 patients a miR-205-5p upregulation compared to controls was observed. Among NMIBC G3, upregulation of miR-21-5p, miR-106b-3p, mir-486-5p, miR-151a-3p, miR-200c-3p, miR-185-5p, miR-185-5p and miR-224-5p and downregulation of miR-30c-2-5p and miR-10b-5p were observed. In MIBCs, miR-205-5p, miR-451a, miR-25-3p and miR-7-1-5p were upregulated, while miR-30a-5p was downregulated compared to controls (97). The application of NGS have increased the diagnostic accuracy. However results obtained in NGS were only partially overlapping with that obtained by qRT-PCR (98) (**Table 2**).

## Long Non Coding RNAs (lncRNAs)

Long non coding RNAs (lncRNAs) regulate gene expression or epigenetic levels. Several findings show lncRNA changes in cancers suggesting a role in the promotion of tumor development and progression (105, 106). The use of lncRNAs as non-invasive BC marker has recently interested (107). Circulating urothelial carcinoma antigen 1 (UCA1) levels in urinary sediments represents a potential diagnostic marker for UC, with 81% sensitivity and 92% specificity (108). Du et al. describe high uc004cox.4 lncRNA level association with poor recurrence-free survival in NMIBCs (102). The retrotrasposome, long interspaced element-1 (LINE-1) has been found to be hypo-methylated and its expression was associated with long recurrence-free and tumor specific survival in BC (109) (**Table 2**).

## Messenger RNAs (mRNAs)

Circulating messenger RNAs (mRNAs) were detected in cancer patients, although the majority of circulating mRNAs are degraded by RNases (110). Given their role in intracellular protein translation, their presence reflects the status of intracellular processes and they are potential cancer biomarkers. Urine Ubiquitin Conjugating Enzyme E2 C (UBE2C) mRNA levels were higher in BC patients, compared to normal and hematuria specimens (111). The expression of isoleucine glutamine motif-containing GTAase-activating proteins (IQGAP3) mRNA in urine was found higher in BC than in controls (112). Further analysis of IQGAP3, with respect to tumor invasiveness and grade also yielded a high diagnostic accuracy, suggesting that IQGAP3 can be used to discriminate BC from non-BC patients with hematuria (112).

In regard to mRNAs extracted by exfoliated urinary cells, the Xpert BC Monitor measuring ABL1, corticotropin releasing hormone (CRH), IGF2, uroplakin 1B (UPK1B), annexin A10 (ANXA10) mRNAs by RT-PCR, increased the overall sensitivity over urinary cytology in low-grade and pTa disease (113).

In addition, the presence of carbonic anhydrase 9 (CAIX) splice variant mRNA in the urine, increased the diagnostic performance for BC (90% sensitivity and 72% specificity) (114). The downregulation of N-Myc downstream-regulated gene 2 (NDRG2) mRNA levels in the urine of BC patients correlated with tumor grade and stage (99) (**Table 2**).

## Transfer RNA Fragments (tRFs)

Elevated levels of transfer RNA fragments (tRF) are found in cancer (115). tRF are 14-32 base long single-stranded RNA derived from mature o precursor tRNA. They are grouped into 3 classes (tRF-1, −3, and −5) and, depending of their cleavage site within a mature RNA, they are further divided in 5 subclasses. The first identified tRF in NMIBCs was miR720/3007a (101) (**Table 2**).

**TABLE 2** | Urinary tumor-derived RNAs as biomarkers in BCs.

| Urinary tumor-derived RNAs | RNA/Protein | Application | References |
|---|---|---|---|
| mRNA | CK20, IGF-II | BC diagnosis | (42) |
| | ABL1, CRH, IGF2, UPK1B and ANXA10 | BC diagnosis | (78) |
| | NDRG2 | Tumor grade and stage | (99) |
| miRNA | miR-146a | BC diagnosis | (77) |
| | miR-126 | BC diagnosis | (82) |
| | miR-200c | Tumor progression | (83) |
| | let-7,miR-1268,−196a,−1,−101,−143 | BC diagnosis | (84) |
| | miR-451a,−16,−486,−92a | Hemolysis | (86) |
| | miR-96,−210 | BC diagnosis | (87) |
| | miR-125b,−30b,−204a,−99a,−532 | BC diagnosis | (89) |
| | miR-9,−182,−200b | aggressiveness, recurrence | (90) |
| | miR-145 | BC diagnosis | (91) |
| | miR-99a,−125b | BC diagnosis | (93) |
| | miR-618,−1255b | BC diagnosis | (94) |
| | miR-21,−106b,−486,−151a,−200c −185,−224, 30c-2,−10b | NMIBC diagnosis | (97) |
| | miR-205,−451a,−25,−7-1,−30a | MIBC diagnosis | (97) |
| | miR-31,−191,−93 | BC diagnosis | (96) |
| miRNA/EVs and Exosomes | miR-375,−146a | BC diagnosis | (100) |
| miRNA/tRF | miR720/3007a | BC diagnosis | (101) |
| lncRNA | uc004cox.4 | Recurrence | (102) |
| lncRNA/exosomes | HOX-AS, ANRIL, and linc-RoR | BC diagnosis | (103, 104) |

*BC, Bladder cancer; NMIBC, muscle non-invasive BC; MIBC, muscle invasive; mRNA, messenger RNA; miR, microRNA; EVs, extracellular vesicles; tRF, transfer RNA fragments; lncRNA, Long non-coding RNA.*

# EXTRACELLULAR VESICLES (EVS) AND EXOSOMES

Extracellular Vesicles (EVs) enrichment was found in BC patient urine. EVs, analyzed by MS based proteomics, demonstrated specific protein and miRNAs pattern in BC patients (116). By using a microarray platform and RT-PCR analysis, miR-375, and miR146a have been found to specifically identify high-grade and low-grade BC, respectively (100). The application of nanowires anchored into a microfluidic substrate will enable the efficiency of EV collection, thus permitting to identify EV harboring miRNAs (117).

Exosomes are membrane vesicles secreted in nearly all body fluids at elevated levels in cancer patients relative to healthy subjects (118, 119). They realize intercellular communication through transferring distinct biologically active molecules (RNAs, DNA, and proteins), thus influencing the therapeutic responses. The HOX transcript antisense RNA (HOTAIR) together with other lncRNA, such as HOX-AS-2, ANRIL, and linc-RoR, were augmented in urinary exosomes from high-grade MIBC patients (103). Loss of HOTAIR expression in BC cells alters the expression of SNA1, TWIST1, ZEB1, ZO1, MMP-1, Laminin Subunit Beta 3 (LAMB3), and Laminin Subunit Gamma 2 (LAMC2) epithelial-to mesenchymal transition genes. Moreover, the tumor-associated calcium-signal transducer 2 (TACSTD2) was found in BC exosomes by proteomic analysis (104). EVs can also promote BC progression by delivering the protein EGF-like repeat and discoidin I-like domain-containing protein-3 (120).

Exosomes in urine also contain miRNAs, in particular miR-1224-3p, miR-135b, and miR15b; in particular, miR-126/miR-152 ratio correlated with positive BC diagnosis (121) (**Table 2**).

Although EVs and exosomes represent an interesting source of cancer biomarkers, the lack of accurate isolation and detection methods affects their utilization in practice. In the next future, the development of sensitive capture platforms for exosomes, likely increases their introduction into clinic.

# URINARY MICROBIOME

Dysbiosis of urinary microbiome has been suggested to be involved in bladder tumorigenesis. Recently, Wu et al. by analyzing DNA extracted by urine pellets, observed specific enrichment of *Acinetobacter*, *Anaerococcus*, and *Sphingobacterium* in BC cohort as respect to controls (122). Moreover, the increase of *Herbaspirillum*, *Porphyrobacter*, and *Bacteroides* in high-risk BC patients suggested that these genera may represent new potential biomarkers (122).

# CONCLUSIONS AND PERSPECTIVES

We provide the state of art into the use of urinary biomarkers as tool to aid diagnosis of BC. Urine cytology, utilized for decades, shows poor sensitivity, particularly for low-grade tumors. The addition of immunoassay and FISH analysis has provided an additional diagnostic armamentarium to determine which patients may need further evaluation. At present, there are growing evidence toward the use of "Liquid Biopsy" to identify urinary biomarkers such as circulating cell-free DNA, DNA methylation, miRNA, cell-free proteins/peptides and exosomes, useful for discriminating NMIBC from MIBC (123). The potential introduction of "smart toilets" working with a more advanced "nano-sensor" able to detect RNA and proteins in urine is close to reality, more that we think (124).

However, now in clinical reality, there is an urgent need to validate the recently discovered extensive proteomic and genomic, epigenomic, transcriptomic and metabolomic data as urinary biomarkers in well-designed multicenter clinical studies (125, 126).

## AUTHOR CONTRIBUTIONS

GS, MM conception and design. GS drafting the manuscript. CA and NB critical revision of the manuscript.

## REFERENCES

1. Siegel RL, Miller KD, Jemal A. Cancer statistics. *CA Cancer J Clin.* (2015) 65:5–29. doi: 10.3322/caac.21254
2. van Rhijn BW, Burger M, Lotan Y, Solsona E, Stief CG, Sylvester RJ, et al. Recurrence and progression of disease in non-muscle-invasive bladder cancer: from epidemiology to treatment strategy. *Eur Urol.* (2009) 56:430–42. doi: 10.1016/j.eururo.2009.06.028
3. Prout GR, Barton BA, Griffin PP, Friedell GH. Treated history of noninvasive grade 1 transitional cell carcinoma. *J Urol.* (1992) 148:1413–9. doi: 10.1016/S0022-5347(17)36924-0
4. Herr HW. Tumor progression and survival of patients with high grade, noninvasive papillary (TaG3) bladder tumors: 15-year outcome. *J Urol.* (2000) 163:60–2. doi: 10.1016/s0022-5347(05)67972-4
5. Sylvester RJ, van der Meijden AP, Oosterlinck W, Witjes JA, Bouffioux C, Denis L, et al. Predicting recurrence and progression in individual patients with stage Ta T1 bladder cancer using EORTC risk tables: a combined analysis of 2596 patients from seven EORTC trials. *Eur Urol.* (2006) 49:466–7. doi: 10.1016/j.eururo.2005.12.031
6. Johnson MI, Merrilees D, Robson WA, Lennon T, Masters J, Orr KE, et al. Oral ciprofloxacin or trimethoprim reduces bacteriuria after flexible cystoscopy. *BJU Int.* (2007) 100:826–9. doi: 10.1111/j.1464-410X.2007.07093.x
7. Soloway MS. Bladder cancer: lack of progress in bladder cancer—what are the obstacles? *Nat Rev Urol.* (2013) 10:5–6. doi: 10.1038/nrurol.2012.219
8. Türkölmez K, Tokgöz H, Reşorlu B, Köse K, Bedük Y. Muscle-invasive bladder cancer: predictive factors and prognostic difference between primary and progressive tumors. *Urology* (2007) 70:477–81. doi: 10.1016/j.urology.2007.05.008
9. Burke DM, Shackley DC, O'Reilly PH. The community-based morbidity of flexible cystoscopy. *BJU Int.* (2002) 89:347–9. doi: 10.1046/j.1464-4096.2001.01899.x
10. Zuiverloon TCM, de Jong FC, Theodorescu D. Clinical decision making in surveillance of non-muscle-invasive bladder cancer: the evolving roles of urinary cytology and molecular markers. *Oncology* (Williston Park) (2017) 31:855–62.
11. Têtu B. Diagnosis of urothelial carcinoma from urine. *Mod Pathol.* (2009) 22 (Suppl 2):S53–9. doi: 10.1038/modpathol.2008.193
12. Sapre N, Hong MK, Huang JG, Pedersen J, Ryan A, Anderson P, et al. Bladder cancer biorepositories in the "-omics" era: integrating quality tissue specimens with comprehensive clinical annotation. *Biopreserv Biobank* (2013) 11:166–72. doi: 10.1089/bio.2012.0062
13. Yafi FA, Brimo F, Steinberg J, Aprikian AG, Tanguay S, Kassouf W. Prospective analysis of sensitivity and specificity of urinary cytology and other urinary biomarkers for bladder cancer. *Urol Oncol.* (2015) 33:66.e25–31. doi: 10.1016/j.urolonc.2014.06.008
14. Lotan Y, Roehrborn CG. Sensitivity and specificity of commonly available bladder tumor markers versus cytology: results of a comprehensive literature review and meta-analyses. *Urology* (2003) 61:109–18. doi: 10.1016/S0090-4295(02)02136-2
15. Simon MA, Lokeshwar VB, Soloway MS. Current bladder cancer tests: unnecessary or beneficial? *Crit Rev Oncol Hematol.* (2003) 47:91–107. doi: 10.1016/S1040-8428(03)00074-X

16. van der Aa MN, Steyerberg EW, Sen EF, Zwarthoff EC, Kirkels WJ, van der Kwast TH, et al. Patients' perceived burden of cystoscopic and urinary surveillance of bladder cancer: a randomized comparison. *BJU Int.* (2008) 101:1106–10. doi: 10.1111/j.1464-410X.2007.07224.x
17. Shariat SF, Karam JA, Lotan Y, Karakiewizc PI. Critical evaluation of urinary markers for bladder cancer detection and monitoring. *Rev Urol.* (2008) 10:120–35.
18. Lokeshwar VB, Habuchi T, Grossman HB, Murphy WM, Hautmann SH, Hemstreet GP, et al. Bladder tumor markers beyond cytology: international Consensus Panel on bladder tumor markers. *Urology* (2005) 66 (6 Suppl 1):35–63. doi: 10.1016/j.urology.2005.08.064
19. Owens CL, VandenBussche CJ, Burroughs FH, Rosenthal DL. A review of reporting systems and terminology for urine cytology. *Cancer Cytopathol.* (2013) 121:9–14. doi: 10.1002/cncy.21253
20. Ralla B, Stephan C, Meller S, Dietrich D, Kristiansen G, Jung K. Nucleic acid-based biomarkers in body fluids of patients with urologic malignancies. *Crit Rev Clin Lab Sci.* (2014) 51:200–31. doi: 10.3109/10408363.2014.914888
21. Di Meo A, Pasic MD, Yousef GM. Proteomics and peptidomics: moving toward precision medicine in urological malignancies. *Oncotarget* (2016) 7:52460–74. doi: 10.18632/oncotarget.8931
22. Kim WT, Cho NH, Ham WS, Lee JS, Ju HJ, Kwon YU, et al. Comparison of the efficacy of urine cytology, Nuclear Matrix Protein 22 (NMP22), and Fluorescence *in Situ* Hybridization (FISH) for the diagnosis of bladder cancer. *Korean J Urol.* (2009) 50:6–11. doi: 10.4111/kju.2009.50.1.6
23. Hajdinjak T. UroVysion FISH test for detecting urothelial cancers: meta-analysis of diagnostic accuracy and comparison with urinary cytology testing. *Urol Oncol.* (2008) 26:646–51. doi: 10.1016/j.urolonc.2007.06.002
24. Horstmann M, Patschan O, Hennenlotter J, Senger E, Feil G, Stenzl A. Combinations of urine-based tumour markers in bladder cancer surveillance. *Scand J Urol Nephrol.* (2009) 43:461–6. doi: 10.3109/00365590903296837
25. Todenhöfer T, Hennenlotter J, Esser M, Mohrhardt S, Tews V, Aufderklamm S, et al. Combined application of cytology and molecular urine markers to improve the detection of urothelial carcinoma. *Cancer Cytopathol.* (2013) 121:252–60. doi: 10.1002/cncy.21247
26. He H, Han C, Hao L, Zang G. ImmunoCyt test compared to cytology in the diagnosis of bladder cancer: a meta-analysis. *Oncol Lett.* (2016) 12:83–8. doi: 10.3892/ol.2016.4556
27. Deininger S, Hennenlotter J, Rausch S, Docktor K, Neumann E, da Costa IA, et al. No influence of smoking status on the performance of urine markers for the detection of bladder cancer. *J Cancer Res Clin Oncol.* (2018) 144:1367–73. doi: 10.1007/s00432-018-2639-z
28. de Martino M, Shariat SF, Hofbauer SL, Lucca I, Taus C, Wiener HG, et al. Aurora A Kinase as a diagnostic urinary marker for urothelial bladder cancer. *World J Urol.* (2015) 33:105–10. doi: 10.1007/s00345-014-1267-8
29. Siemens DR, Morales A, Johnston B, Emerson L. A comparative analysis of rapid urine tests for the diagnosis of upper urinary tract malignancy. *Can J Urol.* (2003) 10:1754–8.
30. Rosso O, Piazza T, Bongarzone I, Rossello A, Mezzanzanica D, Canevari S, et al. The ALCAM shedding by the metalloprotease ADAM17/TACE is involved in motility of ovarian carcinoma cells. *Mol Cancer Res.* (2007) 5:1246–53. doi: 10.1158/1541-7786.MCR-07-0060

31. Egloff SA, Du L, Loomans HA, Starchenko A, Su PF, Ketova T, et al. Shed urinary ALCAM is an independent prognostic biomarker of three-year overall survival after cystectomy in patients with bladder cancer. *Oncotarget* (2017) 8:722–41. doi: 10.18632/oncotarget.13546

32. Pozzi V, Di Ruscio G, Sartini D, Campagna R, Seta R, Fulvi P, et al. Clinical performance and utility of a NNMT-based urine test for bladder cancer. *Int J Biol Mark.* (2018) 33:94–101. doi: 10.5301/ijbm.5000311

33. Choi S, Shin JH, Lee YR, Joo HK, Song KH, Na YG, et al. Urinary APE1/Ref-1: A Potential bladder cancer biomarker. *Dis Mark.* (2016) 2016:7276502. doi: 10.1155/2016/7276502

34. Mi Y, Zhao Y, Shi F, Zhang M, Wang C, Liu X. Diagnostic accuracy of urine cytokeratin 20 for bladder cancer: a meta-analysis. *Asia Pac J Clin Oncol.* (2018) doi: 10.1111/ajco.13024. [Epub ahead of print].

35. Ecke TH, Weiß S, Stephan C, Hallmann S, Barski D, Otto T, et al. UBC® Rapid Test for detection of carcinoma *in situ* for bladder cancer. *Tumor Biol.* (2017) 39:1010428317701624. doi: 10.1177/1010428317701624

36. Chen YT, Chen CL, Chen HW, Chung T, Wu CC, Chen CD, et al. Discovery of novel bladder cancer biomarkers by comparative urine proteomics using iTRAQ technology. *J Proteome Res.* (2010) 5:5803–15. doi: 10.1021/pr100576x

37. Chen YT, Chen HW, Domanski D, Smith DS, Liang KH, Wu CC, et al. Multiplexed quantification of 63 proteins in human urine by multiple reaction monitoring-based mass spectrometry for discovery of potential bladder cancer biomarkers. *J Proteomics* (2012) 75:3529–45. doi: 10.1016/j.jprot.2011.12.031

38. Schiffer E, Vlahou A, Petrolekas A, Stravodimos K, Tauber R, Geschwend JE, et al. Prediction of muscle-invasive bladder cancer using urinary proteomics. *Clin Cancer Res.* (2009) 15:4935–43. doi: 10.1158/1078-0432.CCR-09-0226

39. Masuda N, Ogawa O, Park M, Liu AY, Goodison S, Dai Y, et al. Meta-analysis of a 10-plex urine-based biomarker assay for the detection of bladder cancer. *Oncotarget* (2018) 9:7101–11. doi: 10.18632/oncotarget.23872

40. Soukup V, Kalousová M, Capoun O, Sobotka R, Breyl Z, Pešl M, et al. Panel of urinary diagnostic markers for non-invasive detection of primary and recurrent urothelial urinary bladder carcinoma. *Urol Int.* (2015) 95:56–64. doi: 10.1159/000368166

41. Shabayek MI, Sayed OM, Attaia HA, Awida HA, Abozeed H. Diagnostic evaluation of urinary angiogenin (ANG) and clusterin (CLU) as biomarker for bladder cancer. *Pathol Oncol Res.* (2014) 20:859–66. doi: 10.1007/s12253-014-9765-y

42. Salomo K, Huebner D, Boehme MU, Herr A, Brabetz W, Heberling U, et al. Urinary transcript quantitation of CK20 and IGF2 for the non-invasive bladder cancer detection. *J Cancer Res Clin Oncol.* (2017) 143:1757–69. doi: 10.1007/s00432-017-2433-3

43. Snell KIE, Ward DG, Gordon NS, Goldsmith JC, Sutton AJ, Patel P, et al. Exploring the roles of urinary HAI-1, EpCAM & EGFR in bladder cancer prognosis & risk stratification. *Oncotarget* (2018) 9:25244–53. doi: 10.18632/oncotarget.25397

44. Yang Y, Xu J, Zhang Q. Detection of urinary surviving using a magnetic paricles-based chemiluminescence immunoassay for the preliminary diagnosis of bladder cancer and renal cell carcinoma combined with LAPTM4B. *Oncol Lett.* (2018) 15:7923–33. doi: 10.3892/ol.2018.8317

45. Santi R, Cai T, Nobili S, Galli IC, Amorosi A, Comperat E, et al. Snail immunohistochemical overexpression correlates to recurrence risk in non-muscle invasive bladder cancer: results from a longitudinal cohort study. *Virchows Arch.* (2018) 472:605–13. doi: 10.1007/s00428-018-2310-8

46. Azevedo R, Soares J, Gaiteiro C, Peixoto A, Lima L, Ferreira D, et al. Glycan affinity magnetic nanoplatforms for urinary glycobiomarkers discovery in bladder cancer. *Talanta* (2018) 184:347–55. doi: 10.1016/j.talanta.2018.03.028

47. Shao CH, Chen CL, Lin JY, Chen CJ, Fu SH, Chen YT, et al. Metabolite marker discovery for the detection of bladder cancer by comparative metabolomics. *Oncotarget* (2017) 8:38802–10. doi: 10.18632/oncotarget.16393

48. Shen C, Sun Z, Chen D, Su X, Jiang J, Li G, et al. Developing urinary metabolomic signatures as early bladder cancer diagnostic markers. *OMICS* (2015) 19:1–11. doi: 10.1089/omi.2014.0116

49. Liu X, Cheng X, Liu X, He L, Zhang W, Wang Y, et al. Investigation of urinary metabolic variations and the application in bladder cancer biomarker discovery. *Int J Cancer* (2018) 143:408–18. doi: 10.1002/ijc.31323

50. Loras A, Trassierra M, Sanjuan-Herráez D, Martínez-Bisbal MC, Castell JV, Quintás G, et al. Bladder cancer recurrence surveillance by urine metabolomics analysis. *Sci Rep.* (2018) 8:9172. doi: 10.1038/s41598-018-27538-3

51. Goessl C, Müller M, Straub B, Miller K. DNA alterations in body fluids as molecular tumor markers for urological malignancies. *Eur Urol.* (2002) 41:668–76. doi: 10.1016/S0302-2838(02)00126-4

52. Brisuda A, Pazourkova E, Soukup V, Horinek A, Hrbáček J, Capoun O, et al. Urinary cell-free DNA quantification as non-invasive biomarker in patients with bladder cancer. *Urol Int.* (2016) 96:25–31. doi: 10.1159/0004 38828

53. Qin Z, Ljubimov VA, Zhou C, Tong Y, Liang J. Cell-free circulating tumor DNA in cancer. *Chin J Cancer* (2016) 35:36. doi: 10.1186/s40880-016-0092-4

54. Su SF, de Castro Abreu AL, Chihara Y, Tsai Y, Andreu-Vieyra C, Daneshmand S, et al. A panel of three markers hyper- and hypomethylated in urine sediments accurately predicts bladder cancer recurrence. *Clin Cancer Res.* (2014) 20:1978–89. doi: 10.1158/1078-0432.CCR-13-2637

55. Pu RT, Laitala LE, Clark DP. Methylation profiling of urothelial carcinoma in bladder biopsy and urine. *Acta Cytol.* (2006) 50:499–506. doi: 10.1159/000326003

56. Hauser S, Kogej M, Fechner G, VON Pezold J, Vorreuther R, Lümmen G, et al. Serum DNA hypermethylation in patients with bladder cancer: results of a prospective multicenter study. *Anticancer Res.* (2013) 33:779–84.

57. Renard I, Joniau S, van Cleynenbreugel B, Collette C, Naômé C, Vlassenbroeck I, et al. Identification and validation of the methylated TWIST1 and NID2 genes through real-time methylation-specific polymerase chain reaction assays for the noninvasive detection of primary bladder cancer in urine samples. *Eur Urol.* (2010) 58:96–104. doi: 10.1016/j.eururo.2009.07.041

58. Fantony JJ, Longo TA, Gopalakrishna A, Owusu R, Lance RS, Foo WC, et al. Urinary NID2 and TWIST1 methylation to augment conventional urine cytology for the detection of bladder cancer. *Cancer Biomark.* (2017) 18:381–7. doi: 10.3233/CBM-160261

59. van der Heijden AG, Mengual L, Ingelmo-Torres M, Lozano JJ, van Rijt-van de Westerlo CCM, Baixauli M, et al. Urine cell-based DNA methylation classifier for monitoring bladder cancer. *Clin Epigenetics.* (2018) 10:71. doi: 10.1186/s13148-018-0496-x

60. Wolff EM, Chihara Y, Pan F, Weisenberger DJ, Siegmund KD, Sugano K, et al. Unique DNA methylation patterns distinguish noninvasive and invasive urothelial cancers and establish an epigenetic field defect in premalignant tissue. *Cancer Res.* (2010) 70:8169–78. doi: 10.1158/0008-5472.CAN-10-1335

61. Wang Y, Yu Y, Ye R, Zhang D, Li Q, An D, et al. An epigenetic biomarker combination of PCDH17 and POU4F2 detects bladder cancer accurately by methylation analyses of urine sediment DNA in Han Chinese. *Oncotarget* (2016) 7:2754–64. doi: 10.18632/oncotarget.6666

62. Roperch JP, Grandchamp B, Desgrandchamps F, Mongiat-Artus P, Ravery V, Ouzaid I, et al. Promoter hypermethylation of HS3ST2, SEPTIN9 and SLIT2 combined with FGFR3 mutations as a sensitive/specific urinary assay for diagnosis and surveillance in patients with low or high-risk non-muscle-invasive bladder cancer. *BMC Cancer* (2016) 16:704. doi: 10.1186/s12885-016-2748-5

63. Pietrusinski M, Kępczyński Ł, Jędrzejczyk A, Borkowska E, Traczyk-Borszyńska M, et al. Detection of bladder cancer in urine sediments by a hypermethylation panel of selected tumor suppressor genes. *Cancer Biomark.* 2017:18:47–59. doi: 10.3233/CBM-160673

64. Peng M, Chen C, Hulbert A, Brock MV, Yu F. Non-blood circulating tumor DNA detection in cancer. *Oncotarget* (2017) 8:69162–73. doi: 10.18632/oncotarget.19942

65. Bosschieter J, Lutz C, Segerink LI, Vis AN, Zwarthoff EC, A van Moorselaar RJ, et al. The diagnostic accuracy of methylation markers in urine for the detection of bladder cancer: a systematic review. *Epigenomics* (2018) 10:673–87. doi: 10.2217/epi-2017-0156

66. Kinde I, Munari E, Faraj SF, Hruban RH, Schoenberg M, Bivalacqua T, et al. TERT promoter mutations occur early in urothelial neoplasia and are biomarkers of early disease and disease recurrence in urine. *Cancer Res.* (2013) 73:7162–7. doi: 10.1158/0008-5472.CAN-13-2498

67. Hosen I, Rachakonda PS, Heidenreich B, de Verdier PJ, Ryk C, Steineck G, et al. Mutations in TERT promoter and FGFR3 and telomere length in bladder cancer. *Int J Cancer* (2015) 137:1621–9. doi: 10.1002/ijc.29526

68. Beukers W, van der Keur KA, Kandimalla R, Vergouwe Y, Steyerberg EW, Boormans JL, et al. FGFR3, TERT and OTX1 as a urinary biomarker combination for surveillance of patients with bladder cancer in a large prospective multicenter study. *J Urol.* (2017) 197:1410–8. doi: 10.1016/j.juro.2016.12.096

69. Christensen E, Birkenkamp-Demtröder K, Nordentoft I, Høyer S, van der Keur K, van Kessel K, et al. Liquid biopsy analysis of FGFR3 and PIK3CA hotspot mutations for disease surveillance in bladder cancer. *Eur Urol.* (2017) 71:961–9. doi: 10.1016/j.eururo.2016.12.016

70. Schneider AC, Heukamp LC, Rogenhofer S, Fechner G, Bastian PJ, von Ruecker A, et al. Global histone H4K20 trimethylation predicts cancer-specific survival in patients with muscle-invasive bladder cancer. *BJU Int.* (2011) 108:E290–6. doi: 10.1111/j.1464-410X.2011.10203.x

71. Liu J, Li Y, Liao Y, Mai S, Zhang Z, Liu Z, et al. High expression of H3K27me3 is an independent predictor of worse outcome in patients with urothelial carcinoma of bladder treated with radical cystectomy. *Biomed Res Int.* (2013) 2013:390482. doi: 10.1155/2013/390482

72. Hussmann D, Hansen LL. Methylation-Sensitive High Resolution Melting (MS-HRM). *Methods Mol Biol.* (2018) 1708:551–71. doi: 10.1007/978-1-4939-7481-8_28

73. Tommasi S, Besaratinia A. A versatile assay for detection of aberrant DNA methylation in bladder cancer. *Methods Mol Biol.* (2018) 1655:29–41. doi: 10.1007/978-1-4939-7234-0_3

74. Seripa D, Parrella P, Gallucci M, Gravina C, Papa S, Fortunato P, et al. Sensitive detection of transitional cell carcinoma of the bladder by microsatellite analysis of cells exfoliated in urine. *Int J Cancer* (2001) 95:364–9. doi: 10.1002/1097-0215(20011120)95:6<364::AID-IJC1064>3.0.CO;2-V

75. García-Baquero R, Puerta P, Beltran M, Alvarez-Mújica M, Alvarez-Ossorio JL, Sánchez-Carbayo M. Methylation of tumor suppressor genes in a novel panel predicts clinical outcome in paraffin-embedded bladder tumors. *Tumour Biol.* (2014) 35:5777–86. doi: 10.1007/s13277-014-1767-6

76. Bryzgunova OE, Laktionov PP. Extracellular nucleic acids in urine: sources, structure, diagnostic potential. *Actanaturae* (2015) 7:48–54.

77. Sasaki H, Yoshiike M, Nozawa S, Usuba W, Katsuoka Y, Aida K, et al. expression level of urinary microrna-146a-5p is increased in patients with bladder cancer and decreased in those after transurethral resection. *Clin Genitourin Cancer* (2016) 14:e493–9. doi: 10.1016/j.clgc.2016.04.002

78. Sethi S, Sethi S, Bluth MH. Clinical Implication of micrornas in molecular pathology: an update for 2018. *Clin Lab Med.* (2018) 38:237–51. doi: 10.1016/j.cll.2018.02.003

79. Liu X, Wu Y, Wu Q, Wang Q, Yang Z, Li L. MicroRNAs in biofluids are novel tools for bladder cancer screening. *Oncotarget* (2017) 8:32370–9. doi: 10.18632/oncotarget.16026

80. Fuessel S, Lohse-Fischer A, Vu Van D, Salomo K, Erdmann K, Wirth MP. quantification of micrornas in urine-derived specimens. *Methods Mol Biol.* (2018) 1655:201–26. doi: 10.1007/978-1-4939-7234-0_16

81. Xiao S, Wang J, Xiao N. MicroRNAs as noninvasive biomarkers in bladder cancer detection: a diagnostic meta-analysis based on qRT-PCR data. *Int J Biol Markers* (2016) 31:e276–85. doi: 10.5301/jbm.5000199

82. Hanke M, Hoefig K, Merz H, Feller AC, Kausch I, Jocham D, et al. A robust methodology to study urine microRNA as tumor marker: microRNA-126 and microRNA-182 are related to urinary bladder cancer. *Urol Oncol.* (2010) 28:655–61. doi: 10.1016/j.urolonc.2009.01.027

83. Wiklund ED, Gao S, Hulf T, Sibbritt T, Nair S, Costea DE, et al. MicroRNA alterations and associated aberrant DNA methylation patterns across multiple sample types in oral squamous cell carcinoma. *PLoS ONE* (2011) 6:e27840. doi: 10.1371/journal.pone.0027840

84. Chen YH, Wang SQ, Wu XL, Shen M, Chen ZG, Chen XG, et al. Characterization of microRNAs expression profiling in one group of Chinese urothelial cell carcinoma identified by Solexa sequencing. *Urol Oncol.* (2013) 31:219–27. doi: 10.1016/j.urolonc.2010.11.007

85. Braicu C, Cojocneanu-Petric R, Chira S, Truta A, Floares A, Petrut B, et al. Clinical and pathological implications of miRNA in bladder cancer. *Int J Nanomed.* (2015) 10:791–800. doi: 10.2147/IJN.S72904

86. Pritchard CC, Kroh E, Wood B, Arroyo JD, Dougherty KJ, Miyaji MM, et al. Blood cell origin of circulating microRNAs: a cautionary note for cancer biomarker studies. *Cancer Prev Res.* (2012) 5:492–7. doi: 10.1158/1940-6207.CAPR-11-0370

87. Eissa S, Matboli M, Essawy NO, Kotb YM. Integrative functional genetic-epigenetic approach for selecting genes as urine biomarkers for bladder cancer diagnosis. *Tumour Biol.* (2015) 36:9545–52. doi: 10.1007/s13277-015-3722-6

88. Sapre N, Macintyre G, Clarkson M, Naeem H, Cmero M, Kowalczyk A, et al. A urinary microRNA signature can predict the presence of bladder urothelial carcinoma in patients undergoing surveillance. *Br J Cancer* (2016) 114:454–62. doi: 10.1038/bjc.2015.472

89. Pospisilova S, Pazourkova E, Horinek A, Brisuda A, Svobodova I, Soukup V, et al. MicroRNAs in urine supernatant as potential non-invasive markers for bladder cancer detection. *Neoplasma* (2016) 63:799–808. doi: 10.4149/neo_2016_518

90. Pignot G, Cizeron-Clairac G, Vacher S, Susini A, Tozlu S, Vieillefond A, et al. MicroRNA expression profile in a large series of bladder tumors: identification of a 3-miRNA signature associated with aggressiveness of muscle-invasive bladder cancer. *Int J Cancer* (2013) 132:2479–91. doi: 10.1002/ijc.27949

91. Yun SJ, Jeong P, Kim WT, Kim TH, Lee YS, Song PH, et al. Cell-free microRNAs in urine as diagnostic and prognostic biomarkers of bladder cancer. *Int J Oncol.* (2012) 41:1871–8. doi: 10.3892/ijo.2012.1622

92. Matsushita R, Seki N, Chiyomaru T, Inoguchi S, Ishihara T, Goto Y, et al. Tumour-suppressive microRNA-144-5p directly targets CCNE1/2 as potential prognostic markers in bladder cancer. *Br J Cancer* (2015) 113:282–9. doi: 10.1038/bjc.2015.195

93. Zhang DZ, Lau KM, Chan ES, Wang G, Szeto CC, Wong K, et al. Cell-free urinary microRNA-99a and microRNA-125b are diagnostic markers for the non-invasive screening of bladder cancer. *PLoS ONE* (2014) 9:e100793. doi: 10.1371/journal.pone.0100793

94. Tölle A, Jung M, Rabenhorst S, Kilic E, Jung K, Weikert S. Identification of microRNAs in blood and urine as tumour markers for the detection of urinary bladder cancer. *Oncol Rep.* (2013) 30:1949–56. doi: 10.3892/or.2013.2621

95. Chen L, Cui Z, Liu Y, Bai Y, Lan F. MicroRNAs as biomarkers for the diagnostics of bladder cancer: a meta-analysis. *Clin Lab.* (2015) 61:1101–8.

96. Juracek J, Peltanova B, Dolezel J, Fedorko M, Pacik D, Radova L, et al. Genome-wide identification of urinary cell-free microRNAs for non-invasive detection of bladder cancer. *J Cell Mol Med.* (2018) 22:2033–8. doi: 10.1111/jcmm.13487

97. Pardini B, Cordero F, Naccarati A, Viberti C, Birolo G, Oderda M, et al. MicroRNA profiles in urine by next-generation sequencing can stratify bladder cancer subtypes. *Oncotarget* (2018) 9:20658–69. doi: 10.18632/oncotarget.25057

98. Matullo G, Naccarati A, Pardini B. MicroRNA expression profiling in bladder cancer: the challenge of next-generation sequencing in tissues and biofluids. *Int J Cancer* (2016) 138:2334–45. doi: 10.1002/ijc.2989

99. Zhang M, Ren H, Li Z, Niu W, Wang Y. Expression of N-Myc Downstream-Regulated Gene 2 in bladder cancer and its potential utility as a urinary diagnostic biomarkers. *Med Sci Monit.* (2017) 23:4644–9. doi: 10.12659/MSM.901610

100. Andreu Z, Otta Oshiro R, Redruello A, López-Martín S, Gutiérrez-Vázquez C, Morato E, et al. Extracellular vesicles as a source for non-invasive biomarkers in bladder cancer progression. *Eur J Pharm Sci.* (2017) 98:70–9. doi: 10.1016/j.ejps.2016.10.008

101. Armstrong DA, Green BB, Seigne JD, Schned AR, Marsit CJ. MicroRNA molecular profiling from matched tumor and bio-fluids in bladder cancer. *Mol Cancer* (2015) 14:194. doi: 10.1186/s12943-015-0466-2

102. Du L, Duan W, Jiang X, Zhao L, Li J, Wang R, et al. Cell-free lncRNA expression signatures in urine serve as novel non-invasive biomarkers for diagnosis and recurrence prediction of bladder cancer. *J Cell Mol Med.* (2018) 22:2838–45. doi: 10.1111/jcmm.13578

103. Berrondo C, Flax J, Kucherov V, Siebert A, Osinski T, Rosenberg A, et al. Expression of the long non-coding rna hotair correlates with disease progression in bladder cancer and is contained in bladder

cancer patient urinary exosomes. *PLoS ONE* (2016) 11:e0147236. doi: 10.1371/journal.pone.0147236

104. Chen CL, Lai YF, Tang P, Chien KY, Yu JS, Tsai CH et al. Comparative and targeted proteomic analyses of urinary microparticles from bladder cancer and hernia patients. *J Proteome Res.* (2012) 11:5611–29. doi: 10.1021/pr3008732

105. Martens-Uzunova ES, Böttcher R, Croce CM, Jenster G, Visakorpi T, Calin GA. Long noncoding RNA in prostate, bladder, and kidney cancer. *Eur Urol.* (2014) 65:1140–51. doi: 10.1016/j.eururo.2013.12.003

106. Terracciano D, Ferro M, Terreri S, Lucarelli G, D'Elia C, Musi G, et al. Urinary long noncoding RNAs in nonmuscle-invasive bladder cancer: new architects in cancer prognostic biomarkers. *Transl Res.* (2017) 184:108–17. doi: 10.1016/j.trsl.2017.03.005

107. Fan Y, Shen B, Tan M, Mu X, Qin Y, Zhang F, et al. Long non-coding RNA UCA1 increases chemoresistance of bladder cancer cells by regulating Wnt signaling. *FEBS J.* (2014) 281:1750–8. doi: 10.1111/febs.12737

108. Peter S, Borkowska E, Drayton RM, Rakhit CP, Noon A, Chen W, et al. Identification of differentially expressed long noncoding RNAs in bladder cancer. *Clin Cancer Res.* (2014) 20:5311–21. doi: 10.1158/1078-0432.CCR-14-0706

109. Neuhausen A, Florl AR, Grimm MO, Schulz WA. DNA methylation alterations in urothelial carcinoma. *Cancer Biol Ther.* (2006) 5:993–1001. doi: 10.4161/cbt.5.8.2885

110. Deligezer U, Erten N, Akisik EE, Dalay N. Circulating fragmented nucleosomal DNA and caspase-3 mRNA in patients with lymphoma and myeloma. *Exp Mol Pathol.* (2006) 80:72–6. doi: 10.1016/j.yexmp.2005.05.001

111. Kim WT, Jeong P, Yan C, Kim YH, Lee IS, Kang HW, et al. UBE2C cell-free RNA in urine can discriminate between bladder cancer and hematuria. *Oncotarget* (2016) 7:58193–202. doi: 10.18632/oncotarget.11277

112. Kim WT, Kim YH, Jeong P, Seo SP, Kang HW, Kim YJ, et al. Urinary cell-free nucleic acid IQGAP3: a new non-invasive diagnostic marker for bladder cancer. *Oncotarget* (2018) 9:14354–65. doi: 10.18632/oncotarget

113. Pichler R, Fritz J, Tulchiner G, Klinglmair G, Soleiman A, Horninger W, et al. Increased accuracy of a novel mRNA-based urine test for bladder cancer surveillance. *BJU Int.* (2018) 121:29–37. doi: 10.1111/bju.14019

114. Malentacchi F, Vinci S, Melina AD, Kuncova J, Villari D, Nesi G, et al. Urinary carbonic anhydrase IX splicing messenger RNA variants in urogenital cancers. *Urol Oncol.* (2016) 34:292.e9-292.e16. doi: 10.1016/j.urolonc.2016.02.01

115. Haussecker D, Huang Y, Lau A, Parameswaran P, Fire AZ, Kay MA. Human tRNA-derived small RNAs in the global regulation of RNA silencing. *RNA* (2010) 16:673–95. doi: 10.1261/rna.2000810

116. Lee J, McKinney KQ, Pavlopoulos AJ, Niu M, Kang JW, Oh JW, et al. Altered proteome of extracellular vesicles derived from bladder cancer patients urine. *Mol Cells* (2018) 41:179–87. doi: 10.14348/molcells.2018.2110

117. Yasui T, Yanagida T, Ito S, Konakade Y, Takeshita D, Naganawa T, et al. Unveiling massive numbers of cancer-related urinary-microRNA candidates via nanowires. *Sci Adv.* (2017) 3:e1701133. doi: 10.1126/sciadv.1701133

118. Yu S, Cao H, Shen B, Feng J. Tumor-derived exosomes in cancer progression and treatment failure. *Oncotarget* (2015) 6:37151–68. doi: 10.18632/oncotarget.6022

119. Rosell R, Wei J, Taron M. Circulating MicroRNA signatures of tumor-derived exosomes for early diagnosis of non-small-cell lung cancer. *Clin Lung Cancer* (2009) 10:8–9. doi: 10.3816/CLC.2009.n.001

120. Beckham CJ, Olsen J, Yin PN, Wu CH, Ting HJ, Hagen FK, et al. Bladder cancer exosomes contain EDIL-3/Del1 and facilitate cancer progression. *J Urol.* (2014) 192:583–92. doi: 10.1016/j.juro.2014.02.035

121. Huang X, Liang M, Dittmar R, Wang L. Extracellular microRNAs in urologic malignancies: chances and challenges. *Int J Mol Sci.* (2013) 14:14785–99. doi: 10.3390/ijms140714785

122. Wu P, Zhang G, Zhao J, Chen J, Chen Y, Huang W, et al. Profiling the urinary microbiota in male patients with bladder cancer in China. *Front Cell Infect Microbiol.* (2018) 8:167. doi: 10.3389/fcimb.2018.00167

123. Ward DG, Bryan RT. Liquid biopsies for bladder cancer. *Transl Androl Urol.* (2017) 6:331–5. doi: 10.21037/tau.2017.03.08

124. Wald C. Diagnostics: a flow of information. *Nature* (2017) 551:S48–50. doi: 10.1038/551S48a

125. Piao XM, Byun YJ, Kim WJ, Kim J. Unmasking molecular profiles of bladder cancer. *Invest Clin Urol.* (2018) 59:72–82. doi: 10.4111/icu.2018.59.2.72

126. Soria F, Droller MJ, Lotan Y, Gontero P, D'Andrea D, Gust KM, et al. An up-to-date catalog of available urinary biomarkers for the surveillance of non-muscle invasive bladder cancer. *World J Urol.* (2018). doi: 10.1007/s00345-018-2380-x. [Epub ahead of print].

# 20

# Emerging Biomarkers for Predicting Bladder Cancer Lymph Node Metastasis

Chunyu Zhang[1], Jiao Hu[1], Huihuang Li[1], Hongzhi Ma[2], Belaydi Othmane[1],
Wenbiao Ren[1,3], Zhenglin Yi[1], Dongxu Qiu[1], Zhenyu Ou[1], Jinbo Chen[1*] and Xiongbing Zu[1*]

[1] Department of Urology, Xiangya Hospital, Central South University, Changsha, China, [2] Department of Radiation Oncology,
Hunan Cancer Hospital, Central South University, Changsha, China, [3] George Whipple Lab for Cancer Research, University
of Rochester Medical Institute, Rochester, NY, United States

*Correspondence:
Xiongbing Zu
zuxbxyyy@126.com
Jinbo Chen
chenjinbo1989@yahoo.com

Bladder cancer is one of the leading causes of cancer deaths worldwide. Early detection of lymph node metastasis of bladder cancer is essential to improve patients' prognosis and overall survival. Current diagnostic methods are limited, so there is an urgent need for new specific biomarkers. Non-coding RNA and m6A have recently been reported to be abnormally expressed in bladder cancer related to lymph node metastasis. In this review, we tried to summarize the latest knowledge about biomarkers, which predict lymph node metastasis in bladder cancer and their mechanisms. In particular, we paid attention to the impact of non-coding RNA on lymphatic metastasis of bladder cancer and its specific molecular mechanisms, as well as some prediction models based on imaging, pathology, and biomolecules, in an effort to find more accurate diagnostic methods for future clinical application.

Keywords: lymph node metastasis, bladder cancer, biomarkers, oncogenes, tumor suppressor genes

## INTRODUCTION

Bladder cancer (BCa) is the 10th most common cancer form, causing an estimated 549,000 new cases and 200,000 deaths in 2018. The incidence of BCa in men is four times that of women, and smoking is the most important risk factor for BCa in the population (1). More than 90% of bladder cancers are urothelial carcinoma, and the rest are squamous cell carcinoma and adenocarcinoma.

The most common metastatic manner of BCa is lymph node metastasis (LNM), which is more common in pelvic lymph nodes. LNM has a great influence on the prognosis and survival rate of BCa patients. For BCa patients with positive LNM, the 5-year CSS rate was 27.7%, which is significantly lower than that of patients without lymph node metastasis (2). CT or MRI is commonly used in clinical practice to diagnose pelvic LNM, but it is often difficult to accurately detect metastatic lymph nodes less than 6.8 mm in diameter (3). Many studies have recently reported the correlation between molecular markers and BCa metastasis, indicating a direct link between LNM and abnormal expression of specific biomarkers. Therefore, high-risk LNM patients can be diagnosed by detecting specific biomarkers to achieve early detection and early treatment, thereby achieving timely treatment and improving the survival rate.

Moreover, some predictive models, including imaging, pathology, and molecular markers, have been gradually developed and verified. In this review, we summarized the markers for LNM in BCa from different aspects, including genes, non-coding RNA, and some predictive models (**Figure 1**). The downstream genes of non-coding RNA are specifically listed here (**Table 1**). Generally, mechanisms for LNM in cancers mainly include cell proliferation, cell invasion and migration, inhibition of cell apoptosis, and chemosensitivity. Based on this, we also elaborated on the regulation mechanism of these biomarkers.

## THE MOLECULAR FUNCTION OF GENES IN BCA WITH LNM

There have been many studies on genes as markers for lymph node metastasis in bladder cancer. These genes act as oncogenes or tumor suppressor genes to influence the progression of cancer (**Figure 2**).

### Genes as Oncogenes

VEGF-C (vascular endothelial growth factor C) is the first discovered lymphangiogenesis factor. It contains the mature form of the VEGF homology region. Our team's studies found that the expression of VEGF-C in BCa patients with LNM was significantly higher than that in BCa patients without LNM (57). Simultaneously, we also found that VEGF-C can promote proliferation, invasion, metastasis, and mitomycin C resistance of BCa cells. The mechanisms for that are thought to be related to the increased ratio of Bcl-2/Bax, inactivation of Caspase-3, and increased expression of MMP-9. Also, phosphorylated p38 MAPK and Akt, Keratin 8, Serpin B5, and Annexin A8 may be involved (58, 59). VEGF-C can promote the formation of tumor lymphatic vessels and the metastasis of tumor cells to regional lymph nodes. The combination of the activated VEGF-C and VEGFR-3 can induce phosphorylation of tyrosine kinase, causing the proliferation of lymphatic endothelial cells, thereby promoting the proliferation or expansion of lymphatic vessels (60). VEGF-C also positively affected primary tumor cells' invasiveness since it changed the adhesion of tumor cells to the extracellular matrix, thereby providing the necessary environmental conditions for tumor cells to more easily transfer to the surrounding extracellular matrix. VEGF-C can stimulate lymphatic endothelial cells to release proteolytic enzymes, such as uPA, which facilitate the invasion and infiltration of cancer cells into the matrix, making cancer cells more easily detached from the original tissue (61). The up-regulation of VEGF-C may be the reason for BCa cells' resistance to cisplatin, and the inhibition of VEGF-C reverses the resistance by increasing the expression level of maspin (62). Therefore, we suggest that VEGF-C and VEGFR-3 expression may serve as new indicators for early detection and diagnosis of BCa lymphatic metastasis in the future. Additionally, COX-2 may stimulate VEGF-C secretion to promote the formation of lymphatic vessels (63). COX-2, a subtype enzyme in the COX family, is an inducible enzyme. COX (Cyclooxygenase) is a rate-limiting enzyme in prostaglandin synthesis, which can catalyze arachidonic acid metabolites to prostaglandins. Previous

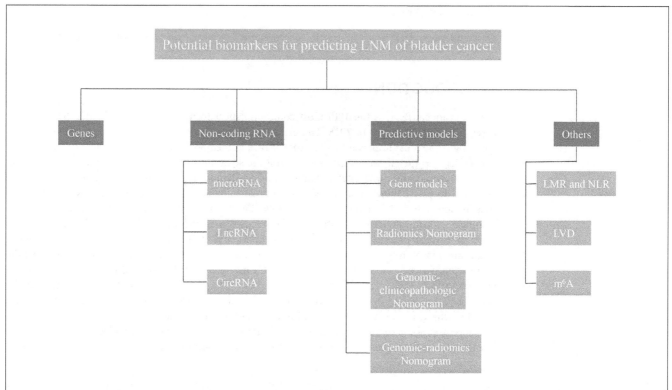

**FIGURE 1** | Potential biomarkers for predicting lymph node metastasis of bladder cancer. Biomarkers for predicting lymphatic metastasis of bladder cancer can be divided into different categories, such asgenes, non-coding RNA, prediction models.

**TABLE 1 |** Downstream genes of non-coding RNA in bladder cancer.

| Marker | Relationship with downstream genes | Downstream genes | Reference |
|---|---|---|---|
| miR-101 | Negative | FZD4 | (4) |
| | | c-FOS | (5) |
| | | c-Met | (6) |
| | | VEGF-C | (7) |
| | | COX-2 | (8) |
| miR-143 | Negative | COX-2 | (9) |
| | | MSI2 | (10) |
| miR-133b | Positive | DUSP1 | (11) |
| | Negative | Bcl-w, Akt1 | (12) |
| | | Epidermal growth factor receptor | (13) |
| | | TAGLN2 | (14) |
| miR-539 | Negative | IGF-1R, AKT, ERK | (15) |
| miR-497 | Positive | E-cadherin | (16) |
| | Negative | Vimentin | |
| | | BIRC5, WNT7A | (17) |
| | | E2F3 | (18) |
| miR-154 | Negative | RSF1, RUNX2 | (19) |
| | | ATG7 | (20) |
| miR-223 | Positive | Caspase-3/7 | (21) |
| | Negative | WDR62 | |
| | | ANLN | (22) |
| | | Nuclear receptor co-activator 1 | (23) |
| miR-148a | Negative | DNMT1 | (24) |
| miR-3658 | Positive | LASS2 | (25) |
| LncRNA MALAT1 | Negative | E-cadherin | (26) |
| | Positive | ZEB1, ZEB2 | |
| | | VEGF-C | (27) |
| | | Bcl-2, MMP-13 | (28) |
| | | Foxq1 | (29) |
| | | Cyclin D1 | (30) |
| LncRNA PVT1 | Positive | VEGF-C | (31) |
| | | CDK1 | (32) |
| LncRNA OXCT1-AS1 | Positive | JAK1 | (33) |
| LncRNA BLACAT2 | Positive | VEGF-C | (34) |
| LncRNA LNMAT1 | Positive | CCL-2, VEGF-C | (35) |
| LncRNA SNHG16 | Positive | ZEB1, ZEB2 | (36) |
| | | TIMP3 | (37) |
| | | STAT3 | (38) |
| LncRNA ZFAS1 | Positive | ZEB1, ZEB2 | (39) |
| | Negative | KLF2, NKD2 | |
| LncRNA DLX6-AS1 | Positive | HSP90B1 | (40) |
| | | Wnt/β-catenin | (41) |
| LINC01296 | Positive | EMT | (42) |
| LncRNA DANCR | Positive | CCND1, PLAU | (43) |
| | | MSI2 | (44) |
| LncRNA SPRY4-IT1 | Positive | EZH2 | (45) |
| LncRNA NNT-AS1 | Positive | HMGB1 | (46) |
| | | PODXL | (47) |
| LncRNA LNMAT2 | Positive | PROX1 | (48) |
| LncRNA HOXA-AS2 | Positive | Smad2 | (49) |
| LncRNA HNF1A-AS1 | Positive | Bcl-2 | (50) |
| CircHIPK3 | Negative | HPSE, MMP-9, VEGF | (51) |
| CircFNDC3B | Negative | G3BP2/SRC/FAK | (52) |
| CircFUT8 | Positive | KLF10 | (53) |
| CircACVR2A | Positive | EYA4 | (54) |
| CircPICALM | Positive | STEAP4, EMT | (55) |
| cTFRC | Positive | TFRC | (56) |

studies have shown that COX-2 expression was significantly increased in BCa tissues and was associated with LNM (64).

Another well-known gene that functions as an oncogene in BCa is PCMT1. PCMTl gene is located at 6p22.3-6q24, about 60kb in length, and contains eight exons and seven introns. Studies have shown that the expression of PCMT1 in BCa tissue was higher than that in normal urothelial tissue, and its expression was significantly associated with LNM. PCMT1 regulated the migration and invasion of BCa cells by regulating the expression of epithelial-mesenchymal transition (EMT) related genes, such as E-cadherin, vimentin, Snail, and Slug (65). Sonic Hedgehog (Shh) also activated EMT to promote tumorigenicity and stemness in BCa (66). Shh is a member of the Hedgehog (HH) family. The study found that the expression of Shh protein was significantly correlated with LNM (67). Shh can promote the migration and invasion of BCa cells. The Shh pathway's activation through the binding of the Shh ligand to the transmembrane protein Patched1 eliminates the inhibitory effect on smoothened (SMO). The activation of SMO produced a downstream signaling cascade that led to the nuclear translocation of the transcription factor Gli1, which further induce the transcription of target genes (68).

The overexpression of CXCL5 can promote the progression of BCa. CXCL5, known as epithelial-derived neutrophil-activating peptide 78 (ENA78), is a small (8-14 kDa) protein belonging to the CXC-type chemokine family. CXCL5 (chemokine C-X-C motif ligand 5) was expressed higher in BCa tissues than normal tissues, which was associated with LNM (69). It is also related to promoting mitomycin resistance by activating EMT and NF-κB pathway (70). Moreover, CXCL5 increased BCa cells proliferation, migration, and decreased cell apoptosis through Snail, PI3K-AKT, and ERK1/2 signaling pathways. In addition, CXCL5 combined with CXCR2 induces the expression of MMP-2 and MMP-9 and activates the PI3K/AKT signaling pathway (71, 72). Matrix metalloproteinases (MMPs) are a family of structurally related zinc-dependent endopeptidases that can substantially degrade all components of the extracellular matrix (ECM). MMP2, MMP7, and MMP9 are important members of the matrix metalloproteinase family. MMP-2 can physiologically degrade type IV collagen. Mohammad et al. (73) found that the higher the MMP-2 activity level in BCa, the higher the positive rate of LNM. MMP-7, also known as matrilysin, is the smallest MMP. It is produced by the tumor cells themselves, unlike other MMPs which are solely produced by stromal cells. Studies have shown that high expression of MMP-7 was significantly associated with LNM of BCa (74). Studies have shown that MMP-9 genes and proteins' expression levels in urine and blood of patients with BCa were significantly increased (75). These genes can also decompose the extracellular matrix, make cancer cells easily pass through the extracellular matrix, and promote tumor metastasis.

In addition, Zhao et al. (76) identified a new oncogene candidate, IPO11, in BCa, which is located on chromosome 5q12. Importin-11, a 116 kD protein, is encoded by IPO11. It is a karyopherin family member, which mediates the nucleocytoplasmic transport of proteins and nucleic acids

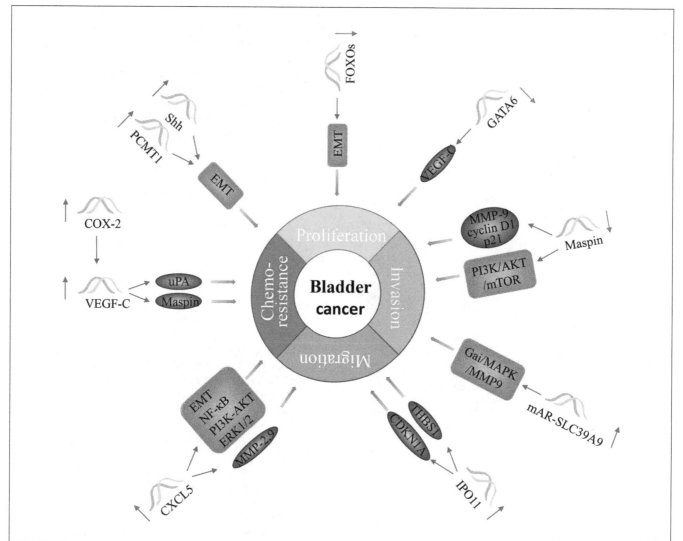

**FIGURE 2** | The molecular function of genes in bladder cancer with lymph node metastasis. Genes can predict lymph node metastasis in bladder cancer. Some of them can promote the progression of cancer, and some can inhibit it.

through the nuclear pore complexes. Studies have shown that IPO11 mRNA was highly expressed in invasive BCa cell lines. The overexpression of importin-11 was positively correlated with LNM. Importin-11 can promote BCa cells' invasiveness, which may be related to the abnormal expression of CDKN1A and THBS1 (77). Presler et al. (78) found that SCD1 was overexpressed in BCa, which was related to LNM. SCD-1 (Stearoyl-CoA desaturase-1) can convert SFA (saturated fatty acids) to MUFA (monounsaturated fatty acids). It is located on chromosome 10q24.31. SCD inhibitors and SCD gene interference reduced the proliferation and invasion of BCa cells (79). FGFR3 (fibroblast growth factor receptor 3) stimulated SCD1 activity to promote tumor growth in BCa cells (80).

The studies of our team also found some new oncogenes. ISYNA1 (Inositol-3-phosphate synthase 1) was positively associated with tumor T stage and LNM of BCa patients. It is an important regulatory factor in promoting proliferation and inhibiting apoptosis in BCa cells (81). The high expression of mAR-SLC39A9 was directly associated with BCa pathological

stage, pathological grade, and lymph node metastasis presence. It also increased BCa metastasis through Gαi/MAPK/MMP9 signaling (82).

## Genes as Tumor Suppressors

Maspin (mammary sefine protease inhibitor) is an important member of the serin protease inhibitor (serpin) superfamily. It is located at 18q21.3-q23. Our team's previous studies found that Maspin expression in BCa tissue was significantly down-regulated in comparison with normal tissues adjacent to the cancer and was related also to LNM. The negative correlation between the protein expression level and VEGF-C is statistically significant (83, 84). Maspin can inhibit the invasion of BCa cells, and its growth-inhibiting properties were related to its localization in cells. The surface-bound Maspin directly controlled the adhesion of BCa cells to the blood vessel wall (85). The combination of nuclear-localized maspin and chromatin can effectively prevent cell migration. Mapsin mainly promoted the development of BCa through DNA methylation and histone deacetylation to cause low expression of genes (86). Maspin modulated HDAC1 target genes, including cyclin D1, p21, MMP9, and vimentin (87). In our previous study, maspin could enhance Cisplatin chemosensitivity through the PI3K/AKT/mTOR signaling pathway in MIBC T24 and 5637 cell lines (88).

Another gene that functions as a tumor suppressor in BCa is GATA6. GATA6 (GATA-binding factor 6), a zinc-finger transcription factor, is located at 18q11.2. It regulates transcription cofactors and RNA polymerase II to the proximal promoter to regulate target genes' transcription. Wang et al. (89) found that GATA6 decreased in BCa, and further decreased in patients with positive LNM. GATA6 was significantly down-regulated in BCa through frequent promoter methylation. GATA6 mainly inhibited LNM of BCa by regulating VEGF-C. Down-regulation of GATA6 promoted VEGF-C transcription, which promoted lymphangiogenesis, resulting in an increased lymphatic spread of BCa. This increased spread shows that it is of great significance to check the methylation status of the GATA6 promoter in the urine of BCa patients. The low expression of FOXOs was also associated with LNM in BCa (90). FOXO (Forkhead box class O) is the subgroup O of forkhead box (FOX) transcription factors, which has four members, FOXO1, FOXO3, FOXO4 and FOXO6. FOXOs have a highly conserved forkhead DNA binding domain. FOXOs can inhibit the invasion of BCa cells by down-regulating Twist2 and YB-1 and up-regulating E-cadherin (91).

## REGULATION OF MICRORNAS FOR BCA PATIENTS WITH LYMPH NODE METASTASIS

MiRNA is a type of 21-23nt small RNA, which can complement mRNA and either silence it or degrade it. Most miRNAs are down-regulated in bladder cancer. Moreover, they inhibit the lymph node metastasis of bladder cancer (**Figure 3**).

MiR-101 can suppress the progression of BCa. Studies have shown that the expression of miR-101 in BCa patients was down-regulated and significantly associated with LNM (92). Moreover, it can inhibit the proliferation, migration, and invasion of BCa cells by directly targeting FZD4 (frizzled class receptor 4), c-FOS, and c-Met (4–6). MiR-101 increased Cisplatin sensitivity by inhibiting the expression of VEGF-C and COX-2 in BCa cells (7, 8). MiR-143 also inhibited the growth and migration of BCa cells by targeting COX-2 (9). MiR-143 was reported to suppress the progression of BCa as well and it is located on chromosome 5q32. Liu et al. (93) found that miR-143 was down-expressed in the serum of BCa patients with LNM. It also directly affected the expression of MSI2 through its RNAi effect, which also effectively inhibited the KRAS network, thereby regulating BCa cells (10).

Another gene, miR-133b, is located on chromosome 6p12.2. Studies have shown that the expression level of miR-133b in BCa tissues is significantly reduced, which was significantly correlated with LNM (94). MiR-133b may inhibit the proliferation of BCa by up-regulating dual-specificity protein phosphatase 1 (DUSP1) (11). It inhibited angiogenesis and enhanced BCa cells'

chemosensitivity to Gemcitabine by targeting transgelin 2 (TAGLN2) (14). MiR-133b can regulate the proliferation, migration, and invasion of BCa cells by down-regulating Bcl-w, Akt1, and epidermal growth factor receptor along with its downstream effector protein (12, 13). Liao et al. (15) found that miR-539 was down-regulated in BCa, and was related to LNM. MiR-539 is located on chromosome 14q32.31, and it can inhibit the proliferation and invasion of BCa cells by directly targeting IGF-1R and inactivating the AKT and ERK signaling pathways.

MiR-497 is also known as a tumor suppressor in BCa, and it is located on chromosome 17p13.1. Studies have revealed that the expression of miR-497 in BCa tissue was lower than that of adjacent non-cancer tissues, and it was correlated with LNM (16). MiR-497 can inhibit the proliferation, migration, and invasion of BCa by up-regulating E-cadherin and down-regulating vimentin, α-smooth muscle actin, BIRC5, WNT7A, and E2F3 (16–18). Previous studies have found that miR-154 was significantly down-regulated in BCa tissues and was associated with LNM. MiR-154 is located in the human imprinted 14q32 domain. MiR-154 inhibited the proliferation, migration, and invasion of BCa cells by regulating the expression of RSF1, RUNX2, and ATG7 (19, 20). MiR-223 is located on chromosome Xq12. Sugita et al. (21) found that the expression level of miR-223 was significantly reduced in BCa tissues, which was related to LNM. MiR-223 inhibited cell invasion and promoted cell apoptosis in BCa via caspase-3/7 activation and negatively regulating WDR62 (WD repeat domain 62), ANLN, and nuclear receptor coactivator 1 (21–23). MiR-148a, with 68 nucleotide sequences, locates to 7p15.2, and is confirmed by Ma et al. (95) that its expression level in BCa tissue is lower than that of adjacent normal tissues, and that its low expression level is associated with advanced tumor progression and LNM. Also, Lombard et al. (24) found that miR-148a increased the apoptosis of BCa cells by reducing the expression of DNA methyltransferase 1 (DNMT1).

MiR-3658 is known as an oncogene in BCa. The expression of miR-3658 in BCa tissue was up-regulated, and its expression was significantly related to the lymph node infiltration, distant metastasis, and TNM stage (96). It can also promote cell proliferation, migration, and invasion by targeting LASS2 (25).

## LNCRNAS REGULATE LYMPH NODE METASTASIS IN BCA

LncRNA is a non-coding RNA with a length of more than 200 nucleotides and is closely related to cancer occurrence and development. It can directly bind to proteins to block its functions or change its cellular location, regulate mRNA translation and act as a miRNA sponge. Most lncRNAs act as oncogenes to promote lymphatic metastasis of bladder cancer (**Figure 4**).

Our team's studies found several lncRNAs as oncogenes, such as MALAT1, PVT1, and OXCT1-AS1. The expression of MALAT1 was positively associated with LNM in BCa. It

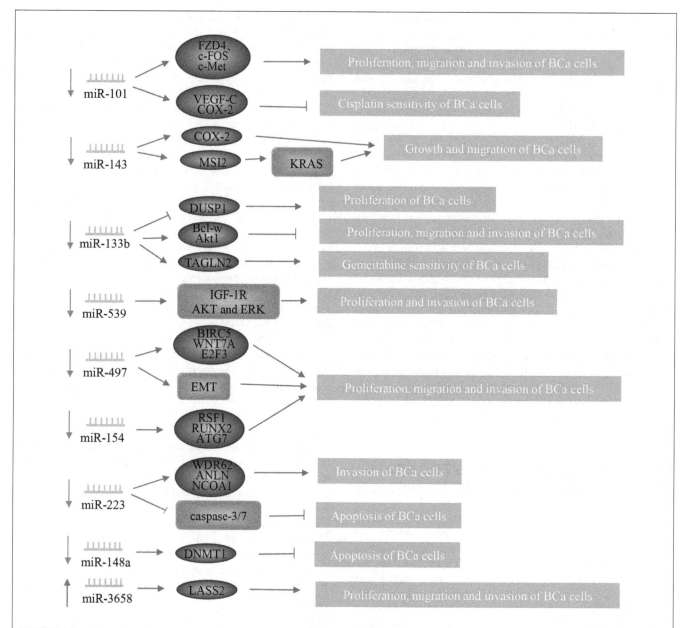

**FIGURE 3** | Regulation of microRNAs in bladder cancer patients with lymph node metastasis. MiRNAs play a vital role in the lymph node metastasis of bladder cancer. They can promote or inhibit the metastasis of bladder cancer by regulating downstream genes or proteins.

enhanced the Cisplatin resistance of the BCa cells by regulating the miR-101-3p/VEGF-C pathway (27, 97). MALAT1 promoted proliferation and invasion by miR-125b-Bcl-2/MMP-13, miR-124/foxq1 and microRNA-34a/cyclin D1 in BCa cells (28–30). It also up-regulated EMT-associated ZEB1, ZEB2, and Slug and downregulated E-cadherin levels (26). LncRNA PVT1 is located at 8q24, downstream of MYC. High PVT1 expression is associated with higher tumor stage and positive lymph node metastasis (98). PVT1 directly interacted with miR-128, reducing the binding of miR-128 to VEGF-C, thereby inhibiting the degradation of VEGFC mRNA by miR-128 (31). Moreover, PVT1 down-regulated miR-31 to enhance CDK1 expression

and promote the proliferation, migration, and invasion of BCa cells (32). LncRNA OXCT1-AS1 (OXCT1 antisense RNA 1) is located on chromosome 5p13.1 and was also significantly up-regulated in BCa cell lines with LNM and was found to be inhibiting miR-455-5p in order to up-regulate the expression of JAK1, thus promoting the invasion of BCa (33).

Some lncRNAs regulate VEGF-C to promote the progression of BCa. BLACAT2 (bladder cancer-associated transcript 2) was significantly overexpressed in BCa patients with LNM. It combines with the VEGF-C promoter by forming triplexes to up-regulate VEGF-C expression, thereby promoting lymphangiogenesis and lymphatic metastasis. BLACAT2

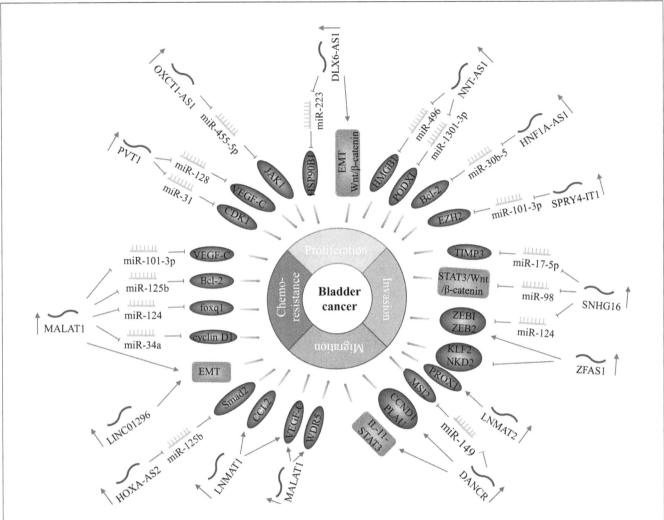

**FIGURE 4 |** LncRNAs regulate lymph node metastasis in bladder cancer. In bladder cancer, the expression level of some lncRNAs is related to lymph node metastasis and regulates lymph node metastasis by regulating cancer cell proliferation, metastasis, invasion, and chemosensitivity.

directly interacted with WDR5 (the core component of the histone H3K4 methyltransferase complex) to epigenetically induce lymphangiogenesis and invasion (34). LNMAT1 (lymph node metastasis-associated Transcript 1) was significantly up-regulated in BCa with LNM. LNMAT1 recruited hnRNPL to the CCL2 promoter to activate CCL2 expression, resulting in increased H3K4 trimethylation, thereby ensuring hnRNPL binding and enhancing transcription. In addition, LNMAT1-induced CCL2 regulated the tumor microenvironment in BCa tissues through tumor-associated macrophages (TAMs) infiltration and VEGF-C upregulation, which ultimately led to lymphangiogenesis and lymphatic metastasis (35).

Several lncRNAs promote the progression of BCa by regulating ZEB1 and ZEB2. LncRNA SNHG16 (small nucleolar RNA host gene 16) is encoded by a 7571-bp region at chromosome 17q25.1. Previous studies have found that SNHG16 was highly expressed in BCa tissues and was positively correlated with LNM (37). SNHG16 can regulate the

proliferation, apoptosis, EMT, invasion, and migration of BCa by directly acting on the miR-17-5p/metalloproteinase 3 (TIMP3) axis, miR-200a-3p/ZEB1/ZEB2 axis, and miR-98/STAT3/Wnt/β-catenin pathway axis (36–38). LncRNA ZFAS1 (zinc finger antisense 1), located on the antisense strand of the ZNFX1 promoter region, is transcript antisense to the 5′- end of the gene zinc finger NFX1-type containing 1 (ZNFX1). Yang et al. (39) found that the expression level of ZFAS1 in BCa was increased and positively correlated with LNM. ZFAS1 can promote the proliferation, migration and invasion of BCa by down-regulating the expression of KLF2 and NKD2, and at the same time, up-regulating the expression of ZEB1 and ZEB2. It also promotes tumorigenesis of BCa through sponging miR-329 (99).

Also, some lncRNAs regulate EMT to promote BCa progression. LncRNA DLX6-AS1 (distal-less homeobox 6 antisense 1) is regulatory of members in the DLX gene family, which is localized on chromosome 7q21.3. DLX6-AS1 was up-regulated in BCa, which was related to LNM. Overexpression of DLX6-AS1 promoted the proliferation, invasion, and migration of BCa cells by regulating EMT and Wnt/β-catenin signaling pathway activity (41). DLX6-AS1-mediated miR-223 silencing can promote the growth and invasion of BCa through the up-regulation of HSP90B1 (40). LINC01296 is a novel intergenic lncRNA located at 14q11.2. The expression of LINC01296 was positively correlated with lymph node-positive BCa, and its up-regulated expression can promote BCa cells metastasis by activating the EMT pathway (42).

Another lncRNA, DANCR (differentiation antagonizing non-protein coding RNA), is located on chromosome 4q12.5, which is mainly distributed in the cytoplasm. Chen et al. (43) found that DANCR was significantly up-regulated in BCa tissues and positively correlated with LNM. DANCR promoted the LNM and BCa cells' proliferation *via* DANCR guided LRPPRC (leucine-rich pentatricopeptide repeat containing) to stabilize its mRNA, then to activate IL-11-STAT3 signaling and increase CCND1 and PLAU expression. Zhan et al. (44) found that DANCR positively regulated the expression of MSI2 (musashi RNA binding protein 2) through sponging miR-149 to promote the malignant phenotype of BCa cells. Zhao et al. (100) found that the expression level of SPRY4-IT1 in BCa tissue was also higher than that of adjacent non-tumor tissues and was associated with LNM. SPRY4-IT1 is derived from the intron region of the SPRY4 gene and may contain several long hairpin secondary structures, which are located in 5q31.3. SPRY4-IT1 can promote proliferation and metastasis of BCa cells by sponging miR-101-3p to actively regulate the expression of EZH2 (45). Wu et al. (46) found that lncRNA NNT-AS1 was up-regulated in BCa, which was significantly associated with LNM. NNT-AS1 (nicotinamide nucleotide transhydrogenase antisense RNA 1) is located on chromosome 5p12 with 3 exons. NNT-AS1 promoted the proliferation, migration, and invasion of BCa cells by acting as a competing endogenous RNA for miR-496 to enhance the expression level of HMGB1. NNT-AS1 also targeted the miR-1301-3p/PODXL axis and activated the Wnt pathway, thereby enhancing BCa cells' growth (47). LncRNA LNMAT2 (lymph node metastasis-associated transcript 2) was overexpressed in urinary-EXO and serum-EXO of patients with BCa, which was related to LNM. LNMAT2 was found to bind to the prospero homeobox 1 (PROX1) promoter by inducing H3K4 trimethylation, which enhanced PROX1 transcription, thus promoting lymphangiogenesis and lymph node metastasis in bladder cancer (48).

Additionally, several lncRNAs positively correlated with LNM, including: (1) HOXA-AS2, which inhibited the expression of miR-125b to promote the expression of Smad2, thus promoting the migration and invasion of BCa cells (49); (2) HNF1A-AS1, which positively regulated the expression of Bcl-2 by sponging miR-30b-5 to promote the proliferation of bladder cancer and inhibited its apoptosis (50, 101); (3) ROR1-AS1, which promoted the growth and migration of bladder cancer by regulating miR-504 (102); (4) RMRP, which promoted the proliferation, migration, and invasion of bladder cancer cells by regulating miR-206 as a sponge (103).

# THE ROLE OF CIRCRNAS FOR BCA LYMPH NODE METASTASIS

CircRNA is a type of non-coding RNA that forms a circular structure by covalent bonds but does not have a 5'-end cap and a 3'-end poly(A) tail. It is closely related to the occurrence and development of cancer. It can act as an mRNA 'sponge', regulate transcription and splicing, and interact with RNA-binding proteins (104). Most circRNA negatively regulates lymph node metastasis of bladder cancer, and some molecules positively regulate this process (**Figure 5**).

CircHIPK3 (circRNA ID: hsa_circ_0000284), also known as bladder cancer-related circular RNA-2 (BCRC-2), was significantly down-regulated in BCa and was negatively correlated with LNM. It originates from the second exon of the Homeodomain-interacting protein kinase 3 (HIPK3) gene. CircHIPK3 sponged miR-558 and prevented miR-558 from being transported into the nucleus to bind the promoter of heparanase (HPSE) gene in BCa cells, thereby down-regulating the expression of HPSE and its downstream targets such as MMP-9, and VEGF, thus weakening the migration, invasion and angiogenesis of BCa cells (51). Additionally, Liu et al. (52) confirmed that circFNDC3B was significantly down-regulated in BCa tissue, and its low expression was significantly correlated with LNM. It is originated from exons 5 and 6 of the FNDC3B gene. CircFNDC3B acted as a sponge of miR-1178-3p to inhibit G3BP2 and further inhibit the downstream SRC/FAK signaling pathway, thereby inhibiting the proliferation, migration, and invasion of BCa cells.

By screening RNA sequencing data generated from human BCa tissues and matched adjacent normal bladder tissues, two novel tumor suppressors were separately identified, which are circFUT8 and circACVR2A. CircFUT8 (circBase: hsa_circ_0003028) was originated from exon 3 of the FUT8 gene. CircACVR2A was derived from exons 3, 4, and 5 of the ACVR2A gene. These two tumor suppressors were down-regulated in BCa tissues and were related to LNM (53, 54). CircFUT8 regulated the expression of Slug by sponging miR-570-3p to promote the expression of Krüpple-like-factor 10 (KLF10), thus inhibiting the metastasis and invasion of BCa cells (54). CircACVR2A can inhibit the proliferation, migration, and invasion of BCa cells by directly interacting with miR-626 and acting as a miRNA sponge to regulate EYA4 expression (53). In addition, circPICALM was found to suppress cancer progression. It is generated from exons 9-12 of PICALM. It was down-regulated in BCa tissues and associated with LNM. CircPICALM acted as a miR-1265 sponge to regulate STEAP4 and further affect FAK phosphorylation and EMT, thereby inhibiting the metastasis of BCa (55).

Serval other circRNAs were found to be possibly promoting cancer progression by inducing the malignant proliferation or migration and invasion of cancer cells. Su et al. identified a novel circular RNA called cTFRC. His study has shown that cTFRC was up-regulated in BCa tissues and was associated with LNM. The study also revealed that cTFRC might act as a sponge for miR-107 to up-regulate the expression of TFRC (transferrin

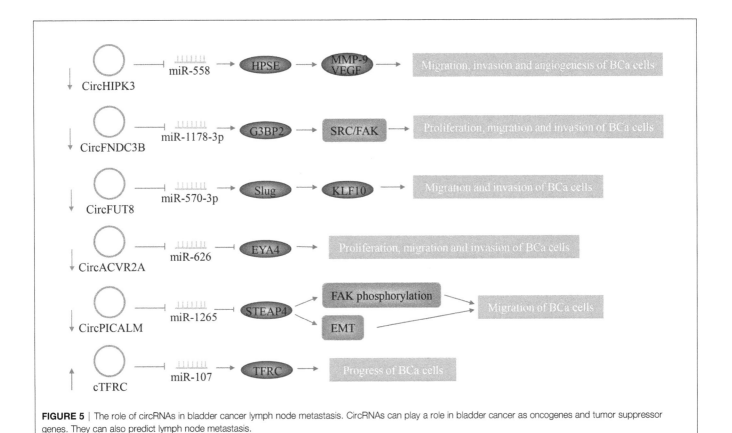

**FIGURE 5** | The role of circRNAs in bladder cancer lymph node metastasis. CircRNAs can play a role in bladder cancer as oncogenes and tumor suppressor genes. They can also predict lymph node metastasis.

receptor), further promoting the transitional phenotype of BCa cells from epithelial to mesenchymal, thereby promoting the progress of BCa. (56) Another circRNA, circPTK2, was significantly increased in BCa, and its expression level is closely related to LNM. CircPTK2 can promote the proliferation and migration of BCa cells, but its specific mechanisms are still unclear (105).

## OTHER MOLECULES AS PREDICTIVE BIOMARKERS

In addition to the molecules described above, studies on the tumor microenvironment and genetic modification can also help predict the lymphatic metastasis of bladder cancer.

Tumors often form a microenvironment that allows inflammatory cells to proliferate and produce large amounts of mediators. D'Andrea et al. (106) found that LMR (lymphocyte-to-monocyte ratio) and NLR (neutrophil-to-lymphocyte ratio) can be used as independent factors to predict the preoperative LNM and postoperative recurrence rate of BCa patients. Zhou et al. (107) found that lymphatic vessel density (LVD) within and around the tumor increases, and lymph node metastasis of bladder cancer also increase significantly. LVD is also related to the patient's prognosis.

$m^6A$ (N6-methyladenosine) refers to methylation of the N6 position of adenosine bases. m6A RNA modification is a reversible posttranscriptional modification process maintained by a multicomponent methyltransferase 'writer' complex (KIAA1429, METTL3, METTL14, RBM15, WTAP, and ZC3H13) and removed by demethylases 'erasers' (FTO and ALKBH5). The function of $m^6A$ in mRNA metabolism primarily depends on reader proteins, which include HNRNPC, YTHDC1, YTHDC2, YTHDF1, and YTHDF2. These regulators were differentially associated with different clinicopathological variables of BCa patients. The expression of WTAP was significantly correlated with LNM (108). Han et al. (109) found that METTL3 was significantly increased in bladder cancer and correlated with high histological grade and poor prognosis. METTL3 interacted with the microprocessor protein DGCR8 and positively modulated the pri-miR221/222 processes, resulting in the reduction of PTEN, which ultimately leads to the progression of bladder cancer.

## PREDICTIVE MODELS AS BIOMARKERS FOR BCA LNM

The prediction model includes many aspects, such as molecules, imaging, and pathology. With the advent of models, the predictive results of bladder cancer lymphatic metastasis have become more and more reliable.

### Gene Expression Model

Smith et al. (110) developed a 20-GEM (gene expression model) for predicting pathological node status, which is evaluable on primary tumor tissue from clinically node-negative (cN0) patients. The predictive efficacy of the model is modest. Seiler et al. (111) invented a KNN51 (K-nearest neighbor classifier 51) to predict pathological lymph node metastases, but the lack of external validation limited its application. Lu et al. (112) presented a preoperative nomogram incorporating the LNM signature and a genomic mutation of MLL2. The LNM signature consists of 48 selected features. The model demonstrated good discrimination and good calibration. KNN51 included 24 non-coding features from the 51 gene signature, but the LN20 signature was based only on coding genes. Clinical factors were not incorporated into the predictive models for evaluation.

## Radiomics Nomogram

Wu et al. (113, 114) developed and validated two types of radiomics nomograms incorporating the radiomics signature and CT/MRI-reported LN status for the preoperative prediction of LNM in patients with BCa, which was a non-invasive preoperative prediction tool. It shows favorable predictive accuracy, especially for cN0 patients. Multicenter validation should be performed to acquire high-level evidence for its clinical application.

## Genomic-Clinicopathologic Nomogram

Wu et al. (115) constructed an inclusive nomogram that incorporated the five-mRNA-based classifier, image-based LN status, transurethral resection (TUR) T stage, and TUR lymphovascular invasion (LVI) to predict LNM in BCa patients. Five LN-status-related mRNAs include ADRA1D, COL10A1, DKK2, HIST2H3D, and MMP11. It shows favorable discriminatory ability and may aid in clinical decision-making, especially for cN-patients. However, it requires multicenter prospective clinical trials to provide high-level evidence for clinical application.

## Genomic-Radiomics Nomogram

Chen et al. (116) validated a genomic-radiomics nomogram incorporating CCR7 and CT to predict LNM in patients with BCa. The combined evaluation of CCR7 and CT appeared to be a more reliable marker for lymph node metastasis in BCa than the diagnosis by CT or CCR7 alone. However, these results require further confirmation by large sample and multi-center prospective studies.

## OTHER FACTORS AFFECTING THE PROGNOSIS OF BCA

### Systemic Diseases

In recent years, studies have found that some systemic diseases were closely related to tumor occurrence and development. Metabolic syndrome (MetS) was defined as the presence of three of the following: hypertension, hyperlipidemia, diabetes, or body mass index >30. Previous studies have proved that MetS cannot predict higher pathological stages and the risks of LVI

and LNM, but a single component of metabolic syndrome was related to them. Body mass index, waist circumference, and hypertension were positively correlated with the risk of higher pathological stages. And higher BMI value was related to lymphatic invasion and lymph node metastasis (117, 118). Obesity was significantly related to recurrence-free survival, cancer-specific survival, and overall mortality. Adipose tissue can produce a variety of inflammatory factors, including leptin, adiponectin, and cytokines. Leptin played an anti-tumor effect by promoting the proliferation and activation of natural killer cells (119, 120). Nonalcoholic fatty liver was positively correlated with

**TABLE 2 |** The relationship between biomarkers and prognosis in bladder cancer.

| Reference | Marker | Relationship with LNM | Prognosis |
|---|---|---|---|
| 57 | VEGF-C | Positive | DFS |
| 64 | COX-2 | Positive | OS |
| 65 | PCMT1 | Positive | OS |
| 67 | Sonic Hedgehog | Positive | No |
| 69 | CXCL5 | Positive | OS, PFS, RFS |
| 75 | MMPs | Positive | OS, RFS |
| 76 | IPO11 | Positive | OS |
| 79 | SCD1 | Positive | OS |
| – | ISYNA1 | Positive | – |
| 82 | mAR-SLC39A9 | Positive | OS, DFS |
| 88 | Maspin | Negative | OS, PFS |
| 89 | GATA6 | Negative | OS |
| 90 | FOXO | Negative | OS |
| Chen et al. (4) | miR-101 | Negative | OS |
| 93 | miR-143 | Negative | OS |
| 94 | miR-133b | Negative | OS, PFS |
| – | miR-539 | Negative | – |
| 18 | miR-497 | Negative | OS |
| 19 | miR-154 | Negative | OS |
| 21 | miR-223 | Negative | No |
| 95 | miR-148a | Negative | OS |
| – | miR-3658 | Positive | – |
| 97 | LncRNA MALAT1 | Positive | OS |
| 98 | LncRNA PVT1 | Positive | OS |
| – | LncRNA OXCT1-AS1 | Positive | – |
| 34 | LncRNA BLACAT2 | Positive | OS |
| 35 | LncRNA LNMAT1 | Positive | OS, DFS |
| Peng et al. (37) | LncRNA SNHG16 | Positive | OS |
| 99 | LncRNA ZFAS1 | Positive | OS, PFS |
| – | LncRNA DLX6-AS1 | Positive | – |
| 42 | LINC01296 | Positive | OS |
| 43 | LncRNA DANCR | Positive | OS, DFS |
| 100 | LncRNA SPRY4-IT1 | Positive | OS |
| 46 | LncRNA NNT-AS1 | Positive | OS |
| | LncRNA LNMAT2 | Positive | |
| – | LncRNA HOXA-AS2 | Positive | – |
| Wang et al. (101) | LncRNA HNF1A-AS1 | Positive | OS |
| Cheng et al. (102) | LncRNA ROR1-AS1 | Positive | OS |
| 103 | LncRNA RMRP | Positive | OS |
| – | CircHIPK3 | Negative | – |
| 52 | CircFNDC3B | Negative | OS |
| He et al. (53) | CircFUT8 | Negative | OS |
| Dong et al. (54) | CircACVR2A | Negative | OS |
| 55 | CircPICALM | Negative | OS |
| 56 | cTFRC | Positive | OS |
| – | CircPTK2 | Positive | – |

*OS, overall survival; DFS, disease free survival; PFS, progression-free survival; RFS, relapse free survival.*

BCa, and it was a poor prognostic factor for BCa. Patients with nonalcoholic fatty liver disease had elevated vascular endothelial growth factor, interleukin 6, TNF-$\alpha$, and IGF-1. These factors may increase the risk of BCa recurrence and lead to a poor prognosis (121). Studies have shown that patients with BCa had higher insulin resistance than those without cancer but with bladder disease (122). DM was associated with elevated BCa or cancer mortality risk, especially in men (123). Metformin is the most commonly used drug for patients with t2DM. Our team's study found that the intake of metformin was positively associated with RFS, which improved PFS and cancer-specific survival (124). Metformin targeted a YAP1-TEAD4 complex *via* AMPK$\alpha$ to regulate CCNE1/2 in BCa cells (125). It can suppress cyclin D1, cyclin-dependent kinase 4 (CDK4), E2F1, and mammalian target of rapamycin (mTOR) (126). The use of insulin can increase the risk of BCa progression (127). High-dose human insulin and insulin glargine similarly promoted T24 BCa cell proliferation *via* PI3K-independent activation of Akt (128).

## Environmental Toxins

Environmental toxins are closely related to cancer occurrence and development, and arsenic is the most reported in BCa. Dimethylarsinic acid (DMAV) is a methylated metabolite of arsenicals found in most mammals, and long-term exposure to DMAV can lead to BCa. Previous studies have found that recurrent BCa with high arsenic levels in tissues was more aggressive and had a higher stage and grade, and recured earlier than people with low levels of arsenic (129). Zhou et al. found that chronic arsenic exposure can upregulate HER2 in human and rat bladder epithelial cells and promote the proliferation, migration, epithelial-mesenchymal transition, and angiogenesis of cancer cells by activating the MAPK, PI3K/AKT, and STAT3 pathways (130). Moreover, sodium arsenite can reduce the human urothelial WIF1 gene expression, increase its DNA methylation level, and promote cancer cells' migration. The WIF1 gene expression and its DNA methylation can be considered as potential biomarkers for the diagnosis of human BCa (131).

## CONCLUSIONS

For the LNM in BCa, three mechanisms are mainly involved: tumor cell proliferation, tumor cell migration and invasion, and chemosensitivity. Most biomarkers are related to the

proliferation, migration, and invasion of BCa cells. Several biomarkers are involved in chemosensitivity. MiR-143, miR-101, miR-133b, MALAT1, CXCL5, and VEGF-C are related to all three of the above mechanisms. These biomarkers are more likely to be prognostic factors for BCa with LNM, but a large number of retrospective studies are still needed for further verification. Previous studies have shown that most biomarkers have a clear relationship with the prognosis of BCa patients (**Table 2**). However, the relationship between these eight biomarkers: ISYNA1, miR-539, miR-3658, OXCT1-AS1, DLX6-AS1, HOXA-AS2, circHIPK3, and circPTK2 and prognosis is still unclear; therefore, further research is needed to tap into their potential for the prognosis of BCa patients. Many biological assessment methods are economical and accurate. For example, peripheral blood can detect MMP, LMR, and NLR. Urine can detect the methylation status of GATA6 promoter, CXCL5, and MMP. Genetic testing for LNM is more sensitive and specific than traditional pathological examinations and is particularly suitable for micrometastasis diagnosis. Those test samples are easy to obtain before surgery, with strong reproducibility and high clinical feasibility. Recently, the research on SNP and m6A is also a hot spot. The relationship between them and bladder cancer with lymph node metastasis is not yet clear, and further investigation is needed, but it provides new directions for our future research. As for imaging, pathology, and molecular composition models, they are more accurate in terms of predicting lymphatic metastasis for bladder cancer, which should be studied in-depth and applied to clinical practice.

## AUTHOR CONTRIBUTIONS

CZ contributed to reading the literature, preparing figures and the table, and writing the manuscript. JH, HL, HM, BO, WR, ZY, DQ, ZO, JC, and XZ assisted with writing and revised the manuscript. All authors contributed to the article and approved the submitted version.

## ACKNOWLEDGMENTS

We sincerely thank You-e He for editing the language of this article.

## REFERENCES

1. Bray F, Ferlay J, Soerjomataram I, Siegel RL, Torre LA, Jemal A. Global cancer statistics 2018: GLOBOCAN estimates of incidence and mortality worldwide for 36 cancers in 185 countries. *CA Cancer J Clin* (2018) 68:394–424. doi: 10.3322/caac.21492

2. Zhang ZL, Dong P, Li YH, Liu ZW, Yao K, Han H, et al. Radical cystectomy for bladder cancer: oncologic outcome in 271 Chinese patients. *Chin J Cancer* (2014) 33:165–71. doi: 10.5732/cjc.012.10312

3. Li Y, Diao F, Shi S, Li K, Zhu W, Wu S, et al. Computed tomography and magnetic resonance imaging evaluation of pelvic lymph node metastasis in bladder cancer. *Chin J Cancer* (2018) 37:3. doi: 10.1186/s40880-018-0269-0

4. Hu Z, Lin Y, Chen H, Mao Y, Wu J, Zhu Y, et al. MicroRNA-101 suppresses motility of bladder cancer cells by targeting c-Met. *Biochem Biophys Res Commun* (2013) 435:82–7. doi: 10.1016/j.bbrc.2013.04.042

5. Long Y, Wu Z, Yang X, Chen L, Han Z, Zhang Y, et al. MicroRNA-101 inhibits the proliferation and invasion of bladder cancer cells *via* targeting c-FOS. *Mol Med Rep* (2016) 14:2651–6. doi: 10.3892/mmr.2016.5534

6. Chen L, Long Y, Han Z, Yuan Z, Liu W, Yang F, et al. MicroRNA-101 inhibits cell migration and invasion in bladder cancer *via* targeting FZD4. *Exp Ther Med* (2019a) 17:1476–85. doi: 10.3892/etm.2018.7084

7. Bu Q, Fang Y, Cao Y, Chen Q, Liu Y. Enforced expression of miR-101 enhances cisplatin sensitivity in human bladder cancer cells by modulating

the cyclooxygenase-2 pathway. *Mol Med Rep* (2014) 10:2203–9. doi: 10.3892/mmr.2014.2455

8. Lei Y, Li B, Tong S, Qi L, Hu X, Cui Y, et al. miR-101 suppresses vascular endothelial growth factor C that inhibits migration and invasion and enhances cisplatin chemosensitivity of bladder cancer cells. *PloS One* (2015) 10:e0117809. doi: 10.1371/journal.pone.0117809

9. Song T, Zhang X, Wang C, Wu Y, Dong J, Gao J, et al. Expression of miR-143 reduces growth and migration of human bladder carcinoma cells by targeting cyclooxygenase-2. *Asian Pac J Cancer Prev* (2011) 12:929–33.

10. Tsujino T, Sugito N, Taniguchi K, Honda R, Komura K, Yoshikawa Y, et al. MicroRNA-143/Musashi-2/KRAS cascade contributes positively to carcinogenesis in human bladder cancer. *Cancer Sci* (2019) 110:2189–99. doi: 10.1111/cas.14035

11. Cai X, Qu L, Yang J, Xu J, Sun L, Wei X, et al. Exosome-transmitted microRNA-133b inhibited bladder cancer proliferation by upregulating dual-specificity protein phosphatase 1. *Cancer Med* (2020) 9:6009–19. doi: 10.1002/cam4.3263

12. Zhou Y, Wu D, Tao J, Qu P, Zhou Z, Hou J. MicroRNA-133 inhibits cell proliferation, migration and invasion by targeting epidermal growth factor receptor and its downstream effector proteins in bladder cancer. *Scand J Urol* (2013) 47:423–32. doi: 10.3109/00365599.2012.748821

13. Chen XN, Wang KF, Xu ZQ, Li SJ, Liu Q, Fu DH, et al. MiR-133b regulates bladder cancer cell proliferation and apoptosis by targeting Bcl-w and Akt1. *Cancer Cell Int* (2014) 14:70. doi: 10.1186/s12935-014-0070-3

14. Zhao F, Zhou LH, Ge YZ, Ping WW, Wu X, Xu ZL, et al. MicroRNA-133b suppresses bladder cancer malignancy by targeting TAGLN2-mediated cell cycle. *J Cell Physiol* (2019) 234:4910–23. doi: 10.1002/jcp.27288

15. Liao G, Chen F, Zhong J, Jiang X. MicroRNA–539 inhibits the proliferation and invasion of bladder cancer cells by regulating IGF–1R. *Mol Med Rep* (2018) 17:4917–24. doi: 10.3892/mmr.2018.8497

16. Wei Z, Hu X, Liu J, Zhu W, Zhan X, Sun S. MicroRNA-497 upregulation inhibits cell invasion and metastasis in T24 and BIU-87 bladder cancer cells. *Mol Med Rep* (2017) 16:2055–60. doi: 10.3892/mmr.2017.6805

17. Itesako T, Seki N, Yoshino H, Chiyomaru T, Yamasaki T, Hidaka H, et al. The microRNA expression signature of bladder cancer by deep sequencing: the functional significance of the miR-195/497 cluster. *PloS One* (2014) 9: e84311. doi: 10.1371/journal.pone.0084311

18. Zhang Y, Zhang Z, Li Z, Gong D, Zhan B, Man X, et al. MicroRNA-497 inhibits the proliferation, migration and invasion of human bladder transitional cell carcinoma cells by targeting E2F3. *Oncol Rep* (2016) 36:1293–300. doi: 10.3892/or.2016.4923

19. Zhao X, Ji Z, Xie Y, Liu G, Li H. MicroRNA-154 as a prognostic factor in bladder cancer inhibits cellular malignancy by targeting RSF1 and RUNX2. *Oncol Rep* (2017) 38:2727–34. doi: 10.3892/or.2017.5992

20. Zhang J, Mao S, Wang L, Zhang W, Zhang Z, Guo Y, et al. MicroRNA–154 functions as a tumor suppressor in bladder cancer by directly targeting ATG7. *Oncol Rep* (2019) 41:819–28. doi: 10.3892/or.2018.6879

21. Sugita S, Yoshino H, Yonemori M, Miyamoto K, Matsushita R, Sakaguchi T, et al. Tumor–suppressive microRNA–223 targets WDR62 directly in bladder cancer. *Int J Oncol* (2019) 54:2222–36. doi: 10.3892/ijo.2019.4762

22. Guo J, Cao R, Yu X, Xiao Z, Chen Z. MicroRNA-223-3p inhibits human bladder cancer cell migration and invasion. *Tumour Biol* (2017) 39:1010428317691678. doi: 10.1177/1010428317691678

23. Sugawara S, Yamada Y, Arai T, Okato A, Idichi T, Kato M, et al. Dual strands of the miR-223 duplex (miR-223-5p and miR-223-3p) inhibit cancer cell aggressiveness: targeted genes are involved in bladder cancer pathogenesis. *J Hum Genet* (2018) 63:657–68. doi: 10.1038/s10038-018-0437-8

24. Lombard AP, Mooso BA, Libertini SJ, Lim RM, Nakagawa RM, Vidallo KD, et al. miR-148a dependent apoptosis of bladder cancer cells is mediated in part by the epigenetic modifier DNMT1. *Mol Carcinog* (2016) 55:757–67. doi: 10.1002/mc.22319

25. Luan T, Zou R, Huang L, Li N, Fu S, Huang Y, et al. Hsa-miR-3658 Promotes Cell Proliferation, Migration and Invasion by Effecting LASS2 in Bladder Cancer. *Clin Lab* (2018) 64:515–25. doi: 10.7754/Clin.Lab.2017.171026

26. Ying L, Chen Q, Wang Y, Zhou Z, Huang Y, Qiu F. Upregulated MALAT-1 contributes to bladder cancer cell migration by inducing epithelial-to-mesenchymal transition. *Mol Biosyst* (2012) 8:2289–94. doi: 10.1039/c2mb25070e

27. Liu P, Li X, Cui Y, Chen J, Li C, Li Q, et al. LncRNA-MALAT1 mediates cisplatin resistance *via* miR-101-3p/VEGF-C pathway in bladder cancer. *Acta Biochim Biophys Sin (Shanghai)* (2019b) 51:1148–57. doi: 10.1093/abbs/gmz112

28. Xie H, Liao X, Chen Z, Fang Y, He A, Zhong Y, et al. LncRNA MALAT1 Inhibits Apoptosis and Promotes Invasion by Antagonizing miR-125b in Bladder Cancer Cells. *J Cancer* (2017) 8:3803–11. doi: 10.7150/jca.21228

29. Jiao D, Li Z, Zhu M, Wang Y, Wu G, Han X. LncRNA MALAT1 promotes tumor growth and metastasis by targeting miR-124/foxq1 in bladder transitional cell carcinoma (BTCC). *Am J Cancer Res* (2018) 8:748–60.

30. Liu Y, Gao S, Du Q, Zhao Q. Knockdown of long non-coding RNA metastasis associated lung adenocarcinoma transcript 1 inhibits the proliferation and migration of bladder cancer cells by modulating the microRNA-34a/cyclin D1 axis. *Int J Mol Med* (2019c) 43:547–56. doi: 10.3892/ijmm.2018.3959

31. Yu C, Longfei L, Long W, Feng Z, Chen J, Chao L, et al. LncRNA PVT1 regulates VEGFC through inhibiting miR-128 in bladder cancer cells. *J Cell Physiol* (2019) 234:1346–53. doi: 10.1002/jcp.26929

32. Tian Z, Cao S, Li C, Xu M, Wei H, Yang H, et al. LncRNA PVT1 regulates growth, migration, and invasion of bladder cancer by miR-31/CDK1. *J Cell Physiol* (2019) 234:4799–811. doi: 10.1002/jcp.27279

33. Chen JB, Zhu YW, Guo X, Yu C, Liu PH, Li C, et al. Microarray expression profiles analysis revealed lncRNA OXCT1-AS1 promoted bladder cancer cell aggressiveness *via* miR-455-5p/JAK1 signaling. *J Cell Physiol* (2019b) 234:13592–601. doi: 10.1002/jcp.28037

34. He W, Zhong G, Jiang N, Wang B, Fan X, Chen C, et al. Long noncoding RNA BLACAT2 promotes bladder cancer-associated lymphangiogenesis and lymphatic metastasis. *J Clin Invest* (2018) 128:861–75. doi: 10.1172/JCI96218

35. Chen C, He W, Huang J, Wang B, Li H, Cai Q, et al. LNMAT1 promotes lymphatic metastasis of bladder cancer *via* CCL2 dependent macrophage recruitment. *Nat Commun* (2018) 9:3826. doi: 10.1038/s41467-018-06152-x

36. Feng F, Chen A, Huang J, Xia Q, Chen Y, Jin X. Long noncoding RNA SNHG16 contributes to the development of bladder cancer *via* regulating miR-98/STAT3/Wnt/β-catenin pathway axis. *J Cell Biochem* (2018) 119:9408–18. doi: 10.1002/jcb.27257

37. Peng H, Li H. The encouraging role of long noncoding RNA small nuclear RNA host gene 16 in epithelial-mesenchymal transition of bladder cancer *via* directly acting on miR-17-5p/metalloproteinases 3 axis. *Mol Carcinog* (2019) 58:1465–80. doi: 10.1002/mc.23028

38. Chen W, Jiang T, Mao H, Gao R, Zhang H, He Y, et al. SNHG16 regulates invasion and migration of bladder cancer through induction of epithelial-to-mesenchymal transition. *Hum Cell* (2020b) 33:737–49. doi: 10.1007/s13577-020-00343-9

39. Yang H, Li G, Cheng B, Jiang R. ZFAS1 functions as an oncogenic long non-coding RNA in bladder cancer. *Biosci Rep* (2018) 38(3):BSR20180475. doi: 10.1042/BSR20180475

40. Fang C, Xu L, He W, Dai J, Sun F. Long noncoding RNA DLX6-AS1 promotes cell growth and invasiveness in bladder cancer *via* modulating the miR-223-HSP90B1 axis. *Cell Cycle* (2019) 18:3288–99. doi: 10.1080/15384101.2019.1673633

41. Guo J, Chen Z, Jiang H, Yu Z, Peng J, Xie J, et al. The lncRNA DLX6-AS1 promoted cell proliferation, invasion, migration and epithelial-to-mesenchymal transition in bladder cancer *via* modulating Wnt/β-catenin signaling pathway. *Cancer Cell Int* (2019b) 19:312. doi: 10.1186/s12935-019-1010-z

42. Wang X, Wang L, Gong Y, Liu Z, Qin Y, Chen J, et al. Long noncoding RNA LINC01296 promotes cancer-cell proliferation and metastasis in urothelial carcinoma of the bladder. *Onco Targets Ther* (2019a) 12:75–85. doi: 10.2147/OTT.S192809

43. Chen Z, Chen X, Xie R, Huang M, Dong W, Han J, et al. DANCR Promotes Metastasis and Proliferation in Bladder Cancer Cells by Enhancing IL-11-STAT3 Signaling and CCND1 Expression. *Mol Ther* (2019c) 27:326–41. doi: 10.1016/j.ymthe.2018.12.015

44. Zhan Y, Chen Z, Li Y, He A, He S, Gong Y, et al. Long non-coding RNA DANCR promotes malignant phenotypes of bladder cancer cells by modulating the miR-149/MSI2 axis as a ceRNA. *J Exp Clin Cancer Res* (2018) 37:273. doi: 10.1186/s13046-018-0921-1

45. Liu D, Li Y, Luo G, Xiao X, Tao D, Wu X, et al. LncRNA SPRY4-IT1 sponges miR-101-3p to promote proliferation and metastasis of bladder cancer cells through up-regulating EZH2. *Cancer Lett* (2017) 388:281–91. doi: 10.1016/j.canlet.2016.12.005

46. Wu D, Zhang T, Wang J, Zhou J, Pan H, Qu P. Long noncoding RNA NNT-AS1 enhances the malignant phenotype of bladder cancer by acting as a competing endogenous RNA on microRNA-496 thereby increasing HMGB1 expression. *Aging (Albany NY)* (2019a) 11:12624–40. doi: 10.18632/aging.102591

47. Liu Y, Wu G. NNT-AS1 enhances bladder cancer cell growth by targeting miR-1301-3p/PODXL axis and activating Wnt pathway. *Neurourol Urodyn* (2020) 39:547–57. doi: 10.1002/nau.24238

48. Chen C, Luo Y, He W, Zhao Y, Kong Y, Liu H, et al. Exosomal long noncoding RNA LNMAT2 promotes lymphatic metastasis in bladder cancer. *J Clin Invest* (2020c) 130:404–21. doi: 10.1172/JCI130892

49. Wang F, Wu D, Chen J, Chen S, He F, Fu H, et al. Long non-coding RNA HOXA-AS2 promotes the migration, invasion and stemness of bladder cancer *via* regulating miR-125b/Smad2 axis. *Exp Cell Res* (2019b) 375:1–10. doi: 10.1016/j.yexcr.2018.11.005

50. Wang YH, Liu YH, Ji YJ, Wei Q, Gao TB. Upregulation of long non-coding RNA HNF1A-AS1 is associated with poor prognosis in urothelial carcinoma of the bladder. *Eur Rev Med Pharmacol Sci* (2018c) 22:2261–5.

51. Li Y, Zheng F, Xiao X, Xie F, Tao D, Huang C, et al. CircHIPK3 sponges miR-558 to suppress heparanase expression in bladder cancer cells. *EMBO Rep* (2017b) 18:1646–59. doi: 10.15252/embr.201643581

52. Liu H, Bi J, Dong W, Yang M, Shi J, Jiang N, et al. Invasion-related circular RNA circFNDC3B inhibits bladder cancer progression through the miR-1178-3p/G3BP2/SRC/FAK axis. *Mol Cancer* (2018) 17:161. doi: 10.1186/s12943-018-0908-8

53. Dong W, Bi J, Liu H, Yan D, He Q, Zhou Q, et al. Circular RNA ACVR2A suppresses bladder cancer cells proliferation and metastasis through miR-626/EYA4 axis. *Mol Cancer* (2019) 18:95. doi: 10.1186/s12943-019-1025-z

54. He Q, Yan D, Dong W, Bi J, Huang L, Yang M, et al. circRNA circFUT8 Upregulates Krüpple-like Factor 10 to Inhibit the Metastasis of Bladder Cancer *via* Sponging miR-570-3p. *Mol Ther Oncolytics* (2020) 16:172–87. doi: 10.1016/j.omto.2019.12.014

55. Yan D, Dong W, He Q, Yang M, Huang L, Kong J, et al. Circular RNA circPICALM sponges miR-1265 to inhibit bladder cancer metastasis and influence FAK phosphorylation. *EBioMedicine* (2019) 48:316–31. doi: 10.1016/j.ebiom.2019.08.074

56. Su H, Tao T, Yang Z, Kang X, Zhang X, Kang D, et al. Circular RNA cTFRC acts as the sponge of MicroRNA-107 to promote bladder carcinoma progression. *Mol Cancer* (2019) 18:27. doi: 10.1186/s12943-019-0951-0

57. Zu X, Tang Z, Li Y, Gao N, Ding J, Qi L. Vascular endothelial growth factor-C expression in bladder transitional cell cancer and its relationship to lymph node metastasis. *BJU Int* (2006) 98:1090–3. doi: 10.1111/j.1464-410X.2006.06446.x

58. Zhang HH, Qi F, Shi YR, Miao JG, Zhou M, He W, et al. RNA interference-mediated vascular endothelial growth factor-C reduction suppresses malignant progression and enhances mitomycin C sensitivity of bladder cancer T24 cells. *Cancer Biother Radiopharm* (2012a) 27:291–8. doi: 10.1089/cbr.2010.0919

59. Zhang HH, Qi F, Zu XB, Cao YH, Miao JG, Xu L, et al. A proteomic study of potential VEGF-C-associated proteins in bladder cancer T24 cells. *Med Sci Monit* (2012b) 18:Br441–9. doi: 10.12659/MSM.883537

60. Mccoll BK, Baldwin ME, Roufail S, Freeman C, Moritz RL, Simpson RJ, et al. Plasmin activates the lymphangiogenic growth factors VEGF-C and VEGF-D. *J Exp Med* (2003) 198:863–8. doi: 10.1084/jem.20030361

61. Pepper MS, Mandriota SJ, Jeltsch M, Kumar V, Alitalo K. Vascular endothelial growth factor (VEGF)-C synergizes with basic fibroblast growth factor and VEGF in the induction of angiogenesis *in vitro* and alters endothelial cell extracellular proteolytic activity. *J Cell Physiol* (1998) 177:439–52. doi: 10.1002/(SICI)1097-4652(199812)177:3<439::AID-JCP7>3.0.CO;2-2

62. Zhu H, Yun F, Shi X, Wang D. VEGF-C inhibition reverses resistance of bladder cancer cells to cisplatin *via* upregulating maspin. *Mol Med Rep* (2015) 12:3163–9. doi: 10.3892/mmr.2015.3684

63. Liu J, Yu HG, Yu JP, Wang XL, Zhou XD, Luo HS. Overexpression of cyclooxygenase-2 in gastric cancer correlates with the high abundance of vascular endothelial growth factor-C and lymphatic metastasis. *Med Oncol* (2005) 22:389–97. doi: 10.1385/MO:22:4:389

64. Al-Maghrabi B, Gomaa W, Abdelwahed M, Al-Maghrabi J. Increased COX-2 Immunostaining in Urothelial Carcinoma of the Urinary Bladder Is Associated with Invasiveness and Poor Prognosis. *Anal Cell Pathol (Amst)* (2019) 2019:5026939. doi: 10.1155/2019/5026939

65. Dong L, Li Y, Xue D, Liu Y. PCMT1 is an unfavorable predictor and functions as an oncogene in bladder cancer. *IUBMB Life* (2018) 70:291–9. doi: 10.1002/iub.1717

66. Islam SS, Mokhtari RB, Noman AS, Uddin M, Rahman MZ, Azadi MA, et al. Sonic hedgehog (Shh) signaling promotes tumorigenicity and stemness *via* activation of epithelial-to-mesenchymal transition (EMT) in bladder cancer. *Mol Carcinog* (2016) 55:537–51. doi: 10.1002/mc.22300

67. Nedjadi T, Salem N, Khayyat D, Al-Sayyad A, Al-Ammari A, Al-Maghrabi J. Sonic Hedgehog Expression is Associated with Lymph Node Invasion in Urothelial Bladder Cancer. *Pathol Oncol Res* (2019) 25:1067–73. doi: 10.1007/s12253-018-0477-6

68. Syed IS, Pedram A, Farhat WA. Role of Sonic Hedgehog (Shh) Signaling in Bladder Cancer Stemness and Tumorigenesis. *Curr Urol Rep* (2016) 17:11. doi: 10.1007/s11934-015-0568-9

69. Zhu X, Qiao Y, Liu W, Wang W, Shen H, Lu Y, et al. CXCL5 is a potential diagnostic and prognostic marker for bladder cancer patients. *Tumour Biol* (2016) 37:4569–77. doi: 10.1007/s13277-015-4275-4

70. Wang C, Li A, Yang S, Qiao R, Zhu X, Zhang J. CXCL5 promotes mitomycin C resistance in non-muscle invasive bladder cancer by activating EMT and NF-κB pathway. *Biochem Biophys Res Commun* (2018a) 498:862–8. doi: 10.1016/j.bbrc.2018.03.071

71. Zheng J, Zhu X, Zhang J. CXCL5 knockdown expression inhibits human bladder cancer T24 cells proliferation and migration. *Biochem Biophys Res Commun* (2014) 446:18–24. doi: 10.1016/j.bbrc.2014.01.172

72. Gao Y, Guan Z, Chen J, Xie H, Yang Z, Fan J, et al. CXCL5/CXCR2 axis promotes bladder cancer cell migration and invasion by activating PI3K/AKT-induced upregulation of MMP2/MMP9. *Int J Oncol* (2015) 47:690–700. doi: 10.3892/ijo.2015.3041

73. Mohammad MA, Ismael NR, Shaarawy SM, El-Merzabani MM. Prognostic value of membrane type 1 and 2 matrix metalloproteinase expression and gelatinase A activity in bladder cancer. *Int J Biol Markers* (2010) 25:69–74. doi: 10.1177/172460081002500202

74. Szarvas T, Becker M, Vom Dorp F, Gethmann C, Tötsch M, Bánkfalvi A, et al. Matrix metalloproteinase-7 as a marker of metastasis and predictor of poor survival in bladder cancer. *Cancer Sci* (2010) 101:1300–8. doi: 10.1111/j.1349-7006.2010.01506.x

75. Vasala K, Pääkko P, Turpeenniemi-Hujanen T. Matrix metalloproteinase-9 (MMP-9) immunoreactive protein in urinary bladder cancer: a marker of favorable prognosis. *Anticancer Res* (2008) 28:1757–61.

76. Zhao J, Xu W, He M, Zhang Z, Zeng S, Ma C, et al. Whole-exome sequencing of muscle-invasive bladder cancer identifies recurrent copy number variation in IPO11 and prognostic significance of importin-11 overexpression on poor survival. *Oncotarget* (2016) 7:75648–58. doi: 10.18632/oncotarget.12315

77. Zhao J, Shi L, Zeng S, Ma C, Xu W, Zhang Z, et al. Importin-11 overexpression promotes the migration, invasion, and progression of bladder cancer associated with the deregulation of CDKN1A and THBS1. *Urol Oncol* (2018) 36:311.e311–13. doi: 10.1016/j.urolonc.2018.03.001

78. Presler M, Wojtczyk-Miaskowska A, Schlichtholz B, Kaluzny A, Matuszewski M, Mika A, et al. Increased expression of the gene encoding stearoyl-CoA desaturase 1 in human bladder cancer. *Mol Cell Biochem* (2018) 447:217–24. doi: 10.1007/s11010-018-3306-z

79. Piao C, Cui X, Zhan B, Li J, Li Z, Li Z, et al. Inhibition of stearoyl CoA desaturase-1 activity suppresses tumour progression and improves prognosis in human bladder cancer. *J Cell Mol Med* (2019) 23:2064–76. doi: 10.1111/jcmm.14114

80. Du X, Wang QR, Chan E, Merchant M, Liu J, French D, et al. FGFR3 stimulates stearoyl CoA desaturase 1 activity to promote bladder tumor growth. *Cancer Res* (2012) 72:5843–55. doi: 10.1158/0008-5472.CAN-12-1329

81. Guo X, Li HH, Hu J, Duan YX, Ren WG, Guo Q, et al. ISYNA1 is overexpressed in bladder carcinoma and regulates cell proliferation and

apoptosis. *Biochem Biophys Res Commun* (2019a) 519:246–52. doi: 10.1016/j.bbrc.2019.08.129

82. Chen J, Chou F, Yeh S, Ou Z, Shyr C, Huang C, et al. Androgen dihydrotestosterone (DHT) promotes the bladder cancer nuclear AR-negative cell invasion *via a* newly identified membrane androgen receptor (mAR-SLC39A9)-mediated Gαi protein/MAPK/MMP9 intracellular signaling. *Oncogene* (2020a) 39:574–86. doi: 10.1038/s41388-019-0964-6

83. Tang Y, Zu X, Xiong Y, Zhang X. [Expression of Maspin in bladder carcinoma and the relationship between Maspin and lymph node metastasis]. *Zhong Nan Da Xue Xue Bao Yi Xue Ban* (2015) 40:1306–12. doi:10.11817/j.issn.1672-7347.2015.12.004

84. Zhang HH, Qi F, Cao YH, Zu XB, Chen MF. Expression and clinical significance of microRNA-21, maspin and vascular endothelial growth factor-C in bladder cancer. *Oncol Lett* (2015) 10:2610–6. doi: 10.3892/ol.2015.3540

85. Juengel E, Beecken WD, Mundiyanapurath S, Engl T, Jonas D, Blaheta RA. Maspin modulates adhesion of bladder carcinoma cells to vascular endothelium. *World J Urol* (2010) 28:465–71. doi: 10.1007/s00345-010-0539-1

86. Sugimoto S, Maass N, Takimoto Y, Sato K, Minei S, Zhang M, et al. Expression and regulation of tumor suppressor gene maspin in human bladder cancer. *Cancer Lett* (2004) 203:209–15. doi: 10.1016/j.canlet.2003.09.010

87. Lin YH, Tsui KH, Chang KS, Hou CP, Feng TH, Juang HH. Maspin is a PTEN-Upregulated and p53-Upregulated Tumor Suppressor Gene and Acts as an HDAC1 Inhibitor in Human Bladder Cancer. *Cancers (Basel)* (2019) 12(1):10. doi: 10.3390/cancers12010010

88. Chen J, Wang L, Tang Y, Gong G, Liu L, Chen M, et al. Maspin enhances cisplatin chemosensitivity in bladder cancer T24 and 5637 cells and correlates with prognosis of muscle-invasive bladder cancer patients receiving cisplatin based neoadjuvant chemotherapy. *J Exp Clin Cancer Res* (2016a) 35:2. doi: 10.1186/s13046-015-0282-y

89. Wang C, Liu Q, Huang M, Zhou Q, Zhang X, Zhang J, et al. Loss of GATA6 expression promotes lymphatic metastasis in bladder cancer. *FASEB J* (2020) 34:5754–66. doi: 10.1096/fj.201903176R

90. Zhang Y, Jia L, Zhang Y, Ji W, Li H. Higher expression of FOXOs correlates to better prognosis of bladder cancer. *Oncotarget* (2017) 8:96313–22. doi: 10.18632/oncotarget.22029

91. Shiota M, Song Y, Yokomizo A, Kiyoshima K, Tada Y, Uchino H, et al. Foxo3a suppression of urothelial cancer invasiveness through Twist1, Y-box-binding protein 1, and E-cadherin regulation. *Clin Cancer Res* (2010) 16:5654–63. doi: 10.1158/1078-0432.CCR-10-0376

92. Chen X. MiR-101 acts as a novel bio-marker in the diagnosis of bladder carcinoma. *Med (Baltimore)* (2019) 98:e16051. doi: 10.1097/MD.0000000000016051

93. Liu X, Zhao W, Wang X, Zhu Y, Zhou Z, Shi B. Expression of mir-143 in serum of bladder cancer patients and its correlation with clinical features and prognosis. *J Buon* (2019a) 24:791–6.

94. Chen X, Wu B, Xu Z, Li S, Tan S, Liu X, et al. Downregulation of miR-133b predict progression and poor prognosis in patients with urothelial carcinoma of bladder. *Cancer Med* (2016b) 5:1856–62. doi: 10.1002/cam4.777

95. Ma L, Xu Z, Xu C, Jiang X. MicroRNA-148a represents an independent prognostic marker in bladder cancer. *Tumour Biol* (2016) 37:7915–20. doi: 10.1007/s13277-015-4688-0

96. Chen YJ, Wang HF, Liang M, Zou RC, Tang ZR, Wang JS. Upregulation of miR-3658 in bladder cancer and tumor progression. *Genet Mol Res* (2016c) 15(4). doi: 10.4238/gmr15049048

97. Li C, Cui Y, Liu LF, Ren WB, Li QQ, Zhou X, et al. High Expression of Long Noncoding RNA MALAT1 Indicates a Poor Prognosis and Promotes Clinical Progression and Metastasis in Bladder Cancer. *Clin Genitourin Cancer* (2017a) 15:570–6. doi: 10.1016/j.clgc.2017.05.001

98. Li B, Guo LH, Ban ZQ, Liu L, Luo C, Cui TY. Upregulation of lncRNA plasmacytoma variant translocation 1 predicts poor prognosis in patients with muscle-invasive bladder cancer. *Med (Baltimore)* (2020) 99:e21059. doi: 10.1097/MD.0000000000021059

99. Wang JS, Liu QH, Cheng XH, Zhang WY, Jin YC. The long noncoding RNA ZFAS1 facilitates bladder cancer tumorigenesis by sponging miR-329.

*BioMed Pharmacother* (2018b) 103:174–81. doi: 10.1016/j.biopha.2018.04.031

100. Zhao XL, Zhao ZH, Xu WC, Hou JQ, Du XY. Increased expression of SPRY4-IT1 predicts poor prognosis and promotes tumor growth and metastasis in bladder cancer. *Int J Clin Exp Pathol* (2015) 8:1954–60.

101. Zhan Y, Li Y, Guan B, Wang Z, Peng D, Chen Z, et al. Long non-coding RNA HNF1A-AS1 promotes proliferation and suppresses apoptosis of bladder cancer cells through upregulating Bcl-2. *Oncotarget* (2017) 8:76656–65. doi: 10.18632/oncotarget.20795

102. Chen Q, Fu L. Upregulation of long non-coding RNA ROR1-AS1 promotes cell growth and migration in bladder cancer by regulation of miR-504. *PloS One* (2020) 15:e0227568. doi: 10.1371/journal.pone.0227568

103. Cao HL, Liu ZJ, Huang PL, Yue YL, Xi JN. lncRNA-RMRP promotes proliferation, migration and invasion of bladder cancer *via* miR-206. *Eur Rev Med Pharmacol Sci* (2019) 23:1012–21.

104. Liang Z, Guo W, Fang S, Zhang Y, Lu L, Xu W, et al. CircRNAs: Emerging Bladder Cancer Biomarkers and Targets. *Front Oncol* (2020) 10:606485. doi: 10.3389/fonc.2020.606485

105. Xu ZQ, Yang MG, Liu HJ, Su CQ. Circular RNA hsa_circ_0003221 (circPTK2) promotes the proliferation and migration of bladder cancer cells. *J Cell Biochem* (2018) 119:3317–25. doi: 10.1002/jcb.26492

106. D'andrea D, Moschini M, Gust KM, Abufaraj M, Özsoy M, Mathieu R, et al. Lymphocyte-to-monocyte ratio and neutrophil-to-lymphocyte ratio as biomarkers for predicting lymph node metastasis and survival in patients treated with radical cystectomy. *J Surg Oncol* (2017) 115:455–61. doi: 10.1002/jso.24521

107. Zhou M, He L, Zu X, Zhang H, Zeng H, Qi L. Lymphatic vessel density as a predictor of lymph node metastasis and its relationship with prognosis in urothelial carcinoma of the bladder. *BJU Int* (2011) 107:1930–5. doi: 10.1111/j.1464-410X.2010.09725.x

108. Chen M, Nie ZY, Wen XH, Gao YH, Cao H, Zhang SF. m6A RNA methylation regulators can contribute to malignant progression and impact the prognosis of bladder cancer. *Biosci Rep* (2019d) 39(12): BSR20192892. doi: 10.1042/BSR20192892

109. Han J, Wang JZ, Yang X, Yu H, Zhou R, Lu HC, et al. METTL3 promote tumor proliferation of bladder cancer by accelerating pri-miR221/222 maturation in m6A-dependent manner. *Mol Cancer* (2019) 18:110. doi: 10.1186/s12943-019-1036-9

110. Smith SC, Baras AS, Dancik G, Ru Y, Ding KF, Moskaluk CA, et al. A 20-gene model for molecular nodal staging of bladder cancer: development and prospective assessment. *Lancet Oncol* (2011) 12:137–43. doi: 10.1016/S1470-2045(10)70296-5

111. Seiler R, Lam LL, Erho N, Takhar M, Mitra AP, Buerki C, et al. Prediction of Lymph Node Metastasis in Patients with Bladder Cancer Using Whole Transcriptome Gene Expression Signatures. *J Urol* (2016) 196:1036–41. doi: 10.1016/j.juro.2016.04.061

112. Lu X, Wang Y, Jiang L, Gao J, Zhu Y, Hu W, et al. A Pre-operative Nomogram for Prediction of Lymph Node Metastasis in Bladder Urothelial Carcinoma. *Front Oncol* (2019) 9:488. doi: 10.3389/fonc.2019.00488

113. Wu S, Zheng J, Li Y, Yu H, Shi S, Xie W, et al. A Radiomics Nomogram for the Preoperative Prediction of Lymph Node Metastasis in Bladder Cancer. *Clin Cancer Res* (2017) 23:6904–11. doi: 10.1158/1078-0432.CCR-17-1510

114. Wu S, Zheng J, Li Y, Wu Z, Shi S, Huang M, et al. Development and Validation of an MRI-Based Radiomics Signature for the Preoperative Prediction of Lymph Node Metastasis in Bladder Cancer. *EBioMedicine* (2018a) 34:76–84. doi: 10.1016/j.ebiom.2018.07.029

115. Wu SX, Huang J, Liu ZW, Chen HG, Guo P, Cai QQ, et al. A Genomic-clinicopathologic Nomogram for the Preoperative Prediction of Lymph Node Metastasis in Bladder Cancer. *EBioMedicine* (2018b) 31:54–65. doi: 10.1016/j.ebiom.2018.03.034

116. Chen J, Cui YU, Liu L, Li C, Tang Y, Zhou XU, et al. CCR7 as a predictive biomarker associated with computed tomography for the diagnosis of lymph node metastasis in bladder carcinoma. *Oncol Lett* (2016d) 11:735–40. doi: 10.3892/ol.2015.3939

117. Cantiello F, Cicione A, Autorino R, Salonia A, Briganti A, Ferro M, et al. Visceral obesity predicts adverse pathological features in urothelial bladder cancer patients undergoing radical cystectomy: a retrospective cohort study. *World J Urol* (2014) 32:559–64. doi: 10.1007/s00345-013-1147-7

118. Garg T, Young AJ, O'keeffe-Rosetti M, Mcmullen CK, Nielsen ME, Murphy TE, et al. Association between metabolic syndrome and recurrence of nonmuscle-invasive bladder cancer in older adults. *Urol Oncol* (2020) 38:737.e717–23. doi: 10.1016/j.urolonc.2020.04.010

119. Chromecki TF, Cha EK, Fajkovic H, Rink M, Ehdaie B, Svatek RS, et al. Obesity is associated with worse oncological outcomes in patients treated with radical cystectomy. *BJU Int* (2013) 111:249–55. doi: 10.1111/j.1464-410X.2012.11322.x

120. Kwon T, Jeong IG, You D, Han KS, Hong S, Hong B, et al. Obesity and prognosis in muscle-invasive bladder cancer: the continuing controversy. *Int J Urol* (2014) 21:1106–12. doi: 10.1111/iju.12530

121. Chiang CL, Huang HH, Huang TY, Shih YL, Hsieh TY, Lin HH. Nonalcoholic Fatty Liver Disease Associated With Bladder Cancer. *Am J Med Sci* (2020) 360:161–5. doi: 10.1016/j.amjms.2020.04.031

122. Tarantino G, Crocetto F, Di Vito C, Creta M, Martino R, Pandolfo SD, et al. Association of NAFLD and Insulin Resistance with Non Metastatic Bladder Cancer Patients: A Cross-Sectional Retrospective Study. *J Clin Med* (2021) 10(2):346. doi: 10.3390/jcm10020346

123. Xu Y, Huo R, Chen X, Yu X. Diabetes mellitus and the risk of bladder cancer: A PRISMA-compliant meta-analysis of cohort studies. *Med (Baltimore)* (2017) 96:e8588. doi: 10.1097/MD.0000000000008588

124. Hu J, Chen JB, Cui Y, Zhu YW, Ren WB, Zhou X, et al. Association of metformin intake with bladder cancer risk and oncologic outcomes in type 2 diabetes mellitus patients: A systematic review and meta-analysis. *Med (Baltimore)* (2018) 97:e11596. doi: 10.1097/MD.0000000000011596

125. Wu Y, Zheng Q, Li Y, Wang G, Gao S, Zhang X, et al. Metformin targets a YAP1-TEAD4 complex *via* AMPKα to regulate CCNE1/2 in bladder cancer cells. *J Exp Clin Cancer Res* (2019b) 38:376. doi: 10.1186/s13046-019-1346-1

126. Zhang T, Guo P, Zhang Y, Xiong H, Yu X, Xu S, et al. The antidiabetic drug metformin inhibits the proliferation of bladder cancer cells *in vitro* and *in vivo*. *Int J Mol Sci* (2013) 14:24603–18. doi: 10.3390/ijms141224603

127. Newton CC, Gapstur SM, Campbell PT, Jacobs EJ. Type 2 diabetes mellitus, insulin-use and risk of bladder cancer in a large cohort study. *Int J Cancer* (2013) 132:2186–91. doi: 10.1002/ijc.27878

128. Liu S, Li Y, Lin T, Fan X, Liang Y, Heemann U. High dose human insulin and insulin glargine promote T24 bladder cancer cell proliferation *via* PI3K-independent activation of Akt. *Diabetes Res Clin Pract* (2011) 91:177–82. doi: 10.1016/j.diabres.2010.11.009

129. Pal DK, Agrawal A, Ghosh S, Ghosh A. Association of arsenic with recurrence of urinary bladder cancer. *Trop Doct* (2020) 50:325–30. doi: 10.1177/0049475520930155

130. Zhou Q, Jin P, Liu J, Li S, Liu W, Xi S. Arsenic-induced HER2 promotes proliferation, migration and angiogenesis of bladder epithelial cells *via* activation of multiple signaling pathways *in vitro* and *in vivo*. *Sci Total Environ* (2021) 753:141962. doi: 10.1016/j.scitotenv.2020.141962

131. Jou YC, Wang SC, Dai YC, Chen SY, Shen CH, Lee YR, et al. Gene expression and DNA methylation regulation of arsenic in mouse bladder tissues and in human urothelial cells. *Oncol Rep* (2019) 42:1005–16. doi: 10.3892/or.2019.7235

# Permissions

All chapters in this book were first published by Frontiers; hereby published with permission under the Creative Commons Attribution License or equivalent. Every chapter published in this book has been scrutinized by our experts. Their significance has been extensively debated. The topics covered herein carry significant findings which will fuel the growth of the discipline. They may even be implemented as practical applications or may be referred to as a beginning point for another development.

The contributors of this book come from diverse backgrounds, making this book a truly international effort. This book will bring forth new frontiers with its revolutionizing research information and detailed analysis of the nascent developments around the world.

We would like to thank all the contributing authors for lending their expertise to make the book truly unique. They have played a crucial role in the development of this book. Without their invaluable contributions this book wouldn't have been possible. They have made vital efforts to compile up to date information on the varied aspects of this subject to make this book a valuable addition to the collection of many professionals and students.

This book was conceptualized with the vision of imparting up-to-date information and advanced data in this field. To ensure the same, a matchless editorial board was set up. Every individual on the board went through rigorous rounds of assessment to prove their worth. After which they invested a large part of their time researching and compiling the most relevant data for our readers.

The editorial board has been involved in producing this book since its inception. They have spent rigorous hours researching and exploring the diverse topics which have resulted in the successful publishing of this book. They have passed on their knowledge of decades through this book. To expedite this challenging task, the publisher supported the team at every step. A small team of assistant editors was also appointed to further simplify the editing procedure and attain best results for the readers.

Apart from the editorial board, the designing team has also invested a significant amount of their time in understanding the subject and creating the most relevant covers. They scrutinized every image to scout for the most suitable representation of the subject and create an appropriate cover for the book.

The publishing team has been an ardent support to the editorial, designing and production team. Their endless efforts to recruit the best for this project, has resulted in the accomplishment of this book. They are a veteran in the field of academics and their pool of knowledge is as vast as their experience in printing. Their expertise and guidance has proved useful at every step. Their uncompromising quality standards have made this book an exceptional effort. Their encouragement from time to time has been an inspiration for everyone.

The publisher and the editorial board hope that this book will prove to be a valuable piece of knowledge for researchers, students, practitioners and scholars across the globe.

# List of Contributors

**Han Zhang**
Department of Nephrology, The First Affiliated Hospital of Chongqing Medical University, Chongqing, China
Department of Oncology, Chongqing University Three Gorges Hospital, Chongqing, China

**Hua Gan**
Department of Nephrology, The First Affiliated Hospital of Chongqing Medical University, Chongqing, China

**Hua Wen Liu**
Department of Oncology, Chongqing University Three Gorges Hospital, Chongqing, China

**Chuan Qin**
Department of Gastrointestinal Surgery, Chongqing University Three Gorges Hospital, Chongqing, China

**Xiong Guo**
Department of Gastrointestinal Surgery, The First Affiliated Hospital of Chongqing Medical University, Chongqing, China

**Huaru Zhang and Xiaofu Qiu**
The Second School of Clinical Medicine, Southern Medical University, Guangzhou, China
Department of Urology, Guangdong Second Provincial General Hospital, Guangzhou, China

**Guosheng Yang**
The Second School of Clinical Medicine, Southern Medical University, Guangzhou, China
Department of Urology, Guangdong Second Provincial General Hospital, Guangzhou, China
Department of Urology, Shanghai East Hospital, Tongji University School of Medicine, Shanghai, China

**JunJie Yu, WeiPu Mao, Si Sun, Qiang Hu, Can Wang, ZhiPeng Xu, RuiJi Liu and SaiSai Chen**
Medical College, Southeast University, Nanjing, China

**Bin Xu**
Department of Urology, Affiliated Zhongda Hospital of Southeast University, Nanjing, China

**Ming Chen**
Department of Urology, Affiliated Zhongda Hospital of Southeast University, Nanjing, China
Department of Urology, Affiliated Lishui People's Hospital of Southeast University, Nanjing, China

**Sung Han Kim and Jinsoo Chung**
Department of Urology, Urologic Cancer Center, Research Institute and Hospital of National Cancer Center, Goyang, South Korea

**Boram Park**
Statistics and Data Center, Research Institute for Future Medicine, Samsung Medical Center, Seoul, South Korea

**Eu Chang Hwang**
Department of Urology, Chonnam National University Medical School, Gwangju, South Korea

**Sung-Hoo Hong**
Department of Urology, Seoul St. Mary's Hospital, Seoul, South Korea

**Chang Wook Jeong and Cheol Kwak**
Department of Urology, Seoul National University College of Medicine and Hospital, Seoul, South Korea

**Seok Soo Byun**
Department of Urology, Seoul National University Bundang Hospital, Seongnam, South Korea

**Xi Yu, Mingrui Pang, Yang Du, Tao Xu, Kang Yang, Juncheng Hu, Shaoming Zhu, Lei Wang and Xiuheng Liu**
Department of Urology, Renmin Hospital of Wuhan University, Wuhan, China

**Shenglan Li**
Department of Radiography, Renmin Hospital of Wuhan University, Wuhan, China

**Tao Bai**
Department of Urology, Wuhan No. 1 Hospital, Tongji Medical College, Huazhong University of Science and Technology, Wuhan, China

**Yaxin Hou, Junyi Hu, Lijie Zhou, Lilong Liu and Ke Chen**
Department of Urology, Union Hospital, Tongji Medical College, Huazhong University of Science and Technology, Wuhan, China
Shenzhen Huazhong University of Science and Technology Research Institute, Shenzhen, China

**Yi Li and Xiangyang Guo**
Department of Anesthesiology, Peking University Third Hospital, Beijing, China

**Lihui Sun**
Core Facility for Protein Research, Institute of Biophysics, Chinese Academy of Sciences, Beijing, China

**Na Mo**
Department of Pathology, Beijing Obstetrics and Gynecology Hospital, Capital Medical University, Beijing, China

**Jinku Zhang**
Department of Pathology, First Central Hospital of Baoding, Baoding, China
Key Laboratory of Molecular Pathology and Early Diagnosis of Tumor in Hebei Province, First Central Hospital of Baoding, Baoding, China

**Chong Li**
Core Facility for Protein Research, Institute of Biophysics, Chinese Academy of Sciences, Beijing, China
Key Laboratory of Molecular Pathology and Early Diagnosis of Tumor in Hebei Province, First Central Hospital of Baoding, Baoding, China
Department of Immunology, Beijing Jianlan Institute of Medicine, Beijing, China
Department of Immunology, Beijing Zhongke Jianlan Biotechnology Co., Ltd., Beijing, China

**Lin Gao, Ru Zhao, Wenbo Zhang, Feifei Sun, Wenjie Cai, Qianni Li, Xin Wang, Meng Wang, Hanchen Dong, Xueqing Chen and Tingting Feng**
The Key Laboratory of Experimental Teratology, Ministry of Education and Department of Pathology, School of Basic Medical Sciences, Cheeloo College of Medicine, Shandong University, Jinan, China

**Junmei Liu and Weiwen Chen**
Department of Biochemistry and Molecular Biology, School of Basic Medical Sciences, Cheeloo College of Medicine, Shandong University, Jinan, China

**Qianshuo Yin**
School of Basic Medical Sciences, Shandong University, Jinan, China

**Yiming Qin**
College of Chemical Engineering and Materials Science, Shandong Normal University, Jinan, China

**Xueting Xiong**
Department of Molecular Genetics, University of Toronto, Toronto, ON, Canada

**Hui Liu, Jing Hu and Bo Han**
The Key Laboratory of Experimental Teratology, Ministry of Education and Department of Pathology, School of Basic Medical Sciences, Cheeloo College of Medicine, Shandong University, Jinan, China
Department of Pathology, Qilu Hospital, Cheeloo College of Medicine, Shandong University, Jinan, China

**Ao Liu, Hai Huang, Chuanjie Zhang, Xiaohao Ruan, Wenhao Lin, Lu Chen and Danfeng Xu**
Department of Urinary Surgery, Ruijin Hospital, Shanghai Jiaotong University School of Medicine, Shanghai, China

**Miao Zhang and Biao Li**
Department of Nuclear Medicine, Ruijin Hospital, Shanghai Jiaotong University School of Medicine, Shanghai, China

**Zhongru Fan, Zhe Zhang, Chiyuan Piao, Zhuona Liu, Zeshu Wang and Chuize Kong**
Department of Urology, The First Affiliated Hospital of China Medical University, China Medical University, Shenyang, China

**Jian Zhang and Yawei Yuan**
Department of Radiation Oncology, Affiliated Cancer Hospital & Institute of Guangzhou Medical University, State Key Laboratory of Respiratory Diseases, Guangzhou Institute of Respiratory Disease, Guangzhou, China

**Chunning Zhang**
The First Tumor Department, Maoming People's Hospital, Maoming, China

**Huali Jiang**
Department of Cardiovascularology, Tungwah Hospital of Sun Yat-sen University, Dongguan, China

**Hualong Jiang**
Department of Urology, Tungwah Hospital of Sun Yat-sen University, Dongguan, China

**Jiayin Wang, Lili Su, Changxi Wang, Xuanping Zhang and Xiaoyan Zhu**
School of Electronic and Information Engineering, Xi'an Jiaotong University, Xi'an, China

**Xiaolong Zhang**
School of Electronic and Information Engineering, Xi'an Jiaotong University, Xi'an, China
Sun Yat-sen University Cancer Center, State Key Laboratory of Oncology in South China, Collaborative Innovation Center for Cancer Medicine, Guangzhou, China
School of Medicine, Shenzhen University, Shenzhen, China

**Yuhua Huang**
Sun Yat-sen University Cancer Center, State Key Laboratory of Oncology in South China, Collaborative Innovation Center for Cancer Medicine, Guangzhou, China
Department of Pathology, Sun Yat-sen University Cancer Center, Guangzhou, China

**Jiabin Lu**
Department of Pathology, Sun Yat-sen University Cancer Center, Guangzhou, China

**Jiasheng Chen**
Department of Urology, The Affiliated Changzhou No.2 People's Hospital of Nanjing Medical University, Changzhou, China
Department of Urology, Shanghai Jiao Tong University Affiliated Sixth People's Hospital, Shanghai Eastern Institute of Urologic Reconstruction, Shanghai Jiao Tong University, Shanghai, China

**Shouchun Li**
Department of Urology, The Affiliated Changzhou No.2 People's Hospital of Nanjing Medical University, Changzhou, China

**Nailong Cao and Ying Wang**
Department of Urology, Shanghai Jiao Tong University Affiliated Sixth People's Hospital, Shanghai Eastern Institute of Urologic Reconstruction, Shanghai Jiao Tong University, Shanghai, China

**Yongying Zhou, Weibing Zhang, Daoquan Liu, Ping Chen, Deqiang Xu, Jianmin Liu, Yan Li, Guang Zeng, Mingzhou Li, Zhonghua Wu, Yingao Zhang, Xinghuan Wang and Xinhua Zhang**
Department of Urology, Zhongnan Hospital of Wuhan University, Wuhan, China

**Xiao Wang**
Department of Rehabilitation Medicine, Renmin Hospital of Wuhan University, Wuhan, China

**Huiyong Liu**
Department of Urology, Huanggang Central Hospital, Huanggang, China

**Michael E. DiSanto**
Department of Surgery and Biomedical Sciences, Cooper Medical School of Rowan University, Camden, NJ, United States

**Mehmet A. Bilen, Jacqueline T. Brown, Omer Kucuk and Bradley Carthon**
Department of Hematology and Medical Oncology, Emory University, Atlanta, GA, United States
Winship Cancer Institute of Emory University, Atlanta, GA, United States

**Viraj A. Master**
Winship Cancer Institute of Emory University, Atlanta, GA, United States
Department of Urology, Emory University, Atlanta, GA, United States

**James F. Jiang, Caroline S. Jansen and Haydn Kissick**
Department of Urology, Emory University, Atlanta, GA, United States

**Lara R. Harik**
Department of Pathology, Emory University, Atlanta, GA, United States

**Aarti Sekhar**
Department of Radiology, Emory University, Atlanta, GA, United States

**Shishir K. Maithel**
Department of Surgery, Emory University, Atlanta, GA, United States

**Yongbiao Cheng, Gong Cheng, Tianbo Xu, Yuzhong Ye, Qi Miu, Qi Cao, Xiong Yang and Hailong Ruan**
Department of Urology, Union Hospital, Tongji Medical College, Huazhong University of Science and Technology, Wuhan, China
Institute of Urology, Union Hospital, Tongji Medical College, Huazhong University of Science and Technology, Wuhan, China

**Xiaoping Zhang**
Department of Urology, Union Hospital, Tongji Medical College, Huazhong University of Science and Technology, Wuhan, China
Shenzhen Huazhong University of Science and Technology Research Institute, Shenzhen, China
Institute of Urology, Union Hospital, Tongji Medical College, Huazhong University of Science and Technology, Wuhan, China

**Sen Li**
Department of Urology, Union Hospital, Tongji Medical College, Huazhong University of Science and Technology, Wuhan, China
Institute of Urology, Union Hospital, Tongji Medical College, Huazhong University of Science and Technology, Wuhan, China
Key Lab for Biological Targeted Therapy of Education Ministry and Hubei Province, Union Hospital, Tongji Medical College, Huazhong University of Science and Technology, Wuhan, China

**Jiaju Xu, Yuenan Liu, Jingchong Liu, Yi Shou, Zhiyong Xiong, Qi Wang, Di Liu and Huageng Liang**
Department of Urology, Union Hospital, Tongji Medical College, Huazhong University of Science and Technology, Wuhan, China

**Hairong Xiong and Hongmei Yang**
Department of Pathogenic Biology, School of Basic Medicine, Huazhong University of Science and Technology, Wuhan, China

**Anze Yu**
Department of Urology, Xiangya Hospital, Central South University, Changsha, China
Immunobiology & Transplant Science Center, Houston Methodist Research Institute, Texas Medical Center, Houston, TX, United States

**Giorgio Santoni**
Immunopathology Laboratory, School of Pharmacy, University of Camerino, Camerino, Italy

**Maria B. Morelli**
Immunopathology Laboratory, School of Pharmacy, University of Camerino, Camerino, Italy
Immunopathology Laboratory, School of Biosciences, Biotechnology and Veterinary Medicine, University of Camerino, Camerino, Italy

**Consuelo Amantini**
Immunopathology Laboratory, School of Biosciences, Biotechnology and Veterinary Medicine, University of Camerino, Camerino, Italy

**Nicola Battelli**
Oncology Unit, Macerata Hospital, Macerata, Italy

**Chunyu Zhang, Jiao Hu, Huihuang Li, Belaydi Othmane, Zhenglin Yi, Dongxu Qiu, Zhenyu Ou, Tao Guo, Jinhui Liu, Chunliang Cheng, Jinbo Chen and Xiongbing Zu**
Department of Urology, Xiangya Hospital, Central South University, Changsha, China

**Hongzhi Ma**
Department of Radiation Oncology, Hunan Cancer Hospital, Central South University, Changsha, China

**Wenbiao Ren**
Department of Urology, Xiangya Hospital, Central South University, Changsha, China
George Whipple Lab for Cancer Research, University of Rochester Medical Institute, Rochester, NY, United States

# Index